Orofacial Pain

Guidelines for Assessment, Diagnosis, and Management, Seventh Edition

American Academy of Orofacial Pain

Editors

Gary D. Klasser, DMD
Marcela Romero Reyes, DDS, PhD

Contributors

Simon Akerman, PhD
Rony K. Aouad, MD, MS
Jennifer Bassiur, DDS
Vanessa Benavent Anderson, DDS, MSD
Steven D. Bender, DDS
Charles R. Carlson, PhD
Heidi Crow, DMD, MS
Rob Delcanho, BDSc, MS
Paul Dorman, MD
Justin Durham, BDS, PhD
Paul L. Durham, PhD
Yoly M. Gonzalez-Stucker, DDS, MS
Jean-Paul Goulet, DDS, MSD
Steve Hargitai, DDS, MS
James Hawkins, DDS, MS
Willem de Hertogh, PT, PhD
Pei Feng Lim, BDS, MS
Isabel Moreno Hay, DDS, PhD
Mariona Mulet Pradera, DDS MS
Richard Ohrbach, DDS, PhD
Tara Renton, PhD, MDSc, BDS
Jonathan H. Smith, MD
Tom Weber, DDS, MS
Corine M. Visscher, PT, PhD
Edward F. Wright, DDS, MS

Orofacial Pain

Guidelines for Assessment, Diagnosis, and Management

SEVENTH EDITION

The American Academy of Orofacial Pain

Edited by

Gary D. Klasser, DMD

Professor
Department of Diagnostic Sciences
School of Dentistry
Louisiana State University Health Sciences Center
New Orleans, Louisiana

Marcela Romero Reyes, DDS, PhD

Clinical Professor
Director, Brotman Facial Pain Clinic
Department of Neural and Pain Sciences
School of Dentistry
University of Maryland, Baltimore
Baltimore, Maryland

QUINTESSENCE PUBLISHING

Berlin | Chicago | Tokyo
Barcelona | London | Milan | Mexico City | Paris | Prague | Seoul | Warsaw
Beijing | Istanbul | Sao Paulo | Zagreb

One book, one tree: In support of reforestation worldwide and to address the climate crisis, for every book sold Quintessence Publishing will plant a tree (https://onetreeplanted.org/).

Library of Congress Control Number: 2022949615

A CIP record for this book is available from the British Library.
ISBN: 978-1-64724-037-0

QUINTESSENCE PUBLISHING
USA

Quintessence Publishing Co, Inc
411 N Raddant Rd
Batavia, IL 60510
www.quintpub.com

5 4 3 2 1

Editor: Zach Kocanda
Design: Sue Zubek
Production: Sue Robinson

Printed in the USA

Contents

The glossary is available online and can be accessed by scanning this QR code.

Preface

The American Academy of Orofacial Pain (AAOP), a membership organization, was founded in 1975 with the goal to improve the understanding and quality of education in temporomandibular disorders (TMDs) and orofacial pain. The stated mission of the AAOP is to be an organization of health care professionals dedicated to alleviating pain and suffering through the promotion of excellence in education, research, and patient care in the field of orofacial pain and associated disorders. The AAOP has also been the sponsoring organization for orofacial pain to be recognized as a specialty, which was achieved in March 2020 as it is now considered the 12th dental specialty by the American Dental Association.

There have been six previous publications prior to this current edition of what commonly is referred to as the AAOP Guidelines. Dr Charles McNeill spearheaded the first two editions called *Craniomandibular Disorders: Guidelines for Evaluation, Diagnosis, and Management* (Quintessence, 1990) and *Temporomandibular Disorders: Guidelines for Classification, Assessment, and Management* (Quintessence, 1993). These publications focused predominantly on TMDs. As health care professionals and researchers became more conscious of the relationship between TMDs and other disorders of the head and neck, there was a need to expand the Guidelines to include disorders presenting as or related to TMDs. These disorders included not only headaches and neck disorders but several neuropathic pain conditions as well as biobehavioral factors. In 1996, under the editorship of Dr Jeffrey Okeson, the third version of the AAOP Guidelines was published, titled *Orofacial Pain: Guidelines for Assessment, Diagnosis, and Management.* That edition used the term *orofacial pain* to echo the rapidly changing and expanding field of orofacial pain and to reflect the fact that TMDs and orofacial pain should not be regarded as separate conditions, but that TMDs should be considered part of the disorders that fall under the umbrella of orofacial pain. Under the editorship of Dr Reny de Leeuw, the fourth edition of the Guidelines was published, which started to express evidence-based concepts. This edition included a separate chapter on cervical disorders to emphasize the close relationships between some orofacial pain disorders and cervical pain disorders, and—more importantly—to call attention to the differences and similarities associated with these disorders. The fifth edition, published in 2013, adopted the Research Diagnostic Criteria for Temporomandibular Disorders (RDC/TMD) and the expanded TMD taxonomy based on the work of the International RDC-TMD Consortium now known as the International Network of Orofacial Pain and Related Disorders Methodology (INfORM) Consortium. An updated definition of *bruxism* based on another international consensus work group was also adopted. Moreover, a new chapter was added in the fifth edition dedicated to the relationship between pain disorders and sleep. The sixth edition, published in 2018, employed the *International Classification of Diseases, Tenth Revision* (*ICD-10*) diagnostic codes, and several chapters referenced the International Classification of Headache Disorders, third edition (beta version; ICHD).

While the structure of the present work resembles previous editions, significant changes have been implemented in this current edition. All chapters contain essential updates, and some have undergone more changes than others. References have been updated throughout to reflect the most current literature. When available, evidence-based material has been included to provide the reader with scientifically sound and effective diagnostic procedures and treatment options. *ICD-10* diagnostic codes and the new *ICD-11* diagnostic codes have been used throughout the text. Furthermore, the International Classification of Headache Disorders, third edition (ICHD) codes have been used, where appropriate. Chapter 1 has been updated with discussions related to the influence of gut-brain interactions and dysbiosis, nutrition, and stem cell therapies in relation to chronic pain. In chapter 2, the future of potential biomarkers and the need for personalized/precision care are explored. Chapter 3 introduces the Analgesic, Anesthetic, and Addiction Clinical Trial Translations, Innovations, Opportunities, and Networks (ACTTION) and the American Pain Society (APS) pain taxonomy (AAPT) along with the International Classification of Orofacial Pain (ICOP) system. Moreover, the chapter reviews the newly implemented *ICD-11* classification system. Chapter 4 contains general updates in patient assessment, and chapter 5 contains various general updates with greater emphasis placed on headache pathophysiology as well updates to management including new pharmacologic agents. Chapter 6 was updated and expanded in terms of pharmacotherapeutics and recognition of red ear and first bite syndromes. Chapter 7 contains general updates to the management strategies for several disorders in addition to a section on "newer trends" related to electronic cigarettes/vaping and the SARS-CoV-2 global pandemic. In chapter 8, general updates to content and references have been provided with mapping of *ICD-10* to *ICD-11* classification coding changes. Chapters 9 and 10 have been updated to reflect more contemporary knowledge gained in relationship to cervical spinal disorders and associated headaches and extracranial and systemic causes of orofacial pain. Chapter 11 provides expanded information related to bruxism with brief discussions on the topics of pediatric obstructive sleep apnea, myofunctional therapy, and the glymphatic system. Chapter 12 provides updates on the implementation of various screening tools for biobehavioral factors following the recommendations from the Diagnostic Criteria for Temporomandibular Disorders (DC/TMD). The chapter also incorporates updates in the description of several psychiatric diseases in line with the *Diagnostic and Statistical Manual of Mental Disorders, Fifth Edition* (*DSM-5*). Lastly, the glossary has undergone updates to reflect the emerging and expanding field of orofacial pain. New terms have been added, and obsolete and superfluous terms have been removed.

Finally, despite the various chapters contained within the Guidelines and the depth of discussion among the included topics, it must be remembered that research is continuing and rapidly evolving, thus advancing and updating our knowledge and understanding of various conditions and management protocols. This is not intended to be an all-encompassing textbook exploring complete details regarding all aspects of orofacial pain. Instead, it is meant to provide an overview and insights to assist the reader with the procedures of evidence-based assessment, diagnosis, and management of orofacial pain conditions, based on the most current scientific knowledge.

Gary D. Klasser and Marcela Romero Reyes
Co-chairs, AAOP Guidelines Committee

Acknowledgments

Over the years, numerous AAOP members and nonmembers have participated in the evolution of the AAOP Guidelines, resulting in the seventh edition of this publication. The contributors to the current edition of the AAOP Guidelines are listed on a separate page. Each new edition has reflected the emerging and expanding field of orofacial pain. Based on these developments, new and evidence-based materials have been added. However, this ever-evolving work has built on and edited the work others have done in the past. As such, some parts of previous contributions may still be intact. We therefore want to extend our sincere appreciation to all of you who have contributed to any of the past editions, and especially to those of you who laid the foundation of this publication. We also would like to offer much gratitude to the publishers for providing us with timely advice and guidance so that deadlines could be met. The staff support at Quintessence has been incredibly accommodating and meticulous in their efforts and should be applauded. We truly hope that you will get great enjoyment and practical help from this new edition to the benefit of the patients we are privileged to assist.

1

Introduction to Orofacial Pain

Key Points

- Orofacial pain remains a prevalent and debilitating condition that exerts a significant social and economic impact on patients and the health care system.
- Many of the risk factors associated with temporomandibular disorders (TMDs) involve mechanical, chemical, or environmental stressors that increase the likelihood of developing and maintaining a chronic pathologic state.
- Sensitization and activation of trigeminal nerves and the subsequent development of peripheral and central sensitization are key pathophysiologic events leading to allodynia and hyperalgesia.
- Glial cells play an important role in the transition of acute to chronic pain by modulating the excitability state of nociceptive neurons in the trigeminal ganglion and spinal cord.
- Epigenetic influences on gene expression, mediated by our lifestyle and environment, significantly impact the progression of TMD and migraine pathology, necessitating comprehensive therapy.
- In March 2020, the National Commission on Recognition of Dental Specialties and Certifying Boards officially recognized Orofacial Pain as the dental profession's 12th specialty.
- Discoveries from the Orofacial Pain Prospective Evaluation and Risk Assessment (OPPERA) study have helped to clarify specific risk factors and genes implicated in the development of TMDs.
- Given the complex multifactorial etiology of orofacial pain conditions, management may require multiple interventions, such as—but not limited to—pharmaceuticals, physical therapy, oral appliances, behavioral modifications, diet modifications, and forms of exercise that emphasize proper breathing and increasing flexibility.
- The COVID-19 pandemic has had a major impact on the healthcare community and has driven advances in digital technology such as the use of telemedicine, phone apps, and other electronic aids that will forever change the medical landscape.

The Spectrum of Orofacial Pain

Orofacial pain refers to pain disorders of the jaw, mouth, face, head, and neck. These anatomical regions comprise an array of widely diverse structures and tissues ranging from dental pulp to the meninges of the brain. Pain conditions associated with these structures may derive from local factors or involve systemic, autoimmune, infectious, traumatic, or neoplastic pathologies. These conditions include odontogenic and periodontal pains, musculoskeletal disorders such as temporomandibular disorders (TMDs), headache and neurovascular pains, vascular disorders, and neuropathic pains.

Underlying this kaleidoscope of pain possibilities is a unifying system, the trigeminal sensory complex, in which impulses from the head and neck are conveyed by the branches of the trigeminal and upper cervical nerves to the trigeminal sensory nucleus in the brain stem. These impulses are modified by input originating within the trigeminal system and from higher regions of the central nervous system (CNS). Multiple areas of the brain process and interpret this input, giving rise to the sensation of pain and facilitating physiologic/adaptive responses, including behavioral changes.[1]

The diversity and complexity of orofacial pain conditions have led to recognition of the need for a specialized field of dentistry and for collaboration among multiple fields of medicine to improve care for patients afflicted with these disorders.

The Specialty of Orofacial Pain

Orofacial pain as a specialty has made significant strides in recent years. In 2009, the Commission on Dental Accreditation (CODA) approved orofacial pain as an area of advanced education, and since 2011, multiple residency and fellowship programs have been accredited in the United States. The International Association for the Study of Pain (IASP) has recognized the need for orofacial pain education by developing a core curriculum on this subject for health care professionals.[2] In March 2020, the National Academies of Sciences, Engineering, and Medicine released a consensus study report on TMD entitled Priorities for Research and Care.[3] This study, which was supported by the National Institute of Dental and Craniofacial Research, recommended improvements to education and training on TMDs for health care professionals, stating that "Deans of health professional schools ... should ensure that their schools' curricula include attention to TMDs..." and "The Commission on Dental Accreditation (CODA) should amend the accreditation standards for predoctoral dental programs to include screening, risk assessment, and appropriate evidence-based interventions for TMDs." In addition to these educational initiatives, the discipline of orofacial pain has been bolstered by the establishment of board certification processes and by increasing cooperation among advocacy groups, universities, professional organizations, and federal agencies. A landmark event occurred in March 2020 when the National Commission on Recognition of Dental Specialties and Certifying Boards officially recognized Orofacial Pain as the dental profession's 12th specialty.

The material covered in this chapter represents a broad overview of findings reported in peer-reviewed publications spanning the spectrum of conditions at the root of orofacial pain and current management practices. It is intended for health care professionals who evaluate and treat patients with orofacial pain and face the daunting task of keeping up with the literature in the ever-evolving arena of pain management.

Pain

Understanding of orofacial pain conditions must be grounded in principles and concepts of pain in general. The IASP offers the following defi-

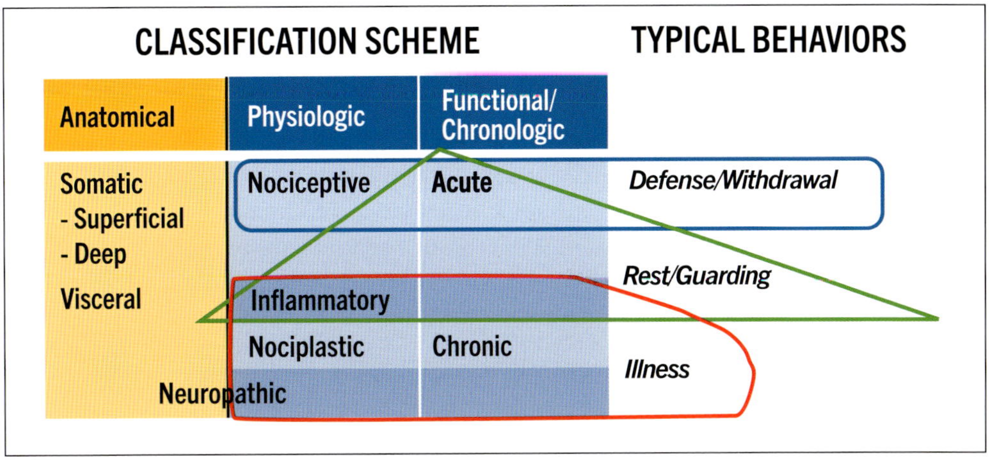

Fig 1-1 Pain classification schemes and typical behaviors.

nition of *pain* (revised in 2020): "An unpleasant sensory and emotional experience associated with, or resembling that associated with, actual or potential tissue damage."[4] The IASP expands upon this definition with these six key notes:

1. Pain is always a personal experience influenced to varying degrees by biologic, psychologic, and social factors.
2. Through their life experiences, individuals learn the concept of pain.
3. A person's report of an experience as pain should be respected.
4. Although pain usually serves an adaptive role, it may have adverse effects on function and social and psychologic well-being.
5. Verbal description is only one of several behaviors to express pain; inability to communicate does not negate the possibility that a human or a nonhuman animal experiences pain.
6. Pain and nociception are different phenomena; pain cannot be inferred solely from activity in sensory neurons.[4]

This final key note highlights an important distinction between the concepts of nociception and pain. *Nociception* has been defined as "information processing triggered by noxious stimuli ... (which) may lead to withdrawal or vegetative responses and/or to the sensation of pain".[5] In simple terms, nociception refers to basic signaling in the nervous system, while pain involves the interpretation and perception associated with those signals.

Classifications of pain

Pain may be viewed through the lenses of different classification schemes, including what may be termed physiologic and anatomical classifications (Fig 1-1). A physiologic classification includes categories of nociceptive and inflammatory pain, as well as a third mechanistic descriptor recently adopted by the IASP and referred to as *nociplastic pain*. Nociceptive pain is momentary, nonpersistent pain that matches its stimulus (does not display an exaggerated response). It acts as a vital defense mechanism, stimulating behavioral and physiologic actions to prevent tissue damage in the face of a noxious stimulus. *Inflammatory pain* occurs in the setting of tissue damage (eg, due to mechanical trauma, heat, or infection).[6] Tissue injury prompts release of a host of inflammatory mediators that interact with sensory neurons to increase the intensity and duration of nociceptive signaling, leading to persistent pain that, in contrast to the momentary experience of nociceptive pain, outlasts its stimulus. This persistence of inflammatory pain encourages protective behaviors ("vegetative responses" such as resting an inflamed body part) intended to limit further injury while healing occurs.[7] *Nociplastic pain* is defined by the IASP as pain that arises from altered nociception despite no clear evidence of actual or threatened tissue damage causing the activation of peripheral nociceptors. The IASP differentiates nociplastic from neuropathic pain (discussed later) with the clarification that nociplastic pain displays no evidence for disease or lesion of the somatosensory system.[4] This type of pain is characteristic of a group of disorders known as chronic overlapping pain conditions (COPCs) that includes, for example, fibromyalgia and irritable bowel syndrome (IBS).

Anatomical classifications include categories of somatic pain and visceral pain (see Fig 1-1). *Somatic pain* encompasses both superficial (eg, cutaneous, mucosal) and deep (musculoskeletal) pain. A site of noxious stimulation in superficial somatic tissues is usually easy for an individual to precisely locate, due at least partly to a relatively high density of free nerve endings in dermal tissue relative to deeper tissues. This ability to localize pain serves as an early warning system to protect against injury to the integrity of the body's outermost protective layers.[8] In contrast, pain arising from musculoskeletal structures is prone to spread or refer beyond the locus of noxious stimulation. *Visceral pain* arises from internal organs and is often diffuse and difficult to localize. Such pain is also prone to refer to areas remote from the source of noxious stimulation, often to superficial somatic areas, as in the classic example of myocardial infarction being perceived in areas such as the chest wall.

The category of neuropathic pain traverses both physiologic and anatomical classification schemes. The IASP defines *neuropathic pain* as "pain caused by a lesion or disease of the somatosensory nervous system."[4] Such pain may be thought of as a faulty or hyperactive alert system, like a smoke alarm (the nervous system) going off even though fire (nonneural tissue damage) is absent.

Probably the most common distinction drawn in classifying pain is between acute and chronic.[9] This distinction is often framed in terms of time, with pain of less than 3 to 6 months duration labeled acute and pain persisting beyond this timeframe as chronic. These labels may be viewed in a slightly different light as functional rather than merely chronologic. In a functional sense, *acute pain* is pain that serves an essential protective function, alerting an organism to potential tissue damage and stimulating behavior to avoid or mitigate that damage. *Chronic pain*, on the other hand, is pain that persists despite the lack of any biologically useful role, potentially becoming a disorder unto itself.

Chronic pain has profound societal effects. The 2016 National Health Interview Survey found a point prevalence of chronic pain in the U.S. adult population of over 20% (50 million people), with 8% (approximately 20 million) having high-impact chronic pain causing frequent limitations to life or work activities. Female sex, lack of current employment, residence in a rural area, low socioeconomic status, and non-Hispanic white ethnicity were associated with higher prevalence of chronic pain after adjusting for age.[10] These findings highlight the need for a better appreciation of the multifactorial nature of pain and the challenge of personalizing treatment to the needs of each individual patient.

Chronic pain is associated with high economic costs. In the United States, billions of dollars are lost annually due to decreased productivity, loss of work, and disability compensation. Chronic pain increases expenses for emergency room

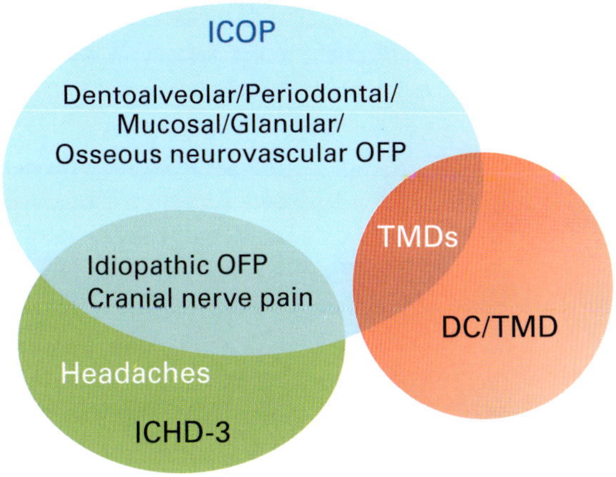

Fig 1-2 Diagnostic criteria for specific pain disorders.

visits, medication costs, and psychologic treatment.[8] The cost of pain is estimated to be similar to the combined annual costs of heart disease, cancer, and diabetes.[11]

Orofacial pain conditions may fit simultaneously within more than one of the pain classification schemes described above. For example, momentary pain elicited in a carious tooth by a cold beverage (reversible pulpitis) is an acute pain from a functional perspective, a nociceptive pain from a physiologic perspective, and a visceral pain from an anatomical perspective. Temporomandibular joint (TMJ) pain of several months' duration that is stimulated by chewing and lasts for several hours after cessation of the stimulus represents a deep somatic pain that is both chronic and inflammatory.

In addition to the general categories of pain outlined above, criteria have been established to guide the diagnosis of specific pain disorders. Three sets of diagnostic criteria focus specifically on orofacial pain:

- The diagnostic criteria for temporomandibular disorders (DC/TMD), developed by the International RDC/TMD Consortium Network (now known as INfORM, the International Network for Orofacial Pain and Related Disorders Methodology) of the International Association for Dental Research and the Orofacial Pain Special Interest Group of the International Association for Dental Research and published in 2014[12]
- The International Classification of Headache Disorders (ICHD-3), published by the International Headache Society and published in its third edition in 2018[13]
- The International Classification of Orofacial Pain (ICOP), also by the International Headache Society and published in its first edition in 2020[14]

Each of these sets of diagnostic criteria includes a taxonomy that arranges pain conditions hierarchically from broad categories of disorders to specific diagnoses based on patient history and examination findings. Specific conditions described by these criteria are more fully elucidated in subsequent chapters. As seen in Fig 1-2, there is overlap among these sets of criteria, and some differences in definitions and terminology exist with respect to specific diagnoses. Hopefully, these differences will be reconciled in the future as the field of orofacial pain continues to evolve to include data from a diverse array of disciplines.

Pathways of Nociception

Peripheral innervation

The progression of a nociceptive impulse from its initiation in peripheral tissues to its transformation in the cerebral cortex into the experience of pain may be visualized as occurring along a simplified pathway of successive sensory neurons (primary, secondary, tertiary). A more accurate picture might be that of a dense urban highway system encompassing a vast number of roads of varying sizes, from multi-lane freeways to one-way back alleys, with a dizzying network of on-ramps, off-ramps and intersections, and a plethora of signs and signals regulating traffic flow.

Nociception from peripheral tissues is initiated by sensory receptors called *nociceptors*, which are free nerve endings located at the peripheral terminals of specialized primary sensory neurons. Nociceptors detect potentially harmful mechanical, thermal, or chemical stimuli. Many nociceptors respond to more than one of these forms of stimuli. This polymodal receptivity is a feature unique to nociceptors; other sensory receptors of the body are specialized to a single modality (eg, innocuous mechanical or thermal stimuli). A sufficiently intense noxious stimulus triggers nociceptors to initiate action potentials that travel centrally along the axons of primary sensory neurons. The frequency of nociceptive action potentials increases as a function of increasing stimulus intensity, causing a summation in signal strength at the neuron's central connection with a secondary neuron.[15]

The vast majority of nociceptive primary neurons have thin axonal fibers that conduct impulses more slowly than the larger-diameter fibers that are responsible for innocuous sensory impulses and initiation of skeletal muscle activity. Classification of peripheral neurons is based on axon diameter, degree of myelination, and the resulting conduction velocity (Table 1-1). Nociceptive primary neurons generally fall within the categories of Aδ fibers (thinly myelinated) and C fibers (unmyelinated), although the borders between categories associating fiber types with types of sensory impulses are not well delineated: some unmyelinated fibers convey innocuous sensory information (eg, C fibers that conduct pleasant stroking sensations[16]), and under conditions of sensitization or demyelination, large-diameter fibers (Aβ fibers) that normally respond to innocuous stimuli convey information that is interpreted as nociceptive (see discussion below).

The cell bodies of primary sensory neurons that carry input from the head and neck reside in the trigeminal ganglion (also referred to as the *Gasserian* or *semilunar ganglion*) at the convergence of the three branches of the trigeminal nerve. Axons travel centrally from the trigeminal ganglion via a single large sensory root to enter the pons. Cell bodies of sensory neurons from the trunk and limbs reside in the dorsal root ganglia, and the axons of these neurons join with the spinal cord via the dorsal roots. Axons of primary sensory neurons synapse with secondary neurons in the trigeminal sensory nucleus (for impulses from the head and neck) or dorsal horn (for impulses from the trunk and limbs).

Trigeminal branches

The ophthalmic nerve branch (V1) transmits only sensory information from its branches in the scalp, forehead, upper eyelid, conjunctiva, cornea, nose (including the tip of the nose), nasal mucosa, frontal sinuses and deep structures in these regions, as well as parts of the meninges (the dura and blood vessels). These branches merge to enter the skull through the superior orbital fissure. The ophthalmic branch

Table 1-1 **Sensory fiber type and known stimulus**

Sensory fiber	Stimulus
Aα and Aβ	Propioception and light touch.
Aδ	Nociception (noxious mechanical, thermal, chemical). Fast, pricking quality of pain.
C	Nociception (noxious mechanical, thermal, chemical). Slower, burning quality of pain.

also carries postganglionic parasympathetic motor fibers to the glands and sympathetic fibers to the pupillary dilator muscles.

The maxillary nerve branch (V2) carries only sensation from the lower eyelid and cheek, the nares and upper lip, the maxillary teeth and gingiva, the nasal mucosa, the palate roof of the pharynx, the uvula, the maxillary and ethmoid and sphenoid sinuses, and parts of the meninges. Peripheral branches converge to enter the skull through the foramen rotundum. The nerve is then joined by the middle meningeal nerve carrying sensation from the middle meningeal artery and part of the dura.

The mandibular nerve branch (V3) transmits both sensory and motor impulses. The sensory component carries information from the lower lip, mandibular teeth and gingiva, floor of the mouth, anterior two-thirds of the tongue, chin and jaw (except the angle of the jaw, which is supplied by C2 and C3), parts of the external ear, parts of the meninges, and deep structures. The auriculotemporal nerve innervates most of the TMJ. Sensory branches merge to enter the skull via the foramen ovale. Motor axons transmit impulses from the trigeminal motor nuclei in the mid-pons to the muscles of mastication (ie, masseter, temporalis, medial pterygoid, lateral pterygoid, anterior digastric, and mylohyoid); the tensor veli palatini, involved with eustachian tube function; and the tensor tympani, which attaches to the malleus bone in the eardrum.

The CNS structures affected by trigeminal nociceptive input are also contacted by secondary neurons from the dorsal horn of the spinal cord. Therefore, potential pain input from regions outside trigeminal receptive fields may excite CNS structures that communicate with trigeminal nuclei and modulate their functions. The trigeminal system is directly or indirectly associated with the other cranial nerves, which are extensions of the brain that innervate tissues of the head and face.[8] The specialized neurons of the olfactory, optic, and vestibulocochlear nerves that send smell, sight, sound, and balance information to the CNS do not travel through the trigeminal nuclei. However, nerves associated with the nose, eye, and ear tissues do transmit proprioceptive, pressure, and potential pain impulses into the trigeminal nuclei. These cranial nerves, along with the oculomotor, trochlear, abducens, and the hypoglossal nerves, will not be reviewed here. However, a comprehensive orofacial pain evaluation should include a basic assessment of the function of all cranial nerves (see chapter 2).

Facial nerve

The seventh cranial nerve is a mixed nerve that has five branches (temporal, zygomatic, buccal, mandibular, and cervical) that course through the parotid gland but do not innervate the gland. Its main function is motor control of most of the muscles of facial expression and the stapedius muscle of the middle ear. The facial nerve supplies parasympathetic fibers to the sublingual and submandibular glands via the chorda tympani and to the lacrimal gland via the pterygopalatine ganglion. In addition, it conveys taste sensations from the anterior two-thirds of the tongue to the solitary tract nucleus and transmits cutaneous sensation from the skin in and around the earlobe via the nervous intermedius.

Glossopharyngeal nerve

The ninth cranial nerve is a mixed nerve comprised of somatic, visceral, and motor fibers. It conveys sensory information from the posterior third of the tongue, tonsils, pharynx, middle ear, and carotid body. Taste sensation from the posterior third of the tongue as well as carotid body baroreceptor and chemoreceptor information is transmitted to the solitary tract nucleus. Nociceptive input from the ear is sent to the spinal trigeminal nucleus. From the inferior salivatory nucleus, the glossopharyngeal nerve delivers parasympathetic control to the parotid and mucous glands throughout the oral cavity while motor fibers from the nucleus ambiguous project to the stylopharyngeus muscle and upper pharyngeal muscles. An altered gag reflex indicates glossopharyngeal nerve damage.

Vagus nerve

The tenth cranial nerve originates in the brain stem and extends to the abdomen and innervates virtually all organs from the neck to the transverse colon except the adrenal glands. It supplies visceral afferent fibers to the mucous membranes of the pharynx, larynx, bronchi, lungs, heart, esophagus, stomach, intestines, and kidneys and distributes efferent or parasympathetic fibers to the heart, esophagus, stomach, trachea, bronchi, biliary tract, and most of the intestine. Also, the vagus nerve affects motor control of the voluntary muscles of the larynx, pharynx, and palate and carries somatic sensory fibers that terminate in the skin of the posterior surface of the external ear and the external acoustic meatus. Through these connections, the vagus affects activities as varied as respiration, cardiac function, sweating, digestion, peristalsis, hearing, and speech.

Spinal accessory nerve

The eleventh cranial nerve innervates the cervical muscles, the sternocleidomastoid and trapezius, which are coactivated during masticatory behaviors. Like the trigeminal motor nucleus, the accessory motor nuclei are rich in norepinephrine receptors, which can facilitate vigilant behaviors. Nociceptive afferents from the cervical muscles converge onto the spinal trigeminal nucleus. It is notable that cervical myofascial pain seems to be prominent in patients with orofacial pain.

Central connections

Trigeminal sensory nuclei

All pressure, proprioception, chemical, and temperature sensory input from the face and all nociceptive inputs from the face, head, and neck are transmitted to the cell bodies of second-

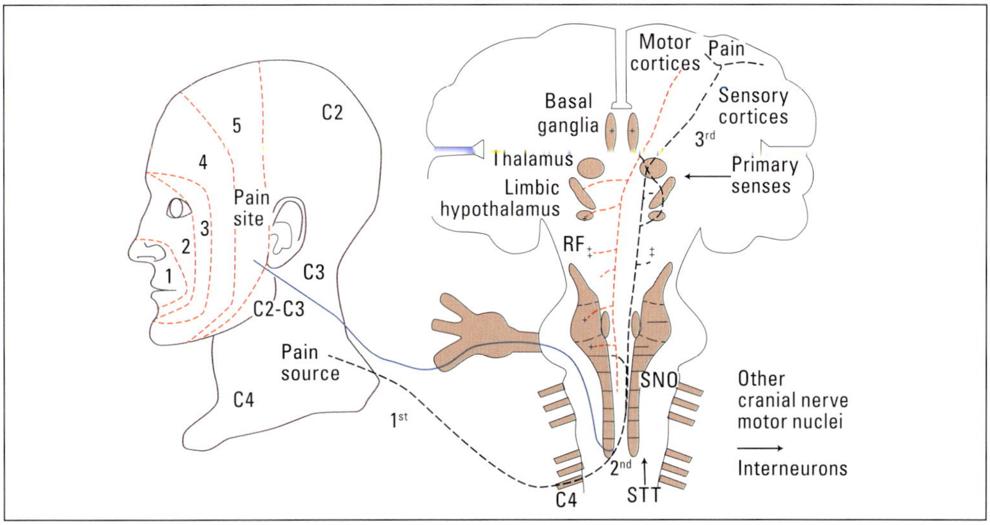

Fig 1-3 Trigeminal sensory pathways and motor response to referred pain. The primary neurons from a pain site in facial lamina 5 and from the pain source in the C4 receptive field each converge on lamina 5 of the subnucleus caudalis and excite the same secondary neurons. As these secondary neurons ascend, they arborize with the subnucleus oralis and subnucleus interpolaris (not shown) and many reticular formation structures before synapsing with tertiary neurons in the thalamus. The tertiary neurons are thalamo-cortico-basal ganglia-limbic circuits that interpret pain and generate the descending motor and pain modulatory reactions to pain interpretation. The descending motor neurons also arborize with reticular formation locations and connect, via interneurons, to the trigeminal motor nucleus and to all cranial nerve motor nuclei. Note that trigeminal input is never analyzed in isolation, as primary sensory and spinal thalamic tract input is also always being presented to the brain for analysis. RF, reticular formation structure; SNO, subnucleus oralis; STT, spinal thalamic tract.

ary neurons in the trigeminal sensory nuclei.[8] These nuclei are located in bilateral columns on either side of the brain stem, stretching from the midbrain rostrally and blending caudally with the dorsal horn of the cervical spinal cord (Fig 1-3). Moving in a rostrocaudal direction, the trigeminal sensory nuclei comprise the mesencephalic nucleus (in the midbrain), which is involved in jaw reflex activity, the main sensory nucleus (in the pons), which receives proprioceptive and pressure input from orofacial structures, and the spinal trigeminal nucleus.[15]

The mesencephalic nucleus, which is functionally more a ganglion than a nucleus, houses the cell bodies of the proprioceptive neurons that convey input from the apical periodontal ligament and the muscle fibers that contract during the jaw-closing reflex. These proprioceptive neurons, and possibly the blink reflex nerves, represent the only peripheral nerves with cell bodies located within the CNS.[8,17] The neurons are monosynaptic and pass through the mesencephalic nucleus to synapse in the trigeminal motor nuclei located medially to the much larger main sensory nucleus. The main sensory nucleus receives the facial proprioceptive and pressure input for orofacial behaviors other than the jaw-closing reflex (eg, chewing, kissing, smiling, and light touch). These neurons have their cell bodies in the trigeminal ganglion and synapse in the main sensory nucleus where input is conveyed to the motor nuclei by arrays of small interneurons.[8]

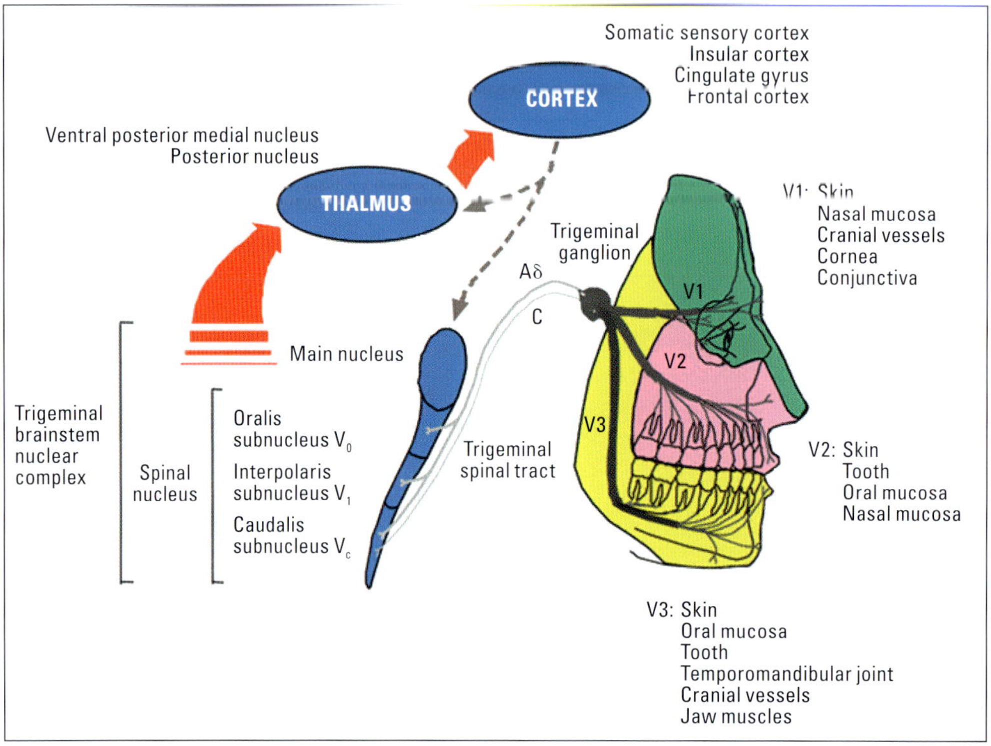

Fig 1-4 The trigeminal (V) complex. (Reprinted from Hu and Wada[8] with permission.)

The spinal trigeminal nucleus (SpV) is located in the medulla and consists of three subnuclei.[18] From rostral to caudal, they are the subnucleus oralis (V_o), subnucleus interpolaris (V_i), and subnucleus caudalis (V_c). Subnuclei oralis and interpolaris receive chiefly temperature information from Aδ fibers and non-nociceptive tactile input from Aβ fibers.[8] They also receive some nociceptive input originating from intraoral structures. The subnucleus caudalis is sometimes referred to as the *medullary dorsal horn*[1] due to the similarity of its cellular organization to that of the dorsal horn of the spinal cord. It receives the bulk of the nociceptive input from trigeminal receptive fields. In response to nociceptor activation, neuropeptides and other inflammatory agents are released in the spinal trigeminal nucleus and can cause excitation of neurons and glial cells that promotes development of central sensitization, allodynia, and hyperalgesia, which are physiologic events associated with acute and chronic pain.[19,20]

Receptive fields in the face are organized somatotopically in an "onion peel" configuration (Fig 1-4) such that, regardless of which trigeminal nerve branch carries their input, nociceptive primary afferent neurons from the most anterior areas of the face synapse with secondary neurons in the most rostral areas of the V_c. Moving outward and posteriorly in a ring-like fashion from the most anterior regions of the face, primary neurons terminate centrally in progressively more caudal areas of V_c (see Fig 1-4).[8] For instance, A and C-fiber neurons

[1] This term is sometimes used to refer to the spinal nucleus in its entirety, ie, all three subnuclei taken together.

Table 1-2 Nociceptive input to spinal nucleus

Peripheral nerve or nerve branch	Structures/areas innervated
Ophthalmic (V1)	Nasal mucosa Cranial vessels Cornea Conjunctiva
Maxillary (V2)	Skin Teeth Oral mucosa Nasal mucosa
Mandibular (V3)	Skin Oral mucosa Temporomandibular joint Jaw muscles Cranial vessels
Nervus intermedius of facial nerve (VII)	Ear lobe
Glossopharyngeal (IX)	Ear Tongue (posterior third) Pharynx Larynx
Vagus (X)	Pharynx Larynx
C2–C4, possibly C5	Posterior head and neck Auricle External acoustic meatus Anterior neck Angle of mandible Shoulders Upper thoracic region (greater occipital nerve [GON] and lesser occipital nerve, greater auricular, transverse cervical, supraclavicular)

from area 5 in the face, whether they start in V1, V2, or V3, all synapse with secondary nociceptive neurons in the most caudal aspect of the subnucleus caudalis, lamina 5. Such convergence means that a dural blood vessel, masseter muscle, or a tooth or tongue nociceptive afferent could excite the same secondary neurons.

This convergence is a probable anatomical basis for referred pain and is not restricted to the trigeminal nerve branches. SpV receives peripheral input from the upper cervical sensory nerves as far caudally as C5. Therefore, nociceptive input from cervical and upper shoulder areas converges onto the same secondary neurons that receive signals from the face, head, and oral cavity, meaning that trapezius or sternocleidomastoid nociceptive afferents can excite secondary neurons that also receive input from facial tissues.[21-23] Nociceptive input carried by branches of the facial, glossopharyngeal, and vagus nerves likewise converges onto SpV neurons (Table 1-2). This neuronal organization may help to explain the high prevalence of painful comorbidities in tissues of the head and face (ie, headache and sinusitis, headache and TMDs, neck pain and facial pain).

All of the CNS structures affected by trigeminal nociceptive input are also contacted by secondary neurons from the dorsal horn of the spinal cord.[24] Therefore, potential pain input from regions outside trigeminal receptive fields may excite CNS structures that communicate with trigeminal nuclei and modulate their functions.

Neurons whose cell bodies are housed within the dorsal horn include projection neurons, whose ascending axons relay sensory input to higher CNS areas, as well as a vast number of interneurons, which modify signals at the level of the brainstem. Some projection neurons are nociceptive specific, ie, they receive input only from nociceptive primary afferent fibers. Other projection neurons receive a variety of signals, including both nociceptive and non-nociceptive sensory input, and are called *wide dynamic range neurons* (WDRs).

Whether and with what frequency a secondary neuron fires action potentials in response to peripheral nociceptive input depends on both spatial and temporal summation, ie, whether incoming signal frequency at a given location within a given time is sufficient to overcome inhibitory influences (see following section, "Modulation of Pain") and reach the threshold required to excite the secondary neuron's membrane and evoke a response. This threshold is not "set in stone" but is dynamic and can be modified as cytokines and other sensitizing molecules induce changes in the type, number, and activity level of receptors and ion channels in the secondary neuron's cell membrane (see discussion of sensitization below).

Axons of secondary neurons that project information for touch and proprioception follow the lemniscal pathway. This pathway ascends via the dorsal column of the spinal cord before decussating in the medulla.[25] Branches from the lemniscal pathway are involved in local inhibition of pain. On the other hand, the pathway responsible for transmitting information about pain and nonpainful temperatures is called the *spinothalamic pathway*.[26] In this pathway, the synapse between a primary and a dorsal horn secondary sensory neuron occurs on the same side of the spinal cord. Secondary neurons have a single axon that crosses the midline to the contralateral side of the spinal cord before ascending as part of the lateral spinothalamic tract. Hence, this pathway follows the side of the body opposite to where the signal originated. The difference between the lemniscal pathway (for touch and proprioception) and the spinothalamic pathway (for pain and temperature) has important clinical implications because some injuries that only affect one side of the spinal cord may interrupt only the sense of touch with respect to one side of the body, while other injuries may only alter pain sensation. In similar fashion to the spinothalamic tract, trigeminal secondary axons originating in the main sensory nucleus and SpV decussate before ascending via the ventral trigeminal lemniscus to higher CNS centers.[25]

As secondary axons carrying information about pain and nonpainful temperatures ascend from the SpV toward the thalamus, they send multiple offshoots (arborizations) to various areas of the reticular formation of the brain stem. The reticular formation plays important roles in the control of baseline processes such as behavioral arousal, consciousness, and motivation and therefore represents an early opportunity in the chain of neuronal transmission for nociception to elicit subconscious physiologic responses.[8,24,27,28] Secondary neurons that are stimulated by glutamate-releasing Aδ fibers arborize less than those receiving impulses from slower-conducting C fibers, which release a wide variety of neurotransmitters and neuropeptides.[8,29,30] Thus, information from Aδ fibers stimulates a much faster nocifensive (ie, protective reflex) response than that elicited by C

Table 1-3 Brain regions associated with dimensions of pain

Cerebral structure/region	Aspect of pain	Dimension of pain (per Melzack and Casey[31])
1° somatosensory cortex	Sensory processing	Sensory-discriminative
Insular cortex	Emotional and arousal response; attentional processing	Motivational-affective
Cingulate cortex	Emotional and arousal response; attentional processing	
Amygdala and hippocampus	Anticipation of pain	
Prefrontal cortex	Reframing/contextual evaluation of event	Cognitive-evaluative
Thalamus	Sensory processing; modulation of input to limbic system	

fiber input, which is important in maintaining persistent pain and coordinating reparative and behavioral responses.

Axons of secondary SpV neurons carry nociceptive impulses to the rostral ventral medulla (RVM) and periaqueductal gray (PAG) and then on to tertiary neurons whose cell bodies reside in the thalamus. These thalamic neurons form connections with higher brain centers, including primary and secondary somatosensory cortices, prefrontal cortex, anterior cortex, amygdala, and nucleus accumbens. The brain contains no single "pain center"; rather, the interplay of multiple cerebral regions transforms the neural activity of nociception into the multidimensional experience of pain.

Three dimensions of this pain experience were described in a 1968 chapter by Melzack and Casey as sensory-discriminative, cognitive-evaluative, and motivational-affective.[31] The sensory-discriminative dimension includes sensation of pain characteristics such as location, intensity, duration, and quality. Motivational-affective refers to the emotion-charged urge to take action to escape the unpleasantness of the pain. The cognitive-evaluative encompasses appraisal of the meaning of the pain experience and may be heavily influenced by cultural factors.

Melzack and Casey[31] provided a useful illustration of these three pain dimensions in action: Imagine someone being given a hot beverage in a mug belonging to her friend. Upon picking up the mug, the individual immediately senses painful, unpleasant heat in the palms and fingers (sensory-discriminative) and feels a strong urge to immediately drop the mug (motivational-affective). However, the individual is simultaneously aware that allowing the mug to shatter on the floor would be socially awkward and might give offense to her friend (cognitive-evaluative) so instead she quickly but carefully sets the mug on the table.

Functional magnetic resonance imaging has provided insights into areas of the cortex that are active during pain and the roles these areas play in different dimensions of pain. Some of these insights are summarized in Table 1-3 and grouped according to the three dimensions of pain described above.

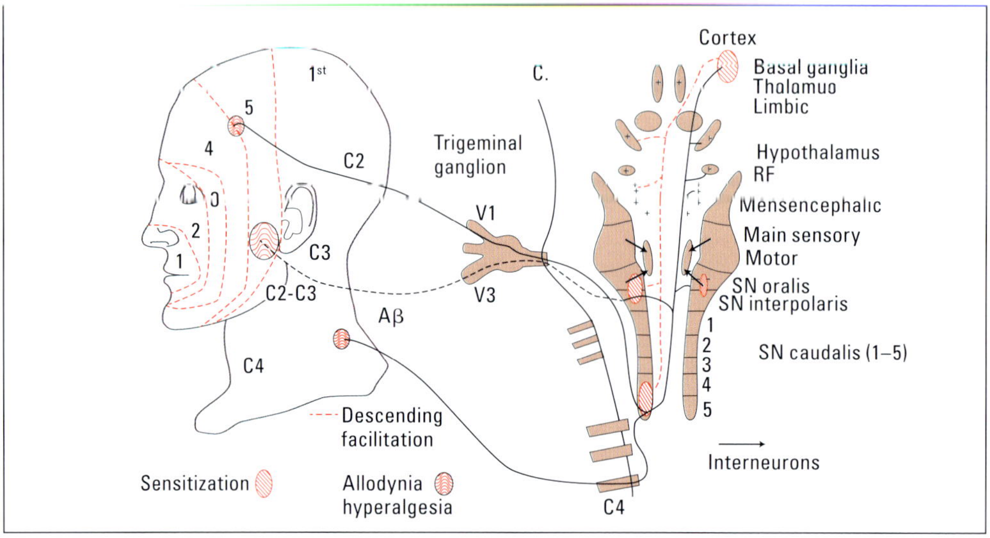

Fig 1-5 Sensitization of trigeminal system. Primary nociceptive neurons from facial lamina 5 transmitted via V1 and C4 converge onto lamina 5 of the subnucleus caudalis. If the pain sources are not controlled, summation exceeds descending inhibition, and progressive levels of central sensitization occur, first at the subnucleus caudalis, then at the ipsilateral subnucleus oralis, where Aβ fibers are carried on V3 synapse. With continued summation, sensitization occurs at higher brain sites and at the contralateral subnucleus oralis. Nonpainful thermal and tactile inputs are experienced as painful (allodynia) or a more intense pain is felt (hyperalgesia) because of the effects of central sensitization. RF, reticular formation structure; SN, subnucleus.

Nociceptive impulses generated by potential or actual tissue damage are one of many types of input that are continually assessed and evaluated throughout the various levels of the CNS. The senses (smell, sight, hearing, touch, and taste) alert the brain to stimuli through thalamic-amygdala and thalamic-cortical-amygdala circuits, and those data streams are analyzed and compared to stored information within the brain to facilitate an efficient behavioral response.[32,33] Ongoing proprioceptive, nociceptive, thermoreceptive, baroreceptive, chemoreceptive, and vestibular input provides sensory information to the brain about how effectively its tissues are responding and enables the brain to make ongoing behavioral adjustments aimed at maintaining efficiency. Pain stimulates CNS-coordinated behavioral responses including motor commands and changes in muscle and glandular activity and also evokes autonomic nervous system modulated cranial nerve responses.[8,34,35] Hence, pain signals provide the brain an opportunity to make behavioral adjustments to avoid further, potentially damaging stimuli.[36] The multilevel complexity of pain processing in the nervous system suggests that in many cases, successful pain control needs to rely on more than an attempt to isolate and control peripheral tissue damage because pain is ultimately an experience generated by the brain, and brain activity must therefore be a focus of treatment.

Table 1-4 Correlation between neuronal sensitization and clinical manifestation

Aspect of neuronal sensitization	Clinical manifestation
↓ AP firing threshold	Pain in response to weaker painful stimuli (hyperalgesia) or normally nonpainful stimuli (allodynia)
↑ AP frequency	Increased pain intensity
Spontaneous AP firing	Spontaneous pain
Expansion of RF (CS)	Increased area of pain

AP = action potential; RF = receptive field; CS = central sensitization.

Neurophysiologic Phenomena and Clinical Correlates

Sensitization

Neurons alter their structural and functional properties in response to conditions in their local environment and to the input they process and receive, a phenomenon called *neuroplasticity*. Neuroplastic changes are essential for normal processes such as learning, development, and memory formation. However, under some conditions, neuroplastic changes may lead to a hyperactive state of nociception and pain perception that can be difficult to reverse.[37]

Sensitization refers to an increase in neuronal activity characterized by lower thresholds for initiation of action potentials, increased action potential frequency in response to a given stimulus, spontaneous action potential firing, and expansion of receptive fields (Fig 1-5). All other factors being equal, such changes in nociceptive neurons lead to corresponding increases in pain perception and associated clinical manifestations (Table 1-4). Sensitization may occur in primary afferent neurons (peripheral sensitization) or in neural structures farther along the pathway of impulse transmission, eg, SpV neurons and higher (central sensitization). While central sensitization has been demonstrated in nonhuman animal models, its influence on pain in humans cannot be verified experimentally but is inferred based on clinical evidence that is in agreement with physiologic, cellular, and molecular findings in animal models.[38]

Peripheral and central neurons may be sensitized by a barrage of persistent nociceptive signals and/or by inflammatory mediators. Inflammation plays a key role in peripheral sensitization.[26] Injury will activate cells and tissue to release a host of inflammatory mediators. These immune modulations, such as macrophages, endothelial cells, mast cells, and Schwann cells (to name a few), will release a cascade of cytokines and other mediators that sensitize peripheral neurons.[6,38] Once sensitized, peripheral neurons require lower levels of inflammatory mediators to generate nociception, and cytokines that once acted merely as sensitizers can directly initiate firing of action potentials. Aspects of nociception in some peripheral neurons become active only under conditions of peripheral sensitization, as in the case of "silent nociceptors," a population of C fibers that display little response to mechanical stimuli under normal conditions but respond robustly to mechanical stimuli in the setting of inflammation.[39]

The term *receptive field* refers to the peripheral anatomical area from which a secondary neuron (eg, SpV) receives sensory input of sufficient magnitude to initiate a response (such as transmission of action potentials to higher CNS areas). Sensitization may "awaken" responsiveness in a secondary neuron to neural connections that previously failed to elicit a response, such as connections with peripheral input from beyond the secondary neuron's normal receptive field as well as input from peripheral primary neurons that signal non-noxious stimuli (eg, Aβ fibers). Axonal sprouting by secondary neurons may also create new synaptic connections within the SpV (see "Mechanisms of Sensitization" below).

Mechanisms of Sensitization

The development of sensitization is a time- and intensity-dependent process. Initially, low intensity nociceptive volleys carried on Aδ neurons release glutamate and activate post-synaptic alpha-amino-3-hydroxy-5-methyl-4-isoxazole-propionic acid (AMPA) and N-methyl-D-aspartate (NMDA) ion channel receptors in the SpV. Activation of these receptors is implicated in the induction and maintenance of central sensitization and likely contributes to peripheral sensitization and visceral pain. In addition, C fibers release neuropeptides such as calcitonin gene-related peptide (CGRP) and other inflammatory mediators (eg, cytokines, nitric oxide) that cause changes in the expression and activity of membrane receptors and ion channels, resulting in lower activation thresholds in secondary neurons.[40,41] As sensitization develops, peripheral Aδ fibers can sprout additional axons within the SpVc[42,43] while SpVc neurons arborize to the SpVo and SpVi.[19,20] This reorganization of synaptic connectivity contributes to the field expansion and nociceptive interpretation of Aβ input that were described earlier.

Peripheral and central sensitization also involves changes in the activity of non-neuronal cells known as *glial cells*, which actually are more abundant in the brain, spinal cord, and ganglia than neuronal cells. Glial cells include satellite glial cells and Schwann cells in ganglia as well as astrocytes, microglia, and oligodendrocytes in the CNS. The importance of glial cells in the underlying pathology of many inflammatory diseases is now recognized given their prominent roles in regulating the extracellular environment around neurons and modulating neuronal excitability of neural circuits. Thus, glial cells have emerged as potential cellular targets for therapeutic intervention.[44]

Under normal conditions, satellite glia in the trigeminal ganglion are involved in information processing, neuroprotection, and regulation of neuronal activity, including the basal rate of spontaneous firing and the activation threshold (Fig 1-6). Peripheral tissue injury or inflammation leads to increased interactions between satellite glia and neuronal cell bodies via formation of gap junctions and altered paracrine signaling.[45] These increased cell-to-cell interactions are thought to play an important role in the induction and maintenance of peripheral sensitization of trigeminal nociceptive neurons. These changes may be transient as part of a response to acute inflammation, but if inflammation persists then these gap junctions stabilize, a process that has been implicated in preclinical models of TMD.[46] This increase in neuron-glia signaling facilitates cross-excitation among parallel fibers in the ganglion such that cellular changes in one trigeminal nerve branch can cause sensitization or activation in other branches. In this way, inflammation in the TMJ could contribute to the high rates of comorbidity reported among trigeminal pain conditions (eg, TMD and migraine).

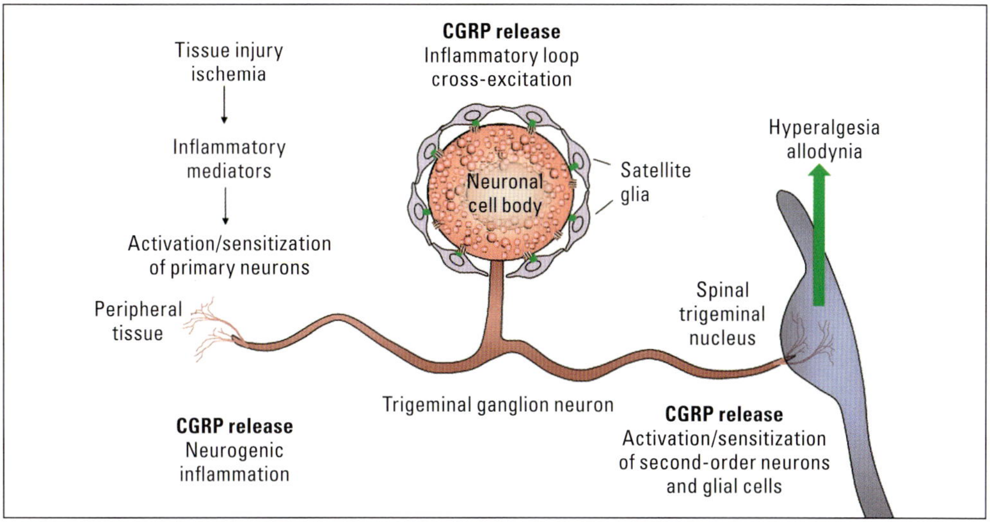

Fig 1-6 Key role of CGRP in trigeminal-mediated pathologies. During CGRP involvement in promoting peripheral and central sensitization of trigeminal nociceptive neurons in response to tissue injury or ischemia, inflammatory mediators cause activation of primary nociceptive neurons and subsequent CGRP release *(1)* in peripheral tissues to promote neurogenic inflammation, *(2)* from the cell body in the ganglion to facilitate development of an inflammatory loop and cross-excitation, and *(3)* in the spinal trigeminal nucleus to cause activation of secondary neurons and glial cells resulting in hyperalgesia and allodynia. While CGRP release in the peripheral tissue and ganglion initiate and sustain peripheral sensitization of primary trigeminal neurons, elevated CGRP levels in the upper spinal cord promote development of central sensitization via activation of astrocytes and microglia. As described in the text, bidirectional signaling can occur within the trigeminal system in which central sensitization mediated by CGRP can promote peripheral sensitization of peripheral nociceptive neurons.

Astrocytes and microglia in the CNS perform functions similar to those of satellite glia in the peripheral nervous system.[47] Astrocytes are the most abundant cell type in the CNS and perform a diverse array of important functions including regulation of neuronal development, synaptic coupling, repair, and nutritional support. In addition, astrocytes are known to monitor and control concentrations of ions, neurotransmitters, and metabolites, as well as water movement around neurons, and thus play a key role in modulating the excitability of neurons both in the brain and spinal cord.[48] Microglia function as immune cells, removing cellular debris and dead cells and releasing inflammatory mediators to promote healing.[49,50]

Traditionally, peripheral sensitization is proposed to precede and facilitate development of central sensitization in response to peripheral tissue injury. However, there is evidence from an animal study that elevated spinal cord levels of the neuropeptide CGRP, which is implicated in central sensitization,[51] could promote peripheral sensitization of trigeminal nociceptive neurons in the absence of tissue injury.[52] An elevated level of CGRP in the cerebrospinal fluid was found to increase mechanical sensitivity of trigeminal neurons and mediate increased gap junction communication between trigeminal neurons and satellite glial cells. Following co-injection of CGRP and a fluorescent dye in the spinal cord, the dye was detected in the neuronal cell body and satellite glial cells, which provides evidence of bidirectional signaling in trigeminal neurons. Hence, changes in the levels of inflammatory mediators such as CGRP within the spinal cord, which could be mediated by an increased allostatic load and dysfunction of the descending pain modulation pathway, could facilitate sensitization of primary nociceptive neurons independent of ischemia or tissue damage.

Referred pain

Patients commonly report pain in areas that are remote from the site of nociceptive stimulation, presenting a challenge for accurate diagnosis. Referred sensations (painful and nonpainful) can be evoked experimentally in humans by applying mechanical or chemical (eg, glutamate, capsaicin, hypertonic saline) stimuli to healthy muscle tissue, suggesting that referral is not modality specific, is not limited to any particular class of peripheral sensory receptor, and does not necessarily involve pathology.[53] Referred sensations, including referred pain, are therefore most likely mediated by the CNS and appear to represent a normal response to intense nociception. The CNS mechanisms thought to underlie the clinical phenomenon of referred pain include *(1)* convergence and unmasking of silent synapses as well as *(2)* priming of central connections from areas of prior pain experience.

Convergence and unmasking of silent synapses

Primary sensory neurons carrying input from the head and neck converge in the trigeminal spinal nucleus, where their signals overlap as they synapse with some of the same secondary neurons. Some of these synaptic connections are quiescent until they become activated by persistent or especially strong nociceptive stimuli.[53] In theory, unmasking of such "silent synapses" expands the receptive field of the secondary neuron such that sensory input from the newly active synapse triggers the secondary neuron to transmit sensory information to higher centers as though the information had originated through both the older and the newly active synapses. This state of activation and referred pain expansion may persist if the secondary neuron becomes chronically sensitized (ie, central sensitization).

For the sake of illustration, imagine a secondary neuron whose cell body in the SpVc receives synaptic input from two primary C fibers: one carrying nociceptive signals from the dental pulp of a mandibular right molar, the other from the right masseter muscle. Under baseline conditions, the synapse from this hypothetical pulpal neuron is silent and makes no contribution to perceived sensation. However, following a lengthy streak of ill-advised and gluttonous energy drink consumption by the patient, the pulp of the molar becomes infected, leading to irreversible pulpitis and stimulating the pulpal C fiber to bombard the secondary neuron with repeated volleys of high-frequency action potentials. The secondary neuron in the SpVc becomes responsive to this enhanced sensory input, converting its silent synapse with the pulpal neuron to an active synapse. Nociception from this newly active synapse triggers the secondary neuron to transmit these signals on to higher centers, where these signals are interpreted as though they had originated from both the molar and the masseter muscle, and the patient experiences pain not only in the tooth but also in the neighboring muscle. WDR neurons probably play a particularly important role in referred pain at this first level of convergence in the trigeminal nucleus because these neurons receive converging input from both superficial and deep tissues, and from both nociceptive and non-nociceptive primary neurons.

As discussed earlier, central sensitization contributes to pain referral by creating new synaptic connections and unmasking previously silent connections. The increase in frequency of outbound signals that is a feature of sensitization may also play a role in referral. For example, a sensitized WDR neuron in the SpVc that receives both nociceptive input from the dura and normally innocuous input from cutaneous V2 branches may be excited by input from low-intensity mechanical stimulation of the temple and "pass it on" to higher centers as a robust nociceptive signal, leading to pain from light contact of the skin of the temples. Such activity may help explain the stroking allodynia (eg, to touch or hair brushing) experienced by many patients during a migraine attack. The pattern of convergence is repeated at higher CNS levels as output from secondary neurons of the trigeminal spinal nuclei converges on multiple brainstem locations involved in motor, ANS, and hypothalamic-pituitary-adrenal (HPA) activity.[21,22]

Priming of central connections from areas of prior pain experience

Experimental evidence has shown that sites of referred sensation are relatively stable in individuals undergoing painful stimulation of the masseter muscles and that referred sensations are often perceived in sites involved in tension-type headache and in other body areas where pain has been previously felt.[53] These findings suggest that past experience of pain in an area of the body increases the likelihood that future referred pain will be perceived in that area. It seems that in some cases a volley of nociception may be sufficient not only to unmask previously silent synapses but to durably "prime" those new connections such that they become favored pathways for future pain referral. If this is true, then pain referral may be a more complex phenomenon than a simple source-to-site phenomenon in which pain elicited in a remote site is purely attributable to a source at the area of stimulation.

Autonomic nervous system

The autonomic nervous system (ANS), which is commonly viewed as a largely involuntary motor system, is composed of three peripheral divisions: sympathetic, parasympathetic, and enteric. These three divisions function to maintain homeostasis in all physiologic systems.[54] The peripheral ANS is controlled by the central ANS, which includes cortical, limbic, and reticular formation structures and nuclei.[55] Stimuli that activate the central ANS induce increased sympathetic activity, initially in the brainstem, and then in the periphery.[55,56] The sympathetic division is involved in vigilance, energy expenditure, and the "flight or fight" response, while the role of the parasympathetic division is to counterbalance sympathetic arousal with "rest and digest" actions.[57] Preganglionic sympathetic and parasympathetic neurons originate in different areas of the CNS and release excitatory neurotransmitters at synapses in autonomic ganglia, where cell bodies of postganglionic neurons reside. These postganglionic neurons deliver impulses to target tissues via neurotransmitters: postganglionic sympathetic neurons release norepinephrine and epinephrine, while parasympathetic neurons secrete acetylcholine at the target sites.

The enteric system provides local sensory and motor fibers to the gastrointestinal tract, the pancreas, and the gallbladder. This system can function autonomously but is regulated by CNS reflexes. Its control of gastrointestinal vascular tone, motility, secretions, and fluid transport plays a vital role in homeostasis. Persistent sympathetic arousal that impairs parasympathetic function and leads to disturbances of the enteric system may be relevant to orofacial pain because functional disorders of visceral organs controlled by the ANS seem to be frequently comorbid with orofacial pain conditions.[57-59] For example, migraine is comorbid with irritable bowel syndrome and is associated with dysbiosis, a change in the normal gut bacteria that are responsible for modulating inflammation and aiding in digestive and nutrient absorption.[60,61]

Heart rate variability is a measure of the beat-to-beat time interval that reflects CNS control of ANS tone.[62] Low heart rate variability, in which the beat-to-beat time interval becomes inflexible, occurs when high sympathetic tone impedes parasympathetic (vagal) dampening of cardiac activity.[63] Low heart rate variability is a common finding for conditions seemingly as diverse as cardiovascular disease, diabetes, depression, anxiety, cognitive problems, irritable bowel syndrome, gastroesophageal reflux disease, posttraumatic stress disorder, migraine, fibromyalgia, and sleep apnea. High heart rate variability, when parasympathetic control modulates a variable beat-to-beat time interval, is associated with health and improved cognitive capacity.[64,65]

TMD patients have been differentiated from controls by pain, anxiety, depression, sleep disturbance, and measures of ANS reactivity,[66] and behavioral therapies have been shown to treat these conditions more successfully than traditional dental therapies.[67,68] Orofacial pain patients with TMD and other comorbid conditions such as headaches, gastroesophageal reflux disease, and fibromyalgia demonstrated low heart rate variability compared with controls when subjected to stressors.[69] In response to self-regulated stress reduction techniques for 3 months, patients with orofacial pain reported improved pain scores and heart rate variability measurements became more similar to those of pain-free controls. The improved heart rate variability scores correlated with decreased pain interference scores, suggesting enhanced self-efficacy in the face of stressors. These data suggest that for some patients with orofacial pain who have multiple comorbid conditions, specific self-regulation skills may enable patients to cope with previously unrecognized and therefore uncontrolled physiologic disturbances associated with the pain.

Modulation of pain

Organisms must recognize and avoid tissue damage without being overly distracted from normal activities by transient nociceptive pain. CNS-driven pain modulation, including descending inhibitory mechanisms, help to strike this balance. The impact of minor nociception on cognitive function and task performance is minimized by inhibitory neurons whose axons project from higher to lower areas of the CNS. Any necessary adjustments in motor and vascular behavior that result from this minor nociception can be coordinated almost subconsciously by communication between secondary neurons and structures in the reticular formation.[35] Perception of pain therefore involves not only activation of the ascending nociceptive pathways, but also modulation by descending inhibitory pathways regulated by signals from the cortex and brainstem.

Higher neural networks within the brain must be activated to counteract nociception whose intensity or duration is sufficient to excite tertiary sensory neurons. Important brain stem centers of inhibitory control include the RVM, PAG, and locus coeruleus. Through a process called *stimulation-produced analgesia* (SPA), the brain utilizes both noradrenergic and serotonergic pathways to inhibit nociceptive transmission at multiple sites, beginning at the synapses of primary and secondary neurons in the spinal trigeminal nucleus and dorsal horn.[8] This descending inhibition is mediated by endogenous opioids, GABA, and various inhibitory amino acids produced in the PAG. These same inhibitory compounds are released in response to stressors that induce anxiety, fear, or depression.[70]

Additionally, peripheral nociceptive signals may be inhibited in the spinal cord by input from non-nociceptive neurons (Aα and Aβ fibers). Melzack and Wall's 1965 gate control theory of pain provided the seminal model of endogenous pain inhibition via interneuron-mediated modulation of sensory input in the dorsal horn.[71] In this model, interneurons excite non-nociceptive neuronal fibers while inhibiting activation of nociceptive neuronal fibers. Pain signaling is therefore a balance between the ascending spinothalamic pathway and the descending inhibitory modulation pathway. A well-known correlate is the instinctive urge to rub an area of the body that has just been injured. The vigorous rubbing activates Aβ fibers that respond to touch while also activating interneurons that inhibit nociception. Transcutaneous electrical nerve stimulation (TENS) may be a clinical application of this physiologic response, inhibiting pain by stimulating non-nociceptive cutaneous neuronal fibers.

Data from human and animal studies demonstrate the ability of organisms to inhibit pain throughout the body in response to a painful stimulus applied anywhere in the body.[46,47] In other words, "pain inhibits pain." The neural activity that underlies this response and that has been observed experimentally in animals is named *diffuse noxious inhibitory control* (DNIC).[72] Behavior in humans that is inferred to result from similar neural processes and is observable during psychophysical testing is called *conditioned pain modulation* (CPM).[53,54] DNIC occurs at the level of the spinal cord and is activated when secondary neurons are strongly inhibited in response to a nociceptive stimulus applied to a remote part of the body outside their own receptive fields. Dysfunction in these inhibitory mechanisms may predispose some individuals to progress to a chronic pain state following tissue injury or infection in the orofacial region.[73] However, results from a recent study provided evidence that neuropathic pain may facilitate a decrease in CPM over time, thus posing a "chicken and egg" question about relationships between inefficient CPM/DNIC and chronic pain.[74]

Brain circuits that interpret pain and direct descending inhibition also direct alterations in motor behavior. In response to severe pain, the CNS alters patterns of movement and recruits alternative motor pathways to minimize continued nociceptive barrages. These descending commands reach structures throughout the reticular formation and travel through vast pools of interneurons to affect all cranial nerve motor nuclei.[75-77] Trigeminal premotor interneurons deliver messages to the main sensory nucleus, the SpVo, and the SpVi, which, through further interneurons, alter activity in the motor nuclei.[24,26,27]

As in the case of inhibition of nociception via conditioned pain modulation, changes in orofacial motor behavior may occur in response to stimulation in distant body areas. For example, stimulation in other more remote areas of the body is reported to induce inhibitory reflex movements in the jaw and tongue in response to noxious craniofacial stimulation.[78,79] Neck or shoulder pain may result in impaired jaw or neck movement just as a sore tooth alters chewing and swallowing or a severe headache that accompanies migraine forces retreat from light (photophobia), sound (phonophobia), and touch (allodynia). Reduced jaw range of motion in response to pain in the sternocleidomastoid is an example of such adaptive behavior that is familiar to orofacial pain practitioners. In addition to causing adaptations in motor behavior, brain circuits involved in descending inhibition induce alterations in ANS activity in response to pain. Such alterations include changes in respiration and cardiovascular mechanisms.[80]

Placebo effects provide striking and clinically consequential examples of endogenous pain modulation. The definition of *placebo* as merely an inert substance or sham procedure employed in a control group has been revised in light of the growing recognition of the active roles that psychosocial and therapeutic contexts play in patient responses to therapy.[81] A 2020 review offered the following definitions of terms:[82]

- *Placebo effects*, including placebo analgesia, are "clinical outcomes patients derive from participation in the rituals, symbols, and behaviors of medical treatment."
- *Placebo responses* constitute a wider category of findings from randomized controlled trials (RCTs) that include both "genuine placebo effects" as defined above as well as "such non-specific effects as regression to the mean, spontaneous improvement, and normal fluctuations in illness."
- *Nocebo effects* can alter the outcome of a given therapy in a negative way, in contrast to placebo effects. The way in which adverse events are presented to patients can not only affect risk perception, but, more importantly, can influence clinical outcomes.

The magnitude of placebo effects varies greatly among patients and may be influenced by prior experiences and expectations[83] (though data in support of a role for conscious expectations are surprisingly sparse). Verbal suggestions by clinicians may be a powerful contributing factor in many settings (see migraine labeling study summarized below). Placebo effects are also idiosyncratic: different individuals respond differently to placebo interventions.[83]

Placebo analgesia involves both endogenous opioid mechanisms, as evidenced by studies demonstrating complete or partial reversal by naloxone, and opioid-independent mechanisms, as shown in a study in which naloxone failed to reverse drug-conditioned placebo effects conditioned by a non-opioid medication.[76] Some placebo mechanisms involve endogenous cannabinoid activity.[83]

Placebo effects and responses contribute significantly to pain-related outcomes. Data from several studies of medication effects on pain suggest that in many cases as much as 50% to 75% of a drug's effect may be attributable to placebo responses.[82] A study of the effects of drug labeling and clinician-provided information provides an intriguing example of placebo response in an orofacial pain context:[84] Subjects with episodic migraine were given either rizatriptan 10 mg or placebo over the course of six headache attacks following an initial attack in which no abortive treatment was provided. A different label-substance combination was used for each treatment episode: for either substance, the subject was told they were receiving placebo, rizatriptan, or rizatriptan or placebo. Effects of active drug and placebo were both lowest when the "placebo" label was applied. Placebo mislabeled rizatriptan" reduced headache intensity as effectively as rizatriptan mislabeled placebo. Placebo reduced pain intensity even when correctly labeled "placebo" as opposed to the no treatment episode, during which pain intensity increased, adding to a body of evidence suggesting that even open-label placebos have an impact; concealment or deceit seem not to be essential to placebo effects. The main conclusion was that clinician-provided information may be as important as an active drug for successful analgesia.[82,84]

Administering a concealed or deceitful placebo treatment to a patient outside an approved research study is outside the boundaries of ethical practice. However, placebo effects are probably an integral component of all treatments, whether those treatments are generally considered "traditional" or "complementary/alternative." Clinician behaviors that may tap into placebo effects, such as active, empathic listening and striving to build a relationship of trust, are ethical imperatives.

The Biopsychosocial Model and Allostatic Load

Mind/body dualism is a concept that views the mind and mental activity as nonphysical entities separate from the physical body. Descartes presented his views on dualism in 1641 and they have cast a long shadow: Many physicians and patients still believe that disease and pain must be the result of a detectable physical malady or injury.[8] Such a strictly mechanistic or biomedical model of disease regards the effects of the mind and society as being outside the scope of medicine. It views pain as the result of tissue damage, and if such organic disease or injury cannot be detected, then pain is explained as psychosomatic.

Engel[85] challenged the traditional biomedical model, which he regarded as too narrowly focused on correcting the somatic parameters of illness. He rejected the notion that psychosocial elements of human malfunction lie outside the domain of medicine's responsibility and authority and instead proposed a biopsychosocial model of disease. This model views biologic, psychologic, and sociologic dimensions as body systems that are just as integral to healthy human functioning as the musculoskeletal or cardiovascular systems. Mounting discoveries using imaging techniques[86] and biologic and genetic markers confirm the adverse effects of psychologic and sociologic factors on physiology, thus broadening our understanding of the meaning of disease.[87,88] The mechanisms of central sensitization and the modification of neuroendocrine parameters that characterize abuse victims, who often suffer from comorbid illnesses, are examples of markers for conditions previously considered to lack a biological basis.[89,90] Pain arises from biopsychosocial factors that occur in combinations and to degrees that are unique to each individual. These factors may contribute to an individual's resilience and adaptive capacity, protecting an individual from pain, or they may predispose a patient to develop chronic pain in the face of stressors.

The processes undertaken by neural, neuroendocrine, and immune mechanisms to adapt to biopsychosocial stressors is called *allostasis*. A simplified shorthand distinction between the terms "homeostasis" and "allostasis" might associate these terms with "survival" and "adaptation" respectively, ie, homeostasis involves processes that maintain stability for survival, and allostasis involves adapting the parameters of physiologic activity to handle changes and the stresses that accompany them.[91,92] Allostasis requires significant physiologic effort and exacts substantial energy demands. *Allostatic load* refers to the cumulative lifetime burden of the effects and consequences that organisms incur as they make the physiologic adaptations necessary for allostasis.[93] In other words, allostatic load is the result of accumulated wear and tear on an organism through exposure to repeated or chronic stressors. Migraine pathology is thought to be a disease of allostatic load that leads to a maladaptive stress response.[94-96] The changes in HPA axis function and brain cytokine activities that underlie cardiac disease, diabetes, and migraine are examples of allostatic load.[91,94-97] With greater allostatic load, there is the risk of the development of persistent central sensitization characterized by enhanced ascending spinothalamic pain track and suppressed descending inhibitory pain modulation pathways.

Our modern-day environment presents us with multiple challenges toward the allostatic load. This lifestyle may contribute to an imbalanced state of sympathetically mediated hyperexcitability or hyperresponsiveness that can lead to a state of mental exhaustion and perceived helplessness in which parasympathetic function is suppressed.

For these patients, investigating only "physical" biomedical parameters will lead to an incomplete clinical picture, and failure to address psychosocial factors may contribute to a deepening state of illness as pathologic processes such as central sensitization persist in the absence of comprehensive diagnosis and treatment. A biopsychosocial approach, often involving interdisciplinary care coordinated among multiple specialists, may prevent increased allostatic load and help patients restore balance between their excitatory and inhibitory neural circuits. Behavioral modifications may help patients manage their allostatic load by shifting the balance of autonomic activity toward lower sympathetic drive and enhanced parasympathetic tone. Activities that encourage proper breathing and tissue flexibility and that naturally evoke a parasympathetic response, such as walking, swimming, yoga, tai chi, Pilates, meditation, or mindfulness training may be helpful.[98] Including such activities in a patient's daily routine may reduce the negative effects of key risk factors that increase allostatic load and help empower the patient to actively participate in managing his or her pain.

Contributing Factors to Chronic Orofacial Pain

Clinicians are very familiar with the fact that different patients react in radically different ways to similar nociceptive stimuli. Many dentists have had the experience of treating a patient who insisted on not receiving local anesthesia for a dental restoration and who sat through the procedure without flinching despite significant mechanical trauma to the dentin (an experience that is probably more disconcerting for the dentist than for the patient). Dentists are equally familiar with patients who exhibit signs of extreme agitation with very little nociceptive provocation.

As noted previously, pain is impacted by a multitude of biopsychosocial variables that are unique to each patient, confer varying degrees of resilience and vulnerability, and give rise to an experience that is idiosyncratic in its sensory-discriminative, motivational-affective, and cognitive-evaluative dimensions.

Major objectives of the longitudinal, multidisciplinary studies known as the Orofacial Pain: Prospective Evaluation and Risk Assessment (OPPERA) studies included determining psychologic and physiologic risk factors, clinical characteristics, and associated genetic/cellular mechanisms that influence the development of TMD.[99,100] Based on findings from those studies, the investigators have presented a model that includes genetic, physiologic, and environmental factors that increase the risk of an individual experiencing TMD pathology (Fig 1-7).

The following section provides an overview of factors that may contribute to chronic orofacial pain, organized in categories analogous to Engel's model: biologic, psychologic/behavioral, and social/environmental (Fig 1-8).[85] Such categorization is to some extent artificial because many factors extend across all these domains, and concepts of "psychologic" versus "sociologic" are often impossible to tease apart. Despite these limitations, it is hoped that this method of presentation will further emphasize the importance of a comprehensive biopsychosocial approach to understanding orofacial pain conditions.

Biologic factors

Genetics

Emerging data from human genetic linkage analysis and genome-wide association studies support the notion that mutations in genes involved in modulation of our nervous system predispose individuals to a hyperexcitable nervous system and thus play an important role in the initiation and maintenance of chronic pain.[101-104] Not surprisingly, all the chronic pain conditions examined thus far, including TMD and migraine, exhibit an augmentation of genes responsible for regulating neurotransmission in both the ascending and descending nociceptive pathways. For example, mutations have been identified in ion channels and receptors on neurons and glial cells that are associated with increased neuronal excitability and an enhanced sensitized state of nociceptors. Collectively, results from these studies have begun to provide a clearer understanding of how genetic variants influenced by environmental factors lead to the development of multifactorial pathologic conditions that share overlapping etiologies. Findings from these genetic studies may help to direct

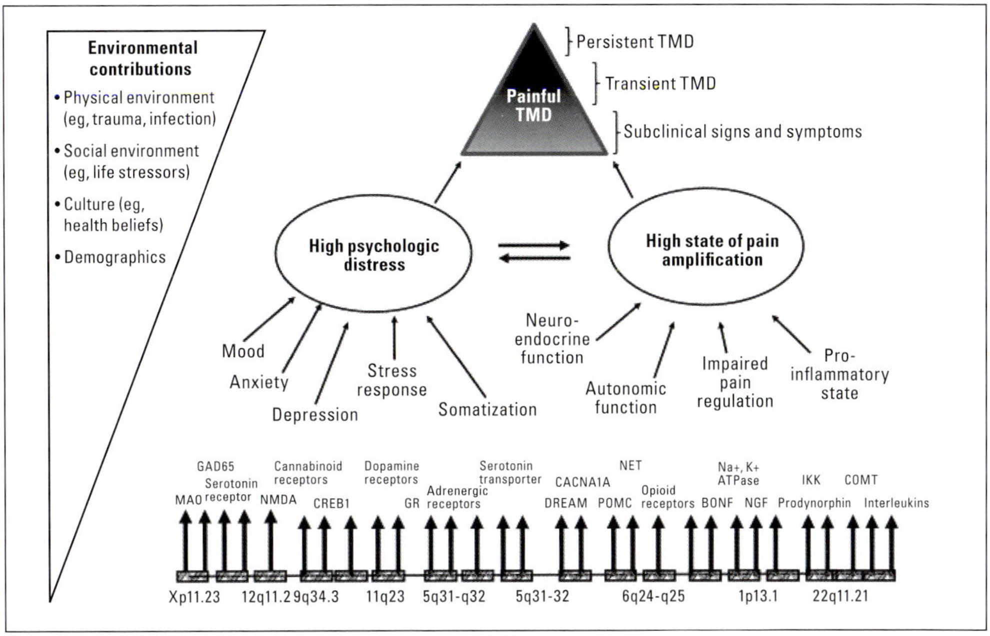

Fig 1-7 Overview of major factors that contribute to development of TMD pathology and the associated genes.

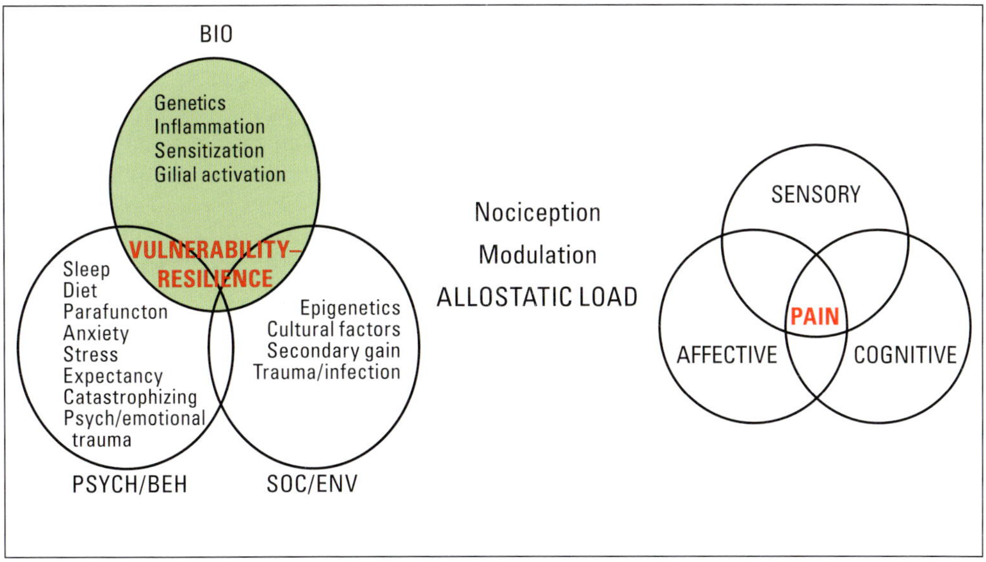

Fig 1-8 Relationships among nociception, biopsychosocial factors such as those noted in text, and the dimensions of pain as described by Melzack and Casey.[31]

development of more personalized strategies including pharmacologic and nonpharmacologic methods for managing chronic pain patients.

Results from multiple genetic studies have demonstrated that TMDs are not caused by a single gene mutation but are associated with changes in the expression of many genes that contribute to the pathology and pain characteristic of this prevalent medical condition. For example, associations have been demonstrated between chronic TMD and single-nucleotide polymorphisms in genes coding for a glucocorticoid receptor (*NR3C1*), a serotonin receptor (*HTR2A*), and a G protein-coupled receptor kinase (*GRK5*).[105] As documented in the OPPERA study, many of the risk factors associated with TMD involve mechanical, chemical, or environmental stressors that increase the likelihood of developing and maintaining a chronic pathologic state.[103,104]

Epigenetics

Although a great deal of effort is dedicated toward understanding genetic predisposition to disease, it is equally if not more important to realize that environmental stressors alter the expression of genetic codes and behavior. An animal model has shown that placing an identical twin in a harsher environment causes downregulation of GABA receptors and increases locus cerulean (noradrenergic) modulated stress behaviors, which leads to persistent central sensitization and a hyperresponsive nervous system.[106]

The field of epigenetics focuses on understanding the impact of environmental factors on genetic expression and thus on our overall health.[107] Areas of interest include determining how changes in our diet, quantity and quality of sleep, amount of exercise, tobacco use, and exposure to drugs and toxins influence the packaging of our DNA and the genetic controls that can either protect us from or render us more susceptible to disease progression.[108-110]

Sex

Reviews published in 2013[111] and 2019[112] highlight sex-based disparities in pain experience. Women are more likely than men to report or experience chronic pain, to report chronic widespread pain, and to seek treatment for pain. Women show higher population prevalence than men in chronic overlapping pain conditions such as fibromyalgia, IBS, and interstitial cystitis. This difference is no secret to orofacial pain practitioners given that common orofacial pain conditions including migraine, chronic tension-type headache, and TMDs are also more prevalent among women than men.

Like most aspects of pain, the mechanisms underlying these sex-associated differences are complex and incompletely understood.[113] These mechanisms may include the effects of sex hormones, differences in activity of the endogenous opioid system, sexual dimorphism in immune and glial cell function, tendencies for women and men to engage different coping mechanisms, and sociocultural beliefs including gender role expectations.

Gut-brain interactions

Disturbances in commensal bacteria of the gastrointestinal tract have been demonstrated in chronic pain conditions such as fibromyalgia, chronic pelvic pain, and osteoarthritis.[114] Associations between chronic pain and dysbiosis of the gut microbiome may be mediated in part by changes in the activation and proliferation of symbiotic bacteria. Interactions between the gut microbiome and the CNS may involve mechanisms such as vagus nerve signaling from the gut to the CNS and by leakage of pro-inflammatory compounds through a compromised intestinal barrier into the systemic circulation and across the blood-brain barrier.[114]

Experimental findings suggest an important role of the gut microbiome in TMD.[115] Induction of TMJ inflammation in mice has been shown to decrease levels of short-chain fatty acids (SCFAs) in the gut. In the same study, mice with inflamed TMJs that received transplanted gut microbiota from other mice that had been treated with the antioxidant resveratrol displayed both reversal of these SCFA changes as well as reduced pain behavior in response to mechanical stimulation of the face. Such findings hold out hope that future studies may demonstrate efficacy of gut-focused interventions for patients with orofacial pain.

Psychologic/behavioral factors

Sleep

The importance of a good night's sleep to our overall health is obvious. With respect to orofacial pain and other chronic pain conditions, it is well established that pain can cause poor sleep quality, which leads to greater pain and worsening sleep patterns, thus creating a vicious cycle. However, poor quality and/or quantity of sleep also can contribute to pain chronification following an injury. For example, sleep disturbances and sleep disorders such as insomnia, obstructive sleep apnea (OSA), restless leg syndrome (RLS), and sleep bruxism are known to frequently be comorbid with chronic pain conditions. Sleep deprivation is a major health issue and has been referred to by the U.S. Centers for Disease Control and Prevention as a pandemic. Unfortunately, we live in a culture that does not place value on the importance of sleep, even in children. Why is sleep so essential to human health? One answer may involve the role of sleep in the clearance of metabolic waste from the brain through a specialized system comprised of glia and lymph vessels known as the *glymphatic system*. Disruption of this system is implicated in migraine pathology because normal glymphatic and meningeal lymphatic activity plays a key role in regulating neuronal excitability and brain inflammation.[116] The relationship between sleep and orofacial pain is further discussed in chapter 11.

Nutrition

A diet rich in fruits and vegetables has been shown to be beneficial in managing many inflammatory diseases that are comorbid with TMD and migraine, including cardiovascular disease, diabetes, IBS, and obesity. Unfortunately, too much attention is paid to calories and not enough to nutrition. Human nutrition should not only provide macronutrients and micronutrients for the health of our cells but also needs to include natural fiber that serves as a nutrient source for our gut bacteria. Given the emerging evidence of the interdependency of the gut-brain axis, it is becoming clear that to have a healthy nervous system, one needs to have a healthy digestive system. Consider the impact of chronic stress on our physiologic systems. The ill effects of severe and chronic stress become manifest in diseases of both the digestive and nervous systems independent of age. One goal in managing patients should be to increase parasympathetic tone while reducing allostatic load and sympathetic tone through behavioral modifications and lifestyle changes. While no one refutes that a poor diet can make you unhealthy, it is more difficult to convince patients that eating a healthier diet enriched with natural fiber and minerals (fruits and vegetables) and containing potent antioxidants (fruits and nuts) is key to managing cellular stress in the digestive and nervous system, hence promoting overall health. A healthy diet enriched with natural fiber provides an essential food source to maintain the commensal gut bacteria and as such functions as a prebiotic. In some cases, it may be advisable to recommend the inclusion of probiotic supplements because they contain living strains of bacteria that can be beneficial in supporting and maintaining a healthy gut microbiome.

Mental health and psychiatric disorders

Of the minority of TMD cases that become chronic,[117] one-third seem to resolve over an 8-to-10-year period.[118] TMD patients who significantly improve may have minimal psychologic issues,[119] while patients with chronic TMD[120,121] have psychologic comorbidity similar to other chronic pain patients.[122,123]

Although this is a delicate subject to broach, clinicians must be able to open the door to skilled therapists for patients with problematic psychosocial histories if pain improvement is to be achieved. Chapter 12 provides a detailed discussion of psychobehavioral considerations in orofacial pain.

Social/environmental factors

Psychologic/emotional trauma

In patients with chronic pain, exposure to physical, emotional, and sexual abuse may be three times greater than that experienced in the general population.[124] Patients with orofacial pain report a high degree of exposure to traumatic events. The taboos associated with abuse, or the repression induced by the sheer horror of a catastrophic event, can prevent patients from revealing these experiences. Severe pain and comorbid conditions associated with maladaptive CNS function may therefore be the only clinical indications of psychosocial distress.

The biopsychosocial factors outlined previously, among many others, may contribute in various ways to the experience and chronification of pain: They may act as predisposing factors, making an individual susceptible to developing chronic pain when certain circumstances arise; they may be initiating factors that act as a direct trigger for the initial onset of pain; they may be maintaining factors, contributing to persistence of pain; or alternatively, they may be protective, guarding against onset of chronic pain in the face of a nociceptive insult.

Familiarity with the range of possible contributing factors enables the orofacial pain practitioner to identify the unique combination of factors that may be in play in the pain experience of an individual patient. These factors may be thought of as "volume control dials" for pain. Some of these dials, such as genetic factors or the existence of a history of traumatic experiences, are locked in place and impossible to modify. But others may be turned down, helping to attenuate pain: Sleep habits can be changed, postural and parafunctional behaviors can be modified, healthy coping strategies for psychologic stress and past trauma can be learned and engaged. Modification of these factors requires primarily the efforts of the patient rather than the clinician. A key component of the orofacial pain practitioner's quest is to collaborate across multiple disciplines with fellow specialists in empowering the patient to put his or her hands on the dials that can ultimately alter the pain experience.

Comorbidities: Orofacial Pain and Chronic Overlapping Pain Conditions

An important subset of chronic pain disorders with relevance to orofacial pain is referred to as *chronic overlapping pain conditions* (COPCs). COPCs include TMD, fibromyalgia, vulvodynia, IBS, interstitial cystitis/painful bladder syndrome, endometriosis, chronic tension-type headache, migraine headache, myalgic encephalomyelitis/chronic fatigue syndrome, and chronic lower back pain.[125]

More than 81% of patients with facial pain also report pain in regions below the head.[126,127] TMD patients frequently have symptoms of fibromyalgia, chronic fatigue syndrome, headaches, panic disorder, gastroesophageal reflux disease, IBS, multiple chemical sensitivity, posttraumatic stress disorder, and interstitial cystitis. Unfortunately, TMD patients may avoid care when symptoms carry psychosomatic stigma.[128] Patient acceptance of a biopsychosocial approach may largely be dependent on previous psychosocial experience.[129]

Persistent elevation of sympathetic tone and impaired parasympathetic tone may contribute to many comorbid conditions that affect orofacial pain patients. Heart rate variability may be a noninvasive measurable parameter that could track the physiology of ANS problems in patients with trigeminal pain and shed light on its cause.[130] Reducing upregulated sympathetic activation, which may drive an imbalanced emotional motor system, may reduce central sensitization that underlies the refractory nature of the spectrum of conditions seen in orofacial pain practice.

Headache and orofacial pain disorders

Recurrent headache may occur in as many as 80% of TMD patients[131,132] compared to a 20% to 23% occurrence rate in a general population.[133-135] One in three persons has been estimated to suffer from severe headache at some point in his or her life,[136] a lifetime incidence similar to the 34% rate estimated for TMD.[137] Yet, only 5% to 10% of the North American population has sought medical advice for severe headache.[135] Although earlier studies have shown associations between TMD and headache,[133,138-142] causal interrelationships have not been demonstrated. However, in a study in which 61% of orofacial pain patients had headache complaints and 38% fulfilled the criteria for migraine, higher migraine disability assessment (MIDAS) scores correlated with masticatory and cervical myalgia but did not correlate with the presence or absence of intracapsular TMJ problems.[143] An association of sleep bruxism and painful TMD was reported to greatly increase the risk for the development of episodic migraine, episodic tension-type headache, and especially chronic migraine.[144] Interestingly, in women experiencing both TMD and migraine, the migraine condition only significantly improved when both conditions were treated. Furthermore, women suffering from migraine are likely to have more muscular and articular TMD,[145] which supports the notion that both disorders are clinically associated and highlights the importance of physical therapy assessment in the multidisciplinary team approach to managing complex pain patients.

Headaches and TMD are major complaints associated with trigeminal pain, leading to significant suffering and absenteeism from work or school.[137,146] Traumatic stressors may play a significant role in this suffering and pain.[147,148] Associations of myalgia with headache[142] suggest that head and neck muscles may modify input that contributes to the ANS dysfunction and central sensitization that may be involved in headache disorders.[34,149-152]

Future Directions for Research and Treatment

Stem cell therapy

The limitations of current therapeutics for TMJ disorders have led to an increased interest in regenerative strategies. Regenerative medicine includes gene therapies, cell therapies, and tissue-engineered products intended to augment, repair, replace or regenerate organs, tissues, cells, genes, and metabolic processes in the body. Hence, the goal of regenerative medicine is to complement current practices by treating the root causes of disease and disorders. Hopefully, future advances will allow tissue engineering to be utilized to repair or replace TMJ structures including the disc, condyle, and glenoid fossa. The goal of tissue engineering of the TMJ is to provide regenerative solutions when surgical management is required. Unfortunately, progress in TMJ regeneration has thus far been challenged by the complex and unique anatomical and functional characteristics of this joint.[153,154] A possible avenue for future progress might include use of stem cells, given their capacity to regenerate tissues such as bone and cartilage, as demonstrated in regeneration of infrabony alveolar defects.[153,154] However, the evidence supporting these specific roles is weak, and further studies are required to evaluate the therapeutic potential of stem cells. Given the prevalence of TMD, regenerative medicine will continue to be an active research area. However, significant challenges must be overcome before the scientific community can determine whether these strategies can effectively treat TMJ pathologies and improve patient outcomes.

New digital technologies

The COVID-19 pandemic has stimulated many changes in the way we engage in business, education, and social meetings as well as how clinicians interact with their patients. A large increase in the use of telemedicine provides support to patients with limited access to care, especially those in rural areas. Hopefully, continued expansion of telemedicine will empower orofacial pain clinicians to improve access to care for the elderly, the disabled, patients in rural settings, and the economically disadvantaged. A wide range of mobile apps can augment telemedicine by assisting with activities such as patient education and self-care instructions, monitoring diet and exercise, guiding relaxation techniques, and tracking vital signs. New options will continue to become available and should provide complementary resources for managing patients experiencing orofacial pain.

References

1. Groenewegen HJ, Uylings HB. The prefrontal cortex and the integration of sensory, limbic and autonomic information. Prog Brain Res 2000;126:3–28.
2. Charlton JE (ed). Core Curriculum for Professional Education in Pain, ed 3. Seattle: IASP, 2005.
3. National Academies of Sciences, Engineering, and Medicine 2020. Temporomandibular disorders: Priorities for research and care. Washington, DC: The National Academies Press. Available at: https://doi.org/10.17226/25652.
4. Terminology. International Association for the Study of Pain website. http://www.iasp-pain.org/resources/terminology. Accessed 6 July 2022.
5. Sandkuhler J. Spinal cord plasticity and pain. In: McMahon SB, Koltzenburg M, Tracey I, Turk DC (eds). Wall and Melzack's Textbook of Pain, ed 6. Philadelphia: Saunders, 2013:94–110.
6. Chichorro JG, Porreca F, Sessle B. Mechanisms of craniofacial pain. Cephalalgia 2017;37:613–626.
7. Woolf CJ. What is this thing called pain? J Clin Invest 2010;120:3742–3744.
8. Hu JW, Wada A. Trigeminal brainstem nuclear complex, physiology. In: Gebhart GF, Schmidt RF (eds). Encyclopedia of Pain. Berlin: Springer, 2013: 4060–4064.
9. Treede RD, Rief W, Barke A, et al. Chronic pain as a symptom or a disease: The IASP classification of chronic pain for the International Classification of Diseases (ICD-11). Pain 2019;160:19–27.
10. Dahlhamer J, Lucas J, Zelaya C, et al. Prevalence of chronic pain and high-impact chronic pain among adults—United States, 2016. MMWR Morb Mortal Wkly Rep 2018;67:1001–1006.
11. Gaskin DJ, Richard P. The economic costs of pain in the United States. J Pain 2012;13:715–724.
12. Schiffman E, Ohrbach R, Truelove E, et al. Diagnostic criteria for temporomandibular disorders (DC/TMD) for clinical and research applications: Recommendations of the International RDC/TMD Consortium Network* and Orofacial Pain Special Interest Group-dagger. J Oral Facial Pain Headache 2014;28:6–27.
13. Headache Classification Committee of the International Headache Society (IHS) The International Classification of Headache Disorders, 3rd edition. Cephalalgia 2018;38:1–211.
14. International Classification of Orofacial Pain, 1st edition (ICOP). Cephalalgia 2020;40:129–221.
15. Sarlani E, Greenspan JD. Why look in the brain for answers to temporomandibular disorder pain? Cells Tissues Organs 2005;180:69–75.
16. Ringkamp M, Srinivasa NR, Campbell JN, Meyer RA. Peripheral mechanisms of cutaneous nociceptrion. In: McMahon SB, Koltzenburg M, Tracey I, Turk DC (eds). Wall and Melzack's Textbook of Pain, ed 6. Philadelphia: Saunders, 2013:1–30.
17. Byers MR, Dong WK. Comparison of trigeminal receptor location and structure in the periodontal ligament of different types of teeth from the rat, cat, and monkey. J Comp Neurol 1989;279:117–127
18. Ren K, Dubner R. The role of trigeminal interpolaris-caudalis transition zone in persistent orofacial pain. Int Rev Neurobiol 2011;97:207–225.

19. Wang H, Wei F, Dubner R, Ren K. Selective distribution and function of primary afferent nociceptive inputs from deep muscle tissue to the brainstem trigeminal transition zone. J Comp Neurol 2006;498:390–402.
20. Ikeda T, Terayama R, Jue SS, Sugiyo S, Dubner R, Ren K. Differential rostral projections of caudal brainstem neurons receiving trigeminal input after masseter inflammation. J Comp Neurol 2003;465:220–233.
21. Marfurt CF, Rajchert DM. Trigeminal primary afferent projections to "non-trigeminal" areas of the rat central nervous system. J Comp Neurol 1991;303:489-511.
22. Saxon DW, Hopkins DA. Efferent and collateral organization of paratrigeminal nucleus projections: An anterograde and retrograde fluorescent tracer study in the rat. J Comp Neurol 1998;402:93–110.
23. Sessle BJ, Hu JW. Mechanisms of pain arising from articular tissues. Can J Physiol Pharmacol 1991;69: 617–626.
24. Olsson KA, Westberg KG. Integration in trigeminal premotor interneurones in the cat. 2. Functional characteristics of neurones in the subnucleus-gamma of the oral nucleus of the spinal trigeminal tract with a projection to the digastric motoneurone subnucleus. Expl Brain Res 1991;84:115–124.
25. Dougherty P. Chapter 4: Somatosensory pathways. In: Neuroscience Online: An electronic textbook for the neurosciences. University of Texas Health Science Center at Houston. https://nba.uth.tmc.edu/neuroscience/m/s2/chapter04.html. Revised 7 Oct 2020. Accessed 6 July 2022.
26. Yam MF, Loh YC, Tan CS, Khadijah Adam S, Abdul Manan N, Basir R. General pathways of pain sensation and the major neurotransmitters involved in pain regulation. Int J Mol Sci 2018;19:2164.
27. Westberg KG, Olsson KA. Integration in trigeminal premotor interneurones in the cat. 1. Functional characteristics of neurones in the subnucleus-gamma of the oral nucleus of the spinal trigeminal tract. Exp Brain Res 1991;84:102–114.
28. Westberg KG, Sandstrom G, Olsson KA. Integration in trigeminal premotor interneurones in the cat. 3. Input characteristics and synaptic actions of neurones in subnucleus-gamma of the oral nucleus of the spinal trigeminal tract with a projection to the masseteric motoneurone subnucleus. Exp Brain Res 1995;104: 449–461.
29. Mannion RJ, Woolf CJ. Pain mechanisms and management: A central perspective. Clin J Pain 2000;16(3 suppl):S144–S156.
30. Bolay H, Moskowitz MA. Mechanisms of pain modulation in chronic syndromes. Neurology 2002;59(5 suppl 2):S2–S7.
31. Melzack R, Casey, KL. Sensory, motivational, and central control determinants of pain: A new conceptual model. In: Kenshalo DR (ed). The Skin Senses: Proceedings of the First International Symposium on the Skin Senses. Springfield, IL: Charles C. Thomas, 1968:423–439.
32. Li XF, Stutzmann GE, LeDoux JE. Convergent but temporally separated inputs to lateral amygdala neurons from the auditory thalamus and auditory cortex use different postsynaptic receptors: In vivo intracellular and extracellular recordings in fear conditioning pathways. Learn Mem 1996;3:229–242.
33. Stutzmann GE, McEwen BS, LeDoux JE. Serotonin modulation of sensory inputs to the lateral amygdala: Dependency on corticosterone. J Neurosci 1998;18: 9529–9538.
34. Yamamura H, Malick A, Chamberlin NL, Burstein R. Cardiovascular and neuronal responses to head stimulation reflect central sensitization and cutaneous allodynia in a rat model of migraine. J Neurophysiol 1999;81:479–493.
35. Benarroch EE. Pain-autonomic interactions: A selective review. Clin Auton Res 2001;11:343–349.
36. Peirs C, Seal RP. Neural circuits for pain: Recent advances and current views. Science 2016;354:578–584.
37. Yang S, Chang MC. Chronic pain: Structural and functional changes in brain structures and associated negative affective states. Int J Mol Sci 2019;20:3130.
38. Shinoda M, Kubo A, Hayashi Y, Iwata K. Peripheral and central mechanisms of persistent orofacial pain. Front Neurosci 2019;13:1227.
39. Cavanaugh DJ, Lee H, Lo L, et al. Distinct subsets of unmyelinated primary sensory fibers mediate behavioral responses to noxious thermal and mechanical stimuli. Proc Natl Acad Sci U S A 2009;106:9075–9080.
40. Sessle BJ. Peripheral and central mechanisms of orofacial inflammatory pain. Int Rev Neurobiol 2011;97:179–206.
41. Woolf CJ. Central sensitization: Implications for the diagnosis and treatment of pain. Pain 2011;152(3 suppl):S2–S15.
42. Woolf CJ, Shortland P, Coggeshall RE. Peripheral nerve injury triggers central sprouting of myelinated afferents. Nature 1992;355:75–78.
43. Coggeshall RE, Lekan HA, Doubell TP, Allchorne A, Woolf CJ. Central changes in primary afferent fibers following peripheral nerve lesions. Neuroscience 1997;77:1115–1122.
44. Ji RR, Berta T, Nedergaard M. Glia and pain: Is chronic pain a gliopathy? Pain 2013;154(suppl 1):S10–S28.
45. Durham PL, Garrett FG. Emerging importance of neuron-satellite glia interactions within trigeminal ganglia in craniofacial pain. TOPAINJ 2010;3:3–13.

46. Garrett FG, Durham PL. Differential expression of connexins in trigeminal ganglion neurons and satellite glial cells in response to chronic or acute joint inflammation. Neuron Glia Biol 2009:1–12.
47. Milligan ED, Watkins LR. Pathological and protective roles of glia in chronic pain. Nat Rev Neurosci 2009;10:23–36.
48. Kimelberg HK, Nedergaard M. Functions of astrocytes and their potential as therapeutic targets. Neurotherapeutics 2010;7:338–353.
49. Davies AJ, Kim YH, Oh SB. Painful neuron-microglia interactions in the trigeminal sensory system. TOPAINJ 2010;3:14–28.
50. Old EA, Clark AK, Malcangio M. The role of glia in the spinal cord in neuropathic and inflammatory pain. Handb Exp Pharmacol 2015;227:145–170.
51. Seybold VS. The role of peptides in central sensitization. Handb Exp Pharmacol 2009;(194):451–491.
52. Cornelison LE, Hawkins JL, Durham PL. Elevated levels of calcitonin gene-related peptide in upper spinal cord promotes sensitization of primary trigeminal nociceptive neurons. Neuroscience 2016;339:491–501.
53. Exposto FG, Udagawa G, Naganawa T, Svensson P. Comparison of masseter muscle referred sensations after mechanical and glutamate stimulation: A randomized, double-blind, controlled, cross-over study. Pain 2018;159:2649–2657.
54. Gray H, Clemente CD. Anatomy of the Human Body, ed 30. Philadelphia: Lea & Febiger, 1985.
55. Thayer JF, Siegle GJ. Neurovisceral integration in cardiac and emotional regulation. IEEE Eng Med Biol Mag 2002;21:24–29.
56. Lachuer J, Gaillet S, Barbagli B, Buda M, Tappaz M. Differential early time course activation of the brainstem catecholaminergic groups in response to various stresses. Neuroendocrinology 1991;53:589–596.
57. Kandel ER, Schwartz JH, Jessell TM. Principles of Neural Science, ed 3. Norwalk, CT: Appleton & Lange, 1991.
58. Aaron LA, Burke MM, Buchwald D. Overlapping conditions among patients with chronic fatigue syndrome, fibromyalgia, and temporomandibular disorder. Arch Intern Med 2000;160:221–227.
59. de Leeuw R, Klasser GD, Albuquerque RJ. Are female patients with orofacial pain medically compromised? J Am Dent Assoc 2005;136:459–468.
60. Arzani M, Jahromi SR, Ghorbani Z, et al. Gut-brain axis and migraine headache: A comprehensive review. J Headache Pain 2020;21:15.
61. van Hemert S, Breedveld AC, Rovers JM, et al. Migraine associated with gastrointestinal disorders: Review of the literature and clinical implications. Front Neurol 2014;5:241.
62. Draghici AE, Taylor JA. The physiological basis and measurement of heart rate variability in humans. J Physiol Anthropol 2016;35:22.
63. Park G, Thayer JF. From the heart to the mind: Cardiac vagal tone modulates top-down and bottom-up visual perception and attention to emotional stimuli. Front Psychol 2014;5:278.
64. Fatisson J, Oswald V, Lalonde F. Influence diagram of physiological and environmental factors affecting heart rate variability: An extended literature overview. Heart Int 2016;11:e32–e40.
65. Thayer JF, Ahs F, Fredrikson M, Sollers JJ 3rd, Wager TD. A meta-analysis of heart rate variability and neuroimaging studies: Implications for heart rate variability as a marker of stress and health. Neurosci Biobehav Rev 2012;36:747–756.
66. Carlson CR, Reid KI, Curran SL, et al. Psychological and physiological parameters of masticatory muscle pain. Pain 1998;76:297–307.
67. Carlson CR, Bertrand PM, Ehrlich AD, Maxwell AW, Burton RG. Physical self-regulation training for the management of temporomandibular disorders. J Orofac Pain 2001;15:47–55.
68. Dworkin SF, Turner JA, Mancl L, et al. A randomized clinical trial of a tailored comprehensive care treatment program for temporomandibular disorders. J Orofac Pain 2002;16:259–276.
69. Chinthakanan S, Laosuwan K, Boonyawong P, Kumfu S, Chattipakorn N, Chattipakorn SC. Reduced heart rate variability and increased saliva cortisol in patients with TMD. Arch Oral Biol 2018;90:125–129.
70. Graeff FG, Guimaraes FS, De Andrade TG, Deakin JF. Role of 5-HT in stress, anxiety, and depression. Pharmacol Biochem Behav 1996;54:129–141.
71. Melzack R, Wall PD. Pain mechanisms: A new theory. Science 1965;150(3699):971–979.
72. Bannister K, Dickenson AH. The plasticity of descending controls in pain: Translational probing. J Physiol 2017;595:4159–4166.
73. Lockwood S, Dickenson AH. What goes up must come down: Insights from studies on descending controls acting on spinal pain processing. J Neural Transm (Vienna) 2020;127:541–549.
74. Gagne M, Cote I, Boulet M, Jutzeler CR, Kramer JLK, Mercier C. Conditioned pain modulation decreases over time in patients with neuropathic pain following a spinal cord injury. Neurorehabil Neural Repair 2020;34:997–1008.
75. Fay RA, Norgren R. Identification of rat brainstem multisynaptic connections to the oral motor nuclei using pseudorabies virus. III. Lingual muscle motor systems. Brain Res Brain Res Rev 1997;25:291–311.

76. Fay RA, Norgren R. Identification of rat brainstem multisynaptic connections to the oral motor nuclei in the rat using pseudorabies virus. II. Facial muscle motor systems. Brain Res Brain Res Rev 1997;25: 276–290.
77. Fay RA, Norgren R. Identification of rat brainstem multisynaptic connections to the oral motor nuclei using pseudorabies virus. I. Masticatory muscle motor systems. Brain Res Brain Res Rev 1997;25:255–275.
78. Dubner R, Sessle BJ, Storey AT. The Beural Basis of Oral and Facial Function. New York: Plenum, 1978.
79. Cadden SW. Modulation of human jaw reflexes: Heterotopic stimuli and stress. Arch Oral Biol 2007; 52:370–373.
80. Lund JP, Donga R, Widmer CG, Stohler CS. The pain-adaptation model: A discussion of the relationship between chronic musculoskeletal pain and motor activity. Can J Physiol Pharmacol 1991;69:683–694.
81. Finniss DG, Kaptchuk TJ, Miller F, Benedetti F. Biological, clinical, and ethical advances of placebo effects. Lancet 2010;375:686–695.
82. Kaptchuk TJ, Hemond CC, Miller FG. Placebos in chronic pain: Evidence, theory, ethics, and use in clinical practice. BMJ 2020;370:m1668.
83. Vase L, Wartolowska K. Pain, placebo, and test of treatment efficacy: A narrative review. Br J Anaesth 2019; 123:e254–e262.
84. Kam-Hansen S, Jakubowski M, Kelley JM, et al. Altered placebo and drug labeling changes the outcome of episodic migraine attacks. Sci Transl Med 2014;6: 218ra5.
85. Engel GL. The need for a new medical model: A challenge for biomedicine. Science 1977;196:129–136.
86. Chugani HT, Behen ME, Muzik O, Juhasz C, Nagy F, Chugani DC. Local brain functional activity following early deprivation: A study of postinstitutionalized Romanian orphans. Neuroimage 2001;14:1290–1301.
87. Monnikes H, Tebbe JJ, Hildebrandt M, et al. Role of stress in functional gastrointestinal disorders. Evidence for stress-induced alterations in gastrointestinal motility and sensitivity. Dig Dis 2001;19:201–211.
88. Mayer EA, Naliboff BD, Chang L. Basic pathophysiologic mechanisms in irritable bowel syndrome. Dig Dis 2001;19:212–218.
89. Kaufman J, Plotsky PM, Nemeroff CB, Charney DS. Effects of early adverse experiences on brain structure and function: Clinical implications. Biol Psychiatry 2000;48:778–790.
90. Heim C, Newport DJ, Bonsall R, Miller AH, Nemeroff CB. Altered pituitary-adrenal axis responses to provocative challenge tests in adult survivors of childhood abuse. Am J Psychiatry 2001;158:575–581.
91. McEwen BS. Stress, adaptation, and disease. Allostasis and allostatic load. Ann N Y Acad Sci 1998;840:33–44.
92. McEwen BS, Wingfield JC. What is in a name? Integrating homeostasis, allostasis and stress. Horm Behav 2010;57:105–111.
93. Guidi J, Lucente M, Sonino N, Fava GA. Allostatic load and its impact on health: A systematic review. Psychother Psychosom 2021;90:11–27.
94. Borsook D, Maleki N, Becerra L, McEwen B. Understanding migraine through the lens of maladaptive stress responses: A model disease of allostatic load. Neuron 2012;73:219–234.
95. Maleki N, Becerra L, Borsook D. Migraine: Maladaptive brain responses to stress. Headache 2012; 52(suppl 2):102–106.
96. Tedeschi G, Russo A, Tessitore A. Functional neuroimaging: The adaptive mechanisms in migraine. J Headache Pain 2015;16(suppl 1):A6.
97. Schulkin J, McEwen BS, Gold PW. Allostasis, amygdala, and anticipatory angst. Neurosci Biobehav Rev 1994;18:385–396.
98. Nicholson RA, Buse DC, Andrasik F, Lipton RB. Nonpharmacologic treatments for migraine and tension-type headache: How to choose and when to use. Curr Treat Options Neurol 2011;13:28–40.
99. Zorina-Lichtenwalter K, Meloto CB, Khoury S, Diatchenko L. Genetic predictors of human chronic pain conditions. Neuroscience 2016;338:36–62.
100. Gormley P, Anttila V, Winsvold BS, et al. Meta-analysis of 375,000 individuals identifies 38 susceptibility loci for migraine. Nat Genet 2016;48:856–866.
101. Kossowsky J, Schuler MS, Giulianini F, et al. Association of genetic variants with migraine subclassified by clinical symptoms in adult females. Front Neurol 2020;11:617472.
102. Anttila V, Winsvold BS, Gormley P, et al. Genome-wide meta-analysis identifies new susceptibility loci for migraine. Nat Genet 2013;45:912–917.
103. Greenspan JD, Slade GD, Bair E, et al. Pain sensitivity risk factors for chronic TMD: Descriptive data and empirically identified domains from the OPPERA case control study. J Pain 2011;12(11 suppl):T61–T74.
104. Ohrbach R, Fillingim RB, Mulkey F, et al. Clinical findings and pain symptoms as potential risk factors for chronic TMD: Descriptive data and empirically identified domains from the OPPERA case-control study. J Pain 2011;12(11 suppl):T27–T45.
105. Slade GD, Ohrbach R, Greenspona JD, Fillingim RB et al. Painful temporomandibular disorder: Decade of discovery from OPPERA studies. J Dent Res 2016;95:1084–1092.

106. Fish EW, Shahrokh D, Bagot R, et al. Epigenetic programming of stress responses through variations in maternal care. Ann N Y Acad Sci 2004;1036:167–180.
107. Berger SL, Kouzarides T, Shiekhattar R, Shilatifard A. An operational definition of epigenetics. Genes Dev 2009;23:781–783.
108. Choi SW, Friso S. Epigenetics: A new bridge between nutrition and health. Adv Nutr 2010;1:8–16.
109. Alvarado S, Tajerian M, Suderman M, et al. An epigenetic hypothesis for the genomic memory of pain. Front Cell Neurosci 2015;9:88.
110. Denk F, McMahon SB. Chronic pain: Emerging evidence for the involvement of epigenetics. Neuron 2012;73:435–444.
111. Bartley EJ, Fillingim RB. Sex differences in pain: A brief review of clinical and experimental findings. Br J Anaesth 2013;111:52–58.
112. Mills SEE, Nicolson KP, Smith BH. Chronic pain: A review of its epidemiology and associated factors in population-based studies. Br J Anaesth 2019;123:e273–e283.
113. Mapplebeck JCS, Beggs S, Salter MW. Sex differences in pain: A tale of two immune cells. Pain 2016;157(suppl 1):S2–S6.
114. Dworsky-Fried Z, Kerr BJ, Taylor AMW. Microbes, microglia, and pain. Neurobiol Pain 2020;7:100045.
115. Ma Y, Liu S, Shu H, Crawford J, Xing Y, Tao F. Resveratrol alleviates temporomandibular joint inflammatory pain by recovering disturbed gut microbiota. Brain Behav Immun 2020;87:455–464.
116. Vgontzas A, Pavlovic JM. Sleep disorders and migraine: Review of literature and potential pathophysiology mechanisms. Headache 2018;58:1030–1039.
117. Von Korff M, Le Resche L, Dworkin SF. First onset of common pain symptoms: A prospective study of depression as a risk factor. Pain 1993;55:251–258.
118. Magni G, Marchetti M, Moreschi C, Merskey H, Luchini SR. Chronic musculoskeletal pain and depressive symptoms in the National Health and Nutrition Examination. I. Epidemiologic follow-up study. Pain 1993;53:163–168.
119. Ohrbach R, Dworkin SF. Five-year outcomes in TMD: Relationship of changes in pain to changes in physical and psychological variables. Pain 1998;74:315–326.
120. Sanders S. Chronic pain: Conceptualization and epidemiology. Ann Behav Med 1985;7:3–5.
121. Kinney RK, Gatchel RJ, Ellis E, Holt C. Major psychological disorders in chronic TMD patients: Implications for successful management. J Am Dent Assoc 1992;123:49–54.
122. Bush FM, Harkins SW. Pain-related limitation in activities of daily living in patients with chronic orofacial pain: Psychometric properties of a disability index. J Orofac Pain 1995;9:57–63.
123. Merskey H. Classification of chronic pain: Descriptions of chronic pain syndromes and definitions of pain terms. Pain 1986;(suppl 3):1–225.
124. Curran SL, Sherman JJ, Cunningham LL, Okeson JP, Reid KI, Carlson CR. Physical and sexual abuse among orofacial pain patients: Linkages with pain and psychologic distress. J Orofac Pain 1995;9:340–346.
125. Maixner W, Fillingim RB, Williams DA, Smith SB, Slade GD. Overlapping chronic pain conditions: Implications for diagnosis and classification. J Pain 2016;17(9 suppl):T93–T107.
126. Turp JC, Kowalski CJ, O'Leary N, Stohler CS. Pain maps from facial pain patients indicate a broad pain geography. J Dent Res 1998;77:1465–1472.
127. Türp JC, Kowalski CJ, Stohler CS. Temporomandibular disorders—Pain outside the head and face is rarely acknowledged in the chief complaint. J Prosthet Dent 1997;78:592–595.
128. Hoge CW, Lesikar SE, Guevara R, et al. Mental disorders among U.S. military personnel in the 1990s: Association with high levels of health care utilization and early military attrition. Am J Psychiatry 2002;159:1576–1583.
129. Browne AL, Schug SA, Ray P, French D. A biopsychosocial approach to pretreatment assessment of patients with persistent pain: Identifying factors associated with pain-related disability. Pain Med 2006;7:466–467.
130. Lewis MJ. Heart rate variability analysis: A tool to assess cardiac autonomic function. Comput Inform Nurs 2005;23:335–341.
131. Magnusson T, Carlsson GE. Comparison between two groups of patients in respect of headache and mandibular dysfunction. Swed Dent J 1978;2:85–92.
132. Andrasik F, Holroyd KA, Abell T. Prevalence of headache within a college student population: A preliminary analysis. Headache 1979;19:384–387.
133. Magnusson T, Carlsson GE. Recurrent headaches in relation to temporomandibular joint pain-dysfunction. Acta Odontol Scand 1978;36:333–338.
134. Rieder CE. The incidence of some occlusal habits and headaches/neckaches in an initial survey population. J Prosthet Dent 1976;35:445–451.
135. Turner DB, Stone AJ. Headache and its treatment: A random sample survey. Headache 1979;19:74–77.
136. Göbel H, Petersen-Braun M, Soyka D. The epidemiology of headache in Germany: A nationwide survey of a representative sample on the basis of the headache classification of the International Headache Society. Cephalalgia 1994;14:97–106.

137. Von Korff M, Dworkin SF, Le Resche L, Kruger A. An epidemiologic comparison of pain complaints. Pain 1988;32:173–183.
138. Schokker RP, Hansson TL, Ansink BJ. The result of treatment of the masticatory system of chronic headache patients. J Craniomandib Disord 1990;4:126–130.
139. Helöe B, Helöe LA. Frequency and distribution of myofascial pain-dysfunction syndrome in a population of 25-year-olds. Community Dent Oral Epidemiol 1979;7:357–360.
140. Wanman A, Agerberg G. Headache and dysfunction of the masticatory system in adolescents. Cephalalgia 1986;6:247–255.
141. Forssell H. Mandibular dysfunction and headache. Proc Finn Dent Soc 1985;81(suppl 1–2):1–91.
142. Schokker RP, Hansson TL, Ansink BJ. Craniomandibular disorders in patients with different types of headache. J Craniomandib Disord 1990;4:47–51.
143. Dando WE, Branch MA, Maye JP. Headache disability in orofacial pain patients. Headache 2006;46:322–326.
144. Fernandes G, Franco AL, Goncalves DA, Speciali JG, Bigal ME, Camparis CM. Temporomandibular disorders, sleep bruxism, and primary headaches are mutually associated. J Orofac Pain 2013;27:14–20.
145. Gonçalves MC, Florencio LL, Chaves TC, Speciali JG, Bigal ME, Bevilaqua-Grossi D. Do women with migraine have higher prevalence of temporomandibular disorders? Braz J Phys Ther 2013;17:64–68.
146. Sternbach RA. Pain and 'hassles' in the United States: Findings of the Nuprin pain report. Pain 1986;27:69–80.
147. De Leeuw R, Bertoli E, Schmidt JE, Carlson CR. Prevalence of post-traumatic stress disorder symptoms in orofacial pain patients. Oral Surg Oral Med Oral Pathol Oral Radiol and Endod 2005;99:558–568.
148. de Leeuw R, Schmidt JE, Carlson CR. Traumatic stressors and post-traumatic stress disorder symptoms in headache patients. Headache 2005;45:1365–1374.
149. Shechter A, Stewart WF, Silberstein SD, Lipton RB. Migraine and autonomic nervous system function: A population-based, case-control study. Neurology 2002;58:422–427.
150. Jensen R. Mechanisms of tension-type headache. Cephalalgia 2001;21:786–789.
151. Bartsch T, Goadsby PJ. The trigeminocervical complex and migraine: Current concepts and synthesis. Curr Pain Headache Rep 2003;7:371–376.
152. Goadsby PJ. Migraine pathophysiology. Headache 2005;45(suppl 1):S14–S24.
153. Serakinci N, Savtekin G. Modeling mesenchymal stem cells in TMJ rheumatoid arthritis and osteoarthritis therapy. Crit Rev Eukaryot Gene Expr 2017;27:205–210.
154. Karic V, Chandran R, Abrahamse H. Laser-induced differentiation of human adipose-derived stem cells to temporomandibular joint disc cells. Lasers Surg Med 2021;53:567–577.

2

General Assessment of the Orofacial Pain Patient

Key Points

- The general assessment of the orofacial pain patient is aimed at identifying the what, where, how, and why of the presenting complaint.
- Diagnosis of orofacial pain requires taking a detailed history, completing a comprehensive clinical examination, and ordering appropriate tests of established validity.
- All dental patients should be screened for temporomandibular disorders (TMDs), and positive screening findings should prompt more comprehensive evaluation.

Successful management of patients who are seeking care for orofacial pain requires the clinician to gain an understanding of the problem and establish a proper diagnosis.[1] Diagnosis (or diagnoses, as there is rarely only one) cannot be based solely on the patient's description of pain; it must also involve taking a detailed pain history, performing a comprehensive physical examination, and ordering and interpreting appropriate diagnostic tests. The orofacial pain clinician must then synthesize the information to determine pain etiology and establish a diagnosis utilizing accepted classification systems.[2] Familiarity with orofacial pain disorders and their classification is essential for targeted assessment and accurate diagnosis. The immediate goal after establishing the diagnosis is to initiate a treatment plan. As such, before commencing any treatment, an evaluation of the patient's overall health status, including their dental, medical and surgical, drug, and psychosocial history, is also required. Collaboration with various specialists (eg, otolaryngology, neurology, rheumatology, psychiatry) is often necessary. The objective of general assessment is to accurately identify the what, where, how, and why of the patient's complaint. This chapter discusses the basic tests and techniques for the assessment of an orofacial pain patient.

Screening Evaluation

It has become integral to current practice that all dental patients be screened for TMDs and other orofacial pain disorders as part of their initial and regular examinations. The results of the screening should help the clinician determine whether a more comprehensive evaluation is necessary.[3] The screening may consist of a short questionnaire (Box 2-1), a brief history, and a limited examination. Although the value of questionnaires may be challenged, a questionnaire can facilitate the clinical examination by focusing on specific complaints.[4] The TMD screener is a three-item questionnaire including questions about duration and timing of pain and aggravating and relieving factors. The questionnaire has a sensitivity of 98% and a specificity of 97% and has been shown to both accurately identify painful TMDs and to discriminate them from other conditions that present with over-

Box 2-1 Example of screening questions for TMDs*

- Do you have difficulty, pain, or both when opening your mouth (eg, when yawning)?
- Does your jaw get stuck, get locked, or go out?
- Do you have difficulty, pain, or both when chewing, talking, or using your jaws?
- Are you aware of noises in the jaw joints?
- Do your jaws regularly feel stiff, tight, or tired?
- Do you have pain in or near the ears, temples, or cheeks?
- Do you have frequent headaches, neck aches, or toothaches?
- Have you had a recent injury to your head, neck, or jaw?
- Have you been aware of any recent changes in your bite?
- Have you been previously treated for unexplained facial pain or a jaw joint problem?

*All dental patients should be screened for TMDs and other orofacial pain disorders. The decision to complete a comprehensive history and clinical examination will depend on the number of positive responses and the apparent severity of the problem for the patient. It should be noted that a positive response to any question may be sufficient to warrant a comprehensive examination if it is of concern to the patient or viewed as clinically significant.

Box 2-2 Example of screening examination procedure for TMDs*

- Measure range of motion of the mandible on opening and right and left lateral movements. (Note any incoordination, deflection, or deviation in the movements.)
- Palpate for preauricular or intrameatal TMJ tenderness.
- Auscultate and/or palpate for TMJ sounds (ie, clicking or crepitation).
- Palpate for tenderness and radiating trigger points in the masseter, temporalis, and cervical muscles.
- Note excessive occlusal wear, excessive tooth mobility, buccal mucosal ridging, or lateral tongue scalloping.
- Inspect symmetry and alignment of the face, jaws, and dental arches.

*All dental patients should be screened for TMDs and other orofacial pains using this or a similar cursory clinical examination. The need for a comprehensive history and clinical examination will depend on the number of positive findings and the clinical significance of each finding. Any single positive finding may be sufficient to warrant a comprehensive examination.

lapping symptoms.[5] The high positive predictive value (> 98%) suggests that the TMD screener can be used to identify patients requiring a more comprehensive evaluation.

The TMD screening examination usually consists of observation of the mandibular range of motion, palpation of the temporomandibular joints (TMJs), and palpation of the masseter and temporalis muscles for pain or tenderness (Box 2-2). Palpation and/or auscultation of the joints for sounds and observation of jaw function can disclose uncoordinated movements that may indicate internal biomechanical problems.[6] Caution should be observed when evaluating the results of the screening process because the clinical findings and the patient's complaints may not be consistent. Positive findings on the screening evaluation may prompt a more comprehensive evaluation. An understanding of the clinical significance of positive findings is essential. For example, a clinical sign such as a clicking TMJ may merely represent a stable, nonpainful condition that does not require treatment.

Comprehensive Evaluation

A comprehensive evaluation should be performed when a patient's complaints of pain are not of dental origin or when a patient's screening evaluation results are positive for an orofacial pain disorder. A comprehensive evaluation starts with a detailed history (Box 2-3). The examination process that follows may include some or all of the components listed in Table 2-1. Many patients present with a list of complaints; if the clinician carefully analyzes the components of each complaint, this can lead to a differential diagnosis. A meticulous history will often guide the clinician to the most likely diagnoses and therefore aid in determining what additional diagnostic procedures may be appropriate, if any.

History Taking

The interview, or history, is usually the first contact between the clinician and the patient, and as such, an empathetic attitude by the clinician can quickly create a bond critical to successful communication.

Chief complaints

The patient must be allowed to comfortably express the symptoms that prompted the consultation, although the clinician must take control of the interview to gather information in an organized manner. Adequate time is necessary to allow the patient to fully describe each

Box 2-3 Comprehensive history format for orofacial pain patients*

1. Chief complaint(s) and history of present illness

- Date and event of onset
- Location
- Quality
- Intensity
- Duration
- Frequency
- Remissions or change over time
- Modifying factors (alleviating, precipitating, or aggravating)
- Previous treatment results

2. Medical history

- Current or preexisting relevant physical disorders or disease (specifically, systemic arthritides or other musculoskeletal or rheumatologic conditions)
- Sleep disorders and sleep-related breathing disorders
- Previous treatments, surgeries, and/ or hospitalizations
- Trauma to the head and face
- Medications (prescription and nonprescription)
- Allergies to medications
- Alcohol and other substances of abuse

3. Dental history

- Current or preexisting relevant physical disorders or diseases
- Previous treatments, including the patient's attitude toward treatment
- History of trauma to the head and neck (including iatrogenic trauma)
- Parafunctional history, both awake and asleep

4. Psychosocial history

- Social, behavioral, and psychologic issues
- Occupational, recreational, and family status
- Litigation, disability, or secondary gain issues

*All dental patients should be screened for TMDs and other orofacial pain disorders. The decision to complete a comprehensive history and clinical examination will depend on the number of positive responses and the apparent severity of the problem for the patient. It should be noted that a positive response to any question may be sufficient to warrant a comprehensive examination if it is of concern to the patient or viewed as clinically significant.

Table 2-1 Comprehensive orofacial pain physical examination procedures

Type of evaluation	Reviewing sequence
General head and neck	1. Note scars; asymmetry; unusual size, shape, consistency, or posture; and involuntary movement or tenderness.
Muscles, TMJ, and cervical spine	1. Palpate the muscles of mastication and cervical muscles. 2. Palpate the TMJ preauricular. 3. Palpate cervical vertebrae. 4. Measure range of motion and its association with pain. 5. Auscultate and palpate for joint noises in all movements. 6. Guide mandibular movement, noting pain, end feel, and joint noise. 7. Note any tenderness, swelling, enlargement, or unusual texture.
Neurologic	1. Perform cranial nerve screening and note signs and symptoms. 2. Note vascular compression of the temporal and carotid arteries.
Ear, nose, and throat	1. Inspect the ears and nose. 2. Inspect the oropharynx and uvula (Mallampati score, tonsillar hypertrophy grade).
Intraoral	1. Assess hard and soft tissue conditions or disease.

of the complaints. The complaints are documented in the order of severity as indicated by the patient, and details of each complaint are elicited in a systematic manner.

History of chief complaints

A description of each chief complaint usually includes its location, onset, quality, intensity, frequency, and duration; triggering, exacerbating and alleviating factors; and associated symptoms. The combination of these features often represents recognizable patterns that can help the clinician to appropriately categorize the complaint, resulting in well-directed interventions.

LOCATION. Very often, the patient will complain of pain in a part of the face or head in terms consistent with how he or she may understand the anatomy. Therefore, it is helpful to have the patient identify the exact location of the pain using a finger to either point to or circumscribe the area of complaint. An important concept to keep in mind is that the location or site of the pain does not always correspond to the source of the pain. Therefore, finding the true source of pain is imperative for both an accurate diagnosis and effective treatment. To assess the extent of pain, asking the patient to draw his or her pain(s) on a whole-body mannequin may be useful.

ONSET. It is important to understand the circumstances that precipitated the pain, if any. Trauma is a frequent cause of pain and should be differentiated from pain secondary to systemic disease or personal stressors. It is also important to know how the pain begins with each episode (ie, whether it arises gradually or suddenly or is spontaneous). The temporal component of pain, be it the time of day, week, or month the pain occurs, may also render important clues regarding diagnosis, contributing factors, and treatment.

QUALITY. Different diagnostic categories of pain may be distinguished based on the quality of pain (Table 2-2). However, the clinician must be cautious when categorizing pain quality because pain related to certain musculoskeletal disorders can mimic neurovascular or neuropathic disorders, and the reverse may also be true. Several clinically validated screening tools with high sensitivity and specificity, although not specifically designed for orofacial pain, are available to help clinicians distinguish between neuropathic pain, nociceptive pain, and mixed pain.[7,8] They include the Leeds Assessment of Neuropathic Symptoms and Signs (LANSS) and S-LANSS (short version), Douleur Neuropathique (DN4), Neuropathic Pain Questionnaire (NPQ), PainDETECT, and ID-Pain.[9–14] The LANSS and DN4 contain clinical items in addition to self-reported symptoms. The self-report items of the DN4 can be used alone with good sensitivity and specificity.[11]

INTENSITY. The intensity of pain is subjective, variable, and often influenced by the psychosocial status of the patient. It is important for clinicians to understand the patient's interpretation of the intensity of his or her pain so that treatment priorities can be established. The intensity of the pain can be rated on a verbal rating scale (ie, mild, moderate, or severe), numeric rating scale (ie, a number between 0 and 10, where 0 represents "no pain" and 10 represents the "most extreme pain"), or a visual analog scale (ie, a 10-cm line labeled at one end with "no pain" and at the other end with "most extreme pain"). Because intensity can vary, it may be rated at the time of presentation in addition to the intensity at worst, best, and average in the preceding week. Sensory changes such as diminished or increased perception of touch or pain can be similarly rated and may relate to neuropathic disorders or centrally mediated pain disorders.

Table 2-2 Pain-quality descriptors and secondary symptoms associated with different pain categories

Pain category	Quality	Secondary symptoms
Musculoskeletal	• Dull • Aching • Pressure • Depressing • Tight • Stiff • Occasionally sharp	• Flushing • Hyperalgesia • Allodynia • Can refer to or be referred from distant sites • Worse with function
Neurovascular	• Throbbing • Stabbing • Pounding • Rhythmic	• Worsened by increasing intracranial pressure (eg, Valsalva, bending over, physical activity) • Sensitivity to light and/or sound • Nausea, vomiting
Neuropathic	• Shooting • Bright • Stimulating • Burning • Itchy • Electric shock–like • Cutting	• Numbness • Hyperalgesia • Paresthesia • Allodynia • Dysesthesia
Psychogenic	• Descriptive	• Complaint patterns often do not match anatomical sensory supply

FREQUENCY AND DURATION. The frequency of painful episodes yields information such as whether the pain comes in clusters, has periods of remission, or is constant. The duration of pain may be recorded in seconds, minutes, hours, days, weeks, or months. The daily duration of pain is rated as continuous or intermittent. If intermittent, the pain can be rated as brief, momentary, or persisting for minutes or hours. The frequency and duration of periods of remission should also be recorded.

MODULATING FACTORS. Precipitating, aggravating, and alleviating factors yield important information. Seemingly minor details that may not strike the patient as important may have tremendous diagnostic value. Examples include *precipitating factors* such as light wind, touch, or shaving initiating the pain and *aggravating factors* such as having increased pain during periods of personal stressors. Similarly, discovering that jaw function does not precipitate or aggravate an individual's pain is of equivalent diagnostic importance. In an injured musculoskeletal system, symptoms tend to aggravate when the system is used. If the masticatory system is the source of pain, then pain should worsen during jaw function. If it does not worsen, the source of the pain may be outside of the masticatory system.

ASSOCIATED SYMPTOMS. Very often, a symptom associated with the patient's pain complaint can help the clinician narrow his or her diagnostic focus. Sensory and motor changes as well as autonomical features may be recorded. For example, the presence of visual and sensory changes or light or sound sensitivity may be indicative of migraine with aura, whereas drooping, redness, and/or tearing of the eye may indicate a trigeminal autonomic cephalalgia.

Previous treatments

Prior medical and dental interventions for each complaint should be listed, along with the patient's perception of results. Results of prior treatment can offer insight into the nature of the complaint. For instance, if an anti-inflammatory drug alleviates the pain complaint, the pain is likely not of neuropathic origin. The patient's recall of medications, dosages, and length of medication trials should also be recorded. This information helps the clinician to evaluate whether previous therapies have been adequately tried and titrated or if they were discontinued due to side effects or adverse events. This part of the interview may also provide insight into patient compliance with previously proposed therapies.

Medical and dental history

Past illnesses, surgeries, developmental or genetic abnormalities, and any sequelae should be documented. Long- and short-term use of medications (including over-the-counter medications and herbal, vitamin, and mineral preparations) and their purpose should also be documented, as they may influence potential treatment options. Use of caffeine, tobacco, alcohol, and recreational drugs should be noted, as well as past or present substance abuse. The patient should be questioned about trauma, both physical and emotional. A complete dental history should be obtained, particularly as it relates to the chief complaint, or as the patient believes it relates to the chief complaint. Complications of therapies are important to document, as are any behaviors such as clenching (while awake or during sleep), bruxism, and other parafunctional activities (eg, gum chewing, nail biting). Because the patient's complaints may be a manifestation of systemic disease, he or she should be questioned regarding any symptoms that might relate to systemic disorders, such as those affecting connective tissue, autoimmune disorders, thyroid or salivary glands, fibromyalgia, diabetes, cardiac disorders, or Lyme disease, as this may influence treatment options and/or prognosis.

Patients must also be questioned about sleep habits and sleep disruptions. Orofacial pain is often associated with difficulties in falling asleep, frequent awakenings, or inadequate sleep quality and/or duration. Sleep disorders may exist as a medical comorbidity or may be directly caused by pain.[2] Pain can disrupt sleep, and sleep loss can increase pain sensation.[15] The orofacial pain clinician must be knowledgeable about normal sleep structure and function and how pain or stressors may disrupt sleep.[2] Psychometric instruments such as the Pittsburgh Sleep Quality Index are useful to assess sleep quality.[16] The Epworth Sleepiness Scale is useful in assessing daytime sleepiness.[17,18] The relationship of pain patterns to the sleep/wake cycle as well as risk factors for sleep-related breathing disorders such as obstructive sleep apnea and sleep-related bruxism should be assessed.[19] The STOP questionnaire, the STOP-Bang questionnaire, the Berlin questionnaire, and the multivariable apnea prediction index (MAPI) are useful tools to assess for obstructive sleep apnea.[20–22] Patients with a suspected sleep disorder should be referred to a sleep physician for full evaluation and diagnosis. The diagnosis of a sleep disorder, including obstructive sleep apnea and other sleep-related breathing disorders, must be made by a physician.[23] The orofacial pain clinician can work with the sleep physician in the management of a patient with obstructive sleep apnea (see chapter 11).

Psychosocial history

For some patients, psychologic and behavioral issues may result in orofacial pain. For others, these problems may be the primary etiologic factor or may play a role in sustaining or amplifying the pain. Therefore, it is advised that the history-gathering portion of the comprehensive evaluation include an evaluation of behavioral, social, emotional, and cognitive factors that can possibly initiate, sustain, or result from the patient's pain complaints (Box 2-4). The psychosocial history may provide insight into the patient's mental status and coping skills, interactions with others, and the presence of any psychologic overlay.

An evaluation for the presence of stressors and the patient's response to stress is important to the diagnostic process. Specific inquiries should be directed to disclose a history of traumatic life events, such as sexual abuse or domestic violence. Litigation, the expectation of monetary reward for disability, or secondary gain can also be complicating factors for the patient's prognosis. It needs to be determined if the patient has depression, anxiety, or both, because these are often comorbid and complicating factors related to chronic pain. A brief screening tool to assess anxiety and depression is the four-item Patient Health Questionnaire (PHQ-4).[24] A more elaborate questionnaire to evaluate anxiety and depression, among other disorders, is the 90-item Symptom Check List Revised (SCL-90-R).[25] In depressed patients, it is especially important to assess and document the risk of suicidal ideation and understand that suicide risk may fluctuate, for example, with increased life stressors.[26]

An appreciation of how pain affects the patient's life can help direct treatment. The Graded Chronic Pain Scale (GCPS) is a brief questionnaire that may be helpful to assess the patient's pain intensity and how the pain interferes with his or her life (see chapter 12 for more details on psychologic disorders, psychometric questionnaires, and suicidal ideation).[27] Referral is recommended when significant factors are identified.

Box 2-4 Checklist of psychologic and behavioral factors

- Inconsistent, inappropriate, and/or vague reports of pain
- Symptoms incompatible with the innervation and function of anatomical structures
- Overdramatization of symptoms
- Symptoms that vary with life events
- Significant pain of greater than 6 months' duration
- Repeated failures with conventional therapies
- Inconsistent response to medications
- History of other stress-related disorders
- Major life events (eg, new job, marriage, divorce, death of a family member or friend)
- Evidence of alcohol and drug abuse
- Clinically significant anxiety, depression, or suicidal or homicidal ideation
- Evidence of secondary gain

Physical Examination

Vital signs

Baseline blood pressure and pulse rate are recorded, and other vital signs (eg, respiration rate, temperature, height, and weight) may be obtained. Evaluating and recording baseline vital signs may provide valuable information for medically compromised patients and patients taking medications. Abnormal findings should prompt a more thorough evaluation with possible referral to a physician.

Neurologic screening

Orofacial pain complaints may be the result of a neurologic problem. As part of the orofacial pain examination, a cranial nerve screening is performed, aimed at assessing the function (ie,

Table 2-3 Overview of cranial nerves and tests to evaluate their functions

No.	Cranial nerve	Test
I	Olfactory	Sense of smell, tested with camphor, coffee, and vanilla
II	Optic	Visual acuity/visual field: pupillary light reflex
III	Oculomotor	Pupillary light reflexes/accommodation, eyelid elevation, most eye movements
IV	Trochlear	Downward gaze during adduction
V	Trigeminal	Sensation of light touch to face in all three divisions; motor innervation of muscles of mastication (strength); corneal reflex
VI	Abducens	Lateral gaze (III, IV, and VI); tested by having the patient follow finger in an H pattern)
VII	Facial	Facial expressions; corneal reflex; taste to the anterior two-thirds of the tongue
VIII	Acoustic vestibulocochlear	Hearing (eg, ability to hear a watch tick); Weber and Rinne tests (tuning fork); observation for nystagmus on extraocular muscle testing; caloric testing
IX	Glossopharyngeal	Gag reflex; taste to posterior one-third of the tongue
X	Vagus	Speech; palatal/uvular elevation; gag reflex
XI	Accessory	Function of sternocleidomastoid and trapezius muscles (press against resistance)
XII	Hypoglossal	Tongue bulk, strength, and movement (protrude and wiggle, press against resistance)

strength, sensation) of the nerves on the right and left sides. Cranial nerve dysfunction may manifest as changes in either motor or sensory function. Abnormal movement of muscles stimulated by one of the cranial nerves can indicate pathosis along the motor pathways. A patient reporting sensory alterations may be tested for anesthesia, paresthesia, dysesthesia, allodynia, and hyperalgesia. Topical and local anesthetic blocking may be part of the neurologic screening. Areas of altered sensation can be mapped at regular intervals, which may help to determine if the patient's condition is progressive or if treatment is effective. However, altered sensations are not pathognomonic for neuropathic pain.

Table 2-3 lists the cranial nerves and the most common methods of screening these nerves for dysfunction. Abnormal findings should prompt a more detailed neurologic evaluation, and if indicated, the patient should be referred to an appropriate medical specialist. Other texts are recommended for a complete review of the components of a neurologic and cranial nerve examination.

General inspection

General inspection of the head and neck includes recording of overall appearance; masses and/or asymmetry of the face, jaws, neck, and thyroid; presence of scars, unusual or abnormal posture, and involuntary movements; and respiration and breathing pattern. It may also be important to observe the overall gait of the individual. This can easily be done when the patient is entering or exiting the examination area.

Palpation

Muscles

The muscles of mastication are palpated in an attempt to reproduce familiar pain or identify tenderness upon palpation and to elicit referral patterns. *Familiar pain* is pain that is described by the patient as being similar to their experienced pain.[28] Reproducing the familiar pain helps to differentiate it from incidental pain provoked by muscle palpation.

The clinician may also palpate for *myofascial trigger points*, which are hyperirritable sites in taut bands of muscle and tendons that, when palpated, cause discomfort and may radiate or refer pain.[29,30] The temporalis, deep and superficial masseter, medial pterygoid, and suprahyoid muscles are often examined. Familiar pain may also be reproduced by asking the patient to clench the teeth while the clinician palpates the patient's masticatory muscles. The inferior lateral pterygoid muscle is difficult to palpate intraorally but can be evaluated by functional manipulation, by challenging the muscle to contract against resistance, or by observing symptom changes from stretching.[31–34] Myalgia may be exacerbated during this maneuver. Similar procedures of functional manipulation may be used for the superior lateral pterygoid and medial pterygoid muscles.[33] Muscles and structures that can be palpated with an intraoral approach include the medial pterygoid muscle, anterior digastric muscle, and the temporal tendon.

It is common for orofacial pain complaints to be caused by, and referred from, primary pain sites among the cervical structures.[34] Therefore, evaluation of the cervical range of motion and palpation of the cervical muscles, including the sternocleidomastoid, splenius capitis, trapezius, levator scapulae, and scalenes should be performed as part of the comprehensive orofacial pain evaluation. The recommended pressure when palpating head and neck muscles is between 0.5 and 4 kg/cm^2, maintained for about 5 to 20 seconds, although there is no universally accepted reference standard for the diagnosis of trigger points.[35–37]

Joints

The TMJs (lateral capsules) are palpated bilaterally for tenderness, pain, swelling, and patterns of movement. Palpation and/or stethoscope auscultation during jaw movements is a common method of detecting joint sounds. The presence and timing of early, middle, or late opening and/or closing sounds or noises (eg, clicking, popping, crepitus) and other interferences with smooth jaw movement should be noted.[38] Joint sounds can be signs of an intracapsular abnormality, such as internal derangement, degenerative processes, or architectural defects of articulating surfaces. They may correlate with pain or pathologic conditions or may be due to functional adaptations not associated with pain or dysfunction. Joint sounds are common in the general population and should be evaluated within the context of other presenting signs and symptoms.[39] While the predictive value of joint palpation is low in nonpatient populations, positive findings may have clinical significance in symptomatic patients.[40–42]

Lymph nodes

As part of the head and neck examination, the clinician should palpate lymph nodes, including the submental, submandibular, superficial, and deep cervical chains. The latter group may be examined with relative ease by palpating the relaxed sternocleidomastoid muscle.

Disease states of the oral cavity are most often reflected in changes of submental and submandibular lymph nodes.[38] Lymph nodes in a healthy individual are soft, nonpalpable structures. Lymph nodes that are palpable, swollen, hard, painful, fixed, or nodular are considered abnormal and potentially indicative of infection, inflammation, or neoplasm. The cause of abnormal nodes requires further investigation.[43]

Arteries

The temporal arteries may be palpated for tenderness, consistency, and provocation of pain in patients over the age of 50 years who complain of headache. Pain on palpation of the temporal artery may be a sign of giant cell arteritis, particularly in elderly patients (see chapter 4). If giant cell arteritis is suspected, additional diagnostic tests are indicated in addition to immediate physician referral.

Range of movement

The recording of mandibular range of movement in opening, lateral, and protrusive excursions with a millimeter ruler is a core examination procedure for TMDs, and the recorded measurements may also serve as a treatment outcome measure. Normal mandibular opening ranges between 40 and 55 mm, whereas excursive movements of at least 7 mm are considered normal.[44] While these are the generally accepted ranges, individual measurements may vary depending on many factors such as stature, craniofacial form, and other variables.[45,46] The normal opening range or active range of motion is lower in women than in men and decreases with increasing age.[46] An international collaborative effort of experts has led to scientifically validated and reliable examination protocols and diagnostic criteria for the most common TMDs. The Diagnostic Criteria for Temporomandibular Disorders (DC/TMD) have been published and are highly recommended in both the clinical and research settings.[28]

Three interincisal mouth opening measurements may be utilized to obtain important information: maximum pain-free opening, maximum unassisted opening, and maximum assisted opening. *Maximal pain-free opening* is that which can be attained without pain. *Maximum unassisted mouth opening,* also called *active range of motion,* is the mouth opening measurement that can be achieved by the patient regardless of the presence of pain. *Assisted mouth opening,* also called *passive range of motion,* is defined as the maximal mouth opening that can be attained with gentle stretching by the examiner after the patient has reached maximum unassisted mouth opening. The "jaw opening pattern" should be noted as either a straight line or deviated to the right, left, or both sides. A *corrected deviation* means that the mandible deviates away from the midline at first but then returns to the midline, while an *uncorrected deviation* means the mandible does not return to the midline. The mandibular lateral and protrusive range of motion should also be measured and recorded as outlined in the DC/TMD.[28] The location and severity of familiar pain elicited by these movements should be recorded. It is important to engage the patient's perception of restricted movement or reduced quality of movement.[46]

Cervical range of movement may also be recorded and includes rotation to the left and right (normal range of motion 65 to 75 degrees), lateral tilt (normal range of motion 35 to 45 degrees), flexion (normal range of motion 50 to 60 degrees), and extension (normal range of motion 60 to 70 degrees). These normal ranges are for middle-aged individuals. The range of motion declines approximately 5 degrees for extension and 3 degrees for all other movements as one ages based upon a 10-year period.[47]

Ear, nose, and throat

Patients who present for assessment of orofacial pain may be suffering from diseases or disorders of the ear, nose, and throat. Given the close and complex anatomical and functional relationship of these structures to the orofacial structures, otolaryngologic problems should be considered as potential causes of orofacial pain and dysfunction. For example, it is common for patients to report ear pain (otalgia) when the pain is primarily due to a TMD. Maxillary tooth pain can be caused by maxillary sinus disease and vice versa. Although aural symptoms are very common in TMD patients, particularly ear fullness and otalgia, symptoms such as ear discharge, hearing loss, tinnitus, dysequilibrium, and vertigo should raise suspicion of possible otologic causes of orofacial pain that require further investigation.[48,49] To date, the cause and background of aural symptoms associated with TMD is not fully understood, and no cause-effect relationship has been identified.[50,51]

In a systematic review inquiring about the effectiveness of conservative TMD therapies on changes to otologic signs and symptoms in adult patients with a TMD and related otologic complaints, the authors concluded there was insufficient evidence for or against the employment of these interventions. Furthermore, it was suggested that further studies with a higher level of evidence and more representative samples should be conducted to increase our understanding regarding the effect of TMD therapy on otologic complaints.[52]

Examination of the external ear, the external auditory canal, and the tympanic membrane is performed using an otoscope.[53] The outer ear may be examined for redness or swelling, which could indicate an infection or inflammatory process. The external auditory canal may be examined by pulling the ear upward and backward to straighten the canal for inspection. The canal is then observed for signs of infection, inflammation, discharge, or blockage. The properly trained clinician can observe the tympanic membrane (ie, eardrum) for any gross pathology that could explain the complaint of ear pain. If the clinician has concerns, then referral to an otolaryngologist is warranted.

When evaluating the nose and sinuses, the skin overlying the nose and maxilla is first inspected for abnormalities, such as unexplained ulcers, dark moles, or tissue growths. The skin over the maxillary and frontal sinuses is palpated and any tenderness is noted. The trained clinician may inspect the nostrils using adequate light and a nasal speculum, looking for swollen turbinates and deviated septa that may be associated with breathing problems.

All major salivary glands, including the parotid, submandibular, and sublingual glands may be palpated. Salivary gland duct exits can be inspected intraorally to confirm salivary flow. If no spontaneous flow is observed after the area of the exit is dried, the gland can be massaged, with the clinician noting color and consistency of any discharged fluid, if any. When indicated, a salivary flow test can be performed, and the saliva may be cultured.[54]

The oropharynx is readily visualized by retraction of the tongue with a tongue depressor or dental mirror. The tonsils and posterior pharyngeal walls should be visualized. Airway patency can be visualized and scored via the modified Mallampati or the Standardized Tonsillar Hypertrophy scales.[55,56]

Dental examination

Depending on the history, the patient may be provided with either a screening or a more thorough dental examination. Particularly where dental or oral mucosal pathosis is suspected as the source of orofacial pain, clinical examination of the oral hard and soft tissues is indicated, possibly in conjunction with radiography. It should always be remembered that the vast majority of orofacial pain is of odontogenic origin or related to the associated structures. Assessment for possible odontogenic pain requires careful inspection for dental caries and cracked teeth as well as the use of pulp vitality testing procedures. In addition to pulp vitality testing, the presence of periapical inflammation can be assessed via tooth percussion and mobility testing, periodontal probing, and periapical radiography. Transillumination may be of assistance in detecting the presence of cracked teeth.

Soft tissue pain or superficial pain may be caused by trauma, oral mucosal infections and disease, and neoplasia. The tongue, floor of the mouth, palate (hard and soft), gingival tissue, and buccal mucosa should be carefully inspected and palpated. The presence of oral ulceration, inflammation, infections, and soft tissue ridging should be noted. Diagnostic anesthesia, either topical and/or local, may assist in the diagnostic process of both odontogenic and soft tissue orofacial pain.

The dental occlusion should be evaluated when indicated, keeping in mind that occlusal variables are of limited use in the diagnosis of TMDs and may be the result of a TMD process rather than its cause.[57,58] A number of occlusal variables have been associated with the presence of various TMDs.[59] Accordingly, extensive tooth wear patterns, anterior open bites, unilateral crossbites, and large slides between the jaw's retruded and maximum intercuspation positions should be recorded. These baseline observations may be of importance in monitoring a progressive disease process.

Diagnostic Tests

The gold standard for diagnosis of orofacial pain, including TMDs, is a thorough history, examination (Axis I), psychosocial assessment (Axis II), and appropriate imaging, when necessary.[60] The clinical diagnostic criteria and examination protocol for the most common TMDs can be obtained via the DC/TMD, which is readily accessible on the website of the International Network for Orofacial Pain and Related Disorders Methodology (INfORM; previously known as the International RDC/TMD Consortium Network). Standardized and validated psychometric tools for assessment of the patient's psychosocial characteristics (Axis II) are also available. Adjunctive diagnostic tests are not necessary in every case; however, there are tests and procedures that may contribute significantly to the diagnostic process for the individual patient. A test should be performed only if it is deemed appropriate for the individual patient to either confirm or rule out a diagnosis and therefore potentially alter the treatment that is being considered.

A selected diagnostic test should have established scientific merit. Reliability and validity are measures that reflect how well a diagnostic test or procedure can measure what it purports to assess. For such a test or procedure to become clinically useful, it must first be proven to consistently, accurately, and reliably identify or measure the specific target. *Reliability* refers to the stability and consistency of measurements, whereas *validity* refers to the test's ability to measure what it is supposed to measure. Additionally, if whatever is measured has no established diagnostic value, then the diagnostic test cannot be considered valid. Several other factors are important in determining the usefulness of certain instruments proposed for use in diagnosis. These include the sensitivity, specificity, and positive and negative predictive values. *Sensitivity* is a measure of how well a certain test is able to identify a disease when the disease is actually present, also called the *true positive rate.* If a highly sensitive test is negative, it rules out the disease. *Specificity* is a measure of how well a test, when negative, identifies those who do not have the disorder, also called the *true negative rate.* A test with high specificity, when positive, can rule in the disease. For appropriate diagnosis, both sensitivity and specificity of the test should be over 70%. The *positive predictive value* is a measure of the probability that a person has the disease, given a positive result. Likewise, the *negative predictive value* is the probability that a person does not have the disease, given a negative result. Many instruments meet the criteria for validity and reliability but demonstrate low sensitivity and specificity and therefore should not be used to establish a diagnosis.[61–69] Relying on these instruments as diagnostic aids could lead to overtreatment and unnecessary increased medical costs.

The lack of scientific validation of many diagnostic tests, especially use of certain technologic devices, may lead to many false positive diagnoses and some false negative diagnoses. Some of these devices are discussed in the next section. There are immediate and implied future health and financial costs related to treating false positives and delayed costs of not treating false negatives. Until well-controlled, double-blind clinical trials are performed on specific subgroups of orofacial pain patients and are compared with control groups, these tests should be considered experimental and should not be used in routine clinical practice.

Electrodiagnostic testing

There are many electronic devices on the market that claim to aid in the diagnosis and treatment of TMDs. Although many of these devices may have the potential to be clinically useful, their reliability, validity, safety, and efficacy have yet to be established.[62,65–69]

Jaw-tracking devices

Observing and recording the range, direction, and quality of various jaw movements is an important aspect of assessing TMDs. Jaw-tracking devices allow jaw movements to be visualized and recorded; however, the utility of these tracings for diagnostic purposes is still unclear.[69–74] Mandibular movement measurements may be obtained with jaw-tracking devices; however, there are no data to demonstrate that this technique is any more useful in measuring mandibular movements than a traditional millimeter ruler.[62] With this in mind, cost efficiency should be considered, and routine use of these devices for TMD diagnosis is currently not supported by the scientific literature.[62]

Although these devices are cleared by the US Food and Drug Administration from a safety standpoint, a special notation was added that documentation for efficacy in diagnosis has to be provided for each device.[60,62] The usefulness of kinesiographic recordings of jaw movements to diagnose TMJ articular disc displacements compared with the use of the gold standard (ie, magnetic resonance imaging [MRI]) has been investigated. The specificity and positive predictive values for all kinesiographic variables were found to be well below acceptable standards to recommend its use.[75] Furthermore, the use of these devices in the diagnosis of myofascial pain as either a standalone measurement or an adjunct to clinical decisions fails to meet the standards of reliability and validity for their usage.[76] A literature review published since the last edition of the AAOP Guidelines failed to identify new articles supporting the use of jaw tracking as a diagnostic aid in TMDs. Therefore, at this time, jaw-tracking devices are not recommended as part of the orofacial pain evaluation.[62]

Electromyography

Electromyography (EMG) is a useful tool for measuring muscle activity and nerve conduction and has been shown to be reliable.[74–80] Although numerous publications have documented the use of EMG testing to establish diagnoses of TMDs, a thorough review of the evidence-based literature concluded that limitations with regard to reliability, validity, sensitivity, and specificity render EMG testing of limited value for TMD diagnosis.[62–69,76,81–83] Furthermore, increased EMG activity correlates poorly with masticatory muscle pain, and it is more likely that long-lasting, low-level contractions may be more relevant.[84–86] A study investigating the diagnostic accuracy of surface EMG for myofascial pain concluded that EMG should not be used clinically to diagnose or monitor the course of TMDs in an individual patient because of the potential risk for overdiagnosis and/or overtreatment.[78] Similar conclusions as to the lack of utility of EMG for diagnosing TMDs have also been described in several systematic reviews.[85,86]

Thermography

The use of thermography to diagnose painful neurologic and musculoskeletal conditions is based on the presence of thermal asymmetries of the skin when comparing normal and abnormal sites. Thermographic assessments of TMDs and other orofacial pain disorders have been published with conflicting results.[87–95] A review from 2004 concluded that there is insufficient evidence to support thermography use in routine clinical practice.[96] Two articles published in 2013 investigated the use of thermography in the diagnosis of TMJ arthralgia and myogenous TMDs, finding low diagnostic accuracy for both.[97,98] To date, the use of thermography for the diagnosis of TMDs or other orofacial pains remains unproven. The available evidence remains insufficient to conclude that thermography has a beneficial impact on either diagnosis or treatment outcomes. Furthermore, standards for image evaluation and cutoff values that may allow clinical decision-making have yet to be established.

Sonography

Doppler sonography data are similar to the data obtained with vibration analysis (see below) but with use of sound recordings instead of joint vibrations. Although Doppler sonography has been suggested for diagnosing TMDs based on the detection of joint sounds, the clinical significance and reproducibility of sounds emanating from the TMJs is not reliable.[82,99] Studies evaluating sonography for the diagnosis of articular disc displacement have found that both clinical and sonographic examination had a high sensitivity but a low specificity compared with MRI findings.[99–101] Since the last edition of the AAOP Guidelines was published, no new data has been published to justify the use of sonography for detection of TMJ sounds and internal derangements in lieu of clinical palpation and auscultation. Hence, there is insufficient evidence to justify the use of sonography for the diagnosis of TMDs.

Vibration analysis

Vibration analysis is similar to sonography in using joint sounds to assist in the diagnosis of TMDs with internal derangements.[102–108] Sensitivity and specificity are less than desired, with many false negatives and false positives.[107] A systematic review investigated the usefulness of joint vibration analysis in the diagnosis of TMD. The authors concluded that the literature failed to establish reliability and validity and that the use of vibration analysis in TMD diagnosis was unconvincing.[108]

Diagnostic imaging of the TMJ

There are a number of diagnostic imaging modalities that may confirm the presence of suspected pathosis, rule out disease, and stage various diseases affecting the orofacial region.[109–111] Imaging should not be done routinely for every patient or as an initial diagnostic test. Appropriate imaging can be used to gather additional information when the clinical diagnosis remains equivocal or unclear. Similarly, the presence of unusual signs and symptoms and the failure of conservative management strategies are indications for the use of appropriate imaging. The optimal type of imaging to be employed depends upon the presenting symptoms and clinical examination findings of the individual patient.[109] When abnormalities that fall outside the scope of an individual's training and experience are suspected or identified, then appropriate referral should be made for medical specialist diagnosis and management.

Panoramic radiography, also known as *orthopantography*, is a type of tomography in which the maxilla and the mandible are depicted on a single film. The panoramic radiograph is useful for screening for gross dental and periodontal pathology, as well as other maxillary and mandibular disorders and diseases. After intraoral dental radiographs, it remains the most common radiographic study performed in a dental office. However, as far as TMJ imaging is concerned, the projected image is inaccurate and cannot be used for diagnostic purposes.[112] Conventional tomography, apart from the panoramic radiograph, has essentially been replaced by computed tomography (CT) procedures.

CT is predominantly used where primary bony pathoses are suspected clinically. CT is particularly useful for evaluating degenerative and arthritic changes, fractures, bony cysts, infection, tumor invasion, and other pathology. The newer multidetector CT (MDCT) also has utility for soft tissues, and using appropriate protocols, the TMJ articular disc and presence of intra-articular effusion can be demonstrated.[113,114] Because soft tissue findings can be critical, this is a significant advantage over CBCT. In general, however, it is considered that soft tissue lesions, the TMJ articular disc, and associated soft tissues are best evaluated with MRI. Relative advantages of CT over MRI include exquisite bone details and three-dimensional assessment of congenital, traumatic, and postsurgical conditions.[109]

CBCT for the maxillofacial region has become readily available and is increasingly used in dentistry.[115,116] The advantages of CBCT over MDCT are lower cost, slightly higher resolution, and lower radiation dose. However, with appropriate protocols, the radiation doses now delivered by modern MDCT scanners are comparable to CBCT. CBCT is useful for evaluation of osseous abnormalities of the orofacial region. However, relative weaknesses include longer imaging times and related potential for motion artifact, low signal-to-noise ratios, beam hardening, and absence of soft tissue detail.

MRI represents the current gold standard of diagnostic imaging technology for soft tissues.[109] MRI does not use radiation and is therefore considered biologically safe. The high resolution and great soft tissue contrast of MRI afford detailed evaluation of TMJ anatomy, as well as TMJ biomechanics, through both open and closed mouth views. MRI enables a determination of the position and morphology of the TMJ articular disc as well as condylar bone morphology. Inflammatory changes such as intra-articular effusion and condylar bone marrow edema are also demonstrated. In consideration of these factors, MRI is considered the imaging modality of choice for the diagnosis of TMJ internal derangements.[117–121] In the comprehensive assessment of orofacial pain, MRI can also be used to rule out intracranial causes of pain in patients with trigeminal neuropathic pain or headaches.

Arthrography of the TMJ involves injection of radiopaque dye into the TMJ that outlines the articular disc under video fluoroscopy. Arthrography is rarely used today, having been replaced by MRI, which noninvasively provides superior information of all the TMJ structures without exposing the patient to radiation.

Nuclear medicine studies involve the intravenous administration of a radioactive isotope (eg, technetium), the uptake of which enters into tissues and is measured via either a scintillation gamma camera or single-photon emission CT (SPECT).[111] These tests have particular utility in identifying fractures, malignancy, infections, and other diseases involving bone.[109] Scintigraphy is useful to determine bone growth activity in hyperplastic TMJ condyles where TMJ surgery is being considered.[122] Scintigraphy is a highly sensitive but very nonspecific test with regard to identifying a specific disease or disorder. A recent study concluded that cross-sectional SPECT is more sensitive than traditional planar scintigraphy in the diagnosis of condylar hyperplasia.[122]

Ultrasonography (US) is generally not considered a conclusive diagnostic tool for TMJ articular disc derangements.[123] A systematic review concluded that US can exclude rather than confirm TMJ articular disc derangements.[124] An evidence-based review of this study confirms these findings.[125] US may also be used for the image-guided injection of medications (eg, corticosteroids, hyaluronic acid, or platelet-rich plasma) into individual muscles and the lower joint space of the TMJ.[126] US is also a very useful technique for evaluating the soft tissues of the head and neck region, especially the salivary glands and masses of uncertain origin and nature on clinical examination. US and US-guided fine-needle aspiration cytology are also excellent diagnostic techniques when indicated.[127]

Functional neuroimaging of orofacial pain and headache has been the focus of many studies over the last few years. Various methods—including functional MRI, magnetoencephalography (MEG), positron emission tomography (PET) and SPECT—record patterns of changes in voltage, current, magnetic fields, neurochemicals, and blood flow spatially in the brain. Magnetic resonance spectroscopy can noninvasively assess different metabolites and neurotransmitters in the brain. Near-infrared spectroscopy can detect changes in blood hemoglobin concentrations associated with neural activity and has great potential in measuring effects of pain upon the brain. Functional neuroimaging studies of migraine, trigeminal neuropathic pain, TMDs, and toothache are furthering our understanding of the anatomical and pathophysiologic mechanisms of these and other orofacial pain disorders.[128]

Neurosensory testing

Neuropathic pain is "caused by a lesion or disease of the somatosensory nervous system."[129] If the patient's history indicates the possibility of a lesion or disease that can affect the peripheral or central somatosensory system, and the pain has a distinct neuroanatomically plausible distribution, then painful neuropathy is likely. Painful neuropathy is characterized by its burning, prickling, electrical, and sharp nature. Painful neuropathy can be spontaneous or evoked with distinctive associated positive (ie, heightened sensation) signs (eg, spontaneous pain, allodynia and hyperalgesia) and/or negative (ie, sensory deficit) signs. There is almost always an area of abnormal sensation.

Neurosensory tests assessing changes in responsiveness to different types of somatosensory stimuli have been adapted for use in the orofacial region and are an important part of the clinical examination. A quick and easy chairside technique can be used, or the patient can be referred to a specialized university setting or pain clinic for comprehensive quantitative sensory testing (QST).[130,131] This type of testing allows noninvasive assessment and quantification of sensory nerve function in patients with suspected neurologic disease or neuropathy. Various mechanical, thermal, and electrical stimuli can be applied to the affected area, and the evoked responses can be measured. The responses can be compared with normal contralateral sites or established normal QST ranges. Alternatively, different stimuli can be applied to establish either pain or other sensory threshold levels. Specific QST modalities can be used to activate different types of sensory nerve fibers, allowing insight into pathologic processes. At this time, the use of QST in the trigeminal system is undergoing research and development and is not yet considered as established for routine clinical practice.[131]

Diagnostic anesthesia

Neural blockade, both somatic and sympathetic nerve blocks, and myoneural (trigger point) injections may be used as diagnostic tools (Table 2-4). Examples of somatic nerve blocks in the head and neck include trigeminal, supraorbital, infraorbital, greater occipital, sphenopalatine ganglion, and cervical plexus nerve blocks. Somatic neural blockade is not only used to determine whether or not pain is emanating from a particular nerve, but it may also be used to determine whether the source of pain is proximal or distal to a particular site along the nerve.[1] In addition to its diagnostic potential, somatic neural blockade may be useful as a therapeutic agent by providing pain relief to the affected area by breaking the cycle of pain.

Lidocaine (1% to 2%, often with epinephrine) is recommended for diagnostic nerve blocks because it produces a prompt, long-lasting, and extensive anesthesia. Neural blockade is of particular prognostic value prior to neurolytic blockade or surgical sympathectomy (neurolysis). When prolonged anesthesia is desired for pain management, bupivacaine (0.25%) can be used.

Primary musculoskeletal pain, meaning pain in an injured or painful muscle or joint that can be provoked, may be arrested by a local or regional anesthetic block. The TMJ can be anesthetized by a lateroposterior and slightly inferior intracapsular approach, a posterior meatal intracapsular approach, or an extracapsular block of the auriculotemporal nerve at the posterior aspect of the neck of the condyle.[1] Myofascial pain may be eliminated only if the anesthetic blocks the source or primary site of pain.[1] Therefore, an equivocal diagnostic injection of a myofascial trigger point suggests that the source of pain has not been discovered, while an effective injection can allow the clinician to be confident that the source of pain has been found.[1] Lidocaine 2% (without epinephrine) or mepivacaine 3% are suitable for this purpose. Bupivacaine appears to be relatively myotoxic and should be avoided for muscle injections.[132] A number of studies have investigated the use of botulinum toxin injections for the treatment of myofascial TMD pain and/or bruxism.[133–137] However, there are no data to suggest that botulinum toxin can be used in a diagnostic sense.

If a regional block, such as a mandibular block, eliminates neuropathic pain distal to the site of injection, the source of pain is located in the region of the anesthetized area. An ineffective diagnostic block suggests that the neuropathic pain is more proximal or central and so may indicate neuroplasticity or involvement of the central nervous system.

Table 2-4 Diagnostic anesthesia

Type of anesthetic block	Type of pain
Dental block	Odontogenic pain or neuropathic pain
Trigger point injections	Myofascial pain and headache
Trigger zone infiltration	Trigeminal neuralgia
Auriculotemporal nerve block	Intracapsular TMJ pain
Intracapsular block	Intracapsular TMJ pain
Greater and lesser occipital block	Cervicogenic pain and headache
Sphenopalatine block	Neuropathic facial pain Neurovascular pain Sympathetically maintained pain
Stellate ganglion block	Sympathetically maintained pain

Stellate ganglion blocks (sympathetic) and sphenopalatine blocks (parasympathetic) are used for diagnosis and treatment of orofacial pain when an autonomic component is suspected. Performing a stellate ganglion block requires special training and is usually done in an operating room by a trained anesthesiologist. Anesthetizing the sphenopalatine ganglion has been described for treatment of orofacial pain, particularly cluster headache. Conventionally, local anesthetic has been delivered to the area by injection into the pterygopalatine fossa under fluoroscopic guidance or transnasal application by cotton-tip applicators. Devices have recently been developed to facilitate the procedure, which may lead to increased utility for this type of block.

Table 2-5 Laboratory testing for nonodontogenic orofacial pain or TMDs

Disease	Tests
Juvenile idiopathic arthritis	• Rheumatoid factor • Antinuclear antibodies • Erythrocyte sedimentation rate
Systemic lupus erythematosus	• Antinuclear antibodies • Other autoantibodies • Complement • Biopsy
Lyme disease	• Indirect fluorescent antibody • Enzyme-linked immunosorbent assay • Immunoblotting • Polymerase chain reaction
Multiple sclerosis	• MRI • Evoked potential studies • Antinuclear antibodies • B12 • Complete blood count • Erythrocyte sedimentation rate • Urinalysis • Elevated myelin levels

Table 2-6 Frequently used hematologic studies

Serologic study	Suspicion of
Full blood count	Predominantly anemias
Hematinics: ferritin, B12, folate	Deficiency states causing secondary burning mouth symptoms
Zinc levels	Fe absorption abnormalities
Hypothyroidism	Cause of headache
HbA1c	Diabetes-related neuropathy
Extractable nuclear antigens	Mixed connective tissue disorders and lupus
Antinuclear antibody	Various autoimmune and connective tissue disorders
Erythrocyte sedimentation rate or C-reactive protein	Inflammatory conditions

Diagnostic casts

Because malocclusion is not a common etiology for TMDs (see chapter 8), diagnostic casts have little value in diagnosis and evaluation in most cases. They are helpful in identifying wear patterns and recording a baseline static occlusion for documentation of occlusal changes during treatment.[138,139] Dental casts also help determine whether or not changes at the level of either the teeth, TMJ, or muscles are responsible for the examination finding of an open bite. If the dental casts are able to achieve maximum intercuspation, it is suggestive that skeletal (TMJ) or muscular changes are the cause rather than the result of tooth movement. If the dental casts do not achieve maximum intercuspation, changes in the occlusion could be due either to dental movement, skeletal changes, muscle contraction, or combinations thereof. Occlusal analysis is often not accurate when the joints or muscles are tender or painful; therefore, any in-depth evaluation of the occlusion should be performed only after the pain is under control.[140] Even the most accurate casts will not provide enough information by themselves for an accurate diagnosis of joint or muscle pathology.[141]

Laboratory testing

A comprehensive assessment may include selective serologic testing, but this should not be a routine part of the orofacial pain examination.[142,143] Blood chemical analysis can rule out hematologic, rheumatologic, metabolic, or other abnormalities suggestive of systemic disease (Table 2-5). The most frequently employed hematologic investigations for orofacial pain are listed in Table 2-6. The clinician should know the appropriate serologic studies and be able to collect and interpret the data to establish a differential diagnosis. If it is established that complaints of orofacial pain are related to a systemic disease, referral to a physician is indicated.

Pretreatment testing and patient monitoring

Specific tests are sometimes necessary before or during certain pharmacotherapeutic treatments.[142] For example, the use of antiepileptic drugs, such as carbamazepine, must be preceded by a baseline complete blood count, a blood differential test, and liver function tests. Tricyclic antidepressant drugs may be preceded by a baseline electrocardiogram for assessment of arrhythmia, especially in older patients.

Renal function

The kidneys are responsible for regulating fluid volume and acid-base balance of the plasma, excreting nitrogenous waste, and synthesizing erythropoietin, hydroxycholecalciferol, and renin. End-stage renal disease occurs when the kidney loses the ability to perform these functions. The early phase of renal disease, which usually is asymptomatic except for some mild laboratory abnormalities, is called *renal insufficiency*. If the proposed medication could exacerbate or initiate renal dysfunction, the patient should be pretested or referred for treatment.

Hepatic function

Some medications can have significant effects on liver function, so knowledge of the status of liver function may be beneficial. In addition, the metabolism of most medications is dependent on liver function. When medications that require monitoring of the liver for hepatocellular damage are prescribed, a liver profile is recommended. Blood chemical analysis is often required prior to and periodically during pharmacologic therapy.

Pharmacogenomics

One of the main challenges in caring for patients with chronic orofacial pain disorders is the large variability and heterogeneity of conditions, with diagnosis and treatment still primarily based on subjective measures that have modest reliability. There is a substantial unmet need for objective markers of various chronic pain disorders to augment the validity of patient self-report, aid diagnosis, treatment, and prognosis—so-called "personalized medicine."[144]

Biologic markers, or *biomarkers*, are defined by the World Health Organization as "any substance, structure or process that can be measured in the body or its products, and influence or predict the incidence or outcome of disease."[145] These measures include neuroimaging (eg, functional MRI, MR spectroscopy, PET), genetic and pharmacogenomic analysis, molecular testing, and psychophysical measures (eg, quantitative sensory testing profiles in neuropathic pain).

Pharmacogenomic testing seeks to personalize pharmacologic therapies to the individual patient's genetic profile, thus assisting clinical decisions regarding choice of medications and doses. Genes code for enzymes involved in metabolizing medications, and knowledge of each patient's genes provides information on the baseline function of associated enzymes. Pharmacogenomic testing provides clinically relevant information that can help predict response to medications, identify medications with greater potential to attain a clinically significant response, and reduce prescription of medications that are unlikely to be effective. It may be particularly useful in patients exhibiting either unwelcome side effects or a poor response to their prescribed class of medication. Potential drug interactions can also be identified; for example, certain medications may induce or inhibit metabolizing enzymes, therefore affecting the response to other medications.

At present, biomarker development for pain disorders is still in its early stages, and there are no universally accepted diagnostic or predictive biomarkers unique to the clinical practice of orofacial pain. Patient self-report, clinical diagnosis, and experience-based treatment decision-making therefore remain the cornerstone of chronic pain management. However, the European Union Innovative Medicines Initiative consortium and the National Institutes of Health Helping to End Addiction Long-term (HEAL) initiative have recently been launched to facilitate the discovery of robust biomarkers for the diagnosis, prognosis, and management of chronic pain disorders.[146]

Scheduled drug agreement

On occasion, the clinician may have no other option than to treat a patient with nonmalignant intractable pain with scheduled drugs such as opioids. If the clinician deems this the best course of treatment for the patient, a thorough evaluation of the patient's mental health status and psychosocial situation is recommended. The clinician should discuss the additional risks associated with these drugs, such as physical and psychologic dependence. It is also recommended that the clinician engage in a scheduled drug agreement, in which the responsibilities of both parties are documented. Such responsibilities could include statements that prescriptions should be taken as prescribed, that prescriptions will not be filled early, that the patient agrees not to receive additional similar medications from other health care providers, that the patient is subject to random urine screens and pill counts, and so on. The agreement could restrict the patient to filling his or her prescription at a predetermined pharmacy and indicate that if the patient breaches the agreement, scheduled drugs will no longer be provided but other forms of treatment will be offered. The goal of treatment is to reduce pain, to improve function, and to increase quality of life. If these goals are not achieved with this type of treatment, the patient should be weaned off the medications and alternative treatments offered. Because cognitive impairment could be a side effect with long-term use of these medications, patients should be routinely tested for such side effects. The clinician may desire the assistance of a qualified health psychologist to provide this assessment.

References

1. Okeson JP. Principles of pain diagnosis. In: Okeson JP. Bell's Oral and Facial Pain, ed 7. Chicago: Quintessence, 2014:135–180.
2. Sharav Y, Benoliel R. The diagnostic process. In: Sharav Y, Benoliel R (eds). Orofacial Pain and Headache. Chicago: Quintessence, 2015:1–29.
3. Heir GM. An organized approach for examining the orofacial pain and craniomandibular patient. Cranio 1993;11:157–159.
4. Heir GM. History taking of the facial pain patient with the assistance of a comprehensive questionnaire. Cranio 1993;11:76–79.
5. Gonzalez YM, Schiffman E, Gordon SM, et al. Development of a brief and effective temporomandibular disorder pain screening questionnaire: Reliability and validity. J Am Dent Assoc 2011;142:1183–1191.
6. Farrar W, McCarty WL. A Clinical Outline of Temporomandibular Joint Diagnosis and Treatment. Montgomery, AL: Normandie Study Group for TMJ Dysfunction, 1982.
7. Cruccu G, Sommer C, Anand P, et al. EFNS guidelines on neuropathic pain assessment: Revised 2009. Eur J Neurol 2010;17:1010–1018.
8. Haanpää M, Attal N, Backonja M, et al. NeuPSIG guidelines on neuropathic pain assessment. Pain 2011;152:14–27.

9. Bennett M. The LANSS Pain Scale: The Leeds assessment of neuropathic symptoms and signs. Pain 2001; 92:147–157.
10. Bennett MI, Smith BH, Torrance N, Potter J. The S-LANSS score for identifying pain of predominantly neuropathic origin: Validation for use in clinical and postal research. J Pain 2005;6:149–158.
11. Bouhassira D, Attal N, Alchaar H, et al. Comparison of pain syndromes associated with nervous or somatic lesions and development of a new neuropathic pain diagnostic questionnaire (DN4). Pain 2005;114: 29–36.
12. Krause SJ, Backonja MM. Development of a neuropathic pain questionnaire. Clin J Pain 2003;19: 306–314.
13. Freynhagen R, Baron R, Gockel U, Tölle TR. PainDETECT: A new screening questionnaire to identify neuropathic components in patients with back pain. Curr Med Res Opin 2006;22:1911–1920.
14. Portenoy R. Development and testing of a neuropathic pain screening questionnaire: ID Pain. Curr Med Res Opin 2006;22:1555–1565.
15. Lautenbacher S, Kundermann B, Krieg JC. Sleep deprivation and pain perception. Sleep Med Rev 2006;10: 357–369.
16. Buysse DJ, Reynolds CF 3rd, Monk TH, Berman SR, Kupfer DJ. The Pittsburgh Sleep Quality Index: A new instrument for psychiatric practice and research. Psychiatry Res 1989;28:193–213.
17. Johns MW. A new method for measuring daytime sleepiness: The Epworth sleepiness scale. Sleep 1991; 14:540–545.
18. Johns MW. Reliability and factor analysis of the Epworth sleepiness scale. Sleep 1992;15:376–381.
19. Almonznino G, Benoliel R, Sharav Y, Haviv Y. Sleep disorders and chronic craniofacial pain: Characteristics and management possibilities. Sleep Med Rev 2017;33: 39–50.
20. Chung F, Yegneswaran B, Liao P, et al. STOP questionnaire: A tool to screen patients for obstructive sleep apnea. Anesthesiology 2008;108:812–821.
21. Netzer NC, Stoohs RA, Netzer CM, Clark K, Strohl KP. Using the Berlin questionnaire to identify patients at risk for the sleep apnea syndrome. Ann Intern Med 1999;109:1902–1907.
22. Maislin G, Pack AI, Kribbs NB, et al. A survey screen for prediction of apnea. Sleep 1995;18:159–166.
23. Lavigne GJ, Heinzer RC, Cistulli PA, Smith MT. Classification of sleep disorders. In: Lavigne GJ, Cistulli PA, Smith MT (eds). Sleep Medicine for Dentists: A Practical Overview. Chicago: Quintessence, 2009:21–31.
24. Kroenke K, Spitzer RL, Williams JB, Löwe B. An ultrabrief screening scale for anxiety and depression: The PHQ-4. Psychosomatics 2009;50:613–621.
25. Derogatis LR. The SCL 90R: Administration, Scoring and Procedure Manual. Baltimore: Clinical Psychology Research, 1977.
26. Bryan CJ, Rudd MD. The importance of temporal dynamics in the transition from suicidal thought to behavior. Clin Psychol Sci Pract 2016:23:21–25.
27. Von Korff M, Ormel J, Keefe FJ, Dworkin SF. Grading the severity of chronic pain. Pain 1992;50:133–149.
28. Schiffman E, Ohrbach R, Truelove E, et al. Diagnostic Criteria for Temporomandibular Disorders (DC/TMD) for Clinical and Research Applications: Recommendations of the International RDC/TMD Consortium Network and Orofacial Pain Special Interest Group. J Oral Facial Pain Headache 2014;28:6–27.
29. Hong CZ, Kuan TS, Chen JT, Chen SM. Referred pain elicited by palpation and by needling of myofascial trigger points: A comparison. Arch Phys Med Rehabil 1997;78:957–960.
30. Simons DG, Travell JC, Simons LS. Travell and Simons' Myofascial Pain and Dysfunction: The Trigger Point Manual. Vol 1. Upper Half of Body, ed 2. Baltimore: Williams & Wilkins, 1999.
31. Johnstone DR, Templeton M. The feasibility of palpating the lateral pterygoid muscle. J Prosthet Dent 1980;44:318–323.
32. Stratmann U, Mokrys K, Meyer U, et al. Clinical anatomy and palpability of the inferior lateral pterygoid muscle. J Prosthet Dent 2000;83:548–554.
33. Okeson JP. Management of Temporomandibular Disorders and Occlusion, ed 7. St Louis: Mosby, 2013.
34. Wright EF. Manual of Temporomandibular Disorders, ed 3. Ames, IA: Wiley Blackwell, 2014.
35. Reeves JL, Jaeger B, Graff-Radford SB. Reliability of the pressure algometer as a measure of myofascial trigger point sensitivity. Pain 1986;24:313–321.
36. Ohrbach R, Gonzalez YM, List T, Michelotti A, Schiffman EL. Diagnostic Criteria for Temporomandibular Disorders (DC/TMD) Clinical Examination Protocol. ubwp.buffalo.edu/rdc-tmdinternational/tmd-assessmentdiagnosis/dc-tmd/. Accessed on 10 November 2022.
37. Lucas N, Macaskill P, Irwig L, Moran R, Bogduk N. Reliability of physical examination for diagnosis of myofascial trigger points: A systematic review of the literature. Clin J Pain 2009;25:80–89.
38. Curl DD. The visual range of motion scale: Analysis of mandibular gait in a chiropractic setting. J Manipulative Physiol Ther 1992;15:115–122.
39. Tallents RH, Hatala M, Katzberg RW, Westesson PL. Temporomandibular joint sounds in asymptomatic volunteers. J Prosthet Dent 1993;69:298–304.
40. Kirveskari P. Prediction of demand for treatment of temporomandibular disorders. J Oral Rehabil 2001; 28:572–575.

41. Brown FF, Robinson ME, Riley JL 3rd, Gremillion HA, McSolay J, Meyers G. Better palpation of pain: Reliability and validity of a new pressure pain protocol in TMD. Cranio 2000;18:58–65.
42. Glaros AG, Glass EG, Williams KB. Clinical examination findings of temporomandibular disorder patients: A factor analytic study. J Orofac Pain 1998;12:193–202.
43. Hiatt JL, Gartner LP. Textbook of Head and Neck Anatomy, ed 3. Philadelphia: Lippincott Williams & Wilkins, 2001.
44. de Wijer A, Lobbezoo-Scholte AM, Steenks MH, Bosman F. Reliability of clinical findings in temporomandibular disorders. J Orofac Pain 1995;9:181–191.
45. Ingervall B. Variation of the range of movement of the mandible in relation to facial morphology in young adults. Scand J Dent Res 1971;79:133–140.
46. Szentpétery A. Clinical utility of mandibular movement ranges. J Orofac Pain 1993;7:163–168.
47. Youdas JW, Garrett TR, Suman VJ, Bogard CL, Hallman HO, Carey JR. Normal range of motion of the cervical spine: An initial goniometric study. Phys Ther 1992;72:770–780.
48. Porto De Toledo I, Stefani FM, Porporatti AL, et al. Prevalence of otologic signs and symptoms in adult patients with temporomandibular disorders: A systematic review and meta-analysis. Clin Oral Investig 2017;21:597–605.
49. Mejersjö C, Näslund I. Aural symptoms in patients referred for temporomandibular pain/dysfunction. Swed Dent J 2016;40:13–20.
50. Salvetti G, Manfredini D, Barsotti S, Bosco M. Otologic symptoms in temporomandibular disorders patients: Is there evidence of an association-relationship? Minerva Stomatol 2006;55:627–637.
51. Lam DK, Lawrence HP, Tenenbaum HC. Aural symptoms in temporomandibular disorder patients attending a craniofacial pain unit. J Orofac Pain 2001;15:146–157.
52. Stechman-Neto J, Porporatti AL, Porto de Toledo I, et al. Effect of temporomandibular disorder therapy on otologic signs and symptoms: A systematic review. J Oral Rehabil 2016;43:468–479.
53. Murtagh J. The painful ear. Aust Fam Physician 1991;20:1779–1783.
54. Scully C, Felix DH. Oral Medicine—Update for the dental practitioner: Dry mouth and disorders of salivation. Br Dent J 2005;199:423–427.
55. Mallampati SR, Gatt SP, Gugino LD, et al. A clinical sign to predict difficult tracheal intubation: A prospective study. Can Anaesth Soc J 1985;32:429–434.
56. Chan J, Edman JC, Koltai PJ. Obstructive sleep apnea in children. Am Fam Physician 2004;69:1147–1154.
57. Pullinger AG, Seligman DA. Quantification and validation of predictive values of occlusal variables in temporomandibular disorders using a multifactorial analysis. J Prosthet Dent 2000;83:66–75.
58. Manfredini D, Lombardo L, Siciliani G. Temporomandibular disorders and dental occlusion. A systematic review of association studies: End of an era? J Oral Rehabil 2017;44:908–923.
59. Seligman DA, Pullinger AG. The role of functional occlusal relationships in temporomandibular disorders. J Craniomandib Disord 1991;5:265–279.
60. Greene CS. Managing the care of patients with temporomandibular disorders: A new guideline for care. J Am Dent Assoc 2010;141:1086–1088.
61. Douglass CW, McNeil BJ. Clinical decision analysis methods applied to diagnostic tests in dentistry. J Dent Educ 1983;47:708–714.
62. Greene CS, Lund JP, Widmer CG. Clinical diagnosis of orofacial pain: Impact of recent FDA ruling on electronic devices. J Orofac Pain 1995;9:7–8.
63. Goulet JP, Clark GT. Clinical TMJ examination methods. J Calif Dent Assoc 1990;18:25–33.
64. Widmer CG, Lund JP, Feine JS. Evaluation of diagnostic tests for TMD. J Calif Dent Assoc 1990;18:53–60.
65. Mohl ND, Crow H. Role of electronic devices in diagnosis of temporomandibular disorders. N Y State Dent J 1993;59:57–61.
66. Mohl ND, Dixon DC. Current status of diagnostic procedures for temporomandibular disorders. J Am Dent Assoc 1994;125:56–64.
67. Mohl ND. Reliability and validity of diagnostic modalities for temporomandibular disorders. Adv Dent Res 1993;7:113–119.
68. Lund JP, Widmer CG, Feine JS. Validity of diagnostic and monitoring tests used for temporomandibular disorders. J Dent Res 1995;74:1133–1143.
69. Baba K, Tsukiyama Y, Yamazaki M, Clark GT. A review of temporomandibular disorder diagnostic techniques. J Prosthet Dent 2001;86:184–194.
70. Theusner J, Plesh O, Curtis DA, Hutton JE. Axiographic tracings of temporomandibular joint movements. J Prosthet Dent 1993;69:209–215.
71. Velasco J, Tasaki T, Gale EN. Study of pantographic tracings of TMD patients and asymptomatic subjects [abstract 843]. J Dent Res 1991;70(special issue):371.
72. Tsolka P, Preiskel HW. Kinesiographic and electromyographic assessment of the effects of occlusal adjustment therapy on craniomandibular disorders by a double-blind method. J Prosthet Dent 1993;69:85–92.
73. Kinuta S, Wakabayashi K, Sohmura T, et al. Measurement of masticatory movement by a new jaw tracking system using a home digital camcorder. Dent Mater J 2005;24:661–666.

74. Sae-Lee D, Wanigaratne K, Whittle T, Peck CC, Murray GM. A method for studying jaw muscle activity during standardized jaw movements under experimental jaw muscle pain. J Neurosci Methods 2006;157:285–293.
75. Manfredini D, Favero L, Federzoni E, Cocilovo F, Guarda-Nardini L. Kinesiographic recordings of jaw movements are not accurate to detect magnetic resonance-diagnosed temporomandibular joint (TMJ) effusion and disk displacement: Findings from a validation study. Oral Surg Oral Med Oral Pathol Oral Radiol 2012;114:457–463.
76. Manfredini D, Cocilovo F, Favero L, Ferronato G, Tonello S, Guarda-Nardini L. Surface electromyography of jaw muscles and kinesiographic recordings: Diagnostic accuracy for myofascial pain. J Oral Rehabil 2011;38:791–799.
77. Gallo LM, Gross SS, Palla S. Nocturnal masseter EMG activity of healthy subjects in a natural environment. J Dent Res 1999;78:1436–1444.
78. Bowley JF, Marx DB. Masticatory muscle activity assessment and reliability of a portable electromyographic instrument. J Prosthet Dent 2001;85:252–260.
79. Cecere F, Ruf S, Pancherz H. Is quantitative electromyography reliable? J Orofac Pain 1996;10:38–47.
80. Ferrario VF, Sforza C, D'Addona A, Miani A Jr. Reproducibility of electromyographic measures: A statistical analysis. J Oral Rehabil 1991;18:513–521.
81. Lund JP, Widmer CG. Evaluation of the use of surface electromyography in the diagnosis, documentation, and treatment of dental patients. J Craniomandib Disord 1989;3:125–137.
82. Mohl ND, Lund JP, Widmer CG, McCall WD Jr. Devices for the diagnosis and treatment of temporomandibular disorders. Part II: Electromyography and sonography. J Prosthet Dent 1990;63:332–336.
83. Klasser GD, Okeson JP. The clinical usefulness of surface electromyography in the diagnosis and treatment of temporomandibular disorders. J Am Dent Assoc 2006;137:763–771.
84. Murray GM, Peck CC. Orofacial pain and jaw muscle activity: A new model. J Orofac Pain 2007;21:263–278.
85. Al-Saleh MA, Armijo-Olivo S, Flores-Mir C, Thie NM. Electromyography in diagnosing temporomandibular disorders. J Am Dent Assoc 2012;143:351–362.
86. Suvinen TI, Kemppainen P. Review of clinical EMG studies related to muscle and occlusal factors in healthy and TMD subjects. J Oral Rehabil 2007;34:631–644.
87. Gratt BM, Sickles EA, Wexler CE. Thermographic characterization of osteoarthrosis of the temporomandibular joint. J Orofac Pain 1993;7:345–353.
88. Swerdlow B, Dieter JN. An evaluation of the sensitivity and specificity of medical thermography for the documentation of myofascial trigger points. Pain 1992;48:205–213.
89. Canavan D, Gratt BM. Electronic thermography for the assessment of mild and moderate temporomandibular joint dysfunction. Oral Surg Oral Med Oral Pathol Oral Radiol Endod 1995;79:778–786.
90. Gratt BM, Sickles EA, Wexler CE, Ross JB. Thermographic characterization of internal derangement of the temporomandibular joint. J Orofac Pain 1994;8:197–206.
91. Gratt BM, Sickles EA, Graff-Radford SB, Solberg WK. Electronic thermography in the diagnosis of atypical odontalgia: A pilot study. Oral Surg Oral Med Oral Pathol 1989;68:472–481.
92. Gratt BM, Sickles EA, Ross JB, Wexler CE, Gornbein JA. Thermographic assessment of craniomandibular disorders: Diagnostic interpretation versus temperature measurement analysis. J Orofac Pain 1994;8:278–288.
93. Gratt BM, Sickles EA, Shetty V. Thermography for the clinical assessment of inferior alveolar nerve deficit: A pilot study. J Orofac Pain 1994;8:369–374.
94. Graff-Radford SB, Ketelaer MC, Gratt BM, Solberg WK. Thermographic assessment of neuropathic facial pain. J Orofac Pain 1995;9:138–146.
95. Gratt BM, Graff-Radford SB, Shetty V, Solberg WK, Sickles EA. A 6-year clinical assessment of electronic facial thermography. Dentomaxillofac Radiol 1996;25:247–255.
96. Fikackova H, Ekberg E. Can infrared thermography be a diagnostic tool for arthralgia of the temporomandibular joint? Oral Surg Oral Med Oral Pathol Oral Radiol Endod 2004;98:643–650.
97. Dibai Filho AV, Packer AC, Costa AC, Rodrigues-Bigaton D. Accuracy of infrared thermography of the masticatory muscles for the diagnosis of myogenous temporomandibular disorder. J Manipulative Physiol Ther 2013;36:245–252.
98. Rodrigues-Bigaton D, Dibai Filho AV, Costa AC, Packer AC, de Castro EM. Accuracy and reliability of infrared thermography in the diagnosis of arthralgia in women with temporomandibular disorder. J Manipulative Physiol Ther 2013;36:253–258.
99. Tanzilli RA, Tallents RH, Katzberg RW, Kyrkanides S, Moss ME. Temporomandibular joint sound evaluation with an electronic device and clinical evaluation. Clin Orthod Res 2001;4:72–78.
100. Puri P, Kambylafkas P, Kyrkanides S, Katzberg R, Tallents RH. Comparison of Doppler sonography to magnetic resonance imaging and clinical examination for disc displacement. Angle Orthod 2006;76:824–829.

101. Motoyoshi M, Hayashi A, Arimoto M, Ohnuma M, Namura S. Studies of temporomandibular joint sounds. Part 3. The clinical usefulness of TMJ Doppler. J Nihon Univ Sch Dent 1995;37:209–213.
102. Christensen LV. Physics and the sounds produced by the temporomandibular joints. Part II. J Oral Rehabil 1992;19:615–627.
103. Paiva G, Paiva PF, de Oliveira ON. Vibrations in the temporomandibular joints in patients examined and treated in a private clinic. Cranio 1993;11:202–205.
104. Wabeke KB, Spruijt RJ, van der Weyden KJ, Naeije M. Evaluation of a technique for recording temporomandibular joint sounds. J Prosthet Dent 1992;68:676–682.
105. Christensen LV, Donegan SJ, McKay DC. Temporomandibular joint vibration analysis in a sample of non-patients. Cranio 1992;10:35–42.
106. Ishigaki S, Bessette RW, Maruyama T. Vibration analysis of the temporomandibular joints with meniscal displacement with and without reduction. Cranio 1993;11:192–201.
107. Widmer CG. Temporomandibular joint sounds: A critique of techniques for recording and analysis. J Craniomandib Disord 1989;3:213–217.
108. Sharma S, Crow HC, McCall WD Jr, Gonzalez YM. Systematic review of reliability and diagnostic validity of joint vibration analysis for diagnosis of temporomandibular disorders. J Orofac Pain 2013;27:51–60.
109. Bag AK, Gaddikeri S, Singhal A, et al. Imaging of the temporomandibular joint: An update. World J Radiol 2014;6:567–582.
110. Brooks SL, Brand JW, Gibbs SJ, et al. Imaging of the temporomandibular joint: A position paper of the American Academy of Oral and Maxillofacial Radiology. Oral Surg Oral Med Oral Pathol Oral Radiol Endod 1997;83:609–618.
111. Hunter A, Kalathingal S. Diagnostic imaging for temporomandibular disorders and orofacial pain. Dent Clin North Am 2013;57:405–418.
112. Poveda-Roda R, Bagan J, Carbonell E, Margaix M. Diagnostic validity (sensitivity and specificity) of panoramic X-rays in osteoarthrosis of the temporomandibular joint. Cranio 2015;33:189–194.
113. Lim MJ, Lee JY. Computed tomographic study of the patterns of osteoarthritic change which occur on the mandibular condyle. J Craniomaxillofac Surg 2014;42:1897–1902.
114. Boeddinghaus R, Whyte A. Computed tomography of the temporomandibular joint. J Med Imaging Radiat Oncol 2013;57:448–454.
115. Krishnamoorthy B, Mamatha N, Kumar VA. TMJ imaging by CBCT: Current scenario. Ann Maxillofac Surg 2013;3:80–83.
116. Larheim,TA, Abrahamsson AK, Kristensen M, Arvidsson LZ. Temporomandibular joint diagnostics using CBCT. Dentomaxillofac Radiol 2015;44:20140235.
117. Lamot U, Strojan P, Šurlan K, Popović K. Magnetic resonance imaging of temporomandibular joint dysfunctioncorrelation with clinical symptoms, age, and gender. Oral Surg Oral Med Oral Pathol Oral Radiol 2013;116:258–263.
118. Emshoff R, Innerhofer K, Rudisch A, Bertram S. Clinical versus magnetic resonance imaging findings with internal derangement of the temporomandibular joint: An evaluation of anterior disc displacement without reduction. J Oral Maxillofac Surg 2002;60:36–43.
119. Haley DP, Schiffman EL, Lindgren BR, Anderson Q, Andreasen K. The relationship between clinical and MRI findings in patients with unilateral temporomandibular joint pain. J Am Dent Assoc 2001;132:476–481.
120. Santos KC, Dutra ME, Warmling LV, Oliveira JX. Correlation among the changes observed in temporomandibular joint internal derangements assessed by magnetic resonance in symptomatic patients. J Oral Maxillofac Surg 2013;71:1504–1512.
121. Koh KJ, List T, Petersson A, Rohlin M. Relationship between clinical and magnetic resonance imaging diagnoses and findings in degenerative and inflammatory temporomandibular joint diseases: A systematic literature review. J Orofac Pain 2009;23:123–139.
122. López B DF, Corral S CM. Comparison of planar bone scintigraphy and single photon emission computed tomography for diagnosis of active condylar hyperplasia. J Craniomaxillofac Surg 2016;44:70–74.
123. Dupuy-Bonafé M, Picot L, Maldonado IL, Lachiche V, Granier I, Bonafé A. Internal derangement of the temporomandibular joint: Is there still a place for ultrasound? Oral Surg Oral Med Oral Pathol Oral Radiol 2012;113:832–840.
124. Li C, Su N, Yang X, Yang X, Shi Z, Li L. Ultrasonography for detection of disc displacement of temporomandibular joint: A systematic review and meta-analysis. J Oral Maxillofac Surg 2012;70:1300–1309.
125. Manfredini D. Ultrasonography has an acceptable diagnostic efficacy for temporomandibular disc displacement. Evid Based Dent 2012;13:84–85.
126. Levorova J, Machon V, Hirjak D, Foltan R. Ultrasound-guided injection into the lower joint space of the temporomandibular joint. Int J Maxillofac Surg 2015;44:491–492.
127. Vilanova JC, Barceló J, Puig J, Remollo S, Nicolau C, Bru C. Diagnostic imaging: Magnetic resonance imaging, computed tomography, and ultrasound. Semin Ultrasound CT MR 2007;28:184–191.

128. de Leeuw R, Davis CE, Albuquerque R, Carlson CR, Andersen AH. Brain activity during stimulation of the trigeminal nerve with noxious heat. Oral Surg Oral Med Oral Pathol Oral Radiol Endod 2006;102:750–757.
129. Finnerup NB, Haroutounian S, Karnerman P, et al. Neuropathic pain: An updated grading system for research and clinical practice. Pain 2016;157:1599–1606.
130. Svensson P, Drangsholt M, Pfau DB, List T. Neurosensory testing of orofacial pain in the dental clinic. J Am Dent Assoc 2012;143:e37–e39.
131. Svensson P, Baad-Hanssen L, Pigg M, et al. Guidelines and recommendations for assessment of somatosensory function in oro-facial pain conditions—A taskforce report. J Oral Rehabil 2011;38:366–394.
132. Foster AH, Carlson BM. Myotoxicity of local anesthetics and regeneration of the damaged muscle fibers. Anesth Analg 1980;59:727–736.
133. Lee SJ, McCall WD Jr, Kim YK, Chung SC, Chung JW. Effect of botulinum toxin injection on nocturnal bruxism: A randomized controlled trial. Am J Phys Med Rehabil 2010;89:16–23.
134. Shim YJ, Lee MK, Kato T, Park HU, Heo K, Kim ST. Effects of botulinum toxin on jaw motor events during sleep in sleep bruxism patients: A polysomnographic evaluation. J Clin Sleep Med 2014;10:291–298.
135. Ernberg M, Hedenberg-Magnusson B, List T, Svensson P. Efficacy of botulinum toxin type A for treatment of persistent myofascial TMD pain: A randomized, controlled, double-blind multicenter study. Pain 2011;152:1988–1996.
136. Nixdorf DR, Heo G, Major PW. Randomized controlled trial of botulinum toxin A for chronic myogenous orofacial pain. Pain 2002;99:465--473.
137. Chen YW, Chiu YW, Chen CY, Chuang SK. Botulinum toxin therapy for temporomandibular joint disorders: A systematic review of randomized controlled trials. J Oral Maxillofac Surg 2015;44:1018–1026.
138. Pullinger AG, Seligman DA. The degree to which attrition characterizes differentiated patient groups of temporomandibular disorders. J Orofac Pain 1993; 7:196–208.
139. Haralur SB. Digital evaluation of functional occlusion parameters and their association with temporomandibular disorders. J Clin Diagn Res 2013;7:1772–1775.
140. Dyer EH. Importance of a stable maxillomandibular relation. J Prosthet Dent 1973;30:241–251.
141. Türp JC, Greene CS, Strub JR. Dental occlusion: A critical reflection on past, present and future concepts. J Oral Rehabil 2008;35:446–453.
142. Little JW, Falace DA, Miller CS, Rhodus N. Dental Management of the Medically Compromised Patient, ed 8. St Louis: Mosby, 2013.
143. Wright EF, Des Rosier KF, Clark MK, Bifano SL. Identifying undiagnosed rheumatic disorders among patients with TMD. J Am Dent Assoc 1997;128:738–744.
144. Doshi TL, Nixdorf DR, Campbell CM, Raja SN. Biomarkers in temporomandibular disorder and trigeminal neuralgia: A conceptual framework for understanding chronic pain. Can J Pain 2020;4:1–18.
145. World Health Organization. Biomarkers in Risk Assessment: Validity and Validation—Environmental Health Criteria 222. Geneva, 2001.
146. David KD, Aghaeepour N, Ahn AH. Discovery and validation of biomarkers to aid the development of safe and effective pain therapeutics: Challenges and opportunities. Nat Rev Neurol 2020;16:381–400.

3

Diagnostic Classification of Orofacial Pain

Key points

- Diagnostic classification systems are needed to assist with management of orofacial pain.
- There are many widely varying classification schemes, which reflects the complexity of pain as a field.
- No diagnostic classification is without shortcomings and criticism, and there is still an urgent need for validation of classification schemes.
- The diagnostic classification presented in this chapter is in accord with internationally accepted standards and should be useful for clinicians attempting to manage patients who are suffering from orofacial pain.

The ability to understand and investigate the pathophysiologic processes underlying a disorder depends on a valid, reliable diagnostic classification system and common terminology to facilitate communication among clinicians, researchers, academics, and patients. Without a universal system of organization in place, discussion, investigation, and ultimately understanding of the disorder are difficult to achieve.

The process of classification entails the grouping of various disorders according to common signs and symptoms and then dividing further by common pathophysiology and treatment approaches. In this manner, the diagnostic classification can assist clinicians in treatment selection. From a clinical perspective, it is not essential to further divide subgroups when all of the disorders within a given subgroup are managed by the same therapy; therefore, from a therapeutic standpoint, subcategories are useful when therapy or the prognosis demand it.

Another purpose of a common or universal diagnostic classification system is to assist researchers in gaining insight into the prevalence, etiology, and natural course of a specific disorder. Knowledge can only be advanced when there is agreement on the case definition of specific disorders so that research efforts can be compared between patients and various research groups. At this time, it is uncertain whether diagnostic criteria for research purposes are compatible with diagnostic criteria for determining therapy. For example, it is quite reasonable to separate muscle disorders from intracapsular joint disorders for the purpose of studying the natural course of these temporomandibular disorders (TMDs). However, merely identifying that a patient is suffering from one of these types of disorders may not be adequate to effectively manage the condition considering the specific etiology and how psychosocial factors may influence treatment response. The most useful classification system would provide both research and diagnostic advantages.

The first step in developing and establishing a classification system is identifying a group of common signs and symptoms. Once these signs and symptoms have been identified, the disorder is named. The disorder is then investigated to learn more about its etiology so that effective treatment may be developed. It is very important that the signs and symptoms used to identify the disorder be unique to the disorder so that other unrelated disorders are not misidentified. It is therefore necessary to develop specific inclusion and exclusion criteria that will permit accurate grouping of similar disorders. To eliminate as much variability in diagnosis as possible, it is very important to be specific, avoiding words such as "usually," "typically," or "sometimes." Testing is then necessary to determine if the diagnostic criteria are valid and reliable for determining the specific disorder. Once diagnostic criteria are proven reliable, research efforts can be directed toward gaining better insight into etiology, eventually leading to more effective and personalized treatment.

In this chapter, past and present terminology and diagnostic classification systems for TMDs and orofacial pain disorders are discussed, and a classification system for orofacial pain disorders is presented. To assist the reader, the codes from the *International Classification of Diseases, Tenth Revision (ICD-10)* and *Eleventh Revision (ICD-11)* will be provided for each diagnosis throughout the next chapters.

Terminology

Over the years, functional disturbances of the masticatory system have been identified by a variety of terms, which likely led to confusion in this area. In 1934, Dr James Costen[1] described a group of symptoms that centered around the ears and temporomandibular joints (TMJs), which became known as *Costen syndrome*. In 1959, Shore[2] used the term *temporomandibular joint dysfunction syndrome* for those symptoms.

Later, the term *functional temporomandibular joint disturbances* was introduced by Ramfjord and Ash.[3] Some earlier terms, such as *occluso-mandibular disturbance* and *myoarthropathy of the temporomandibular joint*, were based on possible etiologic factors.[4,5] Other terminology stressed the featured pain symptom, such as *temporomandibular pain-dysfunction syndrome* and *myofascial pain-dysfunction syndrome*.[6,7]

Because the symptoms are not always isolated to the TMJs, some authors believe that the previously mentioned terms were too limited and a broader, more collective term should be used, such as *craniomandibular disorders*.[8] Bell[9] suggested the term *temporomandibular disorders*, which has gained wide acceptance and popularity. As described in this text, this term includes not only problems related to the TMJ itself, but all functional disturbances of the masticatory system. Any musculoskeletal disorder of the masticatory system can be considered a TMD.

Diagnostic Classification Systems

History of classification systems

A review of the literature regarding the classification of orofacial pain reveals little consensus on the most favorable diagnostic classification system. Many classification systems with varying advantages and disadvantages have been offered. Categories of division included etiologic factors, common signs and symptoms, tissue origin or functional region of the body, or combinations thereof. Perhaps the first classification system for TMJ problems was offered by Weinmann and Sicher.[10] In 1951, they classified TMJ problems into *(1)* vitamin deficiencies, *(2)* endocrine disorders, and *(3)* arthritis. Five years later, Schwartz[11] introduced the term *temporomandibular joint pain-dysfunction syndrome* to distinguish organic disturbances of the joint proper from masticatory muscle disorders. In 1960, Bell[12] developed a classification composed of six groups, recognizing both intracapsular and muscle (ie, extracapsular) disorders. Acknowledging the need for a suitable classification for functional disorders of the masticatory system, the American Academy of Orofacial Pain (AAOP) published a position paper with a suggested classification system.[8] Soon after, the American Dental Association (ADA) organized a national conference in which Bell suggested the term *temporomandibular disorders*, and a revised classification of TMDs consisting of five categories was introduced. Both the term and the classification were accepted by the ADA, but unfortunately, no diagnostic criteria were offered at that time.[13]

In 1985, Eversole and Machado[14] felt it was unrealistic to include all non-arthritic TMJ regional pain disorders as myofascial pain dysfunction syndrome. They thought the diagnosis of the TMJ dysfunctional states should better reflect the tissue source of pain and the spectrum of signs and symptoms observed among patients with arthrographically documented TMJ internal derangement. Therefore, they proposed a classification scheme of functional disorders divided into myogenic facial pain; internal TMJ derangement type 1, 2, or 3; and degenerative joint disease. The classification included specific diagnostic criteria based on subjective and objective findings and allowed dual diagnoses of myogenic facial pain with any of the joint disorders. In 1989, Stegenga et al[15] proposed a system of classification emphasizing TMJ articular disorders. They divided their classification into inflammatory and noninflammatory articular disorders and nonarticular disorders. The subcategories of osteoarthrosis and internal derangements were further divided according to staging over time. Although this classification provided insight into intracapsular disorders, it placed little emphasis on masticatory muscle disorders. No diagnostic criteria were offered with this classification. As the dental profession began to appreciate the similarity between many TMDs and other medical conditions, a need grew to include TMDs in a more inclusive medical classification for pain disorders. In 1986, the International Association for the Study of Pain (IASP)[16] published a classification of pain conditions. Of the 32 categories of pain disorders, category III was designated as "craniofacial pain of musculoskeletal origin." Within this category were two subcategories: *(1)* temporomandibular pain and dysfunction syndrome and *(2)* osteoarthritis of the TMJ. This classification failed to recognize any pain disorders arising from the masticatory muscles.

In 1990, the American Academy of Head, Neck, Facial Pain and TMJ Orthopedics[17] proposed a classification with five TMD categories and two non-TMD categories. The subcategories represented a mixture of both traditional and nontraditional disorders. Brief explanations were offered for most subcategories but not for all. There were 19 subcategories under the main category of "myofascial disorders," some of which were separated by the specific muscle or tendon involved. Some diagnostic categories, such as "bruxism," might better represent a precipitating or contributing factor of muscle pain and not necessarily a muscle pain disorder itself. No diagnostic criteria were offered to assist in classifying these disorders.

In 1992, Truelove et al[18] proposed a classification system for TMDs that allowed for multiple diagnoses within the same subject group. Required operational criteria were listed for each diagnostic group, allowing the researcher to investigate a sample population and determine the types and severity of disorders present. This concept was further elaborated through the research diagnostic criteria (RDC) offered by Dworkin and LeResche.[19]

Another classification suggested a much broader approach. Woda and Pionchon[20] proposed the adoption of a unifying classification for "idiopathic orofacial pain disorders." Most clinicians who treat orofacial pain disorders recognize that there are certain patients who present with clinical symptoms that do not easily fit into the known and generally well-accepted classifications of orofacial pain disorders. The authors suggest that many of these unclassified conditions present with some common clinical symptoms. Because our understanding of these disorders is not complete, the profession has assigned such terms as *atypical facial pain* and *atypical odontalgia*. These atypical cases may present with common clinical symptoms associated with common pathophysiologic mechanisms. If common mechanisms do in fact exist, then it may be useful to group these conditions together. Yet until these mechanisms are better understood, grouping them into a large classification will not likely improve treatment selection. In fact, placing TMDs—with relatively known etiologies and treatment strategies—into a group of idiopathic orofacial pain disorders would be taking a step in the wrong direction.

In 2012, a group of researchers and clinicians attempted a new approach to the classification of orofacial pain, which was based on ontology.[21] *Ontology* is the study of the nature of being, such as whether an entity exists or not, how entities are similar and different as well as how they relate to each other within a hierarchy, and how these differences or similarities define their subgroup.[22] Identifying a disorder or disease is dependent on several levels of evidence, such as reality, observations, interpretations, and/or beliefs. This new endeavor to classify orofacial pain has only attempted to examine a few orofacial pain conditions, and therefore a full classification is not available. This approach to nosology is unique, and its usefulness has yet to be demonstrated.

The International Classification of Headache Disorders (ICHD)

In 1988, the International Headache Society (IHS) proposed their first classification for headache composed of 13 broad categories, called the International Classification of Headache Disorders (ICHD).[23] The 11th category was designated as "headache or facial pain attributed to disorder of cranium, neck, eyes, ears, nose, sinuses, teeth, mouth, or other facial or cranial structures." There were no specific subcategories related to TMDs, despite recommendations by the AAOP.[24] In 2004, the IHS published their second version of the classification, outlining more than 230 types of headaches. TMDs were still minimally addressed in this version under category 11.[25] The AAOP provided diagnostic criteria and subcategories within the third and fourth editions of their organization's Guidelines book in 1996 and 2008, respectively.[26,27] In 2018, the IHS published the third edition of the ICHD, which is the classification system used in this text for headaches and neuropathic pain (ICHD-3).[28] Many clinicians have embraced this classification because of its inclusive considerations for all head pains. Clinically useful diagnostic criteria are provided for more than 300 disorders, all organized in a flexible hierarchy allowing the clinician differing "depths" for ruling in a diagnosis. Section 13 encompasses the multitude of painful cranial neuropathies. Section 11 ("Headache or facial pain attributed to disorder of the cranium, neck, eyes, ears, nose, sinuses, teeth, mouth or other facial or cervical structure") includes both 11.6 "Headache attributed to disorder of the teeth" and 11.7 "Headache attributed to temporomandibular disorder (TMD)." There are no further sub/categories for TMDs in section 11, instead referring to the RDC/TMD. There is also no axis to address the psychosocial dimensions of the various disorders.[29]

The RDC/TMD, DC/TMD, and Expanded TMD Taxonomy

The Research Diagnostic Criteria for Temporomandibular Disorders (RDC/TMD) classification not only provided specific diagnostic criteria for eight TMD subgroups—it also recognized another level or axis that must be considered when evaluating and managing TMD pain: the psychosocial component. For the first time in any classification system, a dual diagnosis was established that recognized the physical conditions (Axis I) and psychosocial status (Axis II) that contribute to the suffering, pain behavior, and disability associated with the patient's pain experience. (This Axis II should not be confused with the designated axis system endorsed by the *Diagnostic and Statistical Manual of Mental Disorders, Fifth Edition [DSM-5]* of the American Psychiatric Association.) This dual-axis classification approach has been incorporated into Bell's classification for all orofacial pain disorders.[30] The RDC/TMD offered what appeared to be reasonable diagnostic criteria, specifically for research purposes.[29] Although some questioned whether these criteria were specific enough to accurately distinguish subgroups of TMD patients, using the RDC/TMD for the most common TMDs has acceptable reliability.[31–34] The former International RDC/TMD Consortium from the International Association for Dental Research and the Special Interest Group on Orofacial Pain from the IASP joined forces to revise the RDC/TMD diagnostic algorithms to produce the dual-axis Diagnostic Criteria (DC/TMD) for the most common pain-related TMDs. These evidence-based clinical criteria have improved diagnostic accuracy for the most common TMDs and are easy for both clinicians and researchers to use.[35] The validation project established high sensitivity and specificity for the painful musculoskeletal TMDs and high specificity for disc derangements in the DC/TMD.[36,37] As of October 2021, the DC/TMD has been translated into 21 languages and 13 more languages are in progress.[38]

The Axis II instruments include inventories to evaluate pain burden (Graded Chronic Pain Scale v 2.0), functional interference (Jaw Functional Limitation Scale – 20), global body pain extent and symptomatology (Pain Drawing, PHQ-15), anxiety and depression (PHQ-9 and GAD-7, or PHQ-4), and parafunction

(Oral Behavior Checklist).[39] These pain maps and scales help evaluate the patient's subjective experience as a biopsychosocial whole and better direct the diagnosis and multidisciplinary management of chronic orofacial pain.

Peck et al[40] expanded on the DC/TMD taxonomy in 2014 to include less common—but still clinically relevant—disorders such as adhesions, ankylosis, idiopathic condylar resorption, synovial chondromatosis, tendonitis, masticatory muscle spasm, movement disorders, and coronoid hyperplasia. This list of 37 disorders featured plausible diagnostic criteria that could be operationalized and further studied.[40] An executive summary of the DC/TMD published in the *Journal of the American Dental Association* in 2016 promoted this evidence-based, biopsychosocial approach to TMD classification with the wider dental audience.[41] Future directions for the DC/TMD may include qualitative research to validate psychosocial phenotypes[42]; additional axes to describe genetics, and neurobiologic plasticity and biomarkers[43]; and clarifying the etiologic, diagnostic, and management overlap of sleep and awake bruxism, orofacial dyskinesia, and oromandibular dystonia. In 2017, the International RDC/TMD Consortium Network changed its name to the International Network for Orofacial Pain and Related Disorders Methodology (INfORM).[45]

The ACTTION-APS Pain Taxonomy (AAPT)

In 2014, the Analgesic, Anesthetic, and Addiction Clinical Trial Translations, Innovations, Opportunities, and Networks (ACTTION) and the American Pain Society (APS) provided a mechanistic framework for the development of chronic pain diagnostic criteria called the ACTTION-APS Pain Taxonomy (AAPT).[46,47] It organizes pain into five dimensions: *(1)* core diagnostic criteria; *(2)* common features; *(3)* common medical and psychiatric comorbidities; *(4)* neurobiological, psychosocial, and functional consequences; and *(5)* putative neurobiologic and psychosocial mechanisms, risk factors, and protective factors. In the AAPT, "temporomandibular disorders" are organized separately in "Orofacial and head pain" even though these could legitimately be classified in "Musculoskeletal pain," and "Headache disorders" refers readers to the classification provided by the ICHD.[25]

The International Classification of Orofacial Pain (ICOP)

An international collaborative effort by the Orofacial and Head Pain Special Interest Group of the IASP, INfORM, AAOP, and IHS culminated in the International Classification of Orofacial Pain, 1st edition (ICOP) published in 2020. The ICOP's hierarchical formatting mirrors the ICHD-3's structure, integrates the painful TMDs classified in the DC/TMD, refers to the ICHD-3 for primary and secondary headaches, and aligns with *ICD-11*/IASP criteria. The ICOP encompasses acute pain (eg, odontogenic, mucosal, salivary gland pain), the myriad of chronic orofacial pains discussed at length in later chapters of this book, and expanded psychosocial instruments for patient assessment.[48] The classification scheme organizes orofacial pain disorders into six mutually exclusive categories: *(1)* orofacial pain attributed to disorders of dentoalveolar and anatomically related structures; *(2)* myofascial orofacial pain; *(3)* TMJ pain; *(4)* orofacial pain attributed to lesion or disease of the cranial nerves; *(5)* orofacial pain resembling presentations of primary headaches; and *(6)* idiopathic orofacial pain. Each category contains subtypes or subforms of orofacial pain disorders, further subdivided based on the pathophysiology and underlying cause. As a tool for enhancing research and clinical management of orofacial pain, the ICOP provides empirically derived diagnostic criteria for individual entities.

International Classification of Diseases, Eleventh Revision

Implementation of *ICD-11* makes considerable advances in the classification of chronic pain, spearheaded by the IASP Task Force for the Classification of Chronic Pain on behalf of the World Health Organization (WHO). Adopted in 2019 with projected implementation to be in 2022, the *ICD-11* is a fully electronic database that allows for cross-referenced categories. Chronic pain disorders are divided into seven groups: one for primary pain (eg, fibromyalgia, migraine, irritable bowel syndrome, TMD)[49] and six secondary pain groups (cancer, neuropathic, visceral, posttraumatic and postsurgical, headache and orofacial, and musculoskeletal).[50] The *ICD-11* organizes chronic pain entities by giving first priority to the pain's etiology, then to the pathophysiologic mechanism underlying the pain, and lastly the location of pain in the body. Organized into 27 chapters, stem codes and extension codes can be combined (called "cluster coding") to give significant diagnostic detail in a standard format: eg, stem code/stem code and extension code. A brand-new chapter categorizes sleep-wake disorders.

Future directions

Remarkable strides have been made in the last 30 years, leading to the *ICD-11*, which distinguishes chronic primary and chronic secondary pain syndromes, and the recent publication of the ICOP, a systematic classification scheme of painful orofacial disorders. Although the ICOP organizes entities into a logical and applicable system, only time will tell its real impact once broadly adopted by the intended users.[51] As classification systems are dynamic tools evolving with the emergence of new knowledge, future efforts could streamline the classification structure, leaving aside empirical approaches to focus on hypothesis-driven descriptions and interrelations of disease entities. Among other endeavors are the need to confirm the psychometric adequacy of the ICOP by beta-testing the classification for reliability, sensitivity, and specificity.[52] In addition to refining clinical phenotyping, the next ICOP edition should follow ontologic principles and incorporate axes for biomarkers, neurobiologic pain processing changes over time (suggested as "nociplastic pain"),[53] and putative psychosocial factors deemed to impact treatment decisions. Finally, there is a need to establish crosswalks (mapping) between the ICOP and other parent classification systems such as the *ICD-11*, the ICHD-3, and the DC/TMD to help unify and streamline clinical diagnosis and care worldwide.[54,55]

Differential Diagnosis of Orofacial Pain

The diagnostic process is a clinical skill joining science and art. The goals are to identify any primary physical (Axis I) diagnoses based on pain mechanisms[56] and to recognize contributing factors, level of complexity, and prognosis. This generates a list of conditions that are most likely responsible for each of the presenting complaints until all pain sources are established. It is essential to exclude serious, life-threatening intracranial or extracranial disorders or diseases early in the diagnostic process because these conditions may require immediate care and input from other health care providers. The tail end of the diagnostic process is to rule in a disorder based on established diagnostic criteria while excluding disorders that can cause similar symptoms. The differential diagnosis is a critical step because an incorrect or omitted diagnosis is one of the most frequent causes of inappropriate and misdirected treatment or treatment failure.[57]

Clinicians should be familiar with the breadth of conditions that cause orofacial pain and understand pain mechanisms and modulating factors. This should be done from a diagnostic classification that provides insights into the range of putative sources of orofacial pain. The recently published ICOP[48] represents the best available tool owing to the proposed operational criteria for the diagnosis of acute and chronic orofacial pain conditions and consensus regarding the denomination of clinical entities.

Orofacial pain mechanisms can fall into one of five main categories: *Nociceptive pain* results from the activation of peripheral nociceptors in nonneuronal tissue; the immune system drives *inflammatory pain* to promote healing; *neuropathic pain* is caused by a lesion or disease of the somatosensory nervous system; *nociplastic pain* reflects an altered function of nociceptive pathways; and *neurovascular pain* shares the pathophysiologic features of migraine and trigeminal autonomic cephalalgias.[53,58]

Establishing the correct Axis I physical diagnosis is usually straightforward for simple orofacial pain. The difficulty arises with the chronic interplay of physiologic, psychologic, and social factors. This dynamic interaction leads to significant heterogeneity among patients with identical Axis I diagnoses and a wide range of responses to treatment. Chronicity and overlap of signs and symptoms of many pain conditions often require a multidisciplinary team approach for diagnosing and managing complex orofacial problems. The pain experience causes psychologic distress, especially when significant comorbidities exist (eg, widespread body pain, irritable bowel syndrome, pelvic pain, chronic headache, and chronic lower back pain).[59–65] Within the context of personalized treatment, clinicians must look beyond the sole Axis I physical diagnoses. Besides comorbidities and putative pain mechanisms, assessing and managing psychosocial factors (Axis II) is crucial.[66] This is especially true when the source of painful symptoms is uncertain and the Axis I diagnosis lies within the ICOP category 6, idiopathic orofacial pain, a group of clinical entities with unknown cause.[48]

These guidelines explore the gamut of orofacial pain and reflect the breadth of pain conditions included in the ICOP, 1st edition.[48] The broad categories included are as follows:

- Vascular and nonvascular intracranial pain disorders
- Primary headache disorders
- Neuropathic pain disorders
- Intraoral pain disorders
- TMDs
- Cervical pain disorders
- Extracranial and systemic causes of orofacial pain

Each of these categories represents a group of Axis I physical orofacial pain conditions frequently accompanied by Axis II psychosocial factors that greatly impact the clinical course and treatment outcomes. The seven broad categories of orofacial pain (Axis I) are briefly introduced in this chapter, along with the Axis II considerations. An additional section includes how sleep disorders may influence these conditions. A more complete description of each is presented in separate chapters.

Vascular and nonvascular intracranial pain disorders

Disorders of the intracranial structures (eg, neoplasm, aneurysm, abscess, hemorrhage or hematoma, and edema) should be considered first in the differential diagnosis because they can be life-threatening and may require immediate attention. The red flags of serious intracranial disorders include new or abrupt onset of pain or progressively more severe pain, interruption of sleep by pain, and pain precipitated by exertion or positional change (ie, coughing, sneezing). Pain-sensitive structures inside the skull subjected to displacement and stretching by a tumor or expansive lesion will refer pain ipsilaterally, to the V_1 and V_3 territories more often than the V_2 and C_2 territories.[67] In addition, tumor-related inflammation may induce local sensitization and contribute to extracranial face pain. Other red flags of intracranial disorders are signs or symptoms of weight loss, ataxia, weakness, fever with pain, neurologic signs or symptoms (eg, seizure, paralysis, vertigo), and neurologic deficits.[68]

Primary headache disorders

Primary headache disorders are a group of pain disorders not caused by another disease but resulting from the activation of a complex brain network. The core of the underlying pathophysiology involves neuronal mechanisms causing sensitization of the trigeminovascular pathways and dysfunction in different brain areas that include the brainstem, diencephalon, hypothalamus, and multiple cortical and subcortical regions.[69,70] Interacting genetic and environmental predisposing factors with sensory processing dysregulation at the brain level give rise to primary headache disorders. According to the ICHD-3, primary headache disorders comprise four categories: migraine, trigeminal autonomic cephalalgias, tension-type headache, and less common primary headache syndromes.[28] The characteristics of these headaches vary. Migraine is described as throbbing, pulsating, and disabling, whereas tension-type headache is characterized as dull, steady, aching pain. The dental profession has become increasingly active in managing some of these pain disorders because headache is the most common pain comorbidity reported by TMD patients.[71] In addition, primary headaches usually perceived solely in the head may spread to the face or coactivate V_1 and V_2 thereby causing orofacial pain. It follows that primary headache pain features, frequently referred to as *neurovascular pain*, may occur explicitly in the orofacial region.[72] The ICOP taxonomy includes neurovascular face pain disorders under category 5, orofacial pains resembling presentations of primary headaches.[48] Whenever the pain is solely in the head area, the major burden of managing primary headache disorders still lies within the medical community.

Neuropathic pain disorders

Neuropathic pain is defined as pain caused by a lesion or disease of the somatosensory nervous system.[73] It is not a diagnosis but refers to painful conditions that arise from neural damage, functional abnormalities, and maladaptive plasticity in the nervous system.[74–76] Because the somatic structures are not affected, the examination fails to reveal any pathology activating the nociceptors. The combined effect of etiologic, genetic, and environmental factors makes the clinical presentation of neuropathic pain heterogenous, and its recognition requires skillful history taking. The level of certainty that the pain is neuropathic may be captured by the three-tier grading system proposed by the IASP Special Interest Group on Neuropathic Pain (NeuPSIG).[77] Possible, probable, and definite neuropathic pain depend on the pain history, neuroanatomic distribution, presence of sensory signs, and testing to confirm the lesion or disease.

An ideal classification for neuropathic pain would be based on the neurobiologic mechanisms responsible for producing the pain condition.[78–80] Unfortunately, our current understanding of these mechanisms has yet to achieve this. Complicating the development of such a classification system is the understanding that both the peripheral and central nervous systems contribute to these pain conditions. Using the Quantitative Sensory Testing (QST) protocol introduced by the German Research Network on Neuropathic Pain (DFNS) to classify patients according to sensory profile—thought to mirror the pain generation mechanism—may assist in advancing this concept.[81,82] The ICOP lists category 4 as "orofacial pain attributed to lesion or disease of the cranial nerves," reflecting the difficulty in developing an encompassing classification for neuropathic pain.[48]

Intraoral pain disorders

Intraoral structures are the most common source of orofacial pain. The dentist plays an important role in the diagnosis of intraoral pain because many of these disorders are solely managed by those in the dental profession. The dentist must be extremely thorough in ruling out nociceptive and inflammatory pain etiologies involving the dental pulp, periodontium, mucogingival tissues, tongue, salivary glands, and the jaw bone, all listed in the ICOP under category 1, orofacial pain attributed to disorders of dentoalveolar and anatomically related structures.[48]

Temporomandibular disorders

TMDs encompass painful and nonpainful disorders that are related to alterations in structure, function, or physiology of the masticatory system.[83] These conditions that involve the masticatory muscles and/or the TMJ may be associated with other systemic and comorbid medical conditions.[84] Painful TMDs are the likeliest cause of nonodontogenic pain in the orofacial region, and these conditions are listed in the ICOP under category 2, myofascial orofacial pain, and category 3, temporomandibular joint pain, which are further subdivided into primary and secondary disorders.[48] General dentists play a pivotal role in the diagnosis and management of common TMDs. However, they must be knowledgeable of the concept that chronic pain related to TMDs is a complex disease best explained by multiple risk determinants that impact the disease course and management.[36]

Cervical pain disorders

The interest in the cervical region comes from the proximity and the complex neurobiologic interconnections with the craniofacial structures. Neck pain is the second most common comorbidity in patients with chronic orofacial pain, and referral to the craniofacial region is common.[71] This may mimic TMD pain due to the convergence of cervical and trigeminal nociceptive afferent inputs in the trigeminocervical complex of the brainstem.[85] It follows that cervical pain disorders represent a group of musculoskeletal conditions that can greatly influence the management of patients with persistent orofacial pain. These disorders are subdivided into those that predominantly originate in the muscles and those that predominantly originate in the cervical spine. Cervical structures deserve a significant diagnostic consideration when assessing orofacial pain.[85]

Extracranial and systemic causes of orofacial pain

There are a variety of associated structures that can cause orofacial pain: ears, eyes, nose, paranasal sinuses, throat, lymph nodes, major vessels, and salivary glands. Many of these structures produce heterotopic (ie, referred) pain felt in the orofacial region, which is often misinterpreted as dental or TMD pain.[86] Although pain from these structures may not be primarily managed by the dentist, a thorough understanding of their characteristics is necessary to establish an accurate diagnosis and avoid inappropriate interventions. Once the diagnosis has been established, proper referral should be considered. Clinicians must be aware that orofacial pain may be related to cardiovascular disease and unusual orofacial pain can occur in medically complex patients.[87,88]

Sleep disorders

Sleep is a vital function, along with the pain signaling system that detects a threat to body integrity or tissue repair in progress. There are instances when pain—especially chronic pain—may lengthen the time to fall asleep, trigger wakefulness, and cause nonrestorative sleep.[89] As will be discussed in chapter 11, good sleep quality is essential for maintaining physical and psychologic health. Sleep disturbances can increase the risk of pain onset or worsen the pain experienced by some individuals.[90] It is very apparent that pain and sleep are often closely associated conditions for many chronic pain patients. The orofacial pain clinician needs to appreciate this relationship, and the chapter on sleep disorders included in this text should help to offer more personalized treatments.

Axis II: Psychologic factors

Abundant evidence supports the biopsychosocial model of health problems and emphasizes how emotion and motivation influence patient behavior. It follows that the mind-body dynamic interplay makes psychologic and social factors significant contributors to the patient's pain experience.[66,91] Rarely does pain exist without some influence of these Axis II factors, especially as pain becomes more chronic. Even common stressful life events, such as conflicts in home or work relationships, financial problems, and cultural readjustment, may contribute to illness and chronic pain.[92–95] These stressors may heighten tensions, insecurities, and dysphoric effects, which may in turn lead to increased strains on the masticatory system by way of unusual parafunctional behaviors. Once established, these adjustment reactions (often with mixed disturbance of emotions and conduct) lead to an upregulation of the autonomic nervous system, which can further exacerbate the physical condition.[96,97]

The major psychologic factors associated with pain disorders are depression, anxiety, catastrophizing, physical symptom reporting, fear avoidance, and prolonged negative feelings. The major social factors include access to care, stigma, and support from family and friends. A mix of these factors is common among chronic pain patients and may make the persistent pain more difficult to tolerate and/or manage. Negative cognitive factors such as counterproductive thoughts or attitudes can make resolution of the illness more difficult. Confusion and misunderstanding are commonly seen in chronic pain patients because they have often received many opposing and varied opinions, diagnoses, and treatment suggestions. This confusion reduces motivation, increases anger or noncompliance, and creates mistrust or skepticism toward health care providers. Also, patients with persistent pain often have unrealistic expectations and may expect complete or immediate pain relief.

It should be emphasized that mental disorders and orofacial pain disorders are not mutually exclusive conditions. When psychologic factors are prominent in the patient's presentation, collaboration with a mental health care professional should be an integral dimension of assessment and management.

References

1. Costen JB. Syndrome of ear and sinus symptoms dependent upon functions of the temporomandibular joint. Ann Otol Rhinol Laryngol 1934;3:1–4.
2. Shore NA. Occlusal Equilibration and Temporomandibular Joint Dysfunction. Philadelphia: JB Lippincott, 1959.
3. Ramfjord SP, Ash MM. Occlusion. Philadelphia: WB Saunders, 1971.
4. Gerber A. Kiefergelenk und Zahnokklusion. Dtsch Zahnärztl 1971;26:119–141.
5. Graber G. Neurologische und psychosomatische Aspekte der Myoarthropathien des Kauorgans. ZWR 1971;80:997–1000.
6. Schwartz L. Disorders of the temporomandibular joint. Philadelphia: WB Saunders, 1959.

7. Laskin DM. Etiology of the pain-dysfunction syndrome. J Am Dent Assoc 1969;79:147–153.
8. McNeill C, Danzig D, Farrar W, et al. Craniomandibular (TMJ) disorders—State of the art. J Prosthet Dent 1980;44:434–437.
9. Bell WE. Clinical Management of Temporomandibular Disorders. Chicago: Year Book Medical Publishers, 1982.
10. Weinmann JP, Sicher H. Pathology of the temporomandibular joint. In: Sarnat BG (ed). The Temporomandibular Joint. Springfield, IL: Charles C Thomas, 1951:65–81.
11. Schwartz LL. A temporomandibular joint pain-dysfunction syndrome. J Chron Dis 1956;3:284.
12. Bell WE. Temporomandibular Joint Disease. Dallas: Egan, 1960.
13. Griffiths RH. Report of the President's Conference on Examination, Diagnosis and Management of Temporomandibular Disorders. J Am Dent Assoc 1983;106:75–77.
14. Eversole LR, Machado L. Temporomandibular joint internal derangements and associated neuromuscular disorders. J Am Dent Assoc 1985;110:69-79.
15. Stegenga B, de Bont L, Boering G. A proposed classification of temporomandibular disorders based on synovial joint pathology. Cranio 1989;7:107–118.
16. Merskey H. Classification of chronic pain: Descriptions of chronic pain syndromes and definitions of pain terms. Pain 1986;(suppl 3):S1–S226.
17. Talley RL, Murphy GJ, Smith SD, Baylin MA, Haden JL. Standards for the history, examination, diagnosis, and treatment of temporomandibular disorders (TMD): A position paper. Cranio 1990;8:60–77.
18. Truelove EL, Sommers EE, LeResche L, Dworkin SF, Von Korff M. Clinical diagnostic criteria for TMD. New classification permits multiple diagnoses [see comments]. J Am Dent Assoc 1992;123:47–54.
19. Dworkin SF, LeResche L. Research diagnostic criteria for temporomandibular disorders: Review, criteria, examinations and specifications, critique. J Craniomandib Disord 1992;6:301–355.
20. Woda A, Pionchon P. A unified concept of idiopathic orofacial pain: Pathophysiologic features. J Orofac Pain 2000;14:196–212.
21. Nixdorf DR, Drangsholt MT, Ettlin DA, et al. Classifying orofacial pains: A new proposal of taxonomy based on ontology. J Oral Rehabil 2012;39:161–169.
22. Smith B, Ceusters W. Ontology as the core discipline of biomedical informatics: Legacies of the past and recommendations for the future direction of research. In: Crnkovic GD, Stuart S (eds). Computing, Philosophy, and Cognitive Science: The Nexus and the Liminal. Cambridge, UK: Scholars Press, 2007:104–122.
23. Oleson J. Classification and diagnostic criteria for headache disorders, cranial neuralgias and facial pain. Cephalalgia 1988;8(suppl 7):1–97.
24. McNeill C. Temporomandibular Disorders: Guidelines for Classification, Assessment, and Management, ed 2. Chicago: Quintessence, 1993.
25. Oleson J. The International Classification of Headache Disorders. Cephalagia 2004;24(suppl):1–160.
26. Okeson JP. Orofacial Pain: Guidelines for Classification, Assessment, and Management, ed 3. Chicago: Quintessence, 1996.
27. de Leeuw R. Orofacial Pain: Guidelines for Assessment, Diagnosis, and Management, ed 4. Chicago: Quintessence, 2008.
28. Headache Classification Committee of The International Headache Society (IHS) The International Classification of Headache Disorders, 3rd edition. Cephalalgia. 2018;38:1–211.
29. Klasser GD, Goulet JP, De Laat A, Manfredini D. Classification of Orofacial Pain. In: Farah CS, Balasubramaniam R, McCullough MJ (eds). Contemporary Oral Medicine: A Comprehensive Approach to Clinical Practice. Cham, Switzerland: Springer International Publishing, 2019:1819–1842.
30. Okeson JP. Bell's Oral and Facial Pain, ed 7. Chicago: Quintessence, 2014.
31. Naeije M, Kalaykova S, Visscher CM, Lobbezoo F. Evaluation of the Research Diagnostic Criteria for Temporomandibular Disorders for the recognition of an anterior disc displacement with reduction. J Orofac Pain 2009;23:303–311.
32. Okeson JP. Critical commentary 1: Evaluation of the Research Diagnostic Criteria for Temporomandibular Disorders for the recognition of an anterior disc displacement with reduction. J Orofac Pain 2009; 23:312–315.
33. Steenks MH, de Wijer A. Validity of the Research Diagnostic Criteria for Temporomandibular Disorders Axis I in clinical and research settings. J Orofac Pain 2009; 23:9–16.
34. John MT, Dworkin SF, Mancl LA. Reliability of clinical temporomandibular disorder diagnoses. Pain 2005; 118:61–69.
35. Schiffman EL, Ohrbach R, Truelove E, et al. Diagnostic Criteria for Temporomandibular Disorders (DC/TMD) for clinical and research applications: Recommendations of the International RDC/TMD Consortium Network and Orofacial Pain Special Interest Group. J Orofac Pain Headache 2014;28:6–27.
36. Ohrbach R, Dworkin SF. The evolution of TMD diagnosis: Past, present, future. J Dent Res 2016;85:1093–1101.

37. Schiffman EL, Ohrbach R, Truelove EL, et al. The research diagnostic criteria for temporomandibular disorders. V: Methods used to establish and validate revised axis I diagnostic algorithms. J Orofac Pain 2010;24:63–78.
38. DC-TMD Translations. International Network for Orofacial Pain and Related Disorders Methodology (INfORM). https://ubwp.buffalo.edu/rdc-tmdinternational/tmd-assessmentdiagnosis/dc-tmd-translations/. Accessed 10 November 2022.
39. Diagnostic Criteria for Temporomandibular Disorders. International Network for Orofacial Pain and Related Disorders Methodology (INfORM). Retrieved from https://ubwp.buffalo.edu/rdc-tmdinternational/tmd-assessmentdiagnosis/dc-tmd/. Accessed 10 November 2022.
40. Peck CC, Goulet JP, Lobbezoo F, et al. Expanding the taxonomy of the diagnostic criteria for temporomandibular disorders. J Oral Rehabil 2014;41:2–23.
41. Schiffman E, Ohrbach R. Executive summary of the Diagnostic Criteria for Temporomandibular Disorders for clinical and research applications. J Am Dent Assoc 2016;147:438–445.
42. Durham J, Raphael KG, Benoliel R, Ceusters W, Michelotti A, Ohrbach R. Perspectives on next steps in classification of orofacial pain—Part 2: Role of psychosocial factors. J Oral Rehab 2015;42:942–955.
43. Ceusters W, Nasri-Heir C, Alnaas D, Cairns BE, Michelotti A, Ohrbach R. Perspectives on next steps in classification of orofacial pain—Part 3: Biomarkers of chronic orofacial pain–from research to clinic. J Oral Rehabil 2015;42:956–966.
44. Michelotti A, Alstergren P, Goulet JP. Next steps in development of the diagnostic criteria for temporomandibular disorders (DC/TMD): Recommendations from the International RDC/TMD Consortium Network workshop. J Oral Rehabil 2016;43:453–467.
45. International Network for Orofacial Pain and Related Disorders Methodology (INfORM). https://www.iadr.org/INfORM. Accessed 10 November 2022.
46. Fillingim RB, Bruehl S, Dworkin RH, et al. The ACTTION-American Pain Society Pain Taxonomy (AAPT): An evidence-based and multidimensional approach to classifying chronic pain conditions. J Pain 2014;15:241–249.
47. Dworkin RH, Bruehl S, Fillingim RB, Loeser JD, Terman GW, Turk DC. Multidimensional diagnostic criteria for chronic pain: Introduction to the ACTTION–American Pain Society Pain Taxonomy (AAPT). J Pain 2016; 17(suppl 2):T1–T9.
48. International Classification of Orofacial Pain, 1st edition (ICOP). Cephalalgia. 2020;40:129–221.
49. Nicholas M, Vlaeyen JW, Rief W, et al. The IASP classification of chronic pain for *ICD-11*: Chronic primary pain. Pain 2019;160:28–37.
50. Treede RD, Rief W, Barke A, et al. Chronic pain as a symptom or a disease: The IASP Classification of Chronic Pain for the *International Classification of Diseases* (*ICD-11*). Pain 2019;160:19–27.
51. Pigg M, Nixdorf DR, Law AS, et al. New international classification of orofacial pain: What is in it for endodontists? J Endod 2021;47:345–357.
52. Ceusters W, Michelotti A, Raphael KG. Review: Perspectives on next steps in classification of orofacial pain—Part 1: Role of ontology. J Oral Rehabil 2015;42:926–941.
53. Kosek E, Cohen M, Baron R, et al. Do we need a third mechanistic descriptor for chronic pain states? Pain 2016;157:1382–1386.
54. Renton T, Durham J, Aggarwal VR. The classification and differential diagnosis of orofacial pain. Expert Rev Neurother 2012;12:569–576.
55. Klasser GD, Manfredini D, Goulet JP, De Laat A. Orofacial pain and temporomandibular disorders classification systems: A critical appraisal and future directions. J Oral Rehabil 2018;45:258–268.
56. Vardeh D, Mannion RJ, Woolf CJ. Toward a mechanism-based approach to pain diagnosis. J Pain 2016; 17(suppl 2):50–69.
57. De Laat A. Differential diagnosis of toothache to prevent erroneous and unnecessary dental treatment. J Oral Rehabil 2020;47:775–781.
58. Goulet JP, Woda A. Orofacial pain: Classification and roadmap to clinical phenotypes. In: Orofacial Pain Biomarkers. Berlin: Springer International, 2017:3–20.
59. Bertoli E, de Leeuw R. Prevalence of suicidal ideation, depression, and anxiety in chronic temporomandibular disorder patients. J Oral Facial Pain Headache 2016;30:296–301.
60. Fricton JR, Kroening RF, Hathaway KW. TMJ and Craniofacial Pain: Diagnosis and Management. St Louis: Ishiyaku EuroAmerica, 1988.
61. Lorduy KM, Liegey-Dougall A, Haggard R, Sanders CN, Gatchel RJ. The prevalence of comorbid symptoms of central sensitization syndrome among three different groups of temporomandibular disorder patients. Pain Practice 2013;13:604–613.
62. Bonato LL, Quinelato V, de Felipe Cordeiro PC, de Sousa EB, Tesch R, Casado PL. Association between temporomandibular disorders and pain in other regions of the body. J Oral Rehabil 2017;44:9–15.
63. Bair E, Gaynord S, Slade GD, et al. Identification of clusters of individuals relevant to temporomandibular disorders and other chronic pain conditions: The OPPERA study. Pain 2016;157:1266–1278.

64. Velly A, Ahmed A, Lenton P, Fricton J. Comorbidities in chronic temporomandibular disorder patients: The links between painful and non-painful conditions. J Pain 2013;14:S12.
65. Velly A, Fricton J. The impact of comorbid conditions on treatment of temporomandibular disorders. J Am Dent Assoc 2011;14:170–172.
66. Cole HA, Carlson CR. Mind-Body considerations in orofacial pain. Dent Clin North Am 2018;62:683–694.
67. Fontaine D, Almairac F, Santucci S, et al. Dural and pial pain-sensitive structures in humans: New inputs from awake craniotomies. Brain 2018;141:1040–1048.
68. Moazzam AA, Habbian M. Patients appearing to dental professionals with orofacial pain arising from intracranial tumors: A literature review. Oral Surg Oral Med Oral Pathol Oral Radiol 2012;114:749–755.
69. Goadsby PJ, Holland PR, Martins-Oliveira M, Hoffmann J, Schankin C, Akerman S. Pathophysiology of migraine: A disorder of sensory processing. Physiol Rev 2017;97:553–622.
70. Hoffmann J, May A. Diagnosis, pathophysiology, and management of cluster headache. Lancet Neurol 2018;17:75–83.
71. Velly A, Fricton J. Orofacial pain comorbidities and their impact on biomarkers. In: Orofacial Pain Biomarkers. Berlin: Springer International, 2017:21–32.
72. Ziegeler C, May A. Facial presentations of migraine, TACs, and other paroxysmal facial pain syndromes. Neurology 2019;93:e1138–e1147.
73. The IASP Taxonomy. https://www.iasp-pain.org/Taxonomy?navItemNumber=576#Neuropathicpain. Accessed 10 November 2022.
74. Costigan M, Scholz J, Woolf CJ. Neuropathic pain: A maladaptive response of the nervous system to damage. Annu Rev Neurosci 2009;32:1–32.
75. Wall P, Melzack R. Textbook of Pain, ed 6. Edinburgh: Churchill Livingstone, 2013.
76. Okeson JP. Principles of pain diagnosis. In: Bell's Oral and Facial Pain, ed 7. Chicago: Quintessence, 2014: 135–180.
77. Finnerup NB, Haroutounian S, Kamerman P, et al. Neuropathic pain: An updated grading system for research and clinical practice. Pain 2016;157:1599–1606.
78. von Hehn CA, Baron R, Woolf CJ. Deconstructing the neuropathic pain phenotype to reveal neural mechanisms. Neuron 2012;73:638–652.
79. Woolf CJ, Mannion RJ. Neuropathic pain: Aetiology, symptoms, mechanisms, and management. Lancet 1999;353:1959–1964.
80. Finnerup NB, Jensen TS. Mechanisms of disease: Mechanism-based classification of neuropathic pain—A critical analysis. Nat Clin Pract Neurol 2006;2:107–115.
81. Baron R, Maier C, Attal N, et al. Peripheral neuropathic pain: A mechanism-related organizing principle based on sensory profiles. Pain 2017;158:261–272.
82. Vollert J, Maier C, Attal N, et al. Stratifying patients with peripheral neuropathic pain based on sensory profiles: Algorithm and sample size recommendations. Pain 2017;158:1446–1455.
83. Bond EC, Mackey S, English R, Liverman CT, Yost O (eds). Temporomandibular Disorders: Priorities for Research and Care. Washington, DC: The National Academies Press, 2020.
84. Costa YM, Conti PC, de Faria FA, Bonjardim LR. Temporomandibular disorders and painful comorbidities: Clinical association and underlying mechanisms. Oral Surg Oral Med Oral Pathol Oral Radiol 2017; 123:288–297.
85. Piovesan EJ, Kowacs PA, Tatsui CE, et al. Referred pain after painful stimulation of the greater occipital nerve in humans: Evidence of convergence of cervical afferences on trigeminal nuclei. Cephalalgia 2001;21:107–109.
86. Renton T. Tooth-related pain or not? Headache 2020;60:235–246.
87. Kreiner M, Okeson JP, Michelis V, Lujambio M, Isberg A. Craniofacial pain as the sole symptom of cardiac ischemia: A prospective multicenter study. J Am Dent Assoc 2007;138:74–79.
88. Shephard MK, Heir G. Orofacial pain in the medically complex patient. In: Farah CS, Balasubramaniam R, McCullough MJ (eds). Contemporary Oral Medicine: A Comprehensive Approach to Clinical Practice. Cham, Switzerland: Springer International, 2019.
89. Lavigne GJ, Sessle BJ. The neurobiology of orofacial pain and sleep and their interactions. J Dent Res 2016;95:1109–1116.
90. Finan PH, Goodin BR, Smith MT. The association of sleep and pain: An update and a path forward. J Pain 2013;14:1539–1552.
91. Campbell CM, Edwards RR. Mind–body interactions in pain: The neurophysiology of anxious and catastrophic pain-related thoughts. Transl Res 2009; 153: 97–101.

92. Bertolotti G, Vidotto G, Sanavio E, Frediani F. Psychological and emotional aspects and pain. Neurol Sci 2003,24(suppl 2):S71–S75.
93. Rollman GB, Gillespie JM. The role of psychosocial factors in temporomandibular disorders. Curr Rev Pain 2000;4:71–81.
94. Korszun A, Papadopoulos E, Demitrack M, Engleberg C, Crofford L. The relationship between temporomandibular disorders and stress-associated syndromes. Oral Surg Oral Med Oral Pathol Oral Radiol Endod 1998;86:416–420.
95. Dworkin SF. Behavioral, emotional, and social aspects of orofacial pain. In: Stohler CS, Carlson DS (eds). Biological and Psychological Aspects of Orofacial Pain. Ann Arbor: University of Michigan, 1994.
96. Carlson C, Bertrand P, Ehrlich A, Maxwell A, Burton RG. Physical self-regulation training for the management of temporomandibular disorders. J Orofac Pain 2001;15:47–55.
97. Curran SL, Carlson CR, Okeson JP.Emotional and physiologic responses to laboratory challenges: Patients with temporomandibular disorders versus matched control subjects. J Orofac Pain 1996;10: 141–150.

4

General Assessment of the Orofacial Pain Patient

Key Points

- Diagnoses of intracranial causes of head, neck, and orofacial pain rely primarily on a careful history, a healthy respect for red flags, and prompt evaluation.
- The SNNOOP10 acronym is a useful mnemonic device for red flags that prompt urgent and extensive investigations to rule out intracranial lesions.
- Intracranial pathologies are numerous and may lead to disability or death if not managed promptly.
- The diagnosis of headaches secondary to intracranial causes can be challenging in the presence of primary headaches. An older adult with migraine who develops a headache with new neurologic signs or symptoms should be considered to have vascular compromise until proven otherwise.

This chapter reviews both vascular and nonvascular intracranial sources of orofacial pain, many of which may be life-threatening and/or associated with significant morbidity if untreated or if treatment is delayed (Box 4-1).

Box 4-1 Intracranial causes of orofacial pain

Vascular disorders

- Ischemic cerebrovascular disease (ICHD 6.1)
- Traumatic intracranial hemorrhage (ICHD 5.5)
- Nontraumatic intracranial hemorrhage (ICHD 6.2)
- Unruptured vascular malformation (ICHD 6.3)
- Arteritis (ICHD 6.4)
- Carotid or vertebral artery pain (ICHD 6.5)
- Venous thrombosis (ICHD 6.6)

Nonvascular disorders

- High cerebrospinal fluid pressure (ICHD 7.1)
- Low cerebrospinal fluid pressure (ICHD 7.2)
- Intracranial noninfectious inflammation (ICHD 7.3)
- Intracranial neoplasm (ICHD 7.4)
- Intracranial infection (ICHD 9.1)

Overview

Although only approximately 1% of patients presenting with a headache will ultimately be found to have a significant abnormality on neuroimaging, the consequences of a missed diagnosis can be catastrophic. In the presence of a normal neurologic examination, the prevalence of vascular, neoplastic, and non-neoplastic findings is low: 6.6 %, 1.4%, and 9.6%, respectively.[1] In the emergency department, the probability of a significant abnormality on neuroimaging is understandably higher at approximately 8%.[2] Predictive factors include acute onset headache, age above 50 years, and an abnormal neurologic examination.[3] According to the American College of Radiology, primary headache disorders with absence of red flag features do not require neuroimaging.[4,5] Further, while neuroimaging is an important diagnostic tool, many secondary headache syndromes (such as giant cell arteritis [GCA] and idiopathic intracranial hypertension) may be overlooked with neuroimaging alone. The mnemonic SNNOOP10 is a useful screener for red flag features (Box 4-2).[6] There are also five headache green flags that seem to suggest a primary rather than a secondary headache (Box 4-3).[7]

Systemic symptoms or disease

Headache associated with systemic features such as fever, weight loss, arthralgia, and/or rashes may indicate an underlying systemic process such as meningoencephalitis, viral illness (eg, COVID-19), vasculitis (eg, GCA), or metastasis. Risk factors such as HIV, cancer, or chronic immunosuppressive therapy may also predispose to systemic disease. To further complicate the diagnostic process, conditions such as HIV are associated with both intracranial infections and cancer.

Neurologic signs or symptoms

Neurologic signs or symptoms ranging from mild confusion or sedation to frank neurologic deficits, such as aphasia or hemiparesis, typically indicate more than a primary pain disorder. Focal neurologic signs and symptoms such as hemiparesis, visual obscuration, diplopia, dizziness/vertigo, imbalance, or numbness definitely warrant further investigation to rule out vascular, infectious, inflammatory, and neoplastic disease of the brain and/or meninges. When migraine attacks are accompanied

Box 4-2 SNNOOP10: Red flags for secondary headaches[6]

Sign or Symptom

1. **S**ystemic symptoms including fever
2. **N**eoplasm in history
3. **N**eurologic deficit or dysfunction (including decreased consciousness)
4. **O**nset of headache is sudden or abrupt
5. **O**lder age (> 50 years)
6. **P**attern change or recent onset of headache
7. **P**ositional headache
8. **P**recipitated by sneezing, coughing, or exercise
9. **P**apilledema
10. **P**rogressive headache in atypical presentations
11. **P**regnancy or puerperium
12. **P**ainful eye with autonomic features
13. **P**osttraumatic onset of headache
14. **P**athology of the immune system such as HIV
15. **P**ainkiller overuse or new drug at onset of headache

Box 4-3 Green flags suggesting primary headaches[7]

1. The current headache has already been present during childhood
2. The headache occurs in temporal relationship with the menstrual cycle
3. The patient has headache-free days
4. Close family members have the same headache phenotype
5. Headache occurred or stopped more than 1 week ago

by neurologic changes such as aphasia, hemisensory symptoms, visual field defects, and/or hemiparesis, an exclusion of secondary causes is necessary. While the temporal profile of an aura is typically gradual and slowly progressive and is associated with positive features (such as scintillating scotoma), a stroke, on the contrary, is associated with an abrupt and static onset of negative features (such as vision loss). In a prospective cohort of patients with transient ischemic attacks (TIA), the ICHD-3 criteria for migraine with aura (unfortunately) demonstrated excellent specificity of between 97% to 100%.[8] There is, therefore, no substitute for clinical diligence and a high index of suspicion.

Onset sudden (thunderclap)

A sudden-onset, severe, and generalized or localized headache must be considered a medical emergency until proven otherwise. The time course of the headache peaking to maximal severity is critical, as opposed to whether the headache is the "worst of one's life." In a prospective series of patients with subarachnoid hemorrhage (SAH), the headache peaked instantly in less than 1 second for 65% of patients and within 1 minute for 80% of the patients.[9] Up to 25% of SAH are unfortunately misdiagnosed.[10] The differential diagnosis for life-threatening acute-onset headaches includes *(1)* vascular

Box 4-4 Differential diagnosis of acute onset secondary headaches[11]

Vascular
Subarachnoid hemorrhage (ICHD 6.2.2)
Saccular aneurysm (ICHD 6.3.1)
Arteriovenous malformation (ICHD 6.3.2)
Carotid or vertebral artery dissection (ICHD 6.5.1)
Cerebral venous thrombosis (ICHD 6.6)
Pituitary apoplexy (ICHD 6.7.4)

Nonvascular
Acute hypertension (ICHD 7.1)
Benign intracranial hypertension (ICHD 7.1.1)
Intermittent hydrocephalus (ICHD 7.1.3)
Intracranial infection (ICHD 9.1)
Pheochromocytoma (ICHD 10.3.1)
Acute glaucoma (ICHD 11.3.1)
Acute mountain sickness (at altitude)
Acute optic neuritis

disorders such as SAH, cerebral infarction, cerebral venous thrombosis, and cervical artery dissection and *(2)* nonvascular disorders such as pituitary apoplexy and central nervous system infections (Box 4-4).

Onset after age 50 years

In patients older than 50 years, new-onset (ie, no prior history) and/or progressive or changing headaches are inherently concerning and likely have a secondary cause.[12] Migraines may begin at any age, but incident migraine after the age of 50 years is uncommon. Contingent on the findings from the history and physical examination, a magnetic resonance imaging (MRI) study of the brain with and without contrast and hematologic tests (such as erythrocyte sedimentation rate [ESR] and C-reactive protein [CRP] to rule out GCA, complete blood count to rule out anemia and blood dyscrasias, free thyroxine and thyroid-stimulating hormone levels to rule out thyroid disease, and a Lyme titer to rule out Lyme disease) may be necessary.

Pattern change

The experience of the first headache or the worst headache of one's life, or a change in attack frequency, severity, associated symptoms, or quality should prompt a review for other red flags and initiation of further investigations. In addition, patients with a history of migraine may also develop secondary headaches, in which case neither a history of migraine nor triptan responsiveness is reassuring. Although chronic and recurrent headaches typically present with similar features over time, patients should be educated to note and report changes in headache pattern. Progressively worsening headaches at any age need to be carefully assessed.

Postural headache

Headaches that are precipitated by sitting upright or standing with improvement on lying down can be a sign of a low-pressure headache due to a cerebrospinal fluid (CSF) leak.[13] In contrast, headaches on lying down can be caused by increased intracranial pressure related to an intracranial mass, cerebral venous thrombosis, meningeal process, or idiopathic intracranial hypertension. Headaches presenting only on awakening may be associated with obstructive sleep apnea, substance overuse or withdrawal, a brain tumor, or oral parafunctional habits such as bruxism. Headaches that awaken a patient from sleep may be attributed to increased intracranial pressure, cervicogenic headache, or primary headaches (such as cluster headache or migraine).

Papilledema

Papilledema is an extremely important neurologic sign of secondary headache. Papilledema indicates swelling of the optic nerve head, which can arise in the context of elevated intracranial pressure.[14] The differential diagnosis of intracranial hypertension includes intracranial mass lesions, cerebral venous sinus thrombosis, meningitis, and idiopathic intracranial hypertension.

Precipitants

Headaches precipitated by a cough, a sneeze, straining, or exertion, although possibly benign, warrant a brain MRI to exclude intracranial structural lesion such as a tumor or Arnold-Chiari malformation. In contrast, headaches that are worsened (not precipitated) by a Valsalva maneuver are typically benign.

Headache Attributed to Cranial or Cervical Vascular Disorder (ICHD-3 Item 6)

Ischemic stroke (ICHD 6.1; *ICD-10* I63; *ICD-11* 8B11) or transient ischemic attack (ICHD 6.1; *ICD-10* G45; *ICD-11* 8B10)

The prevalence of headache associated with acute ischemic cerebrovascular disease is estimated to be between 6% and 44%.[15] This etiology should be suspected when neurologic deficits present in an acute fashion, in a person older than 50 years, and seem temporally related to the head pain. Approximately 11% of patients with cerebellar ischemia had a headache at initial presentation.[16] Headache secondary to ischemic stroke typically affects older individuals with risk factors such as hypertension, atrial fibrillation, and tobacco use. However, stroke can occur at any age. The headache is typically continuous with tension-type features and is only rarely thunderclap in progression.[17] Along with female sex, posterior circulation dysfunction in the vertebral and basilar artery distribution is more likely to cause headache than anterior circulation disease.[15] Neurologic deficits reflect the region of the brain affected and may include vision loss, diplopia, weakness, sensory loss, aphasia, and ataxia. TIAs present in a similar fashion, but the deficits resolve within 24 hours, frequently within 20 minutes.

Migraineurs (especially migraine with aura) are at an increased long-term risk of cerebrovascular events.[18,19] The differential diagnosis of TIA and migraine with aura is extremely challenging.[20] The prevalence of migraine without aura was 20.8% in patients with TIA compared to 7.8% in controls.[21] An older adult with migraine who develops a headache with new neurologic signs or symptoms should be considered to have vascular compromise until proven otherwise.

Signs or symptoms consistent with cerebral ischemia warrant referral to the emergency department. A CT scan of the head is needed to rule out an intracranial hemorrhage. An MRI study with diffusion-weighted imaging has a higher sensitivity and specificity for the detection of acute cerebral ischemia and tissue damage. Treatment for the headache must be individualized. The pain typically lasts a few days at most, and vasoactive drugs are contraindicated.

Traumatic and nontraumatic intracranial hemorrhage

Headache secondary to traumatic intracranial hematoma may be due to an epidural hematoma (ICHD 5.5.1; *ICD-10* S06.4; *ICD-11 NA07.5*) or a subdural hematoma (ICHD 5.5.2; *ICD-10* S06.5; *ICD-11* NA07.6). Headache secondary to nontraumatic intracranial hematoma may be due to an intracerebral hemorrhage (ICHD 6.2.1; *ICD-10* 161; *ICD-11* 8B00) or an SAH

(ICHD 6.2.2; *ICD-10* I60; *ICD-11* 8B01). Similar to pain associated with ischemia, pain stemming from hemorrhage is best diagnosed according to its accompanying symptoms.

Traumatic intracranial hematoma (ICHD 5.5; *ICD-10* S06; *ICD-11* 8B0Z)

An epidural hematoma (ICHD 5.5.1; *ICD-10* S06.4; *ICD-11* NA07.5) is most often caused by severe blunt trauma to the skull and rupture of the middle meningeal artery.[22] A *lucid interval* may be observed wherein the patient appears to mostly recover after head trauma only to become somnolent and then comatose shortly thereafter. This lucid interval is more the exception than the rule. More frequently, patients will continue to have severe pain followed by a change in cognition. Rapid surgical drainage of epidural hematomas is necessary to prevent mortality. A high index of suspicion after head trauma is therefore strongly urged.

A subdural hematoma (ICHD 5.5.2; *ICD-10* S06.5; *ICD-11* NA07.6) may present acutely, subacutely, or even with chronic symptoms.[22] The subdural space fills with blood after the bridging veins coursing through it rupture, usually after a fall or other type of head trauma. Older patients and patients with alcoholism are at greater risk because they are more likely to have gait instability and their bridging veins are not as resistant to trauma. There is often a history of minimal trauma, like a minor motor vehicle accident without direct head trauma in which neurologic symptoms begin several hours or even days later. Patients on anticoagulation therapy and those taking frequent aspirin or nonsteroidal anti-inflammatory drugs (NSAIDs) are particularly at risk, even with seemingly minimal head trauma. Pain is not always the chief complaint. Symptoms may include any neurologic deficit, such as gait disturbance, personality change, somnolence, visual disturbances, or focal changes such as hemiparesis, hemisensory changes, and visual field defects. Surgical evacuation of the hematoma may be necessary, although small subdural hematoma without brain shift or pressure may only require careful observation.

Nontraumatic intracranial hemorrhage (ICHD 6.2; *ICD-10* I62; *ICD-11* 8B0Z)

Head pain associated with a nontraumatic intracerebral hemorrhage (ICHD 6.2.1; *ICD-10* I61; *ICD-11* 8B00) typically presents with acute neurologic deficits.[23] *An intracerebral hematoma* refers to a hematoma within the brain parenchyma and may be caused by hypertension, neoplasm, or arteriovenous malformations. A large hematoma may extend into a ventricle, resulting in coma or death.

Headache due to a subarachnoid hemorrhage (ICHD 6.2.2; *ICD-10* I60; *ICD-11* 8B01)

Headache due to a subarachnoid hemorrhage (SAH) (ICHD 6.2.2; *ICD-10* I60; *ICD-11 8B01*) is associated with a high mortality rate of 40% to 50%. It presents with a very sudden onset and is also known as a *thunderclap headache*.[24] The thunderclap pattern is a very dramatic rise to peak pain within seconds, often under a minute. The Ottawa SAH rule recommends investigation for SAH in the presence of at least one of these symptoms: neck pain or stiffness; age of 40 years or older; witnessed loss of consciousness; headache onset during exertion; thunderclap headache; or limited neck flexion on examination.[25] A ruptured saccular aneurysm is the most common cause of a spontaneous SAH. About 20% of aneurysms leak before they rupture, resulting in a severe headache for several days or 1 to 2 weeks prior. This is known as the *sentinel* or *warning headache*. The sudden or thunderclap onset of the "worst headache of my life" is a medical emergency, and aneurysmal SAH must be excluded with a non-contrast-enhanced CT scan (approximately 90% sensitive for SAH) and a lumbar puncture if the CT scan is negative.[26] Characteristic CSF findings include xanthochromia and an elevated red blood cell count.[27] The fluid-attenuated inversion recovery (FLAIR) MRI has also demonstrated good sensitivity for SAH.[28] Key aspects of treatment include maintaining hemodynamic stability, neurosurgical consultation for either aneurysmal clipping or endovascular coiling, and treatment for avoidance of vasospasm.[29] Many continue to experience headaches for years after the hemorrhage.[30]

Unruptured vascular malformation (ICHD 6.3)

Unruptured vascular malformations include saccular aneurysms (ICHD 6.3.1; *ICD-10* Q28.3; *ICD-11* 8B22.6), arteriovenous malformations (ICHD 6.3.2; *ICD-10* Q28.2; *ICD-11* 8B22.40), dural arteriovenous fistulae (ICHD 6.3.3; *ICD-10* I67.1; *ICD-11* 8B22.42), and venous and cavernous angiomas (ICHD 6.3.4; *ICD-10* D18.0; *ICD-11* XH1GU2). Symptoms may be absent until they rupture, or the patient may present with nonspecific head pain. Patients may present at any age, and a family history is often positive. A magnetic resonance angiogram (MRA) or computed tomography angiography (CTA) is helpful in the diagnostic process.

Saccular aneurysms may be incidental and asymptomatic, and they are present in 3% to 5% of the population.[31] Therefore, assigning causality to these entities as a source for headache can risk inappropriate intervention. Screening with CTA or MRA should be offered to patients who have at least two family members with known aneurysm or prior SAH.[32] Aneurysms that are small (< 7 mm) and in the anterior circulation are unlikely to rupture, whereas large, posterior circulation aneurysms involve a substantially greater risk. While some headaches improve following aneurysmal repair, others unfortunately worsen, the latter being especially likely in the presence of severe headache and trait anxiety.[33]

Arteritis (ICHD 6.4; *ICD-10* M31; *ICD-11* 4A44.2)

Arteritis typically presents with systemic symptoms and/or neurologic deficits, but at times it may present initially with throbbing unilateral pain localized in the temple associated with jaw claudication. GCA, previously known as *temporal arteritis*, is an autoimmune, large-vessel vasculitis preferentially affecting the external carotid artery and the aorta and may rapidly lead to blindness secondary to granulomatous occlusion of the carotid artery vasculature.[34] The incidence of GCA is 77 per 100,000 individuals, and women account for 65% of cases. GCA should be suspected in women over the age of 60 years who present with a sudden onset and persistent headache. GCA is associated with a higher risk of ischemic stroke and dementia and can be comorbid with polymyalgia rheumatica.[35] On examination, an enlarged, indurated, and/or tender temporal artery is often present. Laboratory investigations reveal an elevated ESR (60–100 mm/h), CRP, and platelet count.[36] Temporal artery biopsy or a temporal artery ultrasound (particularly a color-coded duplex sonography) confirms the diagnosis of GCA.[37] An adequate biopsy sample is necessary for diagnosis due to the histopathologic occurrence of skip lesions, where pathologic changes may be interspersed with segments that appear normal. Prompt administration of glucocorticoids (60 to 100 mg of oral prednisolone for 3 days, followed by a 12–18-month taper) is necessary to avoid permanent loss of vision. Tocilizumab, a monoclonal antibody blocker of interleukin (IL)-6, is approved for the treatment of GCA and has shown sustained disease remission.[38]

Cervical carotid or vertebral artery disorder (ICHD 6.5)

In carotid (*ICD-10* I77.71; *ICD-11* BD51.0) or vertebral artery dissection (*ICD-10* I77.74; *ICD-11* BD51.1), blood dissects between the medial and subintimal layers of the artery, which may then fill to form a pseudoaneurysm that causes ischemia by partial occlusion of the lumen. It is a significant cause of stroke or TIA in younger patients but can happen at any age. A traumatic dissection may be caused by blunt trauma to the neck or neck manipulation. Alternatively, a spontaneous dissection occurs without a history of injury. The classic triad of signs include ipsilateral pain in the neck, orbit region, and head; a partial Horner syndrome (due to the intimate association of sympathetic fibers with the internal carotid artery); and cerebral or retinal ischemia.[39,40] Long et al estimated that internal carotid artery dissection accounted for 14.3% of structural pathologies associated with cluster headaches.[41]

Besides checking for ocular manifestations (such as ocular motor nerve palsy), audible bruits should be sought in the neck or over the orbit or temporal bone indicating the presence of turbulent blood flow. Investigations include extracranial duplex ultrasound vascular scanning, MRI, and MRA or CTA of the cervical vessels. The management includes antiplatelet or anticoagulation therapy and endovascular stenting of the affected vessel(s).[42]

Cerebral venous thrombosis (ICHD 6.6; *ICD-10* I63.6; *ICD-11* 8B22.1)

Cerebral venous thrombosis (CVT) is a consequence of thrombosis of the cerebral veins causing obstruction of venous outflow and increased intracranial pressure.[43] It is more common in women under 50 years of age. Risk factors include oral contraceptive use, postpartum state, prothrombotic blood dyscrasias, and infection. COVID-19–associated coagulopathy is also a known cause of CVT.[44] Symptoms are highly variable and include headache without specific features, visual disturbances, signs of increased intracranial pressure (such as vomiting or papilledema), seizures, and frank neurologic deficits. In many, headache is the sole manifestation.[45] Investigations include MR venography or CT venography. In patients with a low pretest probability, a normal serum D-dimer may be helpful in ruling out the diagnosis.[46] The treatment consists of modifying the predisposing factors and at least 6 months of anticoagulation therapy.

Other intracranial arterial disorder (ICHD 6.7)

Reversible cerebral vasoconstriction syndrome (RCVS) (ICHD 6.7.3; *ICD-11* 8B22.2) has a pathognomonic presentation of recurrent thunderclap headache and reversible vasoconstriction of the intracranial arteries.[47,48] It is precipitated by exposure to vasoactive substances, pregnancy or postpartum, and sexual intercourse. RCVS is three times more common in women, with a mean age of about 40 years, and may recur in about 5% of patients. It is typically benign but potentially life-threatening. Complications may include ischemic stroke or hemorrhage (cortical SAH). Investigations via MRA, CTA, or conventional angiography will reveal cerebral vasoconstriction in at least two different arteries.[49] RCVS is treated with calcium channel blockers to reverse the arterial vasospasm. The offending agent (if any) should be discontinued promptly. CSF evaluation is often pursued to exclude angiitis (vasculitis), which may have similar findings on vascular imaging of arterial beading.

Genetic vasculopathy (ICHD 6.8)

Cerebral autosomal dominant arteriopathy with subcortical infarcts and leukoencephalopathy (CADASIL) (ICHD 6.8.1; *ICD-11* 8B22.CO) is a rare hereditary small-vessel angiopathy caused by *Notch3* mutation on chromosome 19.[50,51] It is a cause of recurrent stroke, cerebral small vessel disease, and dementia in young and middle-aged adults. It is strongly associated with migraine with aura. Characteristic white matter hyperintensities involving the anterior temporal poles and external capsule are noted on the MRI. The diagnosis is confirmed with electron microscopy of a skin biopsy and/or genetic testing for the *Notch3* mutations. The management is palliative.[52]

Mitochondrial encephalopathy, lactic acidosis, and stroke-like episodes syndrome (ICHD 6.8.2)

Mitochondrial encephalopathy, lactic acidosis, and stroke-like episodes syndrome (MELAS) (ICHD 6.8.2) is a progressive heterogenous metabolic disorder affecting multiple systems presenting in childhood or adolescence. It is caused by impaired mitochondrial energy production resulting in lactic acidosis. The hallmark feature is stroke-like episodes with symptoms such as hemiplegia, migraine, seizures, vomiting, and/or visual impairment. As implied by the name, lactic acidosis may be evident in the blood or elevated in the brain measured using magnetic resonance spectroscopy. The diagnosis may be confirmed with a muscle biopsy or genetic testing. As with other mitochondrial disorders, the transmission is maternal in origin. Management includes the use of L-arginine and high-dose taurine.[53,54]

Pituitary apoplexy (ICHD 6.9; *ICD-10* E23.6)

Pituitary apoplexy refers to a stroke of the pituitary gland, often associated with a pituitary tumor.[55] Clinical presentation include acute-onset headache and visual field deficits. The diagnosis can be confirmed with MRI. Some patients may require neurosurgery, while others can be managed conservatively. Systemic complications include hypotension and cerebral infarction.[56]

Headache Attributed to Nonvascular Intracranial Disorders (ICHD Item 7)

Increased CSF pressure (ICHD 7.1; *ICD-10* G93.2; *ICD-11* 8D60)

Increased intracranial pressure may yield a nonspecific headache involving any region of the head. Patients may have a mass that exerts pressure or have a process that impairs the normal circulation and egress of CSF, such as venous thrombosis or meningitis. This headache typically worsens with a Valsalva maneuver or recumbence and may be associated with nausea/vomiting, visual problems, and neurologic deficits. Ophthalmologic signs include extraocular movement abnormalities, especially diplopia, and evidence of early papilledema.

Idiopathic intracranial hypertension (*ICD-10* G93.2; *ICD-11* 8D60.Z)

Idiopathic intracranial hypertension (IIH) (*ICD-10* G93.2; *ICD-11* 8D60.Z), previously known as *pseudotumor cerebri*, is more prevalent in young, obese women, although in prepubertal patients there is no association with gender or obesity.[57] It is a rare disorder characterized by raised intracranial pressure (> 250 mm CSF) of unknown cause.[58] Current theories suggest an increased secretion or decreased absorption of CSF, and/or venous sinus stenosis causing obstruction of the cerebral venous outflow.[59] Typically, this condition produces a holocephalic daily headache with intermittent visual disturbances and pulsatile tinnitus. Psychiatric comorbidity is highly prevalent and associated with poorer outcome. Examination may reveal early or frank papilledema and/or bilateral abducens (sixth) nerve palsy.[60] IIH without papilledema is often misdiagnosed as chronic migraine.[61] Slit-like ventricles and sometimes stenosis of both transverse sinuses may be noted on MR venography. Optical coherence tomography has shown to be valuable in imaging the retina.[62] Management together with an ophthalmologist is essential due to blindness secondary to papilloedema if untreated. Fortunately, the increased intracranial pressure can remit with as little as 5% weight loss, which may be the only true disease-modifying therapy.[63] Treatment also includes the use of acetazolamide, which decreases production of CSF and can protect against vision loss. Patients may require multiple lumbar punctures to lower CSF pressure, optic nerve sheath fenestration for relief of papilledema, or ventriculoperitoneal shunting of CSF to reduce headaches and prevent further vision loss.[64] In some, post-dural-puncture headaches can be unfortunate sequelae of the former.[65] Relapse or recurrence following treatment is not unusual.

Low CSF pressure (ICHD 7.2)

Headaches due to low CSF pressure are classically worsened within a few minutes of standing and relieved by recumbence. They may be accompanied by neck stiffness or pain, tinnitus, hypacusia, paresthesia of the neck and arms, photophobia, or nausea. They may be spontaneous, iatrogenic following dural or lumbar punctures, or postoperative.

Spontaneous intracranial hypotension (SIH) (ICHD 7.2.3; *ICD-10* G97.1; *ICD-11* 8D61.0) is a debilitating postural headache resulting from spontaneous CSF leak or CSF hypotension. The CSF leak can occur out of meningeal diverticula, dural tears, or CSF-venous fistulas. Symptoms include orthostatic headache, nausea, vomiting, and neck pain or stiffness.[66] A systematic review and meta-analysis by D'Antona et al reported that brain MRI with contrast revealed diffuse pachymeningeal enhancement in 73% of patients, but was normal in 19% of the cases studied.[67] Localization of the leak is performed with digital subtraction myelography and magnetic resonance myelography. Blood patching completely resolved the symptoms in 60% of the patients.[68] Surgical closure of the leak may be required.

The incidence of post-dural-puncture headache (PDPH) (ICHD 7.2.1; *ICD-10* G97.0; *ICD-11* 8E66) following epidural or spinal anesthesia ranges from 6% to 36%.[69] Unfortunately, there is no evidence that PDPH is associated with low intracranial volume and/or pressure despite its classification as such.[70] PDPH is self-limiting and usually resolves within 1 week without treatment. Bed rest without head elevation for 2 to 3 days, mild analgesics, and caffeine or theophylline is recommended. Severe PDPH may require an epidural blood patch.

Noninfectious inflammatory diseases (ICHD 7.3)

Headaches with inflammatory conditions include neurosarcoidosis (ICHD 7.3.1; *ICD-10* D86.8; *ICD-11* 4B20.3) and aseptic meningitis (ICHD 7.3.2; *ICD-10* A87.9; *ICD-11* 8E40). Neurosarcoidosis is a rare form of sarcoidosis which affects both the peripheral and central nervous system.[71] The signs and symptoms range widely depending on the anatomical involvement. Aseptic meningitis may be caused by medications such as NSAIDs and intravenous immunoglobulin. A red flag implicating aseptic meningitis is a severe headache occurring during or after a viral infection. An MRI scan of the head, CSF examination, and blood studies are needed to diagnose these conditions.

Intracranial neoplasia (ICHD 7.4)

In a cohort of 507 patients with intracranial neoplasms, 52% reported headaches.[72] More often, in addition to the headache, other symptoms include focal neurologic symptoms, seizures, weight loss, personality changes, and neurologic deficits such as focal weakness or numbness. Headaches may be attributed to the increased intracranial pressure or hydrocephalus caused by the neoplasm (ICHD 7.4.1), to the pressure from the neoplasm itself (ICHD 7.4.2), or to carcinomatous meningitis (ICHD 7.4.3; *ICD-10* C79.32; *ICD-11* 8E40.0). Occasionally, neoplastic processes may intermittently occlude normal CSF flow, producing a ball-valve mechanism that manifests as posture-dependent symptoms. The clinical features of brain tumor headaches resemble primary headaches.[73] A contrast-enhanced MRI study of the head is warranted.

Chiari malformation type I (ICHD 7.7; *ICD-10* Q07.0; *ICD-11* LA07.4)

Herniation of the cerebellar tonsils 3 to 5 mm below the foramen magnum or caudal to the C2 level is known as *Arnold-Chiari malformation*. There are several types of this condition, and type 1 is the most common. The estimated incidence is 1 in 1,280. It can be congenital or secondary to downward pressure by a posterior fossa mass, intracranial hypotension, or intracranial hypertension.[74] It may affect children or adults, and cough-associated headache is a common symptom, although some are asymptomatic. More serious complications occur if the medulla or cervical spinal cord is compressed, which could lead to weakness of the limbs and hyperreflexia with extensor plantar responses, thereby necessitating surgical decompression. Milder cases without neurologic symptoms are managed conservatively.[75]

Headache Attributed to Infection (ICHD 9)

Headaches may be attributed to intracranial infections including bacterial meningitis (infection of the meninges) (ICHD 9.1.1; *ICD-10* G00.9; *ICD-11* 1D01.0), lymphocytic meningitis (ICHD 9.1.2; *ICD-10* G03.9; *ICD-11* 1C8F), encephalitis (infection of the brain parenchyma) (ICHD 9.1.3; *ICD-10* G04.90; *ICD-11* 1D00), brain abscess (localized, walled-off infection of the brain substance) (ICHD 9.1.4; *ICD-10* G06.0; *ICD-11* 1D03.3), and subdural empyema (infection localized to the subdural space) (ICHD 9.1.5; *ICD-10* G06.2; *ICD-11* 1D03.1).

Meningococcal meningitis is deadly if not treated within hours. Symptoms include a rash, fever, headache, stiff neck, vomiting, and occasionally positive Kernig and Brudzinski signs. Fever may be absent in the very young, old, or immunocompromised. The progression of symptoms over a few hours or rapid deterioration is the most important clue. An emergency diagnostic lumbar puncture must be performed along with a CT or MRI scan. The use of conjugate vaccines and adjunctive dexamethasone has significantly reduced the mortality of pneumococcal meningitis.[76] Up to 35% of patients suffer long-term neurologic or neurobehavioral consequences.[77]

Viral meningitis has a much lower mortality rate than bacterial meningitis. Aseptic viral meningitis is the most common cause of meningitis in the United States, of which herpes simplex virus type 2 is the most common cause.[78] The clinical presentation includes acute headache, fever, cognitive changes, drowsiness, and focal findings such as hemiparesis and seizures. Early antiviral therapy greatly reduces permanent neurologic sequelae. Another example is the long-COVID headache, which is a persistent headache that is the chronic sequela of the COVID-19 viral infection.[79]

References

1. Kamtchum-Tatuene J, Kenteu B, Fogang YF, Zatack JG, Nyaga UF, Noubiap JJ. Neuroimaging findings in headache with normal neurologic examination: Systematic review and meta-analysis. J Neurol Sci 2020;410:116997.
2. Kopel D, Peeler C, Zhu S. Headache emergencies. Neurol Clin 2021;39:355–372.
3. Locker TE, Thompson C, Rylance J, Mason SM. The utility of clinical features in patients presenting with nontraumatic headache: An investigation of adult patients attending an emergency department. Headache 2006;46:954–961.
4. Expert Panel on Neurologic I, Whitehead MT, Cardenas AM, et al. ACR Appropriateness Criteria Headache. J Am Coll Radiol 2019;16(11 suppl):S364–S377.
5. Evans RW, Burch RC, Frishberg BM, et al. Neuroimaging for migraine: The American Headache Society systematic review and evidence-based guideline. Headache 2020;60:318–336.
6. Do TP, Remmers A, Schytz HW, et al. Red and orange flags for secondary headaches in clinical practice: SNNOOP10 list. Neurology 2019;92:134–144.
7. Pohl H, Do TP, Garcia-Azorin D, et al. Green flags and headache: A concept study using the Delphi method. Headache 2021;61:300–309.
8. Lebedeva ER, Gurary NM, Gilev DV, Olesen J. Prospective testing of ICHD-3 beta diagnostic criteria for migraine with aura and migraine with typical aura in patients with transient ischemic attacks. Cephalalgia 2018;38:561–567.
9. Mac Grory B, Vu L, Cutting S, Marcolini E, Gottschalk C, Greer D. Distinguishing characteristics of headache in nontraumatic subarachnoid hemorrhage. Headache 2018;58:364–370.
10. Ois A, Vivas E, Figueras-Aguirre G, et al. Misdiagnosis worsens prognosis in subarachnoid hemorrhage with good Hunt and Hess score. Stroke 2019;50:3072–3076.
11. Schwedt TJ, Matharu MS, Dodick DW. Thunderclap headache. Lancet Neurol 2006;5:621–631.
12. Robblee J, Singh RH. Headache in the older population: Causes, diagnoses, and treatments. Curr Pain Headache Rep 2020;24:34.
13. Kranz PG, Gray L, Amrhein TJ. Spontaneous intracranial hypotension: 10 myths and misperceptions. Headache 2018;58:948–959.
14. D'Antona L, Asif H, Craven CL, et al. Brain MRI and ophthalmic biomarkers of intracranial pressure. Neurology 2021;96:e2714–e2723.
15. Harriott AM, Karakaya F, Ayata C. Headache after ischemic stroke: A systematic review and meta-analysis. Neurology 2020;94:e75–e86.
16. Altıparmak T, Nazliel B, Çaglayan HB, Tokgoz N, Gurses AA, Ucar M. Headache features of cerebellar ischemic strokes: Clinical and radiological-experiences of a single center. J Clin Neurosci 2021;88:173–177.
17. Lu J, Liu W, Zhao H. Headache in cerebrovascular diseases. Stroke Vasc Neurol 2020;5:205–210.
18. Gupta A, Srivastava MVP. Migraine and vascular risk: An update. Neurol India 2021;69(suppl):S83–S90.
19. Tietjen GE, Maly EF. Migraine and ischemnic stroke in women. A narrative review. Headache 2020;60:843–863.
20. Otlivanchik O, Liberman AL. Migraine as a stroke mimic and as a stroke chameleon. Cur Pain Headache Rep 2019;23:63.
21. Lebedeva ER, Gurary NM, Olesen J. Headache in transient ischemic attacks. J Headache Pain 2018;19:60.
22. Kapoor S. Headache attributed to cranial or cervical vascular disorders. Curr Pain Headache Rep 2013;17:334.
23. O'Carroll CB, Brown BL, Freeman WD. Intracerebral hemorrhage: A common yet disproportionately deadly stroke subtype. Mayo Clin Proc 2021;96:1639–1654.
24. Malhotra A, Wu X, Gandhi D, Sanelli P. The patient with thunderclap headache. Neuroimaging Clin N Am 2018;28:335–351.
25. Perry JJ, Sivilotti MLA, Emond M, et al. Prospective implementation of the Ottawa subarachnoid hemorrhage rule and 6-hour computed tomography rule. Stroke 2020;51:424–430.
26. Lin CM, Wang AY, Chen CC, et al. Warning headache correlates survival rate in aneurysmal subarachnoid hemorrhage. Biomed J 2019;42:352–357.
27. Shahan B, Choi EY, Nieves G. Cerebrospinal fluid analysis. Am Fam Physician 2021;103:422–428.
28. Ashraf R, Akhtar M, Akhtar S, Manzoor I. Diagnostic accuracy of flair in detection of acute subarachnoid hemorrhage in patients presenting with severe headache. J Neuroradiol 2019;46:294–298.
29. Tawk RG, Hasan TF, D'Souza CE, Peel JB, Freeman WD. Diagnosis and treatment of unruptured intracranial aneurysms and aneurysmal subarachnoid hemorrhage. Mayo Clin Proc 2021;96:1970–2000.
30. Huckhagel T, Klinger R, Schmidt NO, Regelsberger J, Westphal M, Czorlich P. The burden of headache following aneurysmal subarachnoid hemorrhage: A prospective single-center cross-sectional analysis. Acta Neurochir (Wien) 2020;162:893–903.
31. Mehta VA, Spears CA, Abdelgadir J, et al. Management of unruptured incidentally found intracranial saccular aneurysms. Neurosurg Rev 2021;44:1933–1941.

32. Thompson BG, Brown RD Jr, Amin-Hanjani S, et al. Guidelines for the management of patients with unruptured intracranial aneurysms: A guideline for healthcare professionals from the American Heart Association/American Stroke Association. Stroke 2015;46:2368–2400.
33. Schwedt TJ, Gereau RW, Frey K, Kharasch ED. Headache outcomes following treatment of unruptured intracranial aneurysms: A prospective analysis. Cephalalgia 2011;31:1082–1089.
34. Dinkin M, Johnson E. One giant step for giant cell arteritis: Updates in diagnosis and treatment. Curr Treat Options Neurol 2021;23:6.
35. Robinette ML, Rao DA, Monach PA. The immunopathology of giant cell arteritis across disease spectra. Front Immunol 2021;12:623716.
36. Weis E, Waite C, Roelofs KA. A predictive model for temporal artery biopsy in the setting of suspected giant cell arteritis: A validation study. Ophthalmic Plast Reconstr Surg 2021;37(3 suppl):S23–S26.
37. Guggenberger KV, Bley TA. Imaging in Vasculitis. Curr Rheumatol Rep 2020;22:34.
38. Song GG, Lee YH. Efficacy and safety of biological agents in patients with giant cell arteritis: A meta-analysis of randomized trials. Int J Clin Pharmacol Ther 2020;58:504–510.
39. Song JX, Lin XM, Hao ZQ, Wu SD, Xing YX. Ocular manifestations of internal carotid artery dissection. Int J Ophthalmol 2019;12:834-839.
40. Marciniec M, Sapko K, Kulczyński M, Popek-Marciniec S, Szczepańska-Szerej A, Rejdak K. Non-traumatic cervical artery dissection and ischemic stroke: A narrative review of recent research. Clin Neurol Neurosurg 2019;187:105561.
41. Long RJ, Zhu YS, Wang AP. Cluster headache due to structural lesions: A systematic review of published cases. World J Clin Cases 2021;9:3294–3307.
42. Serkin Z, Le S, Sila C. Treatment of extracranial arterial dissection: The roles of antiplatelet agents, anticoagulants, and stenting. Curr Treat Options Neurol 2019;21:48.
43. Spadaro A, Scott KR, Koyfman A, Long B. Cerebral venous thrombosis: Diagnosis and management in the emergency department setting. Am J Emerg Med 2021;47:24–29.
44. Ghosh R, Roy D, Mandal A, et al. Cerebral venous thrombosis in COVID-19. Diabetes Metab Syndr 2021;15:1039–1045.
45. Aliprandi A, Borelli P, Polonia V, Salmaggi A. Headache in cerebral venous thrombosis. Neurol Sci 2020; 41(suppl 2):401–406.
46. Heldner MR, Zuurbier SM, Li B, et al. Prediction of cerebral venous thrombosis with a new clinical score and D-dimer levels. Neurology 2020;95:e898–e909.
47. Song TJ, Lee KH, Li H, et al. Reversible cerebral vasoconstriction syndrome: A comprehensive systematic review. Eur Rev Med Pharmacol Sci 2021;25:3519–3529.
48. Ling YH, Chen SP. Narrative review: Headaches after reversible cerebral vasoconstriction syndrome. Curr Pain Headache Rep 2020;24:74.
49. Burton TM, Bushnell CD. Reversible cerebral vasoconstriction syndrome. Stroke 2019;50:2253–2258.
50. Mizuno T, Mizuta I, Watanabe-Hosomi A, Mukai M, Koizumi T. Clinical and genetic aspects of CADASIL. Front Aging Neurosci 2020;12:91.
51. Locatelli M, Padovani A, Pezzini A. Pathophysiological mechanisms and potential therapeutic targets in cerebral autosomal dominant arteriopathy with subcortical infarcts and leukoencephalopathy (CADASIL). Front Pharmacol 2020;11:321.
52. Manini A, Pantoni L. CADASIL from bench to bedside: Disease models and novel therapeutic approaches. Mol Neurobiol 2021;58:2558–2573.
53. Koga Y, Povalko N, Inoue E, et al. Therapeutic regimen of L-arginine for MELAS: 9-year, prospective, multicenter, clinical research. J Neurol 2018;265:2861–2874.
54. Ohsawa Y, Hagiwara H, Nishimatsu SI, et al. Taurine supplementation for prevention of stroke-like episodes in MELAS: A multicentre, open-label, 52-week phase III trial. J Neurol Neurosurg Psychiatry 2019;90:529–536.
55. Muthukumar N. Pituitary apoplexy: A comprehensive review. Neurol India 2020;68(suppl):S72–S78.
56. Jiang Q, Xiao S, Shu L, Huang X, Chen X, Hong H. Pituitary apoplexy leading to cerebral infarction: A systematic review. Eur Neurol 2020;83:121–130.
57. Virdee J, Larcombe S, Vijay V, Sinclair AJ, Dayan M, Mollan SP. Reviewing the recent developments in idiopathic intracranial hypertension. Ophthalmol Ther 2020;9:767–781.
58. Toscano S, Lo Fermo S, Reggio E, Chisari CG, Patti F, Zappia M. An update on idiopathic intracranial hypertension in adults: A look at pathophysiology, diagnostic approach and management. J Neurol 2021;268: 3249–3268.
59. Mondejar V, Patsalides A. The role of arachnoid granulations and the glymphatic system in the pathophysiology of idiopathic intracranial hypertension. Curr Neurol Neurosci Rep 2020;20:20.
60. Elsaid N, Ahmed O, Belal T, Razek A, Azab A. Pathogenesis and evaluation of the effects of idiopathic intracranial hypertension on the optic nerves. Neuroophthalmology 2020;44:281–289.
61. De Simone R, Sansone M, Bonavita V. Headache in idiopathic intracranial hypertension. A CGRP-dependent head pain? Neurol Sci 2020;41(suppl 2):417–421.

62. Moreno-Ajona D, McHugh JA, Hoffmann J. An update on imaging in idiopathic intracranial hypertension. Front Neurol 2020;11:453.
63. Mollan SP, Davies B, Silver NC, et al. Idiopathic intracranial hypertension: Consensus guidelines on management. J Neurol Neurosurg Psychiatry 2018;89:1088–1100.
64. Sunderland GJ, Jenkinson MD, Conroy EJ, Gamble C, Mallucci CL. Neurosurgical CSF diversion in idiopathic intracranial hypertension: A narrative review. Life (Basel) 2021;11:393.
65. Yiangou A, Mitchell J, Markey KA, et al. Therapeutic lumbar puncture for headache in idiopathic intracranial hypertension: Minimal gain, is it worth the pain? Cephalalgia 2019;39:245–253.
66. D'Amico D, Usai S, Chiapparini L, et al. Headache in spontaneous intracranial hypotension: An overview with indications for differential diagnosis in the clinical practice. Neurol Sci 2020;41(suppl 2):423–427.
67. D'Antona L, Jaime Merchan MA, Vassiliou A, et al. Clinical presentation, investigation findings, and treatment outcomes of spontaneous intracranial hypotension syndrome: A systematic review and meta-analysis. JAMA Neurol 2021;78:329–337.
68. Signorelli F, Caccavella VM, Giordano M, et al. A systematic review and meta-analysis of factors affecting the outcome of the epidural blood patching in spontaneous intracranial hypotension. Neurosurg Rev 2021;44:3079–3085.
69. Patel R, Urits I, Orhurhu V, et al. A comprehensive update on the treatment and management of postdural puncture headache. Curr Pain Headache Rep 2020;24:24.
70. Smith JH, Mac Grory B, Butterfield RJ, Khokhar B, Falk BL, Marks LA. CSF pressure, volume, and post-dural puncture headache: A case-control study and systematic review. Headache 2019;59:1324–1338.
71. Voortman M, Stern BJ, Saketkoo LA, Drent M. The burden of neurosarcoidosis: Essential approaches to early diagnosis and treatment. Semin Respir Crit Care Med 2020;41:641–651.
72. Munkvold BKR, Bo HK, Jakola AS, et al. Tumor volume assessment in low-grade gliomas: A comparison of preoperative magnetic resonance imaging to coregistered intraoperative 3-dimensional ultrasound recordings. Neurosurgery 2018;83:288–296.
73. Palmieri A, Valentinis L, Zanchin G. Update on headache and brain tumors. Cephalalgia 2021;41:431–437.
74. Bezuidenhout AF, Chang YM, Heilman CB, Bhadelia RA. Headache in Chiari malformation. Neuroimaging Clin N Am 2019;29:243–253.
75. Chatrath A, Marino A, Taylor D, Elsarrag M, Soldozy S, Jane JA Jr. Chiari I malformation in children—The natural history. Childs Nerv Syst 2019;35:1793–1799.
76. Koelman DLH, Brouwer MC, Ter Horst L, Bijlsma MW, van der Ende A, van de Beek D. Pneumococcal meningitis in adults: A prospective nationwide cohort study over a 20-year period. Clin Infect Dis 2021;74:657–667.
77. Schiess N, Groce NE, Dua T. The impact and burden of neurological sequelae following bacterial meningitis: A narrative review. Microorganisms 2021;9:900.
78. Marshall C, Clark ZT, Minckler MR. Aseptic viral meningitis secondary to herpes simplex virus 2 genital infection. Cureus 2021;13:e14535.
79. Martelletti P, Bentivegna E, Spuntarelli V, Luciani M. Long-COVID headache. SN Compr Clin Med 2021;3:1704–1706.

5

Primary Headache Disorders

Key Points

- Clinicians who treat oral and facial pains should become well versed in primary headache disorders.
- Clinicians should use the most current version of the International Classification of Headache Disorders (ICHD) to accurately diagnose primary headache disorders.
- Clinicians need to be familiar with the most up-to-date, evidence-based care of primary headache disorders. Recent years have been an exciting new era in migraine therapeutics, with the approval of many new classes of treatments. It is the responsibility of the clinician to keep up to date with these new evidence-based migraine therapeutic approaches and to stay informed on updates to dosage, indications, and side effect profiles.
- If the clinician is in any doubt as to a definitive diagnosis and appropriate therapy, they should consider referral to a health care practitioner who is knowledgeable in the diagnosis and management of headache disorders.

Primary headaches are disorders unto themselves and are not attributed to any other cause or condition. The criteria for diagnosis include the descriptors and clinical presentation as well as the exclusion of other disorders. Primary headaches account for approximately 90% of headache cases in patients presenting to primary care.[1] The third edition of the International Classification of Headache Disorders (ICHD) classifies primary headache disorders into four categories[2]:

1. Migraine
2. Tension-type headache (TTH)
3. Trigeminal autonomic cephalalgias (TACs)
4. Other primary headache disorders

A complete listing of primary headache disorders and their classification can be found at the IHS Classification ICHD-3 website (https://ichd-3.org/). This chapter focuses on the most common primary headache presentations: migraine, TTH, and select TACs. Each discussed disorder includes the ICHD codes established by the Headache Classification Committee of the International Headache Society as well as those described in the *International Classification of Diseases, Tenth Revision (ICD-10)* and *Eleventh Revision (ICD-11).*

Migraine (ICHD 1.x.x ; *ICD-10* G43.xxx ; *ICD-11* 8A80.xxx)

Clinical presentation and diagnosis

Globally, as of 2016, migraine is the sixth most prevalent and second most disabling illness after lower back pain, based on years lived with disability (YLDs).[3,4] It is considered an inherited neurobiologic disorder of the central nervous system (CNS) characterized by increased brain sensitivity and mostly episodic pain presentation.[5] Migraine typically presents with recurrent throbbing and mostly unilateral painful attacks of moderate to severe intensity, commonly localized in the periorbital or upper cervical regions and lasting 4 to 72 hours untreated or undertreated. In children and adolescents (aged under 18 years), the attacks may last 2 to 72 hours. Migraine is associated with certain characteristic features, such as nausea, phonophobia, and photophobia, and is typically aggravated by physical activity. A third of migraineurs will experience transient neurologic symptoms such as visual disturbance or other sensory phenomena prior to the onset of the headache event. This is known as *aura*,[2,6] and these symptoms develop gradually over 5 to 20 minutes and last no more than 1 hour. Aura most often takes the form of positive visual phenomena (occurring in over 90% of migraine aura patients) that move across the visual field over minutes. Patients can also experience migrating paresthesias or dysphasic speech. Migraine attacks may occur without aura (ICHD 1.1; *ICD-10* G43.0; *ICD-11* 8A80.0) or with aura (ICHD 1.2; *ICD-10* G43.1; *ICD-11* 8A80.1). Aura may also occur in the absence of a typical migraine headache (ICHD 1.2.1.2; *ICD-10* G43.104; *ICD-11* 8A80-1Y). Some individuals will experience premonitory (prodromal) symptoms such as tiredness, yawning, sensory hypersensitivity, increased food cravings, thirst, and polyuria that tend to be highly predictive of the attack. These symptoms may occur anywhere from 2 to 24 hours prior to the attack and are highly suggestive of CNS etiology.[2,7] These premonitory symptoms should not be mistaken for patient-reported migraine triggers. Growing evidence now suggests that previously, descriptions by patients of triggers of migraine are in fact early premonitory symptoms, occurring before any headache. A recent study reported that subject-reported triggers such as bright light, sounds, certain foods, and skipping meals/hunger were strongly associated with migraine symptoms of photophobia, phonophobia, and food cravings.[8,9] There is also strong evidence to suggest that changes within the brain, including the hypothalamus,

Box 5-1 ICHD-3—Diagnostic criteria for migraine[2]

1.1 Migraine without aura (*ICD-10* G43.0; *ICD-11* 8A80.0)

A. At least five attacks fulfilling criteria B to D
B. Headache attacks last 4 to 72 hours (when untreated or unsuccessfully treated)
C. Headache has at least two of the following characteristics:
   1. Unilateral location
   2. Pulsating quality
   3. Moderate or severe pain intensity
   4. Aggravation by or causing the avoidance of routine physical activity (eg, walking or climbing stairs)
D. During headache at least one of the following:
   1. Nausea and/or vomiting
   2. Photophobia and phonophobia
E. Not better accounted for by another ICHD-3 diagnosis

1.2 Migraine with aura (*ICD-10* G43.1; *ICD-11* 8A80.1)

A. At least two attacks fulfilling criteria B and C
B. One or more of the following fully reversible aura symptoms:
   1. Visual
   2. Sensory
   3. Speech and/or language
   4. Motor
   5. Brainstem
   6. Retinal
C. At least three of the following six characteristics:
   1. At least one aura symptom spreads gradually over ≥ 5 minutes
   2. Two or more aura symptoms occur in succession
   3. Each individual aura symptom lasts 5 to 60 minutes
   4. At least one aura symptom is unilateral
   5. At least one aura symptom is positive
   6. The aura is accompanied, or followed within 60 minutes, by headache
D. Not better accounted for by another ICHD-3 diagnosis

1.3 Chronic migraine (*ICD-10* G43.3; *ICD-11* 8A80.2)

A. Headache (migraine-like or tension-type-like) on ≥ 15 days/month for > 3 months, and fulfilling criteria B and C
B. Occurring in a patient who has had at least five attacks fulfilling criteria B to D for 1.1 Migraine without aura and/or criteria B and C for 1.2 Migraine with aura
C. On ≥ 8 days/month for > 3 months, fulfilling any of the following:
   1. Criteria C and D for 1.1 Migraine without aura
   2. Criteria B and C for 1.2 Migraine with aura
   3. Believed by the patient to be migraine at onset and relieved by a triptan or ergot derivative
D. Not better accounted for by another ICHD-3 diagnosis

1.5 Probable migraine with or without aura (*ICD-10* G43.909)

A. Attacks fulfilling all but one of criteria A–D for 1.1 Migraine without aura, or all but one of criteria A to C for 1.2 Migraine with aura
B. Not fulfilling ICHD-3 criteria for any other headache disorder
C. Not better accounted for by another ICHD-3 diagnosis

are already taking place that are involved in migraine mechanisms and are likely responsible for these premonitory symptoms.[9] Patients also commonly experience a so-called "postdrome," similar to premonitory symptoms, which can include feeling tired or weary, having difficulty concentrating, and experiencing neck stiffness.[10] The ICHD criteria (Box 5-1) may be used to confirm the diagnosis of migraine when the described criteria are met and after organic disease is excluded. If a patient meets the criteria for more than one subtype of migraine, all subtypes should be diagnosed and coded. In the ICHD-3, it is noted for the first time, under the area of comments of migraine without aura, the existence of a facial location of migraine called *facial migraine* that possesses the same characteristics of migraine and is recognized as a subset but not a separate subgroup.[1] Furthermore, the International Classification of Orofacial Pain, 1st edition (ICOP), has incorporated a section of orofacial pains resembling presentations of primary headache disorders including orofacial migraine, tension-type orofacial pain, trigeminal autonomic orofacial pain, and neurovascular orofacial pain.[11] This is very important because it introduces the concept that primary headaches may appear not only in their classical location of the periorbital region (V1) or cervical areas but also in V2 or V3 areas, even involving intraoral structures as a primary location.[12,13]

Individuals who meet the criteria for migraine without aura but have had fewer than five attacks should be coded as probable migraine without aura (ICHD 1.5.1; *ICD-10* G43.909), and individuals who meet the criteria for migraine with aura that have had only one attack should be coded as probable migraine with aura (ICHD 1.5.2; *ICD-10* G43.909). If headache occurs on more than 15 days per month for at least 3 months and fulfills the headache criteria for migraine with or without aura on at least 8 days/month, it is classified as *chronic migraine* (ICHD 1.3; *ICD-10* G43.3; *ICD-11* 8A80.2). A debilitating migraine persisting for more than 72 hours in succession is classified as *status migrainosus* (ICHD 1.4.1; *ICD-10* G43.2; *ICD-11* 8A80.30). Complications of migraines are rare but may include persistent aura without infarction (ICHD 1.4.2; *ICD-10* G43.3; *ICD-11* 8A80.3Y), migrainous infarct (ICHD 1.4.3; *ICD-10* G43.3; *ICD-11* 8A80.3Y), and migraine aura-triggered seizure (ICHD 1.4.4; *ICD-10* G43.3; *ICD-11* 8A80.3Y).

Epidemiology

Migraine is a common condition affecting over a billion adults globally and over 15% of the population in Western countries.[4,14] In the United States, the prevalence of migraine is approximately 18% in females and 6% in males,[14] a female-to-male ratio of 3:1. While the exact reason for this sex bias is not known, a significant proportion of migraine in women is associated with menstruation. It has been reported that greater than 90% of patients presenting with a stable, recurring, severe headache probably have migraine.[15] According to a recent Global Burden of Disease report, migraine is now the second highest cause of disability worldwide,[4] and the most disabling of all headaches and neurologic disorders. In boys, migraine with aura will peak at age 5 years, while migraine without aura tends to peak at age 10 to 11 years.[16] Migraine peaks later in girls than in boys, with migraine with aura occurring at age 12 to 13 years and migraine without aura at age 14 to 17 years.[16] New onset of migraine is an uncommon finding in men in their third decade. The highest prevalence of migraine occurs at ages 30 to 39 years and is at its lowest after the age of 60 years.

Because migraine usually affects people during their most productive years, it is a major burden to the patient and society. Not only does it affect the patient's quality of life by impairing their ability to participate in family, social, and recreational activities, but it also affects society in terms of direct costs (eg, medical care) and indirect costs (eg, absenteeism and reduced effectiveness at work). It is estimated that 23 million US residents have severe migraines.[15] Twenty-five percent of women experience four or more severe attacks per month, and more than 85% of women and more than 82% of men with severe migraine had some migraine-related disability.[17] Furthermore, in the US, severe migraine prevalence is highest in Native Americans (17.7%), then Whites (15.5 %), followed closely by Hispanics (14.5%), Blacks (14.45%),

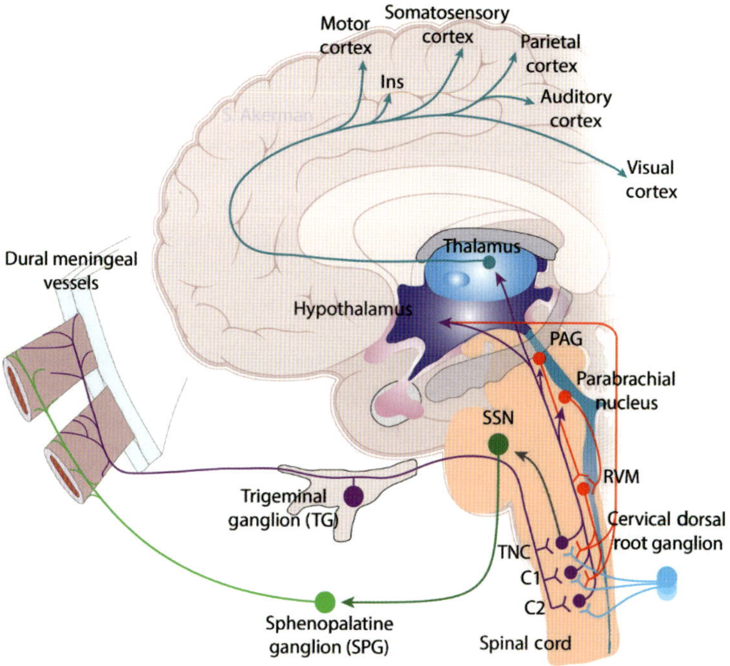

Fig 5-1 Overview of the trigeminovascular system.[19,20] Nociceptive afferents (both unmyelinated C-fiber and myelinated Aδ-fiber axons) that originate in the trigeminal ganglion (TG) innervate the meninges. The densest innervation is found in the dural blood vessels. Projections from upper cervical dorsal root ganglia also innervate the meninges. Together, these contribute to the anatomical and physiologic substrate of ipsilateral intracranial pain in migraine. Central TG axonal projections terminate in the spinal trigeminal nucleus caudalis (TNC) and upper cervical spinal cord (C1-C2). Here, they converge onto neurons that also receive input from the periorbital skin and pericranial muscles. These second-order trigeminovascular neurons convey pain signals to nuclei in the brainstem, hypothalamus, and thalamus, which likely contribute to symptoms associated with autonomic, affective, and homeostatic functions. Trigeminothalamic neurons that relay these pain signals project to somatosensory, insular (Ins), auditory, visual, and olfactory cortices, contributing to the expanded sensory hypersensitivity related to migraine. A reflex connection from the superior salivatory nucleus (SSN), which projects to the cranial vasculature via the sphenopalatine ganglion (SPG), also contributes to the activation of nociceptive trigeminal afferents. Trigeminovascular neurons are also under the control of descending pain-modulatory circuits (in *red*) in the brainstem (including PAG, RVM, and parabrachial nucleus) and hypothalamus, which modulate nociceptive inputs. PAG, periaqueductal gray; RVM, rostral ventromedial medulla.

and Asians (9.2%), and is higher in females of all races and ethnic groups.[18]

Pathogenesis

Based on a large body of evidence, it is now generally accepted that the anatomical and physiologic substrate of intracranial migraine-like headache, as well as the associated cranial hypersensitivity, is *activation and sensitization* of the dural-trigeminovascular system (Fig 5-1[19,20]). This includes primary trigeminal nociceptive projections to the intracranial dural-vasculature and central projections in the medullary dorsal horn (trigeminal nucleus caudalis) and upper cervical spinal cord. From here, neurons ascend via brainstem nuclei to the thalamocortical region where inputs are processed; together this is known as the *trigeminal migraine pain pathway*. Central trigeminovascular neurons are also under the control of pain-modulatory circuits in the brainstem and diencephalon, which also impacts nociceptive processing. They are therefore considered as integrative relay neurons between peripheral and central pain mechanisms.

While the underlying mechanisms in migraine are not completely understood, it is hypothesized that it involves activation of peripheral afferent fibers that innervate dural meningeal vessels[19,20] and dysfunction of central structures, including brain stem and hypothalamic nuclei that normally modulate or gate sensory inputs, including light, sound, touch, and smell. This is supported by imaging studies that demonstrate activation in the hypothalamus and in areas that include the medulla, pontine and midbrain regions before, during, and after a migraine attack.[21–26] The net result is *activation and sensitization* of central trigeminovascular neurons, which are processed as nociceptive in thalamocortical areas involved in pain perception. This leads to its clinical manifestation, intracranial throbbing headache and a generalized increase in sensitivity to all sensory inputs[17] to cause cutaneous allodynia/hyperalgesia, photophobia, and phonophobia.

These peripheral and central mechanisms involve the release of several major neuropeptides and a local dural inflammatory response.[19,20,27] Clinical studies provide strong support for the release of calcitonin gene-related peptide (CGRP) and pituitary adenylate cyclase-activating peptide (PACAP) into the cranial vasculature during migraine.[28,29] These increased levels of CGRP and PACAP were reduced after headache relief with the selective migraine abortive therapy, sumatriptan. Preclinical studies confirm that activation of the trigeminovascular system mediates antidromic release of these vasoactive molecules.[28,29] Confirming their role in migraine, both CGRP and PACAP also trigger delayed migraine-like headache in migraineurs[30,31] and in preclinical studies mediate delayed activation and sensitization of central trigeminovascular neurons.[32,33] Similarly, neuroinflammatory mediators, prostaglandin E1 and I2, trigger migraine-like headache in migraineurs[34,35] and in preclinical studies, when applied to the dura mater, cause activation and sensitization of primary afferent and central trigeminovascular neurons.[36,37] The effectiveness of pharmacologics and biologics that target the CGRP pathway, NSAIDs, and hypothesis-driven PACAP targeting support the role of these neurotransmitters in migraine mechanisms.

Migraine aura is thought to be the clinical manifestation of cortical spreading depression (depolarization; CSD[38]). CSD is characterized by a slowly propagating wave of neuronal excitability and glial activation that is followed by a prolonged period of hyperpolarization.[39] It has been suggested that CSD events, which can mediate the introduction of pro-inflammatory molecules and CGRP to the dura mater, may be the trigger of migraine,[40] as supported by preclinical studies.[41] While this theory fails to explain the development of migraine without aura where CSD-like events are probably absent, it is likely that at the very least, migraine aura exacerbates the consequent headache and associated symptoms.

Currently, it is not known why or how migraine attacks are triggered. We are gaining a better understanding of the mechanisms involved in symptoms, but not what the initial driver might be. An old and now comprehensively rejected theory is that migraine is purely a consequence of dilation of cranial blood vessels. While vascular changes may occur, particularly at the level of the dura mater, these are not causal, neither necessary nor sufficient for symptoms, and at best considered an epiphenomenon to activation of the trigeminovascular system and the release of vasodilatory neuropeptides.[42] Given the growing data from preclinical studies concerning changes in trigeminovascular neurons and imaging studies supporting the importance of the brain, it is perhaps best to consider migraine as a "brain state," involving a failure of brain integration and filtering mechanisms that result in the perception of activation, or hyperactivation, via the trigeminovascular system, of sensory information under normal conditions.[19]

The clustering of migraine in families suggests a genetic component. The exact genomic loci are not clear, and the complex nature and heterogeneity of migraine across individuals suggests it is polygenic. Indeed, one genome-wide association meta-analysis identified 38 genomic loci that affect migraine risk, related to the vasculature.[43] Interestingly, having a family history of migraine alone is likely to increase prevalence of migraine, with earlier onset, migraine aura, and the need to use medications.[44] The impact of these genetic loci is likely due to both gene-gene and gene-environmental interactions, which supports the complex nature of the relationship of genes in migraine pathogenesis. However, identification of causal genes in polygenic subtypes that define mechanisms has been difficult.[44] Rarer forms of migraine identified as monogenic have been identified, and here the causal links are clearer. These include familial hemiplegic migraine (FHM), cerebral autosomal dominant arteriopathy with subcortical infarcts and leukoencephalopathy, retinal vasculopathy with cerebral leukoencephalopathy and systemic manifestations, and familial advanced sleep phase syndrome.[45] Genetic causal links are associated with ion channel upregulation, enhanced neurotransmission—particularly glutamatergic—and increased CSD susceptibility. While there does not appear to be much in the way of overlap of mechanisms between the monogenic or polygenic migraine subtypes, common pathways involving the development and function of neurons and synapses and glutamate transport mechanisms appear to be significant for both.[46]

Management

In addition to pharmacotherapy, migraine management modalities should include educational interventions, lifestyle and behavioral modifications, and trigger-avoidance strategies. Pharmacologic interventions may be abortive or preventive. The most appropriate management approach should be selected based on the frequency of attacks (episodic or chronic), the level of impairment that they cause, previous management history and response, and patient preferences. Abortive medications may only be used for individuals with episodic attacks fewer than 4 headache days per month and no impairment or those with no more than 1 headache day per month regardless of impairment.[14] In cases where frequency increases to above 6 migraine days per month with days of impairment[14] and in cases like those described in ICHD 1.3 Chronic Migraine where the headache occurs on 15 or more days per month for more than 3 months, which, on at least 8 days per month, has the features of migraine,[2] preventive management should be implemented and a rescue modality, such as an abortive medication in case of a breakthrough headache, should be considered. It is also important to recognize during medical history the frequency of medication intake because ICHD 8.2 Medication Overuse Headache can cause symptoms suggestive of chronic migraine. In addition, consideration should also be given to any comorbid conditions such as depression or hypertension. If there is a comorbid illness, a preventive agent that can treat both conditions should be used when possible, and agents that might aggravate a comorbid illness should be avoided. A comorbidity that is important to recognize is temporomandibular disorders (TMDs) and migraine, where each can also potentially exacerbate the other. Migraine has been shown to be the most prevalent primary headache observed in the TMD population,[47] and it has been shown that in migraineurs, the presence of muscular TMD, such as myofascial pain, presents a higher disability impact.[48] In addition, it has been shown that migraine and recurrent headaches may contribute to a risk of developing TMD.[49] From preclinical studies, CGRP also appears to have an important role in TMD pathophysiology.[50,51] When both disorders are present, the presence of TMD may exacerbate the migraine phenotype, and it is postulated that CGRP may be a key modulator of this exacerbated phenotype.[52] Therefore, it is important to recognize that management of both disorders should occur when they present together.

Nonpharmacologic methods such as biofeedback, relaxation techniques, acupuncture, and other behavioral interventions can be used as adjunctive therapy.[53] Neuromodulation for headache disorders is also a very attractive approach as a nonpharmacologic avenue that has shown effectiveness without the side effects that medications may present. This is also a good alternative in cases of medication overuse headache and during pregnancy. Currently, the US Food and Drug Administration (FDA) has approved four noninvasive neuromodulatory devices. Noninvasive vagal nerve stimulation (nVNS) has shown to be effective in the management of acute and chronic migraine,[54] where it appears to directly and indirectly modulate dural-trigeminovascular neurons.[55,56] Supraorbital stimulation (e-TNS)[57] and single-pulse transcranial magnetic stimulation (sTMS)[58] have also been shown to be effective for acute management and prevention. Lastly, remote electrical neuromodulation (REN), which applies the principle of conditioned pain modulation[59] where electrical stimulation is applied in the upper arm to engage endogenous descending analgesic mechanisms to effect remote body regions, has also been shown to have high efficacy for the treatment of episodic migraine.[60] These devices have the advantage of being able to be used independently as a single therapy approach for management or together with pharmacologic treatment.[61] Contraindications include patients with other implanted devices such as cochlear implants and pacemakers.[62]

Abortive treatment

Medications typically used for acute migraine management to alleviate or remove pain should be administered early in the headache phase of an attack (when pain is mild).[63,64] The most commonly used medications are over the counter nonsteroidal anti-inflammatory drugs (NSAIDs), with the most effective being acetylsalicylic acid (aspirin), diclofenac, and naproxen.[65,66] Nonopioid analgesics, such as acetaminophen, can be used for those patients contraindicated for NSAIDs. It is important to emphasize that opioids are not recommended for migraine management because of limited efficacy, increased disability, potential of dependency, risks of overuse, and enhanced risks of medication-overuse headache and opioid-induced hyperalgesia.[67,68] The triptan class of medications, 5-$HT_{1B/1D}$ receptor agonists, have been shown to be effective in aborting an acute migraine attack. If one oral triptan is ineffective in three migraine attacks, patients are advised to switch to another in the same drug class, which may provide adequate pain relief. If oral triptans provide some but not adequate pain relief, they can be combined with a fast-acting NSAID (such as naproxen).[65] Ergot derivatives are a further alternative. Subcutaneous sumatriptan is an option for those patients that struggle to take oral triptans because of vomiting. Likewise, dopamine-antagonists (antiemetics) can be used in the event of severe nausea or vomiting. Triptans are contraindicated in patients with cardiovascular and cerebrovascular disorders limiting their use because of their vasoconstrictive properties.[69] The exploration of the serotonin 5-HT receptor family has led to the development of a new class of migraine abortives that selectively targets the 5-HT_{1F} receptor (ditans), which is not expressed in the vasculature.[70] Lasmiditan, a 5-HT1F receptor agonist, is the first medication of this class that is FDA approved for the management of acute migraine that has shown to be promising for patients with cardiovascular risk factors.[71,72] Furthermore, the FDA has approved two second-generation CGRP

Table 5-1 Acute migraine treatments[65,76,77]

Clinical situation	Treatment	Possible adverse events
Initial therapy—NSAIDs	Aspirin (500–900 mg) Diclofenac (50–100 mg) Ibuprofen (200–800 mg) Naproxen (500–1000 mg) Tolfenamic acid (200 mg) Ketorolac (30–60 mg)	Esophageal/gastric irritation
OTC analgesics	Acetaminophen (500–1000 mg)	Esophageal/gastric irritation
Combination analgesics	Acetaminophen/aspirin/caffeine (500/500/130 mg)	
Failed NSAIDs/analgesics—triptans (PO)	Sumatriptan (50–100 mg) Rizatriptan (5–10 mg Almotriptan (6.25–12.5 mg) Eletriptan (20–40 mg) Zolmitriptan (2.5–5 mg)	Warmth, tightness, and discomfort in torso, head, and neck; sedation (nausea-DHE) Arterial ischemia in patients with coronary disease (rare)
Slower effect triptans	Naratriptan (1–2.5 mg) Frovatriptan (2.5 mg)	
Ergot derivatives	Dihydroergotamine (DHE; 0.5–2 mg nasal spray)	
Headache recurrence	Combination triptan/NSAID (sumatriptan + naproxen)	
Insufficient response to triptans	Gepants (small molecule CGRP receptor antagonists) Rimegepant (75 mg, PO) Ubrogepant (50–100 mg, PO)	Dry mouth, dizziness
	Ditans (5-HT1F agonists) Lasmiditan (50–200 mg, PO)	Sedation, dizziness, impaired driving for 8 h
Nonpharmacologic—neuromodulation	Single-pulse transcranial magnetic stimulation (sTMS) Noninvasive vagus nerve stimulation (nVNS) Remote electrical stimulation Trigeminal nerve stimulation (TNS)	Dizziness (sTMS), hoarseness (nVNS), sedation (TNS) Local discomfort (all)

OTC, over the counter; PO, orally.

receptor antagonists (gepants)—ubrogepant and rimegepant—for the acute management of migraine that have not reported cardiovascular or hepatotoxicity warnings and have shown efficacy and safety and are well tolerated.[73–75]

Pharmacologic agents with evidence-based support of statistical and clinical benefit, according to the American Academy of Neurology, are listed in Table 5-1[65,76,77] and should be given as first-line management.[78]

Table 5-2 Preventive migraine treatments[65,76–80]

Drug or class	Treatment (dose)	Possible adverse events
β-blockers	*Propranolol (40–100 mg, b.i.d.) *Metoprolol (25–100 mg, b.i.d.) *Timolol (10–30 mg)	Reduced energy, tiredness, hypotension, postural symptoms. Contraindicated in asthma
Anticonvulsants	*Vaproate (valproic acid; 400–600 mg, b.i.d.) *Topiramate (50–200 mg/day) Gabapentin (900–3600 mg/ day)	Drowsiness, weight gain, tremor, hair loss, teratogenicity, hematological/liver abnormalities Paresthesia, cognitive dysfunction, weight loss, taste perversion, angle closure glaucoma, teratogenicity Dizziness, sedation
Antidepressants	Amitriptyline (25–75 mg/day) Nortriptyline (25–75 mg/day) Venlafaxine (75–150 mg/day)	Drowsiness, dry mouth, urinary retention, tachycardia, weight gain As above, plus erectile dysfunction, nausea, insomnia, tremor
CGRP monoclonal antibodies	*Eptinezumab (IV; 100 mg or 300 mg quarterly) *Erenumab (SC; 70 mg or 140 mg monthly *Fremanezumab (SC; 225 mg monthly or 675 mg quarterly) *Galcanezumab (SC; 240 mg loading dose then 120 mg monthly)	All: injection site irritation, brief upper respiratory infection-like symptoms Erenumab: constipation, hypertension may occur
Angiotensin receptor blocker	Candesartan (16 mg/day) Lisinopril (10–20 mg/day)	Dizziness, hypotension
Botulinum toxin	**Onabotulinumtoxin type A (155 U every 12 weeks)	Loss of brow furrow, neck pain
Nutraceuticals	Riboflavin (vitamin B2; 400 mg/day) Coenzyme Q10 (100 mg, t.i.d.) Butterbur (50–75 mg, b.i.d.) Magnesium (400–800 mg) Melatonin (3 mg at night)	Orange urine Gastrointestinal upset Elevation of transaminases Gastrointestinal upset Tiredness
Neuromodulatory devices	*Single-pulse transcranial magnetic stimulation (sTMS) *Noninvasive vagus nerve stimulation (nVNS) *Trigeminal nerve stimulation (TNS)	Dizziness (sTMS), tinnitus, tingling, scalp irritation, local pain Lip/facial twitching, local neck/throat pain, hoarseness Drowsiness, uncomfortable scalp feeling

OTC, over the counter; PO, orally; SC, subcutaneous; IV, intravenous; b.i.d, twice daily; t.i.d., three times daily.
*FDA approved/cleared for migraine prevention.
**FDA approved for prevention of chronic migraine only.

Preventive treatment

As a recurrent disorder, long-term management of migraine may be necessary with preventive treatment. These medications include a broad range of agents.[65,66] Much of this is based on the work of the US Headache Consortium Guidelines and the European Headache Federation Aid to Management of Headache Disorders, which recommend evidence-based pharmacologic management for migraine prevention in adults (Table 5-2). The overall aim is to reduce attack frequency, duration, and/or severity. The most widely used medications are anticonvulsants (eg, sodium valproate and topiramate), anti-hypertensives such as β-blockers (eg, metoprolol, propranolol, timolol) and candesartan, and tricyclic anti-depressants (eg, amitriptyline), which have the strongest evidence of benefit for migraine prevention. These medications are started at low doses and gradually titrated to the desired effect to minimize side effects and arrive at the minimal dose necessary for therapeutic effect. In more refractory cases, polypharmacy may be necessary. While a number of NSAIDs are included in the practice guidelines as effective for the prevention of episodic migraine, caution must be exercised about daily use because analgesic overuse can induce medication overuse headache.[81] Botulinum toxin type A is also approved by the FDA, specifically for the preventive management of chronic migraine.[82] For the management of menstrual-related migraine, perimenstrual use of frovatriptan has been recommended.[78] Naratriptan and zolmitriptan have been classified as "probably effective" for this type of migraine presentation.[81] In many cases, patients are able to identify factors that seem to precipitate the onset of a migraine attack. Strategies to identify and cope with or avoid these triggers often prove helpful for these individuals.[83] Some common triggers are environmental factors, including light, noise, allergens, and barometric changes; behavioral factors, such as emotional stress, missing meals, or getting too much or too little sleep; and food/beverage items, such as caffeine, aspartame, monosodium glutamate, nitrites, and nitrates.[84]

The lack of better treatment options to provide relief from migraine has led to the search for new, safer, and effective management methods. Based on both human and preclinical studies, there has been a successful translation from the bench to bedside of new therapies that specifically target the CGRP pathway.[85,86] The FDA has now approved four CGRP monoclonal antibodies: erenumab, which was the first approved, followed by fremanezumab, galcanezumab, and eptinezumab.[87–90] This class of medications was developed for preventitive use against chronic and episodic migraines and was designed to target the CGRP receptor (erenumab) or its ligand, a specificity which has shown to provide good tolerability and a low side effect profile. In addition, the long half-life of these medications improves patient compliance[91,92] (see Table 5-2). Furthermore, the FDA has now approved two CGRP receptor antagonists for migraine prevention: rimegepant and atogepant.

Other management options that are generally well-tolerated procedures and are also a good alternative for the population of patients that presented side effects or failed to respond to preventives include sphenopalatine ganglion blockade for the management of acute and chronic migraine[93] and peripheral nerve blocks such as greater occipital nerve, lesser occipital nerve, and supratrochlear and supraorbital nerve blocks used for acute and preventive headache management.[94]

Tension-Type Headache (ICHD 2.x.x; *ICD-10* G44.2xx; *ICD-11* 8A81.xx)

Clinical presentation and diagnosis

Tension-type headache (TTH) is generally mild-moderate in pain intensity, tending to be bilateral, sometimes described as hat-band/

Box 5-2 ICHD-3—Diagnostic criteria for tension-type headache[2]

2.1 Infrequent episodic tension-type headache (*ICD-10* G44.2; *ICD-11* 8A81.0)

A. At least 10 episodes of headache occurring on < 1 day/month on average (< 12 days/year) and fulfilling criteria B to D
B. Lasting from 30 minutes to 7 days
C. At least two of the following four characteristics:
   1. Bilateral location
   2. Pressing or tightening (non-pulsating) quality
   3. Mild or moderate intensity
   4. Not aggravated by routine physical activity such as walking or climbing stairs
D. Both of the following:
   1. No nausea or vomiting
   2. No more than one of photophobia or phonophobia
E. Not better accounted for by another ICHD-3 diagnosis

2.2 Frequent episodic tension-type headache (*ICD-10* G44.2; *ICD-11* 8A81.1)

A. At least 10 episodes of headache occurring on 1 to 14 days/month on average for > 3 months (> 12 and < 180 days/year) and fulfilling criteria B to D (as above), plus E

2.3 Chronic tension-type headache (*ICD-10* G44.2; *ICD-11* 8A81.2)

A. Headache occurring on ≥ 15 days/month on average for > 3 months (> 180 days/year), fulfilling criteria B to D
B. Lasting hours to days, or unremitting
C. At least two of the following four characteristics:
   1. Bilateral location
   2. Pressing or tightening (non-pulsating) quality
   3. Mild or moderate intensity
   4. Not aggravated by routine physical activity such as walking or climbing stairs
D. Both of the following:
   1. No more than one of photophobia, phonophobia, or mild nausea
   2. Neither moderate or severe nausea or vomiting
E. Not better accounted for by another ICHD-3 diagnosis

band-like in its pattern of distribution. The pain can also occur in the forehead, posterior head regions, and neck. It is often described as pressing or tightening (non-pulsatile) in quality, particularly compared to migraine headache.[2] Temporalis and masseter muscle involvement may be present, and mastication may be affected in some patients. Therefore, it is necessary to consider the possibility of headache due to TMD if it meets the criteria of *(1)* headache localized in the temple area that is changed with jaw movement, function or parafunction and *(2)* provocation of the headache by jaw movement or temporalis muscle palpation.[95] TTH is not accompanied by nausea or vomiting, nor is it aggravated by routine physical activity, but it may be associated with sensitivity to either light or noise.[2] The headaches may last from 30 minutes to 7 days (Box 5-2; ICHD-3). Based on at least 10 episodes of headaches, TTHs are classified as *infrequent episodic* (ICHD 2.1; *ICD-10* G44.2; *ICD-11* 8A81.0) if they occur on fewer than 1 day per month (< 12 days per year) or *frequent episodic* (ICHD 2.2; *ICD-10* G44.2; *ICD-11* 8A81.1) if they occur on 1 to 14 days/month for greater than 3 months (≥ 12 and < 180 days/year. *Chronic TTH* (ICHD 2.3; *ICD-10* G44.2; *ICD-11* 8A81.2) evolves from episodic TTH and is diagnosed when headaches occur on greater than 15 days/month on average for greater than 3 months (≥ 180 days/year). The classification categories are typically subdivided and coded according to the criteria of increased pericranial tenderness upon manual palpation. A new persistent headache that is daily from onset with pain that lacks clear characteristic features—and may be migraine-like or tension-type-headache-like, or both—is classified as *new daily persistent headache* (ICHD 4.10; *ICD-10* G44.52; *ICD-11* 8A83). Sensitivity to light and/or noise and mild nausea may be present with these types of headaches. There may be difficulty distinguishing between chronic migraine and chronic TTH, and these disorders may present simultaneously.

Epidemiology

Based on data from 2016, TTH is the third most prevalent disorder globally, the most prevalent neurologic disorder, and therefore the most common of all primary headaches.[4] The global prevalence of TTH was 26.1% in 2016, in an approximately 3:2 ratio in favor of women, with peak age of suffering between 15 to 50 years.[96] In 2017 in the US, it was estimated that 121.6 million people, more than a third of the population, suffered with TTH,[97] with 1-year prevalence in China of 10.8%, and in European studies of approximately 80%.[98] This suggests variability across countries, but high prevalence throughout. While numbers vary across countries, the global prevalence of chronic TTH is approximately 2% to 3%. TTH carries much less burden with respect to years lived with disability compared to migraine, which reflects how TTH is a milder form of headache and fewer associated symptoms.

Pathogenesis

While long considered a peripheral disorder of the myofascial tissue, largely because of the common occurrence of pericranial tenderness, it is now generally acknowledged that TTH also involves a central component too, particularly chronic TTH. Manual palpation is the common method to evaluate tenderness in patients and both pericranial muscles and tendon insertions have higher tenderness scores in episodic and chronic TTH.[98] However, whether muscular tenderness is a consequence of the pain or involved in the development of TTH is still not known. Myofascial trigger points, hyperexcitable spots associated with bands of muscle fibers with increased tone in skeletal muscles that elicit local and referred pain when compressed, may also be important in TTH pathophysiology. Referred pain from muscles in the regions of the neck, shoulders, and head can mimic TTH.[99,100] Patients with episodic and chronic TTH have a higher frequency of myofascial trigger points compared to controls.[101] Although data supporting this association are inconsistent, suggesting methods to assess this need to be standardized. While muscle tenderness may be present in some individuals, normal electromyographic (EMG) activity was observed in most patients with episodic TTH, and only small trigger point areas showed increased EMG activity in patients with chronic TTH.[102,103] It seems that emotional stressors in TTH patients are more likely to increase EMG activity compared with controls.[104,105] Indeed, in TTH, stress has been shown to trigger higher pericranial muscle pain rating, although there is no evidence linking this to increased EMG activity, and its role in TTH is unclear.

The chronification of TTH also likely involves central sensitization of second-order neurons in the medullary and upper spinal dorsal horns and supraspinal regions, as well as altered modulatory activity from supraspinal structures involved in nociceptive processing.[98] This is supported by the fact that both episodic and chronic TTH patients have lower pain detection thresholds compared to patients with infrequent TTH.[107,108] Overall, studies support the presence of hyperalgesia and allodynia in patients with episodic and chronic TTH, the nature of which is often widespread and non-specific, which is suggestive of an involvement of sensitization of central pain processing. Neuroimaging studies have found both functional and structural changes in cortical regions involved in pain processing,[109,110] including decreased gray matter volume in the insula and anterior cingulate cortex. These findings might be considered a consequence of frequent peripheral nociceptive inputs and central sensitization. A final and controversial point is that with shared anatomical mechanisms in migraine and TTH, the presence of central sensitization in their chronification, the role of potential nitric oxide (NO)–related mechanisms, and overlaps of structural and functional abnormalities (although common to many pain disorders), migrane and TTH are sometimes considered different ends of a headache continuum. However, the difference in clinical phenotypes strongly supports that they are separate disorders.

Management

Most individuals with TTH rarely, if ever, seek medical help, and instead tend to self-medicate with over-the-counter analgesics. While there are no standardized guidelines in the US, the European Federation of Neurological Societies (EFNS) guidelines recommend oral use of acetaminophen and aspirin for the acute treatment of TTH.[111] Ibuprofen and ketoprofen also have high efficacy for acute treatment. Combination analgesic agents with caffeine have been shown to be effective in clinical trials, improving the efficacy of analgesics.[112,113] As with migraine, it is recommended that opioids are avoided, and triptans show no efficacy. Preventive treatment is only recommended for patients with frequent episodic and chronic TTH. Amitriptyline is categorized as a first-choice preventive, with moderate to high efficacy in several studies.[111] Mirtazapine and venlafaxine are second-choice options, and clomipramine, maprotiline, and mianserin third-choice options. The mechanism of action for these is not known but may involve serotoninergic and noradrenergic mechanism pathways. These therapies have common side effects that include drowsiness, weight gain, somnolence, nausea, vomiting, and dizziness, which limit tolerability. Other agents that have been trialed in small-scale or open-label studies that might represent options for prevention when other agents fail include, combination pindolol and amitriptyline, topiramate, valproate, and buspirone.[98] Botulinum toxin type A and ibuprofen do not appear to be effective.[111] No drugs are FDA approved for preventive TTH management. Management may also include behavioral methods such as relaxation training, biofeedback techniques, physical therapy,[114] complementary medicines (acupuncture and massage), and lifestyle enhancement (managing sleep, diet, hydration, stress, and exercise).[98] Of these nonpharmacologic therapies, the most evidenced-based approach is the combination of biofeedback with cognitive behavioral counseling.[115]

Trigeminal Autonomic Cephalalgias (TACs)

Cluster Headache (ICHD 3.1.x; *ICD-10* G44.01x–G44.02x; *ICD-11* 8A82.xxx)

Clinical presentation and diagnosis

Cluster headache is a primary headache disorder that is classified along with similar painful conditions known as TACs.[2] According to the ICHD (Box 5-3), cluster headache is described as "attacks of severe, strictly unilateral pain, which is orbital, supraorbital, temporal, or in any combination of these sites, lasting 15 to 180 minutes"[2] and may also appear in the facial region.[116] In one study, bilateral pain presen-

Box 5-3 International Classification for Headache Disorders (ICHD)-3—Diagnostic criteria for trigeminal autonomic cephalalgias[2]

3.1 Cluster headache (*ICD-10* G44.00; *ICD-11* 8A82.xxx)

A. At least five attacks fulfilling criteria B to D
B. Severe or very severe unilateral orbital, supraorbital, and/or temporal pain lasting 15 to 180 minutes (when untreated)
C. Either or both of the following:
   1. At least one of the following symptoms or signs, ipsilateral to the headache:
      a. Conjunctival injection and/or lacrimation
      b. Nasal congestion and/or rhinorrhoea
      c. Eyelid oedema
      d. Forehead and facial sweating
      e. Miosis and/or ptosis
   2. A sense of restlessness or agitation
D. Occurring with a frequency between one every other day and eight per day
E. Not better accounted for by another ICHD-3 diagnosis

3.1.1 Episodic cluster headache (*ICD-10* G44.01x; *ICD-11* 8A82.xx)

A. Attacks fulfilling criteria for 3.1 Cluster headache and occurring in bouts (cluster periods)
B. At least two cluster periods lasting from 7 days to 1 year (when untreated) and separated by pain-free remission periods of ≥ 3 months

3.1.2 Chronic cluster headache (*ICD-10* G44.02x; *ICD-11* 8A82.xx)

A. Attacks fulfilling criteria for 3.1 Cluster headache, and criterion B below
B. Occurring without a remission period, or with remissions lasting < 3 months, for at least one year

3.2 Paroxysmal hemicrania (*ICD-10* G44.03x–G44.04x; *ICD-11* 8A82.xx)

A. At least 20 attacks fulfilling criteria B to E
B. Severe unilateral orbital, supraorbital, and/or temporal pain lasting 2 to 30 minutes
C. Either or both of the following:
   1. At least one of the following symptoms or signs, ipsilateral to the headache:
      a. Conjunctival injection and/or lacrimation
      b. Nasal congestion and/or rhinorrhea
      c. Eyelid oedema
      d. Forehead and facial sweating
      e. Miosis and/or ptosis
   2. A sense of restlessness or agitation
D. Occurring with a frequency of > 5 per day
E. Prevented absolutely by therapeutic doses of indomethacin
F. Not better accounted for by another ICHD-3 diagnosis

3.3 Short-lasting unilateral neuralgiform headache attacks (*ICD-10* G44.05x; *ICD-11* 8A82.xx)

A. At least 20 attacks fulfilling B to D
B. Moderate or severe unilateral head pain, with orbital, supraorbital, temporal, and/or other trigeminal distribution, lasting for 1 to 600 seconds and occurring as single stabs, series of stabs, or in a saw-tooth pattern
C. At least one of the following five cranial autonomic symptoms or signs, ipsilateral to the pain:
   1. Conjunctival injection and/or lacrimation
   2. Nasal congestion and/or rhinorrhoea
   3. Eyelid oedema
   4. Forehead and facial sweating
   5. Miosis and/or ptosis
D. Occurring with a frequency of at least one day
E. Not better accounted for by another ICHD-3 diagnosis

3.3.1 Short-lasting unilateral neuralgiform headache attacks with conjunctival injection and tearing (SUNCT)

A. Fulfilling criteria for 3.3 (above), and criterion B below
B. Both of the following, ipsilateral to the pain:
   1. Conjunctival injection
   2. Lacrimation (tearing)

3.3.2 Short-lasting unilateral neuralgiform headache attacks with cranial autonomic symptoms (SUNA)

A. Fulfilling criteria for 3.3 (above), and criterion B below
B. Not more than one of the following, ipsilateral to the pain:
   1. Conjunctival injection
   2. Lacrimation (tearing)

Box 5-3 *(cont)* **International Classification for Headache Disorders (ICHD)-3—Diagnostic criteria for trigeminal autonomic cephalalgias**[2]

3.4 Hemicrania continua

A. Unilateral headache fulfilling B to D
B. Present for > 3 months, with exacerbations of moderate or greater intensity
C. Either or both or the following:
   1. At least one of the following symptoms or signs, ipsilateral to the pain:
      a. Conjunctival injection and/or lacrimation
      b. Nasal congestion and/or rhinorrhea
      c. Eyelid oedema
      d. Forehead and facial sweating
      e. Miosis and/or ptosis
   2. A sense of restlessness or agitation, or aggravation of the pain by movement
D. Responds absolutely to therapeutic doses of indomethacin
E. Not better accounted for by another ICHD-3 diagnosis

tation was found in 3% of subjects. Side shifts occurred in approximately 8% of subjects during an individual attack and in approximately 31% of patients between individual headaches or headache cycles.[117] The headache is accompanied by autonomic features, restlessness or agitation, or both. Autonomic features ipsilateral to the headache include conjunctival injection and/or lacrimation, nasal congestion and/or rhinorrhea, forehead and facial sweating, miosis and/or ptosis, and/or eyelid edema.[2] The attacks may occur anywhere from once every other day up to eight times per day, often occurring during sleep. Cluster headache is considered to be one of the most severe pain conditions that humans can experience, with the severity of the pain considered similar in severity to childbirth or bone fracture. Because of the high frequency of attacks and severity of the pain, cluster headache has a significant impact on the patient's quality of life, and in some cases, can lead to suicidal ideation.[117] Most commonly (85% to 90% of patients), cluster patients have *episodic* attacks, which appear as a series of daily or nearly daily attacks lasting for 2 weeks or months. This cluster period will often recur on an annual or biannual basis during the same seasons. Patients report one or two episodes (or clusters; *episodic* cluster headache) a year, commonly in spring or autumn, with more than 1 month of headache-free days per year (ICHD 3.1.1; ICD10 G44.01x; *ICD-11* 8A82.xx). If the episode does not remit within 12 months or with remissions lasting less that 1 month (as occurs in 10% to 15% of patients[118]) the disease is classified as *chronic* cluster headache[2] (ICHD 3.1.2; *ICD-10* G44.02x; *ICD-11* 8A82.xx). Approximately one-third of chronic cluster headache patients will spontaneously remit to an episodic form.

Cluster headache is frequently associated with psychiatric comorbidities, such as depression, anxiety, and aggressive behavior,[119] increasing disease burden and complexity of treatment. It is not clear whether the psychiatric symptoms are a consequence of the psychologic impact of the frequent attacks, paucity of sleep, or more complex interactions. Despite increased awareness and improvements in diagnostic accuracy, the average patient still has to wait many years and visit different physicians before a correct diagnosis is achieved.[120,121] One study reported that only 21% of patients received the correct diagnosis at the time of initial consultation.[117] The presence of nausea or photophobia, more commonly associated with migraine, can occur in cluster headache, thereby contributing to the potential misdiagnosis of cluster headache.[120] However, photophobia and phonophobia associated with cluster headache attacks tend to be unilateral, ipsilateral to the side of the headache as opposed to the bilateral presentation seen in migraine. Because of the location, severity, and abrupt onset of pain, cluster headache is also often mistaken for trigeminal neuralgia, a sinus disorder, or dental pain.[122] The latter is the reason why up to 45% of cluster headache patients are first evaluated for their condition by a dentist.[121] In one survey, 23% of cluster headache patients reported that they received an initial diagnosis of a tooth- or jaw-related issue.[123] In a retrospective study of 14 patients presenting to a dentist with cluster headache symptoms, 6 patients were prescribed oral appliances, 4 had tooth extractions, 3 had occlusal equilibration, and 2 underwent endodontic procedures with unfavorable outcomes.[118]

Epidemiology

Cluster headache affects 0.1% of the general population, based on surveys from the US and Europe.[124] Typical age of onset is about 30 years,[124] but it can develop at any time,[125] and prevalence of the disease decreases substantially with age. Men are typically more affected than women, with a current male-to-female ratio of 3:1. However, this ratio has decreased over the past few decades with more women being diagnosed, suggesting the accuracy of historical estimates is questionable.[126] The reason for this change is not known, although it could reflect improvement in diagnostic accuracy rather than actual ratio change. This might be particularly relevant for women who were frequently misdiagnosed with migraine.[127] Data also suggest that between 70% to 85% of cluster headache patients are smokers or former smokers, although stopping nicotine consumption does not affect the course of the disorder. By contrast, alcohol can trigger an attack during a cluster period,[128] therefore patients tend to avoid alcohol completely.[117]

Pathogenesis

The pathogenesis of cluster headache is related to three key structures in the peripheral and central nervous systems that contribute to its three main symptomatic features: intracranial (in and around the orbit) headache, cranial autonomic features, and circadian periodicity.

The headache in cluster headache is unilateral, and primarily located in and around the orbit, or in the temporal region. Similar to migraine, it likely involves activation of the trigeminovascular system (see Fig 5-1), especially trigeminal afferent neurons that innervate the dural superior sagittal sinus and/or middle meningeal artery; stimulation of these structures in conscious patients mediates ipsilateral pain located in the peri-orbital and temporal regions.[129–131] Curiously, complete trigeminal nerve root section does not seem to reduce attack frequency, or the efficacy of sumatriptan.[132] This might point to a more central mechanistic origin that may modulate or alter the perception of trigeminoavascular responses.

Cranial autonomic symptoms are mediated by activation of the cranial autonomic parasympathetic projection. There is a reflex connection between the trigeminal nerve, restricted to the intracranial ophthalmic division, and the cell bodies of the parasympathetic system, located in the superior salivatory nucleus (SSN), known as the *trigeminal autonomic reflex*[133] (see Fig 5-1). From the SSN, preganglionic parasympathetic nerve fibers synapse with the sphenopalatine ganglion (SPG), traveling with the facial nerve, and postganglionic parasympathetic projections innervate the lacrimal and nasal mucosal glands, as well as the intracranial dural vasculature.[134] Thus, stimulation of the dural-trigeminovascular system, which mediates activation of the trigeminal autonomic reflex to the SSN, stimulates the cranial parasympathetic projection to cause cranial autonomic symptoms, such as lacrimation and conjunctival injection. There is also evidence to suggest that activation of the cranial parasympathetic projection may modulate nociceptive trigeminal neurons[135,136] involved in the headache component of cluster headache. Dural blood vessels are richly innervated by parasympathetic nerve fibers.[137] Activation leads to changes in the dural microenvironment, including dilation of intracranial vessels and release of inflammatory mediators.[138] Stimulation of preganglionic SSN neurons leads to action potential responses of trigeminal neurons.[135,136] This is further supported by the fact that low-frequency stimulation of SPG neurons can provoke cluster-like attacks, which are subsequently alleviated by therapeutic high-frequency SPG stimulation.[139] Therefore, it is likely that each pathway contributes to generation of the other symptoms, and likely exacerbates each by their presence.

Activation of both trigeminovascular and parasympathetic systems leads to the release of neuropeptides that likely contribute to headache and autonomic symptoms. CGRP, vasoactive intestinal peptide (VIP), and PACAP levels are all increased in blood samples that reflect the cranial vasculature during cluster headache.[140,141] CGRP and PACAP are both present in sensory trigeminal neurons, both are potent vasodilators, and each mediates activation of central trigeminovascular neurons.[32,142] VIP and PACAP are contained within postganglionic parasympathetic neurons and released upon activation.[137] Furthermore, they both cause profound cranial autonomic symptoms when given to migraineurs,[143–145] suggesting a role in cranial autonomic symptoms.

Cluster headache is also defined by its circadian periodicity, with attacks occurring at night and following a seasonal pattern. This strongly points to a role of the hypothalamus in its pathogenesis. Imaging studies confirm this, demonstrating hypothalamic activation and structural abnormalities in overlapping regions.[146,147] Acute trigeminal pain does not mediate hypothalamic activation,[148] suggesting these changes may be causative rather than a response to pain itself. Mechanistically, both the central trigeminal nucleus and SSN receive direct projections from hypothalamic nuclei,[149–151] and chemical manipulation of the posterior and paraventricular hypothalamic nuclei in rodents modulates dural-trigeminovascular nociceptive transmission.[149,152] These studies also implicate PACAP, orexins, 5-$HT_{1B/1D}$ receptors, and GABAergic mechanisms. Orexins in particular have gained interest in cluster headache mechanisms. They are synthesized in the hypothalamus, are associated with arousal, and they modulate dural-trigeminal nociception.[152,153] Orexinergic hypothalamic neurons receive inputs for the suprachiasmatic nucleus of the hypothalamus (which maintains circadian regulation) and inputs from areas related to stress, emotion, and autonomic responses.[154] Orexinergic neurons project to areas that regulate wakefulness, attention, motivation, and reward.[154] Orexin A levels are decreased in the CSF in cluster headache patients compared to controls,[155] and a polymorphism in the gene that encodes orexin 2 receptors suggests an increased risk in cluster headache.[156] Together, these human and animal data support that the hypothalamus is positioned to fundamentally influence and potentially trigger both trigeminal sensory and autonomic pathways to mediate symptoms in cluster headache, while under the control of our internal biologic clock. Reports have also described a close relationship between cluster headaches and sleep-disordered breathing.[157] Kudrow[158] postulated that altered hypothalamic influence on the brainstem centers controlling respiration and vasomotor function diminishes carotid chemoreceptor activity.

Management

The management of cluster headache is essentially pharmacologic, with the goal of shortening and alleviating the cluster headache attacks and shortening the cycle of attacks.[159] Similar to migraine therapy, management of cluster

Table 5-3 Clinical features and common treatments of trigeminal autonomic cephalalgias[160–163,196–198,208]

Features	Cluster headache	Paroxysmal hemicrania	SUNCT/SUNA	Hemicrania continua
Sex F:M	1:3	1:1	1:1.5	1:2
Pain quality	Sharp/stabbing/ throbbing	Sharp/stabbing/ throbbing	Sharp/stabbing/ throbbing	Throbbing/sharp/ constant
Pain severity	Very severe	Very severe	Severe	Moderate to severe
Pain distribution	V1 > C2 > V2 > V3	V1 > C2 > V2 > V3	V1 > C2 > V2 > V3	V1 > C2 > V2 > V3
Attack frequency	1–8/day	1–40/day	1–100/day	Continuous
Attack duration	15–180 min	2–30 min	1–600 seconds	30 min–3 days
Autonomic features	Ipsilateral to pain	Ipsilateral to pain	Conjunctival injection and lacrimation (SUNCT)	During worsening and bilateral
Restlessness	90%–95%	80%	65%	69%
Periodicity	Yes	No	No	No
Triggers				
Alcohol	+++	+	-	+
Nitroglycerin	+++	+	-	-
Cutaneous	-	-	+++	-
Migrainous features	Yes	Yes	Infrequently	Yes
Abortive treatments	Sumatriptan, oxygen	Sumatriptan (partial response)	< 10%	Partial
Preventive treatments	Verapamil, methysergide, topiramate, lithium, galcanezumab	Indomethacin (absolute response)	Lamotrigine, topiramate, gabapentin, IV lidocaine	Indomethacin (absolute response)

SUNCT, short-lasting unilateral neuralgiform headache attacks with conjunctival injection and tearing; SUNA, short-lasting unilateral neuralgiform headache attacks with cranial autonomic symptoms; C, cervical; V, trigeminal.

headache can be divided into symptomatic/abortive and prophylactic regimens (Table 5-3[160–163]). Because of the short duration and severe pain experienced in cluster headaches, abortive agents must have a rapid onset to be useful. There are current guidelines by both the American Headache Society (AHS) and the EFNS that are evidence based for the management of cluster headache.[159,164,165] The abortive agents demonstrating the best efficacy were found to be subcutaneous sumatriptan, acting within 15 minutes of injection,[166] and zolmitriptan and sumatriptan nasal spray, which are also highly effective.[167] Sumatriptan is FDA approved in its subcutaneous injection formulation for the abortive management of cluster headache.

High-flow oxygen inhalation delivered via a non-rebreathing mask (12 to 15L/min for approximately 15 to 20 minutes) is effective for two thirds of all cluster headache patients,[168] which is unique for primary headaches. Lidocaine nasal spray is effective in aborting acute attacks in a third of patients. This can be considered for patients unresponsive to oxygen or triptans, or if they are contraindicated. Oral zolmitriptan is also effective[169] but should be avoided because the pain-relieving effect is delayed compared to alternative routes. Additionally, similar to migraine, nonpharmacologic options are also available. Noninvasive VNS has FDA approval for the acute treatment of episodic cluster headache. Two pooled prospective double-blind, sham-controlled randomized trials, conducted in the US and Europe, found nVNS to be well tolerated and effective.[170] SPG stimulation has also been shown to be effective at aborting attacks in chronic cluster headache.[171–173] This approach requires invasive implantation of a miniature SPG stimulator affixed ipsilateral to the side of the attacks. The majority of adverse events are related to implantation rather than actual use, including numbness, swelling, or headache, which resolve within 3 months.[173]

Preventive therapies should ideally be initiated as soon as the cluster period begins. Despite guidelines for evidence-based therapies,[159,164,165] there are currently no agents cleared by the FDA for this indication. Several drugs are considered to be effective at reducing the frequency of attacks in episodic and chronic cluster headache. Verapamil (360 to 560 mg/day) is the most widely prescribed although an electrocardiogram (ECG) should be done before and after each dose increase because of the effects it has on cardiac function.[161] Lithium (900 mg) is also effective in reducing attack frequency in episodic and chronic cluster headache.[164,167] Another effective but more invasive approach is a suboccipital blockade of the greater occipital nerve with a mixture of lidocaine and corticosteroid.[167,174] Evidence related to melatonin is conflicting, putting it in a "possibly effective" category.[175,176]

There are also some emerging treatment options. CGRP is known to be released into the cranial vasculature during cluster headache and other TACs,[140,177] and so it represents an attractive target given the success of CGRP-targeted therapies in migraine. Two monoclonal antibodies that target CGRP have now been trialed in randomized, placebo-controlled trials for episodic and chronic cluster headache: fremanezumab (NCT02945046; episodic, NCT02964338; chronic) and galcanezumab (NCT0239747; episodic, NCT02438826, chronic). Galcanezumab was approved by the FDA in 2019 for prevention in episodic cluster headache, significantly reducing the frequency of weekly attacks compared to placebo.[178] Recent evidence seems to suggest that botulinum toxin may prove beneficial in some cases of cluster headache,[179] although injection protocols over several trials were not standardized.[180]

Surgical interventions should be considered for severe, intractable cases of cluster headache when pharmacologic therapy has failed to provide relief. Deep brain stimulation, occipital nerve stimulation, and γ knife radiation of the hypothalamus in patients with intractable chronic cluster headaches have yielded promising results.[181–186]

Paroxysmal Hemicrania (ICHD 3.2.x; *ICD-10* G44.03x–G44.04x; *ICD-11* 8A82.xx)

Paroxysmal hemicrania is a headache with clinical characteristics similar to those of cluster headache (see Box 5-3), but the attacks are shorter in duration (2 to 30 minutes), more frequent, and equally prevalent in men and women.[2,187] The attacks are likewise strictly unilateral, predominantly presenting in the periorbital region, but also can be present in the orofacial area.[188] Paroxysmal hemicrania is accompanied by either or both of a sense of restlessness and one or more cranial autonomic symptoms: lacrimation, conjunctival injection, rhinorrhea, nasal congestion, forehead and facial sweating and flushing, miosis, ptosis, and eyelid edema. An additional diagnostic criterion is that the headache must be prevented "absolutely" by therapeutic dosages of indomethacin. At least two bouts occurring in periods lasting 7 days to 1 year (when untreated) separated by pain-free remission periods of greater than 3 months are classified as *episodic* (ICHD 3.2.1; *ICD-10* G44.03; *ICD-11* 8A82.xx), and attacks occurring without a remission period, or with remissions lasting less than 3 months, for at least 1 year are classified as *chronic* (ICHD 3.2.2; *ICD-10* G44.04; *ICD-11* 8A82.xx).

Very little is known about the pathophysiologic mechanisms that underlie paroxysmal hemicranias. The similarity in clinical presentations and therapeutic outcomes has led to the suggestion that all TACs may share a common pathophysiology.[189] This is somewhat borne out by the fact that, similar to cluster headache, there is evidence of increased levels of both CGRP and VIP in the cranial circulation in a chronic paroxysmal hemicrania patient[177] and using positron emission tomography (PET) imaging in patients revealed activation of the contralateral posterior hypothalamus, ventral midbrain, red nucleus, and substantia nigra during the attack.[190] There was also activation of the pain matrix ictally and interictally. It is not yet known whether these structures are the actual generators of the headache attacks or simply activated during an attack, but activation outside of attacks does support a potential underlying role in mechanisms. A major difference compared to cluster headache is that paroxysmal hemicrania (and also hemicrania continua) are "absolutely" responsive to indomethacin, and they also seem less associated with circadian rhythms. Indeed, the ICHD diagnostic criteria requires 100% responsiveness to a therapeutic dose of indomethacin,[2] although a few cases of paroxysmal hemicrania have been reported as indomethacin resistant.[2,191,192] Indeed, in a review of 74 paroxysmal hemicrania patients, it was found that as many as 25% did not respond to indomethacin.[193] It is not known why indomethacin is so effective compared to other NSAIDs or why it is particularly responsive in only certain TACs. However, a few preclinical studies suggest that indomethacin may be acting directly on the cranial parasympathetic projection, either via pre or post-ganglionic parasympathetic neurons.[194] It also appears to be specifically responsive to NO-induced trigeminovascular changes, suggesting a potential role of NO in its mechanisms.[195] There is conflicting data on the response of paroxysmal hemicrania to sumatriptan, with some reports citing a good response and others finding only a partial response or no response at all.[196–199] There are also reports of paroxysmal hemicrania responding to topiramate.[117,199]

Short-Lasting Unilateral Neuralgiform Headache Attacks (ICHD 3.3.x; *ICD-10* G44.05x; *ICD-11* 8A82.xx)

Short-lasting unilateral neuralgiform headache attacks with conjunctival injection and tearing (SUNCT) (ICHD 3.3.1; *ICD-10* G44.05x; *ICD-11* 8A82.xx) is a primary headache disorder first described by Sjaastad et al.[200,201] SUNCT attacks (see Box 5-3[2]) are very brief (1 to 600 seconds) and are of moderate to severe pain intensity. The pain is unilateral and often orbital, supraorbital, or temporal, although it may occur throughout the trigeminal distribution. The pain is commonly described as stabbing, jabbing, or saw-tooth-like in character, with 1 to 100 attacks occurring per day. Ipsilateral conjunctival injection and lacrimation must accompany the pain. When conjunctival injection or tearing (but not both) is present, or when other autonomic symptoms such as those listed for paroxysmal hemicranias are present, the condition is known as *short-lasting unilateral neuralgiform headache attacks with cranial autonomic symptoms* (SUNA) (ICHD 3.3.2; *ICD-10* G44.05x; *ICD-11* 8A82.xx). SUNA is reported to occur approximately five times less frequently than SUNCT.[201] The differential diagnosis for SUNCT/SUNA prominently includes trigeminal neuralgia. Compared with trigeminal neuralgia, SUNCT attacks are more likely to be located in the ophthalmic division of the trigeminal nerve (V1). While both trigeminal neuralgia and SUNCT/SUNA may be triggered by cutaneous stimuli, SUNCT/SUNA is less likely to be triggered and is also less likely to demonstrate a refractory period after attacks that are triggered.[161] Some reports based on open-label trials indicate that carbamazepine, lamotrigine, gabapentin, topiramate, and intravenous lidocaine may be effective in some patients with SUNCT/SUNA, but there are no available data from large-scale controlled trials.[162,199–205] Unlike paroxysmal hemicrania and hemicrania continua, SUNCT/SUNA is not responsive to indomethacin.[161] It is also unresponsive to high-flow oxygen and subcutaneous sumatriptan, which are effective for cluster headaches.[161]

Hemicrania Continua (ICHD 3.4; *ICD-10* G44.51; *ICD-11* 8A82.xx)

Hemicrania continua, first described in 1981,[206] is a persistent one-sided headache that fluctuates in intensity but never remits. Ipsilateral autonomic features and/or restlessness/agitation accompany this headache during periods of more intense pain, and it is also aggravated by movement[207] (see Box 5-3[2]). An absolute response to therapeutic dosages of indomethacin is necessary for a definitive diagnosis.[2] Hemicrania continua is considered a rare disorder but is most likely underdiagnosed.[162] Nausea, photophobia, and phonophobia may be present in approximately 50% of patients.[207] Management typically consists of indomethacin, but gastrointestinal disturbances may make this agent unacceptable. Cardiovascular issues may also develop with long-term use of indomethacin.[208] Alternative therapies may include the use of topiramate, greater occipital nerve blocks, and in select cases, greater occipital nerve stimulation.[207,209,210]

Conclusion

Cluster headache, paroxysmal hemicranias, SUNCT/SUNA, and hemicrania continua are disorders considered to be TACs (see Table 5-3). All these disorders, except hemicrania continua, are characterized by relatively short-lasting, moderate to very severe headaches with autonomic features, and all have also been associated with hypothalamic changes on imaging studies.[161,162,210–212] Obtaining brain imaging with a focus on the pituitary region as well as laboratory pituitary function testing is recommended because pathologies in this area have occasionally been associated with TACs.[213]

It is important to recognize that any of the primary headache disorders discussed in this chapter can be present in the orofacial region. The new ICOP is a useful resource to assist in the differential diagnosis.[214]

References

1. Tepper SJ, Dahlöf CG, Dowson A, et al. Prevalence and diagnosis of migraine in patients consulting their physician with a complaint of headache: Data from the landmark study. Headache 2004;44:856–864.
2. Headache Classification Committee of the International Headache Society (IHS) The International Classification of Headache Disorders, 3rd edition. Cephalalgia, 2018;38:1–211.
3. Steiner TJ, Stovner LJ, Birbeck GL. Migraine: The seventh disabler. J Headache Pain 2013;14:1.

4. Global Burden of Disease Study C. Global, regional, and national incidence, prevalence, and years lived with disability for 354 diseases and injuries for 195 countries and territories, 1990–2017: A systematic analysis for the Global Burden of Disease Study 2017. Lancet 2018;392:1789–1858.
5. Maher BH, Griffiths LR. Identification of molecular genetic factors that influence migraine. Mol Genet Genomics 2011;285:433–446.
6. Lipton RB, Bigal ME, Steiner TJ, Silberstein SD, Olesen J. Classification of primary headaches. Neurology 2004;63:427–435.
7. Giffin NJ, Ruggiero L, Lipton RB, et al. Premonitory symptoms in migraine: An electronic diary study. Neurology 2003;60:935–940.
8. Karsan N, Bose P, Newman J, Goadsby PJ. Are some patient-perceived migraine triggers simply early manifestations of the attack? J Neurol 2021;268:1885–1893.
9. Schulte LH, Jurgens TP, May A. Photo-, osmo- and phonophobia in the premonitory phase of migraine: mistaking symptoms for triggers? J Headache Pain 2015;16:14.
10. Giffin NJ, Lipton RB, Silberstein SD, Olesen J, Goadsby PJ. The migraine postdrome: An electronic diary study. Neurology 2016;87:309–313.
11. International Classification of Orofacial Pain, 1st edition (ICOP). Cephalalgia. 2020;40(2):129–221.
12. Obermann M, Mueller D, Yoon M-S, Pageler L, Diener H, Katsarava Z. Migraine with isolated facial pain: A diagnostic challenge. Cephalalgia 2007;27:1278–1282.
13. Daudia AT, Jones MS. Facial migraine in a rhinological setting. Clin Otolaryngol Allied Sci 2002;27:521–525.
14. Lipton RB, Bigal ME, Diamond M, et al. Migraine prevalence, disease burden, and the need for preventive therapy. Neurology 2007;68:343–349.
15. Tepper SJ, Tepper DE (eds). The Cleveland Clinic Manual of Headache Therapy, ed 2. Cham, Switzerland: Springer International Publishing Switzerland, 2014.
16. Younger DS. Epidemiology of migraine. Neurol Clin 2016;34:849–861.
17. Lipton RB, Stewart WF, Diamond S, Diamond ML, Reed M. Prevalence and burden of migraine in the United States: Data from the American Migraine Study II. Headache 2001;41:646–657.
18. Loder S, Sheikh HU, Loder E. The prevalence, burden, and treatment of severe, frequent, and migraine headaches in US minority populations: Statistics from National Survey studies. Headache 2015;55:214–228.
19. Goadsby PJ, Holland PR, Martins-Oliveira M, Hoffmann J, Schankin C, Akerman S. Pathophysiology of Migraine: A Disorder of Sensory Processing. Physiol Rev 2017; 97:553–622.
20. Ashina M, Hansen JM, Do TP, Melo-Carrillo A, Burstein R, Moskowitz MA. Migraine and the trigeminovascular system—40 years and counting. Lancet Neurol 2019;18:795–804.
21. Schulte LH, May A. The migraine generator revisited: Continuous scanning of the migraine cycle over 30 days and three spontaneous attacks. Brain 2016; 139:1987–1993.
22. Maniyar FH, Sprenger T, Monteith T, Schankin C, Goadsby PJ. Brain activations in the premonitory phase of nitroglycerin-triggered migraine attacks. Brain 2014;137:232–241.
23. Borsook D, Burstein R. The enigma of the dorsolateral pons as a migraine generator. Cephalalgia 2012; 32:803–812.
24. Weiller C, May A, Limmroth V, et al. Brain stem activation in spontaneous human migraine attacks. Nat Med 1995;1:658–660.
25. Afridi SK, Giffin NJ, Kaube H, et al. A positron emission tomographic study in spontaneous migraine. Arch Neurol 2005;62:1270–1275.
26. Denuelle M, Fabre N, Payoux P, Chollet F, Geraud G. Hypothalamic activation in spontaneous migraine attacks. Headache 2007;47:1418–1426.
27. Olesen J, Burstein R, Ashina M, Tfelt-Hansen P. Origin of pain in migraine: Evidence for peripheral sensitisation. Lancet Neurol 2009;8:679–690.
28. Goadsby PJ, Edvinsson L. The trigeminovascular system and migraine: Studies characterizing cerebrovascular and neuropeptide changes seen in humans and cats. Ann Neurol 1993;33:48–56.
29. Zagami AS, Edvinsson L, Goadsby PJ. Pituitary adenylate cyclase activating polypeptide and migraine. Ann Clin Transl Neurol 2014;1:1036–1040.
30. Schytz HW, Birk S, Wienecke T, Kruuse C, Olesen J, Ashina M. PACAP38 induces migraine-like attacks in patients with migraine without aura. Brain 2009; 132(Pt 1):16–25.
31. Lassen LH, Haderslev PA, Jacobsen VB, Iversen HK, Sperling B, Olesen J. CGRP may play a causative role in migraine. Cephalalgia 2002;22:54–61.
32. Akerman S, Goadsby PJ. Neuronal PAC_1 receptors mediate delayed activation and sensitization of trigeminocervical neurons: Relevance to migraine. Sci Transl Med 2015;7:308ra157.
33. Akerman S, Romero-Reyes M. Preclinical studies investigating the neural mechanisms involved in the co-morbidity of migraine and temporomandibular disorders: The role of CGRP. Br J Pharmacol 2020;177: 5555–5568.

34. Wienecke T, Olesen J, Ashina M. Prostaglandin I2 (epoprostenol) triggers migraine-like attacks in migraineurs. Cephalalgia 2010;30:179–190.
35. Antonova M, Wienecke T, Olesen J, Ashina M. Prostaglandin E_2 induces immediate migraine-like attack in migraine patients without aura. Cephalalgia 2012;32:822–833.
36. 36. Levy D, Jakubowski M, Burstein R. Disruption of communication between peripheral and central trigeminovascular neurons mediates the antimigraine action of 5HT 1B/1D receptor agonists. Proc Natl Acad Sci U S A 2004;101:4274–4279.
37. Zhang XC, Strassman AM, Burstein R, Levy D. Sensitization and activation of intracranial meningeal nociceptors by mast cell mediators. J Pharmacol Exp Ther 2007;322:806–812.
38. Lauritzen M. Pathophysiology of the migraine aura. The spreading depression theory. Brain 1994;117(Pt 1):199–210.
39. Leao AAP. Pial circulation and spreading activity in the cerebral cortex. J Neurophysiol 1944;7:391–396.
40. Karatas H, Erdener SE, Gursoy-Ozdemir Y, et al. Spreading depression triggers headache by activating neuronal Panx1 channels. Science 2013;339:1092–1095.
41. Zhang X, Levy D, Kainz V, Noseda R, Jakubowski M, Burstein R. Activation of central trigeminovascular neurons by cortical spreading depression. Ann Neurol 2011;69:855–865.
42. Goadsby PJ. The vascular theory of migraine—A great story wrecked by the facts. Brain 2009;132:6–7.
43. Gormley P, Anttila V, Winsvold BS, et al. Meta-analysis of 375,000 individuals identifies 38 susceptibility loci for migraine. Nat Genet 2016;48:856–866.
44. Pelzer N, Louter MA, van Zwet EW, et al. Linking migraine frequency with family history of migraine. Cephalalgia 2019;39:229–236.
45. de Boer I, van den Maagdenberg A, Terwindt GM. Advance in genetics of migraine. Curr Opin Neurol 2019;32:413–421.
46. Sutherland HG, Griffiths LR. Genetics of migraine: Insights into the molecular basis of migraine disorders. Headache 2017;57:537–569.
47. Franco AL, Gonçalves DAG, Castanharo SM, Speciali JG, Bigal ME, Camparis CM. Migraine is the most prevalent primary headache in individuals with temporomandibular disorders. J Orofac Pain 2011;24: 287–292.
48. Mitrirattanakul S, Merrill RL. Headache impact in patients with orofacial pain. J Am Dent Assoc 2006; 137:1267–1274.
49. Tchivileva IE, Ohrbach R, Fillingim RB, Greenspan JD, Maixner W, Slade GD. Temporal change in headache and its contribution to the risk of developing first-onset temporomandibular disorder in the Orofacial Pain: Prospective Evaluation and Risk Assessment (OPPERA) study. Pain 2017;158:120–129.
50. Romero-Reyes M, Pardi V, Akerman S. A potent and selective calcitonin gene-related peptide (CGRP) receptor antagonist, MK-8825, inhibits responses to nociceptive trigeminal activation: Role of CGRP in orofacial pain. Exp Neurol 2015;271:95–103.
51. Cady RJ, Glenn JR, Smith KM, Durham PL. Calcitonin gene-related peptide promotes cellular changes in trigeminal neurons and glia implicated in peripheral and central sensitization. Mol Pain 2011;7:94.
52. Akerman S, Romero-Reyes M. Preclinical studies investigating the neural mechanisms involved in the co-morbidity of migraine and temporomandibular disorders: The role of CGRP. Br J Pharmacol 2020; 177:5555–5568.
53. Holroyd KA, Drew JB. Behavioral approaches to the treatment of migraine. Semin Neurol 2006;26:199–207.
54. Silberstein SD, Yuan H, Najib U, et al. Non-invasive vagus nerve stimulation for primary headache: A clinical update. Cephalalgia 2020;40:1370–1384.
55. Akerman S, Simon B, Romero-Reyes M. Vagus nerve stimulation suppresses acute noxious activation of trigeminocervical neurons in animal models of primary headache. Neurobiol Dis 2017;102:96–104.
56. Hawkins JL, Cornelison LE, Blankenship BA, Durham PL. Vagus nerve stimulation inhibits trigeminal nociception in a rodent model of episodic migraine. Pain Rep 2017;2:e628.
57. Chou DE, Yugrakh MS, Winegarner D, Rowe V, Kuruvilla D, Schoenen J. Acute migraine therapy with external trigeminal neurostimulation (ACME): A randomized controlled trial. Cephalalgia 2019;39:3–14.
58. Lipton RB, Dodick DW, Silberstein SD, et al. Single-pulse transcranial magnetic stimulation for acute treatment of migraine with aura: A randomised, double-blind, parallel-group, sham-controlled trial. Lancet Neurol 2010;9:373–380.
59. Nir RR, Yarnitsky D. Conditioned pain modulation. Curr Opin Support Palliat Care 2015;9:131–137.
60. Rapoport AM, Lin T. Device profile of the Nerivio for acute migraine treatment: Overview of its efficacy and safety. Expert Rev Med Devices 2019;16:1017–1023.
61. Reuter U, McClure C, Liebler E, Pozo-Rosich P. Non-invasive neuromodulation for migraine and cluster headache: A systematic review of clinical trials. J Neurol Neurosurg Psychiatry 2019;90:796–804.
62. Digre KB. What's new in the treatment of migraine? J Neuroophthalmol 2019;39:352–359.

63. Díaz-Insa S, Goadsby PJ, Zanchin G, Fortea J, Falques M, Vila C. The impact of allodynia on the efficacy of almotriptan when given early in migraine: Data from the "act when mild" study. Int J Neurosci 2011;121: 655–661.
64. Goadsby PJ, Zanchin G, Geraud G, et al. Early vs. non-early intervention in acute migraine-"Act when Mild (AwM)." A double-blind, placebo-controlled trial of almotriptan. Cephalalgia 2008;28:383–391.
65. Ashina M. Migraine. N Engl J Med 2020;383:1866–1876.
66. American Headache S. The American Headache Society Position Statement on Integrating New Migraine Treatments into Clinical Practice. Headache 2019; 59:1–18.
67. Johnson JL, Hutchinson MR, Williams DB, Rolan P. Medication-overuse headache and opioid-induced hyperalgesia: A review of mechanisms, a neuroimmune hypothesis and a novel approach to treatment. Cephalalgia 2013;33:52–64.
68. Lipton RB, Buse DC, Friedman BW, et al. Characterizing opioid use in a US population with migraine. Results from the CaMEO study. Neurology 2020; 95:e457–e468.
69. Dodick D, Lipton RB, Martin V, et al. Consensus statement: Cardiovascular safety profile of triptans (5-HT1B/1D Agonists) in the acute treatment of migraine. Headache 2004;44:414–425.
70. Cohen ML, Schenck K. 5-hydroxytryptamine (1F) receptors do not participate in vasoconstriction: Lack of vasoconstriction to LY344864, a selective serotonin (1F) receptor agonist in rabbit saphenous vein. J Pharmacol Exp Ther 1999;290:935–939.
71. Lamb YN. Lasmiditan: First approval. Drugs 2019;79: 1989–1996.
72. Goadsby PJ, Wietecha LA, Dennehy EB, et al. Phase 3 randomized, placebo-controlled, double-blind study of lasmiditan for acute treatment of migraine. Brain 2019;142:1894–1904.
73. Moreno-Ajona D, Pérez-Rodríguez A, Goadsby PJ. Gepants, calcitonin-gene-related peptide receptor antagonists: What could be their role in migraine treatment? Curr Opin Neurol 2020;33:309–315.
74. Rimegepant (Nurtec ODT) for acute treatment of migraine. JAMA 2020;324:890–891.
75. Lipton RB, Dodick DW, Ailani J, et al. Effect of ubrogepant vs placebo on pain and the most bothersome associated symptom in the acute treatment of migraine: The ACHIEVE II randomized clinical trial. JAMA 2019;322:1887–1898.
76. Goadsby PJ. Therapeutic prospects for migraine: Can paradise be regained? Ann Neurol 2013;74:423–434.
77. Robbins MS. Diagnosis and management of headache: A review. JAMA 2021;325:1874–1885.
78. Silberstein SD, Holland S, Freitag F, et al. Evidence-based guideline update: Pharmacologic treatment for episodic migraine prevention in adults: Report of the Quality Standards Subcommittee of the American Academy of Neurology and the American Headache Society. Neurology 2012;78:1337–1345.
79. Evers S, Afra J, Frese A, et al. EFNS guideline on the drug treatment of migraine--revised report of an EFNS task force. Eur J Neurol 2009;16:968–981.
80. 80. Steiner TJ, Jensen R, Katsarava Z, et al. Aids to management of headache disorders in primary care (2nd edition): On behalf of the European Headache Federation and *Lifting the Burden:* The Global Campaign against Headache. J Headache Pain 2019; 20:57.
81. Loder E, Burch R, Rizzoli P. The 2012 AHS/AAN guidelines for prevention of episodic migraine: A summary and comparison with other recent clinical practice guidelines. Headache 2012;52:930–945.
82. Dodick DW, Turkel CC, DeGryse RE, et al. Onabotulinum toxin A for treatment of chronic migraine: Pooled results from the double-blind, randomized, placebo-controlled phases of the PREEMPT clinical program. Headache 2010;50:921–936.
83. Martin PR. Behavioral management of migraine headache triggers: Learning to cope with triggers. Curr Pain Headache Rep 2010;14:221–227.
84. Andress-Rothrock D, King W, Rothrock J. An analysis of migraine triggers in a clinic-based population. Headache 2010;50:1366–1370.
85. Edvinsson L, Haanes KA, Warfvinge K, Krause DN. CGRP as the target of new migraine therapies—Successful translation from bench to clinic. Nat Rev Neurol 2018;14:338–350.
86. Do TP, Guo S, Ashina M, Therapeutic novelties in migraine: New drugs, new hope? J Headache Pain 2019;20:37.
87. Tepper SJ. History and review of anti-calcitonin gene-related peptide (CGRP) Therapies: From translational research to treatment. Headache 2018;58 (suppl 3):238–275.
88. Jain S, Yuan H, Spare N, Silberstein SD. Erenumab in the treatment of migraine. Pain Manag 2018;8:415–426.
89. Lamb YN. Galcanezumab: First Global approval. Drugs 2018;78:1769–1775.
90. Dhillon S. Eptinezumab: First approval. Drugs 2020; 80:733–739.
91. Paemeleire K, MaassenVanDenBrink A. Calcitonin-gene-related peptide pathway mAbs and migraine prevention. Curr Opin Neurol 2018;31:274–280.
92. Hargreaves R, Olesen J. Calcitonin gene-related peptide modulators—The history and renaissance of a new migraine drug class. Headache 2019;59:951–970.

93. Mojica J, Mo B, Ng A. Sphenopalatine ganglion block in the management of chronic headaches. Curr Pain Headache Rep 2017;21:27.
94. Blumenfeld A, Ashkenazi A, Napchan U, et al. Expert consensus recommendations for the performance of peripheral nerve blocks for headaches—A narrative review. Headache 2013;53:437–446.
95. Schiffman E, Ohrbach R, List T, et al. Diagnostic criteria for headache attributed to temporomandibular disorders. Cephalalgia 2012;32:683–692.
96. GBD 2016 Study Headache Collaborators. Global, regional, and national burden of migraine and tension-type headache, 1990–2016: A systematic analysis for the Global Burden of Disease Study 2016. Lancet Neurol 2018;17:954–976.
97. GBD 2017 US Neurological Disorders Collaborators, Feigin VL, Vos T, et al. Burden of neurological disorders across the US from 1990–2017: A Global Burden of Disease Study. JAMA Neurol 2021;78:165–176.
98. Ashina S, Mitsikostas DD, Lee MJ, et al. Tension-type headache. Nat Rev Dis Primers 2021;7:24.
99. Fernández-de-las-Peñas C, Arendt-Nielsen L. Improving understanding of trigger points and widespread pressure pain sensitivity in tension-type headache patients: Clinical implications. Expert Rev Neurother 2017;17:933–939.
100. Schmidt-Hansen PT, Svensson P, Jensen TS, Graven-Nielsen T, Bach FW. Patterns of experimentally induced pain in pericranial muscles. Cephalalgia 2006;26:568–577.
101. Do TP, Heldarskard GF, Kolding LT, Hvedstrup J, Schytz HW. Myofascial trigger points in migraine and tension-type headache. J Headache Pain 2018;19:84.
102. Hubbard DR, Berkoff GM. Myofascial trigger points show spontaneous needle EMG activity. Spine (Phila Pa 1976) 1993;18:1803–1807.
103. Jensen R, Fuglsang-Frederiksen A, Olesen J. Quantitative surface EMG of pericranial muscles in headache. A population study. Electroencephalogr Clin Neurophysiol 1994;93:335–344.
104. Feuerstein M, Bush C, Corbisiero R. Stress and chronic headache: A psychophysiological analysis of mechanisms. J Psychosom Res 1982;26:167–182.
105. Schoenen J, Gerard P, De Pasqua V, Juprelle M. EMG activity in pericranial muscles during postural variation and mental activity in healthy volunteers and patients with chronic tension type headache. Headache 1991;31:321–324.
106. Leistad RB, Sand T, Westgaard RH, Nilsen KB, Stovner LJ. Stress-induced pain and muscle activity in patients with migraine and tension-type headache. Cephalalgia 2006;26:64–73.
107. Buchgreitz L, Lyngberg AC, Bendtsen L, Jensen R. Frequency of headache is related to sensitization: A population study. Pain 2006;123:19–27.
108. Fernández-de-las-Peñas C, Plaza-Manzano G, Navarro-Santana MJ, Olesen J, Jensen RH, Bendtsen L. Evidence of localized and widespread pressure pain hypersensitivity in patients with tension-type headache: A systematic review and meta-analysis. Cephalalgia 2021;41:256–273.
109. Schmidt-Wilcke T, Leinisch E, Straube A, et al. Gray matter decrease in patients with chronic tension type headache. Neurology 2005;65:1483–1486.
110. Wang P, Du H, Chen N, et al. Regional homogeneity abnormalities in patients with tension-type headache: A resting-state fMRI study. Neurosci Bull 2014;30: 949–955.
111. Bendtsen L, Evers S, Linde M, et al. EFNS guideline on the treatment of tension-type headache—Report of an EFNS task force. Eur J Neurol 2010;17:1318–1325.
112. Rabello GD, Forte LV, Galvão AC. Clinical evaluation of the efficacy of the paracetamol and caffeine combination in the treatment of tension headache [in Portuguese]. Arq Neuropsiquiatr 2000;58:90–98.
113. Diamond S, Balm TK, Freitag FG. Ibuprofen plus caffeine in the treatment of tension-type headache. Clin Pharmacol Ther 2000;68:312–319.
114. Penzien DB, Rains JC, Lipchik GL, Creer TL. Behavioral interventions for tension-type headache: Overview of current therapies and recommendation for a self-management model for chronic headache. Curr Pain Headache Rep 2004;8:489–499.
115. Andrasik F. Behavioral treatment approaches to chronic headache. Neurol Sci 2003;24(suppl 2):S80–S85.
116. Bittar G, Graff-Radford SB. A retrospective study of patients with cluster headaches. Oral Surg Oral Med Oral Pathol 1992;73:519–525.
117. Rozen TD, Fishman RS. Cluster headache in the United States of America: Demographics, clinical characteristics, triggers, suicidality, and personal burden. Headache 2012;52:99–113.
118. Manzoni GC, Micieli G, Granella F, Tassorelli C, Zanferrari C, Cavallini A. Cluster headache: Course over ten years in 189 patients. Cephalalgia 1991;11: 169–174.
119. Robbins MS. The psychiatric comorbidities of cluster headache. Curr Pain Headache Rep 2013;17:313.
120. van Vliet JA, Eekers PJ, Haan J, Ferrari MD, Dutch RUSSH Study Group. Features involved in the diagnostic delay of cluster headache. J Neurol Neurosurg Psychiatry 2003;74:1123–1125.
121. Bahra A, Goadsby PJ. Diagnostic delays and mismanagement in cluster headache. Acta Neurol Scand 2004;109:175–179.

122. Balasubramaniam R, Klasser GD, Delcanho R. Trigeminal autonomic cephalalgias: A review and implications for dentistry. J Am Dent Assoc 2008;139: 1616–1624.
123. Van Alboom E, Louis P, Van Zandijcke M, Crevits L, Vakaet A, Paemeleire K. Diagnostic and therapeutic trajectory of cluster headache patients in Flanders. Acta Neurol Belg 2009;109:10–17.
124. Russell MB. Epidemiology and genetics of cluster headache. Lancet Neurol 2004;3:279–283.
125. Zidverc-Trajkovic J, Markovic K, Radojicic A, Podgorac A, Sternic N. Cluster headache: Is age of onset important for clinical presentation? Cephalalgia 2014;34: 664–670.
126. Manzoni GC, Bonavita V, Bussone G, et al. Chronic migraine classification: Current knowledge and future perspectives. J Headache Pain 2011;12:585–592.
127. Ekbom K, Hardebo JE. Cluster headache: Aetiology, diagnosis and management. Drugs 2002;62:61–69.
128. Manzoni GC. Cluster headache and lifestyle: Remarks on a population of 374 male patients. Cephalalgia 1999;19:88–94.
129. Penfield W, McNaughton F. Dural headache and innervation of the dura mater. Arch Neurol Psychiatry 1940;44:43–75.
130. McNaughton FL, Feindel W. Innervation of intracranial structures: A reappraisal. In: Rose FC (ed). Physiological aspects of clinical neurology. Oxford: Blackwell Scientific, 1977:279–293.
131. Ray BS, Wolff HG. Experimental studies on headache. Pain sensitive structures of the head and their significance in headache. Arch Surg 1940;41:813–856.
132. Matharu MS, Goadsby PJ. Persistence of attacks of cluster headache after trigeminal nerve root section. Brain 2002;125:976–984.
133. Goadsby PJ. Pathophysiology of cluster headache: A trigeminal autonomic cephalalgia. Lancet Neurol 2002;1:251–257.
134. Spencer SE, Sawyer WB, Wada H, Platt KB, Loewy AD. CNS projections to the pterygopalatine parasympathetic preganglionic neurons in the rat: A retrograde transneuronal viral cell body labeling study. Brain Res 1990;534:149–169.
135. Akerman S, Holland PR, Lasalandra MP, Goadsby PJ. Oxygen inhibits neuronal activation in the trigeminocervical complex after stimulation of trigeminal autonomic reflex, but not during direct dural activation of trigeminal afferents. Headache 2009;49:1131–1143.
136. Akerman S, Holland PR, Summ O, Lasalandra MP, Goadsby PJ. A translational in vivo model of trigeminal autonomic cephalalgias: Therapeutic characterization. Brain 2012;135:3664–3675.
137. Suzuki N, Hardebo JE, Owman C. Origins and pathways of cerebrovascular vasoactive intestinal polypeptide-positive nerves in rat. J Cereb Blood Flow Metab 1988;8:697–712.
138. Burstein R, Noseda R, Borsook D. Migraine: Multiple processes, complex pathophysiology. J Neurosci 2015;35:6619–6629.
139. Schytz HW, Barlose M, Guo S, et al. Experimental activation of the sphenopalatine ganglion provokes cluster-like attacks in humans. Cephalalgia 2013;33: 831–841.
140. Goadsby PJ, Edvinsson L. Human in vivo evidence for trigeminovascular activation in cluster headache. Neuropeptide changes and effects of acute attacks therapies. Brain 1994;117:427–434.
141. Tuka B, Szabo N, Toth E, et al. Release of PACAP-38 in episodic cluster headache patients—An exploratory study. J Headache Pain 2016;17:69.
142. Akerman S, Romero-Reyes M. Preclinical studies investigating the neural mechanisms involved in the co-morbidity of migraine and temporomandibular disorders: The role of CGRP. Br J Pharmacol 2020; 177:5555–5568.
143. Schytz HW, Birk S, Wienecke T, Kruuse C, Olesen J, Ashina M. PACAP38 induces migraine-like attacks in patients with migraine without aura. Brain 2009; 132:16–25.
144. Rahmann A, Wienecke T, Hansen JM, Fahrenkrug J, Olesen J, Ashina M. Vasoactive intestinal peptide causes marked cephalic vasodilation, but does not induce migraine. Cephalalgia 2008;28:226–236.
145. Amin FM, Hougaard A, Schytz HW, et al. Investigation of the pathophysiological mechanisms of migraine attacks induced by pituitary adenylate cyclase-activating polypeptide-38. Brain 2014;137:779–794.
146. May A, Bahra A, Büchel C, Frackowiak RS, Goadsby PJ. Hypothalamic activation in cluster headache attacks. Lancet 1998;352:275–278.
147. May A, Ashburner J, Buchel C, et al. Correlation between structural and functional changes in brain in an idiopathic headache syndrome. Nat Med 1999;5:836–838.
148. May A, Kaube H, Buchel C, et al. Experimental cranial pain elicited by capsaicin: A PET study. Pain 1998; 74:61–66.
149. Robert C, Bourgeais L, Arreto CD, et al. Paraventricular hypothalamic regulation of trigeminovascular mechanisms involved in headaches. J Neurosci 2013; 33:8827–8840.
150. Hosoya Y, Matsushita M, Sugiura Y. A direct hypothalamic projection to the superior salivatory nucleus neurons in the rat. A study using anterograde autoradiographic and retrograde HRP methods. Brain Res 1983;266:329–333.

151. Hosoya Y, Sugiura Y, Ito R, Kohno K. Descending projections from the hypothalamic paraventricular nucleus to the A5 area, including the superior salivatory nucleus, in the rat. Exp Brain Res 1990;82:513–518.
152. Bartsch T, Levy MJ, Knight YE, Goadsby PJ. Differential modulation of nociceptive dural input to [hypocretin] orexin A and B receptor activation in the posterior hypothalamic area. Pain 2004;109:367–378.
153. Holland PR, Akerman S, Goadsby PJ. Modulation of nociceptive dural input to the trigeminal nucleus caudalis via activation of the orexin 1 receptor in the rat. Eur J Neurosci 2006;24:2825–2833.
154. Scammell TE, Winrow CJ. Orexin receptors: Pharmacology and therapeutic opportunities. Annu Rev Pharmacol Toxicol 2011;51:243–266.
155. Barloese M, Jennum P, Lund N, Knudsen S, Gammeltoft S, Jensen R. Reduced CSF hypocretin-1 levels are associated with cluster headache. Cephalalgia 2015;35:869–876.
156. Schurks M, Kurth T, Geissler I, Tessmann G, Diener HC, Rosskopf D. Cluster headache is associated with the G1246A polymorphism in the hypocretin receptor 2 gene. Neurology 2006;66:1917–1919.
157. Evers S, Barth B, Frese A, Husstedt IW, Happe S. Sleep apnea in patients with cluster headache: A case-control study. Cephalalgia 2014;34:828–832.
158. Kudrow L. A possible role of the carotid body in the pathogenesis of cluster headache. Cephalalgia 1983;3:241–247.
159. May A, Leone M, Afra J, et al. EFNS guidelines on the treatment of cluster headache and other trigeminalautonomic cephalalgias. Eur J Neurol 2006;13:1066–1077.
160. Cohen AS, Matharu MS, Goadsby PJ. Short-lasting unilateral neuralgiform headache attacks with conjunctival injection and tearing (SUNCT) or cranial autonomic features (SUNA): A prospective clinical study of SUNCT and SUNA. Brain 2006;129:2746–2760.
161. Goadsby PJ, Cittadini E, Cohen AS. Trigeminal autonomic cephalalgias: Paroxysmal hemicrania, SUNCT/SUNA, and hemicrania continua. Semin Neurol 2010;30:186–191.
162. Eller M, Goadsby PJ. Trigeminal autonomic cephalalgias. Oral Dis 2016;22:1–8.
163. Wei DY, Yuan Ong JJ, Goadsby PJ. Overview of trigeminal autonomic cephalalgias: Nosologic evolution, diagnosis, and management. Ann Indian Acad Neurol 2018;21:S39–S44.
164. Robbins MS, Starling AJ, Pringsheim TM, Becker WJ, Schwedt TJ. Treatment of cluster headache: The American Headache Society evidence-based guidelines. Headache 2016;56:1093–1106.
165. Francis GJ, Becker WJ, Pringsheim TM. Acute and preventive pharmacologic treatment of cluster headache. Neurology 2010;75:463–473.
166. Sumatriptan Cluster Headache Study Group. Treatment of acute cluster headache with sumatriptan. N Engl J Med 1991;325:322–326.
167. Hoffmann J, May A. Diagnosis, pathophysiology, and management of cluster headache. Lancet Neurol 2018;17:75–83.
168. Cohen AS, Burns B, Goadsby PJ. High flow oxygen for treatment of cluster headache. A randomized trial. JAMA 2009;302:2451–2457.
169. Bahra A, Gawel MJ, Hardebo JE, Millson D, Breen SA, Goadsby PJ. Oral zolmitriptan is effective in the acute treatment of cluster headache. Neurology 2000;54:1832–1839.
170. de Coo IF, Marin JC, Silberstein SD, et al. Differential efficacy of non-invasive vagus nerve stimulation for the acute treatment of episodic and chronic cluster headache: A meta-analysis. Cephalalgia 2019;39:967–977.
171. Ansarinia M, Rezai A, Tepper SJ, et al. Electrical stimulation of sphenopalatine ganglion for acute treatment of cluster headaches. Headache 2010;50:1164–1174.
172. Schoenen J, Jensen RH, Lantéri-Minet M, et al. Stimulation of the sphenopalatine ganglion (SPG) for cluster headache treatment. Pathway CH-1: A randomized, sham-controlled study. Cephalalgia 2013;33:816–830.
173. Goadsby PJ, Sahai-Srivastava S, Kezirian EJ, et al. Safety and efficacy of sphenopalatine ganglion stimulation for chronic cluster headache: A double-blind, randomised controlled trial. Lancet Neurol 2019;18:1081–1090.
174. Villar-Martinez MD, Chan C, Goadsby PJ. Evolving options for the treatment of cluster headache. Curr Opin Neurol 2020;33:323–328.
175. Leone M, D'Amico D, Moschiano F, Fraschini F, Bussone G. Melatonin versus placebo in the prophylaxis of cluster headache: A double-blind pilot study with parallel groups. Cephalalgia 1996;16:494–496.
176. Peres MF, Rozen TD. Melatonin in the preventive treatment of chronic cluster headache. Cephalalgia 2001;21:993–995.
177. Goadsby PJ, Edvinsson L. Neuropeptide changes in a case of chronic paroxysmal hemicrania—Evidence for trigemino-parasympathetic activation. Cephalalgia 1996;16:448–450.
178. Goadsby PJ, Dodick DW, Leone M, et al. Trial of galcanezumab in prevention of episodic cluster headache. N Engl J Med 2019;381:132–141.

179. Sostak P, Krause P, Förderreuther S, Reinisch V, Straube A. Botulinum toxin type-A therapy in cluster headache: An open study. J Headache Pain 2007;8: 236–241.
180. Freund B, Kotchetkov IS, Rao A. The efficacy of botulinum toxin in cluster headache: A systematic review. J Oral Facial Pain Headache 2020;34:129–134.
181. Ford RG, Ford KT, Swaid S, Young P, Jennelle R. Gamma knife treatment of refractory cluster headache. Headache 1998;38:3–9.
182. Kano H, Kondziolka D, Mathieu D, et al. Stereotactic radiosurgery for intractable cluster headache: An initial report from the North American Gamma Knife Consortium. J Neurosurg 2011;114:1736–1743.
183. Burns B, Watkins L, Goadsby PJ. Treatment of medically intractable cluster headache by occipital nerve stimulation: Long-term follow-up of eight patients. Lancet 2007;369:1099–1106.
184. Burns B, Watkins L, Goadsby PJ. Treatment of intractable chronic cluster headache by occipital nerve stimulation in 14 patients. Neurology 2009;72:341–345.
185. Magis D, Gerardy PY, Remacle JM, Schoenen J. Sustained effectiveness of occipital nerve stimulation in drug-resistant chronic cluster headache. Headache 2011;51:1191–1201.
186. Leone M, Franzini A, Cecchini AP, Broggi G, Bussone G. Hypothalamic deep brain stimulation in the treatment of chronic cluster headache. Ther Adv Neurol Disord 2010;3:187–195.
187. Prakash S, Patell R. Paroxysmal hemicrania: An update. Curr Pain Headache Rep 2014;18:407.
188. Benoliel R, Sharav Y. Paroxysmal hemicrania. Case studies and review of the literature. Oral Surg Oral Med Oral Pathol Oral Radiol Endod 1998;85:285–292.
189. Prakash S, Hansen JM. Mechanisms of cluster headache and other trigeminal autonomic cephalalgias. In: Martelletti P, Steiner, TJ (eds). Handbook of Headache Practical Management. New York: Springer, 2011:330–340.
190. Matharu MS, Cohen AS, Frackowiak RS, Goadsby PJ. Posterior hypothalamic activation in paroxysmal hemicrania. Ann Neurol 2006;59:535–545.
191. Kuritzky A. Indomethacin-resistant hemicrania continua. Cephalalgia 1992;12:57–59.
192. Mariano Da Silva H, Alcantara MC, Bordini CA, Speciali JG. Strictly unilateral headache reminiscent of hemicrania continua resistant to indomethacin but responsive to gabapentin. Cephalalgia 2002;22:409–410.
193. Boes CJ, Dodick DW. Refining the clinical spectrum of chronic paroxysmal hemicrania: A review of 74 patients. Headache 2002;42:699–708.
194. Akerman S, Holland PR, Summ O, Lasalandra MP, Goadsby PJ. A translational in vivo model of trigeminal autonomic cephalalgias: Therapeutic characterization. Brain 2012;135:3664–3675.
195. Summ O, Andreou AP, Akerman S, Holland PR, Hoffmann J, Goadsby PJ. Differential actions of indomethacin: Clinical relevance in headache. Pain 2021; 162:591–599.
196. Cittadini E, Matharu MS, Goadsby PJ. Paroxysmal hemicrania: A prospective clinical study of 31 cases. Brain 2008;131:1142–1155.
197. Pascual J, Quijano J. A case of chronic paroxysmal hemicrania responding to subcutaneous sumatriptan. J Neurol Neurosurg Psychiatry 1998;65:407.
198. Dahlöf C. Subcutaneous sumatriptan does not abort attacks of chronic paroxysmal hemicrania (CPH). Headache 1993;33:201–202.
199. Cohen AS, Goadsby PJ. Paroxysmal hemicrania responding to topiramate. J Neurol Neurosurg Psychiatry 2007;78:96–97.
200. Sjaastad O, Russell D, Hørven, I, Bunæs, U. Multiple neuralgiform unilateral headache attacks associated with conjunctival injection and appearing in clusters. A nosological problem. Proceedings of the Scandinavian Migraine Society 1978;31.
201. Sjaastad O, Saunte C, Salvesen R, et al. Short-lasting unilateral neuralgiform headache attacks with conjunctival injection, tearing, sweating, and rhinorrhea. Cephalalgia 1989;9:147–156.
202. Rosselli JL, Karpinski JP. The role of lamotrigine in the treatment of short-lasting unilateral neuralgiform headache attacks with conjunctival injection and tearing syndrome. Ann Pharmacother 2011;45:108–113.
203. Cohen AS, Matharu MS, Goadsby PJ. Suggested guidelines for treating SUNCT and SUNA. Cephalalgia 2005;25:1200.
204. Rossi P, Cesarino F, Faroni J, Malpezzi MG, Sandrini G, Nappi G. SUNCT syndrome successfully treated with topiramate: Case reports. Cephalalgia 2003;23: 998–1000.
205. Matharu MS, Cohen AS, Goadsby PJ. SUNCT syndrome responsive to intravenous lidocaine. Cephalalgia 2004;24:985–992.
206. Medina JL, Diamond S. Cluster headache variant. Spectrum of a new headache syndrome. Arch Neurol 1981;38:705–709.
207. Cittadini E, Goadsby PJ. Hemicrania continua: A clinical study of 39 patients with diagnostic implications. Brain 2010;133:1973–1986.
208. McGettigan P, Henry D. Cardiovascular risk and inhibition of cyclooxygenase: A systematic review of the observational studies of selective and nonselective inhibitors of cyclooxygenase 2. JAMA 2006; 296:1633–1644.

209. Afridi SK, Shields KG, Bhola R, Goadsby PJ. Greater occipital nerve injection in primary headache syndromes: Prolonged effects from a single injection. Pain 2006;122:126–129.
210. Burns B, Watkins L, Goadsby PJ. Treatment of hemicrania continua by occipital nerve stimulation with a bion device: Long-term follow-up of a crossover study. Lancet Neurol 2008;7:1001–1012.
211. Matharu M, May A. Functional and structural neuroimaging in trigeminal autonomic cephalalgias. Curr Pain Headache Rep 2008;12:132–137.
212. Matharu MS, Cohen AS, McGonigle DJ, Ward N, Frackowiak RS, Goadsby PJ. Posterior hypothalamic and brainstem activation in hemicrania continua. Headache 2004;44:747–761.
213. Levy MJ, Matharu MS, Meeran K, Powell M, Goadsby PJ. The clinical characteristics of headache in patients with pituitary tumours. Brain 2005;128:1921–1230.
214. International Classification of Orofacial Pain, 1st edition (ICOP). Cephalalgia 2020;40:129-221.

6

Neuropathic Pain

Key Points

- Clinicians need to recognize and understand that not all "toothaches" are of odontogenic origin.
- Neuropathic pain arises from a lesion in the peripheral or central somatosensory system and may present as hyper- or hypo-esthetic. Some conditions described in this section do not have identifiable neural lesions (idiopathic trigeminal neuralgia or burning mouth syndrome) and hence are often placed in idiopathic domains of various classifications.
- Episodic or continuous neuropathic pains may present with symptoms that mimic odontogenic pain, but these may require medical or surgical intervention instead of routine dental intervention. Repeated surgery and prescription of antibiotics are not indicated for neuropathic pain.
- Clinicians should have an understanding of neuropathic processes to avoid misdirected or incomplete treatment.
- Clinicians should have an understanding of the role of routine anesthetic and surgical techniques in the causation of neuropathic pain.
- Referral to other health care providers should be a consideration when patients present with complex and confusing symptoms.
- Management of neuropathic pain often requires a multidimensional and multidisciplinary approach, and early recognition and treatment of post-traumatic neuropathy may prevent chronic pain.

There are three types of pain: nociceptive pain, neuropathic pain, and nociplastic pain, as well as combinations of the three. *Nociceptive pain* is generally a protective process of transduction and transmission to the sensory cortex whereby pain is registered in the region of tissue where the noxious stimulation has been threatened or has occurred, thereby warning the individual to limit the damage. Nociceptive pain can result from the inflammation caused by tissue damage whereby peripheral and central mechanisms cause sensitization of the damaged tissue and the nearby undamaged tissues. This pain thereby serves a protective purpose in helping facilitate tissue repair.

Chronic or persistent pain is a process where the brain continues to overlay pain in a body region when the tissues are healed for more than 3 to 6 months (the normal duration of healing for the tissue involved). This type of pain no longer serves a protective purpose. Chronic pain can be due to nerve damage (neuropathic pain) or to nociplastic pain, which may be caused by amplification of pain signals in the central nervous system (CNS) and can share some of the signs of neuropathic pain, including wind-up, hyperalgesia, and allodynia.[1] *Nociplastic pain*, a term introduced by the International Association for the Study of Pain (IASP) in 2017,[2] represents a phenomenon where nociceptors are activated, resulting in pain being perceived despite there being no active or threatened tissue damage nor any demonstrable disease/lesion of the somatosensory system. It is important to note that combinations of nociceptive and nociplastic pain are possible within a patient and that nociplastic pain can also present with neuropathic signs.

Neuropathic pain is defined as pain that arises from injury, disease, or dysfunction of the peripheral or CNS, as compared to *somatic pain*, which occurs in response to noxious stimulation of normal neural receptors.[3] Neuropathic pain is generally classified according to the agent of insult and anatomical distribution of the pain. Based on temporal features, neuropathic pain can be episodic or continuous and can be peripherally generated or centrally mediated. Often, both central and peripheral sensitization play a role in the continuation or persistence of the condition. Patients experiencing neuropathic pain may complain of a combination of spontaneous (stimulus-independent) or touch-evoked (stimulus-dependent) pain. Sensory signs and symptoms characteristically accompany neuropathic pain. These signs may be either *positive*, meaning gain in function (eg, hyperalgesia or allodynia to mechanical or thermal stimuli); *negative*, meaning loss of function (eg, numbness); or a combination of both, such as dysesthesia. The clinical presentation of neuropathic pain can be dependent on its origin and the initial insult that caused it.

Throughout this chapter, the codes from the third edition of the International Headache Society's Classification of Headache Disorders (ICHD-3)[4] and *The International Classification of Diseases, Tenth Revision (ICD-10)* and *Eleventh Revision (ICD-11)*, are presented for each disorder wherever available. The International Classification of Orofacial Pain (ICOP[5]) is also presented wherever possible, but the chapter has not yet been converted to this classification due to it being a first edition and in need of additional testing. Table 6-1 compares relevant parts of ICOP and ICHD.

Neuralgia

Head and neck pains are mediated by afferent fibers in the trigeminal nerve, nervus intermedius, glossopharyngeal and vagus nerves, and upper cervical roots via the occipital nerves. Neuralgia can result when these nerves are stimulated by compression (entrapment and/or impingement), distortion, other forms of irritation, or lesions in the peripheral or central pathways. A common characteristic of this pain is a paroxysmal (very short-lasting), sharp,

Table 6-1 Comparison of ICHD and ICOP terminology and classification of relevant (presumed) neuropathic conditions/disorder[4,5]

Previous or other names of condition or group of disorders	ICHD classification	ICOP classification	Accompanying notes
Trigeminal neuralgia	Trigeminal neuralgia (ICHD 13.1.1; *ICD-10* G50.0 *ICD-11* 8B82.0)	Trigeminal neuralgia (ICOP 4.1.1)	
Glossopharyngeal neuralgia	Glossopharyngeal neuralgia (ICHD 13.2.1; *ICD-10* G52.1, *ICD-11* 8B87)	Glossopharyngeal neuralgia (ICOP 4.2.1)	
Nervus intermedius neuralgia	Nervus intermedius neuralgia (ICHD 13.3.1)	Not classified	
	Painful trigeminal neuropathies (ICHD 13.1.2)	Other trigeminal neuropathic pain (ICOP 4.1.2)	
Secondary PDAP, phantom tooth pain, atypical odontalgia	Painful posttraumatic trigeminal neuropathy (PPTTN, ICHD 13.1.2.3)	Posttraumatic trigeminal neuropathic pain (ICOP 4.1.2.3)	Can only make probable diagnosis unless confirmed by advanced testing. Subsumes a large number of previously separate conditions including trauma from surgery to trigeminal nerve, PDAP/atypical odontalgia related to deafferentation injury.
	Trigeminal neuropathy attributed to (acute) herpes zoster (ICHD 13.1.2.1)	Trigeminal neuropathy attributed to (acute) herpes zoster (ICOP 4.1.2.1)	
Postherpetic neuralgia	Trigeminal postherpetic neuropathy (ICHD 13.1.2.2; *ICD-10* B02.22)	Trigeminal postherpetic neuropathy (ICOP 4.1.2.2)	
	Trigeminal neuropathic pain attributed to another disorder (ICHD 13.1.2.4)	Trigeminal neuropathic pain attributed to another disorder (ICOP 4.1.2.4)	
	Central neuropathic pain (ICHD 13.13)	Not classified	

Table 6 1 *(cont)* **Comparison of ICHD and ICOP terminology and classification of relevant (presumed) neuropathic conditions/disorder[4,5]**

Previous or other names of condition or group of disorders	ICHD classification	ICOP classification	Accompanying notes
Postherpetic neuralgia	Central neuropathic pain attributed to MS (ICHD 13.13.1)	Not classified	
	Central poststroke pain (ICHD 13.13.2; *ICD-10* G89.0, *ICD-11* MG30.50)	Not classified	
	Tolosa-Hunt syndrome (ICHD 13.8)	Not classified	
	Burning mouth syndrome (ICHD 13.11; *ICD-10* K14.6, *ICD-11* DA0F.0)	Burning mouth syndrome (ICOP 6.1)	
	Persistent idiopathic facial pain (ICHD 13.12; *ICD-10* G50.9, *ICD-11* 8A85)	Persistent idiopathic facial pain (ICOP 6.2)	
Primary PDAP	Unclassified	Persistent idiopathic dentoalveolar pain disorder (ICOP 6.3)	
CRPS (*ICD-11* 8D8A)	Unclassified	Unclassified	
Occlusal dysesthesia, phantom bite syndrome/occlusion	Unclassified	Unclassified	
Numb chin syndrome	Unclassified	Unclassified	
First bite syndrome	Unclassified	Unclassified	
Red ear syndrome	Unclassified	Unclassified	

stabbing, or electric shock–like quality felt in the area innervated by the involved nerve and hence the so-called neuralgia. The pain is often triggered by mild and innocuous stimuli (allodynia). Neuralgia is named according to the nerve involved, with the most common type being trigeminal neuralgia (TN). Other neuralgias include glossopharyngeal and nervus intermedius (geniculate).

Trigeminal neuralgia (ICHD 13.1.1; *ICD-10* G50.0, *ICD-11* 8B82.0; ICOP 4.1.1)

Trigeminal neuralgia (TN), previously known as *tic douloureux*, is a painful condition affecting the face in the distribution of one or more divisions of the trigeminal nerve, most often unilaterally. The condition is characterized by brief (paroxysmal) electric shock–like or lancinating pains that are typically precipitated by nonpainful stimuli, such as washing or lightly touching the face, shaving, talking, or brushing the teeth. Recent data have shed light on the most frequent trigger zone sites,[6] which include the nasal wing (alar rim region), upper lip, cheek and lower lip, plus—importantly—intraoral trigger sites at the upper and lower lateral incisors. The pain may also be spontaneous (untriggered) in nature.

The paroxysmal pains associated with TN are usually severe, with a duration of seconds to a few minutes. Frequently, there is a refractory period following a paroxysm in which an outburst cannot be provoked. Sometimes, several paroxysms will occur in succession and fuse, with the patient describing a longer duration of pain. In addition, some patients who have frequent attacks of pain will describe a longer-lasting burning sensation in the same distribution.

The condition is marked by remission periods lasting days to years during which minimal or no pain is noted. The pain-free intervals usually become shorter and the exacerbations intensify as the neuralgia progresses.[7,8] Attacks usually occur during waking hours but may also awaken the patient from sleep.[9] Clinically, there do not appear to be any neurologic deficits.[4] Attacks can be accompanied by mild autonomic features (such as lacrimation and/or redness of the ipsilateral eye), but this is not typical and cases with autonomic features tend to have longer (~2 minutes) attacks.[10] These new findings in terms of autonomic symptomatology and duration are both accounted for in the most recent version of ICHD within the classical TN grouping.[4] The second and third divisions of the trigeminal nerve are most commonly affected by TN; the first division is affected in only 1% to 2% of patients. The right side of the face is more often involved than the left; it was hypothesized that the nerve on the right side would be more often subject to entrapment because the right side foramen ovale and foramen rotundum are smaller than the left.[11] The pain does not cross the midline of the face, although the condition may affect the face bilaterally in as many as 3% to 5% of patients. The neurologic examination is normal. The average age of onset is approximately 50 years, and the prevalence has been estimated to be 0.16% to 0.3% and incidence at 12.6 to 27.0 per 100,000 person-years, disproportionally affecting more females (60%) than males (40%).[12] There are few data on the differences between ethnic groups and those that are available produce conflicting results. There are very limited indications that TN is more prevalent in white populations as opposed to Black populations. Clinicians should be mindful of data that suggest there may be lower referral rates for neurosurgical procedures in Black populations as opposed to white populations once insurance and socioeconomic status are accounted for.[13] As is commonplace, all management options and their advantages and disadvantages should be carefully explained and patients' understanding and perspectives explored prior to coming to a shared decision on management.

Trigeminal neuralgia is a broad term that can be misinterpreted and unknowingly misused. The ICHD-3 subdivides trigeminal neuralgia into classical trigeminal neuralgia, secondary trigeminal neuralgia, and idiopathic trigeminal neuralgia. *Classical trigeminal neuralgia* (ICHD 13.1.1.1) is TN with no cause identified other than neurovascular compression of the trigeminal nerve in the area of the dorsal root entry zone. The alternate diagnosis in the ICHD TN grouping ("pain attributed to lesion or disease of trigeminal nerve," 13.1) is *painful trigeminal neuropathy* (13.1.2), which accounts for some conditions that might mimic the signs and symptoms of classic TN and would have previously been known as *symptomatic* or *secondary TN* in the previous ICHD (first and second editions). However, it must be noted that conditions in this group typically produce continuous

Box 6-1 Summary of presenting features of classical purely paroxysmal TN and classical TN with concomitant continuous pain as defined by the ICHD[4]

Classical TN, purely paroxysmal

- Recurrent attacks (paroxysms) of unilateral facial pain occurring in one or more of the trigeminal nerve dermatomes with no radiation outside of the affected dermatome(s) affected.
- Pain must have at least three of the following characteristics:
  - Recurring attacks of a paroxysmal nature (duration of attack: from less than 1 second to up to 2 minutes)
  - Severe intensity
  - Character/quality: electric shock, shooting, stabbing, or sharp
  - Triggered by innocuous stimuli to face (some can be spontaneous, but there must be at least three triggered by innocuous stimuli)
- No clinically evident neurologic deficit. It is extremely rare to have deficit and, if present, further investigation is required to exclude occult pathology mimicking TN.
- No persistent pain between attacks.
- Not better accounted for by another ICHD diagnosis.

Classical TN with concomitant continuous pain

- Recurrent attacks fulfilling criteria for classical TN, purely paroxysmal.
- Between paroxysms of pain, there is a persistent or near persistent pain of moderate intensity in the affected dermatome.
- This group of conditions was previously known as atypical TN or TN type 2.

neuropathic pain as opposed to episodic neuropathic pain and therefore were probably not best grouped under the overarching category of TN in the current ICHD. Notwithstanding, continuous neuropathic pain conditions may occasionally produce some symptoms overlapping with TN. This may be clarified with further research and revised in the next edition of the ICHD. TN may also be more accurately considered a secondary neuropathy because it is diagnosed in relation to vascular compression of the trigeminal nerve's dorsal root entry zone.

The ICHD divides classical TN into two subtypes: paroxysmal classical TN (13.1.1.1.1) and classical TN with concomitant continuous pain (13.1.1.1.2; Box 6-1). This is because a significant proportion of classical TN patients describe brief paroxysmal attacks superimposed on a dull background pain. In a recent study, 30% of patients with typical short-duration attacks reported a persistent background pain in addition to the paroxysmal pain.[14] The same study highlighted a subgroup of patients who report attacks lasting more than 2 minutes (according to ICHD criteria, classical TN has a cutoff at 2 minutes); the authors speculated that these patients may be reporting the paroxysm of neuralgic pain and the after pain as one. Previous studies have suggested a correlation between attack duration and disease duration.[15,16] The wider literature suggests that up to 49% of patients experiencing TN can report persistent pain between attacks.[17]

ICOP[5] mirrors the ICHD classification for TN. ICOP presents this within group 4, "Orofacial pain attributed to lesion or disease of the cranial nerves," and is divided into the following three categories: *(1)* classical (4.1.1.1; no other cause better than neurovascular compression), which can either be purely paroxysmal

(4.1.1.1.1) or with concomitant persistent pain (4.1.1.1.2); *(2)* secondary (4.1.1.2), attributable to MS (4.1.1.2.1), space-occupying lesion (4.1.1.2.2), or another cause (4.1.1.2.3); and *(3)* idiopathic (4.1.1.3) with no MRI or electrophysiologic abnormalities demonstrated but presenting as either purely paroxysmal (4.1.1.3.1), or paroxysmal with continuous pain (4.1.1.3.2).

In previous classifications of TN, there had been a defined entity of pretrigeminal neuralgia, but this is now subsumed into the two categories of classical TN in the ICHD and ICOP. However, practitioners should still be aware that it may be possible for patients to present for several months in an almost "prodromal" phase of dull continuous toothache before developing symptoms consistent with classical TN or classical TN with concomitant continuous pain. Successful management of this prodromal state prior to classical TN (with or without concomitant continuous pain) is possible with similar medications as used for classical TN.

Any of the presentations of TN discussed here can present a challenge to the clinician's diagnostic process because they may mimic odontogenic pain, depending on the state of the dentition and the clarity of the patient's history. This might cause clinicians to be led away from a diagnosis of TN. The opposite is also true in that many other conditions can also mimic TN, including painful trigeminal neuropathies arising from infection (eg, herpes zoster) or trauma. According to the ICHD, pathology or disorders producing painful neuropathic symptoms that mimic TN are now classified in a group listed as *painful trigeminal neuropathy* (ICHD 13.1.2) and the ICOP largely mirrors this in group 4 under 4.1.2, "Other trigeminal neuropathic pain": trigeminal neuropathic pain attributed to herpes zoster (4.1.2.1); trigeminal postherpetic neuralgia (4.1.2.2); posttraumatic trigeminal neuropathic pain (4.1.2.3); trigeminal neuropathic pain attributed to another disorder (4.1.2.4); and idiopathic trigeminal neuropathic pain (4.1.2.5).

Pathogenesis

The pathogenesis of classical TN is not completely understood, but there are many hypotheses. Classical TN has been investigated as a result of *demyelination*, the loss of the insulating myelin sheath that separates individual nerve fibers. The cause of the demyelination is most frequently compression of the trigeminal nerve root close to its entry into the pons by overlying blood vessels.[18] This compression and resultant deformation of the trigeminal nerve root and some of its insulating myelin are thought to allow for spontaneous and ectopic nerve firing with ephaptic cross-talk among adjacent fibers (cross-stimulation of C-fibers).[19] This hypothesis may account for the presentation of innocuous stimuli resulting in the spontaneous perception of pain. Some researchers have reported familial TN, suggesting that there are genetic traits that are autosomal dominant. For instance, Charcot-Marie-Tooth disease is an autosomal-dominant sensory motor type I neuropathy that is associated with peripheral demyelination and can therefore produce TN-like symptoms.[20]

Although there appears to be a strong association between demyelination and TN, demyelination theories alone do not account for many of the characteristics of this particular neuropathy. Devor et al[21] proposed the ignition hypothesis, which takes the demyelination theories several steps further. The ignition hypothesis attempts to explain the following phenomena:

- *Triggering:* How a trigger stimulus such as light touch can cause severe pain that long outlasts the stimulus.
- *Amplification:* How the innocuous stimulus results in a response spreading far beyond the area innervated by the originally stimulated nerve fibers.
- *Stop mechanism:* How the pain response is sustained for a period of time and then actually stops itself.

Rappaport and Devor[22] explained 13 out of 14 key features of TN based on neuronal abnormalities related to nerve injury. In most cases, this injury is related to nerve root compression, but other forms of injury may apply. Nerves that are injured become hyperexcitable and therefore may fire with little or no stimulus. These so-called ectopic pacemaker sites may actually be at points of demyelination or at the ends of severed nerves.[21] Some sites may fire continuously at a low level and produce a dull, background, burning pain, and others may require only the slightest stimulation to produce a long-lasting burst of impulses that result in severe pain lasting long beyond the initial stimulus.[23] Nerve fibers may recruit other adjacent fibers and so on, causing short-lasting shooting pain from one point to another. Once ignited, there can be further amplification of the pain by ephaptic transmission or electrical cross-talk between nerve fibers at a site of injury or compression, whereby the adjacent nerve fibers have lost their insulating neural sheaths, allowing direct "short circuit" stimulation. The stop mechanism can be explained by hyperpolarization of the neuron. This stops the burst, and until the ionic imbalance returns to its prestimulation levels, the nerve fiber can no longer be stimulated. Not only is the burst of pain stopped, but it also cannot be triggered again for a period of time. This period is called the *refractory period*.

In the majority of patients who have undergone surgical treatment for TN, microvascular compression of the trigeminal nerve root was identified. These patients mostly responded well to microvascular decompression (MVD) surgery. Compressive damage of trigeminal ganglion has been found in patients as well.[24] If no pathologic factor other than vascular compression is identifiable, the neuralgia is classified as classical TN, previously known as *primary* or *idiopathic TN*. The vast majority (> 85%) of TN patients are diagnosed with classical TN. If the neuralgia is caused by a verifiable lesion—such as a tumor, epidermoid cyst (eg, acoustic neurilemoma or meningioma), cholesteatoma, osteoma, aneurysms, or vascular malformations—it is not classified as TN, but as secondary TN (ICHD 13.1.1.2).[4] Classical TN must therefore also be differentiated from other extracranial causes of facial pain, including local dental disorders, sinus disease, head and neck neoplasms, and infections and headache (or facial pain) associated with a temporomandibular disorder (TMD; ICHD 11.7).

Additionally, three other pain conditions that must be considered in the differential diagnosis are short-lasting unilateral neuralgiform headache attacks with conjunctival injection and tearing (SUNCT; ICHD 3.3), short-lasting unilateral neuralgiform headache attacks with cranial autonomic features (SUNA; ICHD 3.3), and primary stabbing headache (ICHD 4.7). These three conditions predominantly affect the first division of the trigeminal nerve in contrast to classical TN, which mostly involves the second and third divisions. Moreover, autonomic symptoms would usually be a more prominent feature for SUNCT/SUNA. Primary stabbing headache can be distinguished from any form of TN as follows: The frequency of stabbing sensations is usually low; the location of the stabbing sensations often varies; and stab attacks are not precipitated by innocuous stimuli such as touch, cold wind, etc. Imaging studies of the head and brain may be indicated as part of identifying other causes of the pain.

It is important to note that there have been recent data in the form of case reports of familial TN that may offer promise for future therapeutic avenues as well as explain some "tendencies" within families that are anecdotally referred to through generations of the same family. Ion channel mutation has been implicated in the etiology in familial tendencies to TN. A cross-sectional study of 88 patients with TN found 12 patients with a positive family history.[25] Whole exome sequencing was carried out in 11 of these 12 patients and revealed multiple variants in ion channels, including 1 patient who had a gain-of-function mutation in SCN10A (Nav1.8, p.Ala1304Thr), previously reported in a patient with an episodic pain syndrome.

Treatment

The treatment for classical TN can be divided into two modalities: medical and surgical.

MEDICAL MANAGEMENT. Carbamazepine is the most effective medication for classical TN, with a number to treat of 1.9 (95% confidence interval [CI]: 1.6 to 2.5) for > 50% pain relief.[26] The initial response to carbamazepine is good (70%) but drops dramatically (20%) after 5 to 16 years of use.[27] The starting dosage is 100 mg/day, then the dosage is increased by 100 mg every 2 weeks to a maximum of 1,200 mg/day in a divided-dose regimen. A beneficial effect is often apparent within hours to a couple of days after starting this medication. The most common side effects include drowsiness, dizziness, unsteadiness, nausea, and anorexia. These are often transient and can be reduced by starting with a low dose and increasing the dose slowly. Aplastic anemia is a rare side effect, while a transient elevation in liver enzymes may occur in 5% to 10% of patients, and transient leukopenia may manifest in 5% of patients (persistent in 2%). Therefore, patients taking this drug need to have their blood levels carefully monitored for these potential complications. One suggested protocol for monitoring for the side effects of carbamazepine is given by Reisner and Pettengill[28]:

- Perform a complete (full) blood count (CBC) and urea and electrolytes (U&E) pre-administration and every 2 to 4 weeks for the first 3 months. If the total white cell count decreases, then stop usage (this is most likely in the first 3 months).
- Perform liver function tests at baseline and then every 6 weeks. If they are normal for two intervals, then discontinue the tests.
- After close monitoring over the first 3 months, consider checking CBC and U&E every 3 months or twice per year.

A rare complication of carbamazepine use in a white population is Stevens-Johnson syndrome (SJS) or toxic epidermal necrosis (TEN; 0.01% to 0.06% incidence). SJS and TEN are differentiated by the extent of skin detachment, with < 10% body surface involvement for SJS and > 30% for TEN. There is a strong association between a human leucocyte antigen (HLA) allele HLA-B*15:02 and carbamazepine-induced SJS. Only 1% to 2% of white populations are genetic carriers of this allele as opposed to Han Chinese or Thai (Southeast Asian) populations, where 15% of the population are carriers. This results in a much greater risk of SJS in these populations; HLA screening has shown to be cost-effective and is recommended for these populations prior to prescription of carbamazepine by both the US Food and Drug Administration (FDA) in the United States and the Medicines and Healthcare Products Regulatory Agency in the United Kingdom.[29–31] HLA screening (HLA-A*31:01) has also been shown recently to be effective in reducing the incidence of cutaneous adverse reactions to carbamazepine in the Japanese population.[32] As a result, there may be more of a move to global screening for HLA alleles of risk including HLA-A*31:01 and HLA-B*1502 when prescribing carbamazepine for any individual in the future as recommended by the FDA, who added the need for HLA-B*1502 screening to the labeling of carbamazepine.[33]

Sustained or slow-release preparations of carbamazepine have improved compliance and reduce the sedating side effects of the drug. A Cochrane Database systematic review of the efficacy of carbamazepine for the treatment of classical TN revealed only five placebo and three active randomized controlled trials (RCTs). The numbers in the studies that could be evaluated were small but showed that there is evidence that carbamazepine is effective in the treatment of TN.[26]

Oxcarbazepine, a 10-keto-analog of carbamazepine, may be equally effective in the treatment of TN.[34,35] Oxcarbazepine can be started at 150 mg twice daily, increasing the daily dose as tolerated up to 300 to 600 mg twice daily with a maximum dose of 2,400 mg/day. The side effect profile of oxcarbazepine is less severe than that of carbamazepine; however, hyponatremia occurs more frequently when using oxcarbazepine. Oxcarbazepine is now becoming the most likely second drug of choice after carbamazepine and may replace it as the first-choice drug as new evidence emerges.[36] However, it too can cause SJS, and the FDA has also added screening for HLA-B*1502 to its labeling in the United States similar to that for carbamazepine.

Alternatives to oxcarbazepine include augmenting carbamazepine through the use of baclofen, which has a synergistic effect when co-prescribed with carbamazepine.[37] Following this, the next best alternative is lamotrigine, which has been validated for refractory cases, especially in TN due to MS, with doses between 100 and 400 mg daily.[37–39] Side effects may include diplopia, dizziness, headache, and gastrointestinal symptoms. Dermatologic reactions, including SJS, occur in around 0.1% of patients and often present within 2 to 9 weeks of beginning treatment, so lamotrigine should be discontinued as soon as possible at the first sign of any form of rash.[39]

To help prevent rash from escalating, the dose of lamotrigine should not be increased too quickly; a very slow upward taper should be used, eg, 25-mg increments every 2 weeks building toward a target dose of twice daily. Other anticonvulsants lack sufficient evidence to trial them as first- or second-line medications in the absence of specific indications:

- Phenytoin has been prescribed for the treatment of TN. However, long-term success was achieved in only 25% of cases when used alone. The combination of phenytoin and baclofen appears to be more effective.[40] Common side effects are drowsiness, dizziness, and gastrointestinal symptoms.
- Gabapentin may be an alternative treatment. Compared with carbamazepine and phenytoin, gabapentin has minimal side effects and is better tolerated by older patients.[41] However, there are no RCTs specifically investigating the efficacy of phenytoin or gabapentin for TN.[42,43]
- Pregabalin, an antiepileptic drug structurally related to gabapentin, has shown to be efficacious in the treatment of TN in an open-label study and according to patient-reported outcomes.[44,45]
- Topiramate has shown initial promise, and in a meta-analysis comparing topiramate with carbamazepine, it was reported that there seemed to be no differences in the overall effectiveness and tolerability between these two medications in the treatment of classical TN; however, a favorable effect of topiramate was present after a 2-month duration.[46–48] Topiramate can be started at 25 mg once daily, increasing it slowly by 25 mg every 2 weeks, toward a daily dosage of 100 to 400 mg divided twice daily. Side effects include weight loss, somnolence, anxiety, psychomotor disturbance, urinary/renal calculi, and glaucoma. There is also a higher risk of teratogenicity with topiramate, so in the unusual circumstance of prescribing for TN in females of child-bearing age, it is advisable to discuss this and the need for adequate contraception while using the medication.

Cochrane Database systematic reviews concluded that there is insufficient evidence from RCTs to advocate the use of non-seizure medications—including tizanidine, tocainide, proparacaine hydrochloride, pimozide, clomipramine, and amitriptyline—for the treatment of TN. Overall, the methodologic quality of the studies was considered poor, and side effects associated with the medications were common.[49]

EMERGING AND IMPORTANT CONSIDERATIONS ON MEDICAL MANAGEMENT. Botulinum toxin is one locally applied management technique for TN that is gaining interest. This interest has arisen simultaneously with the more general interest in its use for neuropathic pain. In brief, botulinum toxin is thought to exert its therapeutic effect for neuropathic pain through a variety of mechanisms: blocking release of CGRP, substance P, and glutamate both peripherally and centrally (nociceptors, dorsal root ganglia, and spinal cord neurons); decreasing inflammation locally present around nerve terminals; deactivating sodium channels; and decreasing sympathetic nervous system transmission. In vitro cultured trigeminal neurons demonstrate a marked reduction in CGRP release from stimulated neurons when exposed to onabotulinum toxin A (Botox). This is thought to be mediated through botulinum toxin's action on TRPV1 and may account for some of botulinum toxin's effects when used locally in TN.[50]

Current systematic reviews have identified that there are few reproducible studies that substantiate the routine use of botulinum toxin in TN.[51,52] Presently, it might be considered a useful adjunct or alternative to pharmacologic therapy when surgical options are contraindicated due to absence of vascular compression or comorbidities that would complicate the peri- or postoperative course.[53] Most data[51,52] point toward effect on pain intensity being between 30% to 50% reduction beginning within 1 to 2 weeks and lasting from 5 to 24 weeks; intra- or subdermal injections of onabotulinum toxin A of between 20 U to 50 U per trigger site and limit injections to the local trigger site. It is important to inform the patient that it is likely they will have a reversible facial asymmetry as a result of the injections, as this occurs in up to 25% of those receiving treatment. Hu et al[52] suggest this asymmetry reverses quickly, in around 2 weeks, but could last up to 12 weeks.

Novel and target-specific sodium channel blockers are also gaining interest in the management of TN. A targeted Nav1.7 state-dependent selective blocker (Vixotrigine) has recently completed a Phase IIa trial with encouraging results (45% reduction in number of paroxysms; 26% reduction in intensity of paroxysms) and no severe or serious adverse effects.[54] It is now undergoing a Phase III trial in order to fully evaluate its efficacy.[55]

Cannabinoids have been a recent area of interest for the management of a number of chronic pain disorders, including TN. Medical cannabis was studied in a case series of 42 patients with trigeminal neuralgia[56]; 81% of these patients reported improvement in their TN symptoms; adverse effects were reported in 40% of patients, and two patients discontinued the intervention. There is also an anecdotal report of refractory TN responsive to nabiximols in a patient with multiple sclerosis.[57] Given media reporting on cannabis derivatives' efficacy in epilepsy—which is refractory to conventional anti-convulsants—as well as the growth and availability of over-the-counter cannabidiol/cannabis oil, there is growing awareness and public interest in the potential role of cannabis and its derivatives in the management of TN. There is urgent need for randomized controlled studies of cannabidiols for TN.

Tapentadol is a novel analgesic with a dual mechanism of action that combines the complimentary agonism of μ-opioid receptor with inhibition of norepinephrine reuptake. It does possess the potential for dependence and abuse, but the World Health Organization (WHO) concluded that although this was lower than oxycodone, appropriate care must still be taken when prescribing for pain.[58] There has been interest in the use of tapentadol for the management of neuropathic pain. It has demonstrated efficacy for diabetic peripheral neuropathy but so far requires further clinical evaluation in neuropathic facial pain.[59]

Gabapentinoids such as gabapentin and pregabalin can be used for second- or third-line pharmacologic management of TN. They are also recommended as first-line medication for other trigeminal neuropathic pains. In recent years, however, their potential for misuse, abuse, and/or addiction has risen. This has led some countries to recategorize gabapentinoids as controlled drugs similar to benzodiazepines and opioids. In addition, some countries have also restricted the number of days that can be dispensed at any one time. The potential for abuse is believed to be related to concurrent opioid use/abuse and augmenting the euphoria experienced.[60]

Physical dependence on gabapentinoids is known and therefore withdrawal of gabapentinoids is "low and slow." That is a very gradual taper off the medications over weeks/months. There are a number of variations on how to approach this. The authors' slow approach, informed by varying National Health Service guidance in the United Kingdom, is as follows: pregabalin 25 mg decrease in total daily dose every 2 weeks; gabapentin > 900 mg total daily dose decrease total daily dose by 300 mg every 2 weeks, ≤ 900 mg reduce total daily dose by 100 mg every 2 weeks. The risk of abuse is greater with pregabalin than gabapentin due to greater bioavailability which creates a greater euphoric feeling when abused. The at-risk population is those with previous/current substance misuse disorders, especially opioid misuse. The abuse usage usually exceeds therapeutic dosages. The lifetime general population prevalence of nonprescribed pregabalin or gabapentin misuse is estimated at 0.5% to 1%.[61] In pharmacovigilance studies, spontaneous misuse or abuse ranges from 1.5% to 10%.[62] Clinicians must be aware of at risk groups and counsel more generally when prescribing to patients without risk factors. Equally important, clinicians must continue to carefully monitor prescription requests/fulfilment as well as exercising substantial caution when prescribing gabapentinoids in addition to opioids, both in relation to abuse or misuse potential and the cumulative sedative and respiratory effects of co-prescribing.

SURGICAL MANAGEMENT. A number of peripheral and central surgical procedures have been suggested as management techniques for TN.[36] Peripheral surgical techniques include neurectomy, cryotherapy, and alcohol injection. Surgical techniques aimed at the trigeminal (gasserian) ganglion often aim to disrupt or destroy nervous tissue and include radiofrequency thermocoagulation, percutaneous glycerol rhizotomy, and percutaneous balloon microcompression. The central surgical techniques include MVD and stereotactic radiosurgery (gamma knife) surgery.

Neurectomy is a peripheral ablative procedure in which the offending trigeminal nerve branch is avulsed under local or general anesthesia. Success rates for neurectomy are conflicting (50% to 64%), and available studies involve relatively small series with short-term follow-up.[63] Common side effects are hypoesthesias and paresthesias, and pain recurrence is frequent.[64,65]

Cryotherapy is a peripheral ablative procedure in which the offending trigeminal branch is frozen under general or local anesthesia. A specially designed probe allows the procedure to be performed without surgical exposure of the nerve.[66] Generally, the effects of cryotherapy are short lasting (6 to 12 months), although longer pain relief has been reported.[66,67] Side effects may include dysesthesia and/or sensory deficits.

Alcohol injections are performed under local anesthesia. After the affected branch of the trigeminal nerve is anesthetized, a small amount of absolute alcohol is deposited. Compared with neurectomy and radiofrequency thermocoagulation, alcohol blocks result in a higher percentage of recurrence but fewer side effects.[65] Side effects typically include hypoesthesia, paresthesia, and dysesthesia as well as the potential for tissue fibrosis, reactivation of herpes zoster, and bony necrosis.[63] Duration of pain relief is generally less than 1 year. However, the procedure can be repeated without impact on the extent or duration of pain relief. Because of the risk of developing neuropathic pain, peripheral procedures should only be used for patients with significant medical comorbidities that would make other surgical treatments or management techniques unsafe.[63]

Three types of trigeminal ganglion procedures are available for treatment of TN. Percutaneous radiofrequency thermocoagulation and percutaneous glycerol rhizotomy are neurosurgical procedures in which a fluoroscopically guided needle is inserted through the foramen ovale of the patient under sedation. After careful manipulation of the needle and feedback from the patient, the selected nerve fibers are destroyed by thermal lesioning or by injection of anhydrous glycerol. Corneal numbness and masseter weakness are the most common complications of radiofrequency thermocoagulation (10% to 12%). Corneal numbness and dysesthesia are the most common complications of percutaneous glycerol rhizotomy (8% each).[68]

Percutaneous balloon microcompression is a neurosurgical procedure in which the trigeminal nerve is compressed by inflating a tiny balloon in the area of the involved nerve fibers. The needle placement is similar to that of the other two procedures. Reports show high rates of immediate pain relief with balloon compression (91% to 100%), and the recurrence rates at 12 to 18 months were low (2.5% to 5%).[69] A retrospective study with an average follow-up time of almost 11 years reported 19% recurrence within a 5-year period and 32% recurrence over a 20-year period.[70] Side effects of this procedure include numbness and dysesthesia, the severity of which may be related to the amount of compression applied.[69] Transient masseter weakness is also reported frequently. Other complications include arterial and cranial nerve injuries.

An alternative to rhizotomy is MVD of the trigeminal ganglion and dorsal root, first described in 1952 by Taarnhøj[71] in Denmark and by Love[72] in the United States. Jannetta[73] refined and popularized this procedure, which involves a postauricular craniotomy into the posterior fossa, allowing its exploration. The cortex is carefully lifted, exposing the root entry zone of the trigeminal nerve while the offending vessel or lesion responsible for compressing the nerve root is located. The superior cerebellar artery is the most common offending vessel. The vessel is carefully dissected from the trigeminal nerve, and a separator (often some form of sponge) is placed between the structures, often resulting in immediate success. Although MVD appears to have great long-term success in terms of duration of effect and decreased neuropathic adverse effects, a major surgical procedure is required, along with its accompanying morbidity (0.3% to 3%) and mortality.[74] Patient selection is therefore extremely important. Relatively young, healthy patients are the best candidates.

The identification and then selection of patients with sufficiently significant vascular contact for MVD procedures is also problematic. In a recent prospective study from the Danish Headache Centre, 135 patients with classical TN were assessed by high-quality blinded magnetic resonance imaging (MRI).[75] These investigators found that on both the symptomatic and asymptomatic sides (89% and 78%, respectively), some form of contact between the adjacent vasculature and trigeminal dorsal root entry zone was common. However, severe displacement or atrophy of the trigeminal nerve occurred more often on the symptomatic side.

A more minimally invasive method to treat TN is stereotactic neurosurgery (gamma knife surgery). Precisely focused radiation of 40 to 90 Gy emitted from 201 photo beams is applied to the trigeminal root entry zone in the posterior fossa. Compared with other procedures, onset of pain relief is delayed.[76] Reports of pain relief vary from 61% to 92%, while recurrence rates vary from 10% to 27%.[76–79] Dysesthesia is the most prominent side effect related to stereotactic radiosurgery (9%), and this appears to be inversely related with pain control. Repeat surgeries seem to be as efficacious as initial surgeries.[68,80–83] The safety and efficacy of the procedure after more than one repeat surgery have not yet been definitively established, and repeat surgery should be used selectively because limited data are available on the effects of cumulative radiation dose.[84,85] Furthermore, data are also lacking about which patients to treat with a repeat surgery and, when treated with a repeat surgery, which target to aim for and with which dose.[86] From the limited data available, results may suggest that those who developed facial numbness following the first surgery along with a good pain response are more likely to benefit from a second surgery, if required.[83,87]

There are no RCTs comparing different types of surgeries or comparing surgeries with medications for TN. A thorough systematic review including only high-quality studies with actuarial data evaluated the treatment efficacy of radiofrequency thermocoagulation, percutaneous glycerol rhizotomy, percutaneous balloon compression, and stereotactic radiosurgery.[68] This review revealed that, whereas radiofrequency thermocoagulation showed the longest pain relief, the complications, though transient, were also the most frequent. Radiofrequency thermocoagulation and percutaneous glycerol rhizotomy yielded higher percentages of complete pain relief at 6, 12, and 24 months than stereotactic radiosurgery. However, the pain-relieving effects of glycerol rhizotomy rapidly declined after 2 years. It has been reported that MVD and balloon compression have the best prospects to improve the quality of the patient's life. Percutaneous glycerol rhizotomy and radiofrequency thermocoagulation also yielded favorable results, whereas medications were the least likely to improve the patient's quality of life.[88] A systematic review concluded that there is a paucity of high-quality evidence for the efficacy of most neurosurgical procedures (no studies of MVD met inclusion criteria). All the surgical techniques examined in the review produced variable pain relief, but several also resulted in sensory side effects.[89]

The American Academy of Neurology and the European Federation of Neurological Societies have both published guidelines regarding TN management (medical and surgical), and the International Association for the Study of Pain (IASP) neuropathic pain special interest group has also published a review of interventional management in neuropathic pain.[53,90,91] The IASP review concluded that, on the basis of the current evidence, either peripheral procedures are ineffective or there is a lack of evidence of their effectiveness. Based on the current literature, there is inconclusive, low-quality evidence for recommending MVD, radiofrequency or glycerol rhizotomy, balloon compression, or stereotactic radiosurgery; however, consideration should be given to using these in cases of classical TN refractory to medical management because patients seem to benefit from them. The choice between these surgical strategies is based on a level of certainty of diagnosis of TN, sociodemographics, patient preference, patient general health, local expertise, and the presence or absence of vascular compression on MRI. Recent European guidance[53] suggests MVD should be preferred over stereotactic radiosurgery in classical TN patients who have failed pharmacotherapy, have not had previous surgery, and are willing and able to undergo MVD.

Glossopharyngeal neuralgia (ICHD 13.2.1; *ICD-10* G52.1, *ICD-11* 8B87; ICOP 4.2.1)

Glossopharyngeal neuralgia (ICHD 13.2.1) is similar in character to TN but is present in the distribution of the glossopharyngeal nerve and may be present in the distribution of the auricular and pharyngeal branches of the vagus nerve.

The pain is typically severe; transient; stabbing or burning; and located in the ear, base of the tongue, tonsillar fossa, or beneath the angle of the jaw. Estimates of its incidence are fraught with methodologic difficulty but are thought to be about 0.7/100,000 per annum with little sex differentiation, and there are no data available to the authors' knowledge on variations between ethnic groups.[92] The pain is unilateral, although 1% to 2% of patients may experience asynchronous bilateral pain. The paroxysms of pain usually last seconds to 2 minutes and are provoked by swallowing, chewing, talking, or yawning. There may also be concomitant vagal symptoms given the neuroanatomy of the glossopharyngeal and vagus nerves. Glossopharyngeal neuralgia may relapse and remit like TN. The co-occurrence of TN and glossopharyngeal neuralgia is common and expected to occur in 10% to 12% of glossopharyngeal neuralgia patients.[93] The neurologic examination is normal. The pathophysiology is thought to be similar to that of idiopathic TN.

The evaluation of a patient with glossopharyngeal neuralgia should include flexible nasoendoscopy and an MRI scan with contrast to exclude a glossopharyngeal neuralgia secondary to other pathology either centrally or peripherally arising from such pathology as posterior fossa tumors, fusiform (dolichoectatic) vertebral or basilar arterial pathology, vascular anomalies, infection affecting the course of the glossopharyngeal nerve peripherally, and nasopharyngeal tumors. Effective treatment can often be accomplished with the same anticonvulsant medications used for the treatment of TN, such as carbamazepine, oxcarbazepine, baclofen, phenytoin, and lamotrigine, either alone or in combination.[35,94] Surgical procedures include intracranial sectioning of the glossopharyngeal nerve and the upper rootlets of the vagus nerve and MVD of the glossopharyngeal nerve or gamma knife surgery.[95,96]

Nervus intermedius neuralgia (ICHD 13.3.1; *ICD-10* G51.9)

Nervus intermedius neuralgia is a rare condition characterized by unilateral paroxysms of pain felt in the depth of the ear and lasting seconds or minutes. An alternative term used for this condition is *geniculate neuralgia* because the cell bodies of the sensory afferents are located in the geniculate ganglion. There is often a trigger zone in the posterior wall of the auditory canal. Disorders of lacrimation, salivation, and taste are sometimes present. Nervus intermedius neuralgia is now subclassified in the ICHD into classical (13.3.1.1) and secondary nervus intermedius neuropathy (13.3.1.2) An idiopathic version of the diagnosis is also possible within ICHD (13.3.1.3). ICHD also defines painful nervus intermedius neuropathy for patients with a predominant dull deep pain in the ear that is continuous or near continuous (13.3.2). This contrasts with the aforementioned sub-forms for which brief paroxysmal pain is predominant. Painful nervus intermedius neuropathy attributed to herpes zoster (ICHD 13.3.2.1)—previously known as *Ramsay Hunt syndrome*—requires evidence of causation by herpes zoster. The evidence for causation by herpes zoster includes a vesicular eruption in the ear and/or oral mucosa that may have been preceded by pain less than a week before the eruption.[97]

Medications used for TN may be trialed. Surgical section of the nervus intermedius or chorda tympani may relieve the pain. Local ear disorders must be ruled out.

Painful trigeminal neuropathies (ICHD 13.1.2) or other trigeminal neuropathic pain (ICOP 4.1.2)

Consolidated efforts have been made to develop and implement more accurate diagnostic classification of trigeminal neuropathies. ICOP has made this task more transparent, but given that it has been published more recently than ICHD, there are subtle differences in the descriptions by which ICOP classifies these types of pain. These differences mainly relate to the use of "probable" diagnoses under posttraumatic trigeminal neuropathic pain and under trigeminal neuropathic pain attributed to another disorder. Trigeminal neuropathic pain attributed to herpes zoster (ICOP 4.1.2.1) and trigeminal postherpetic neuralgia (4.1.2.2) both simply mirror their counterparts in ICHD (13.1.2.1; 13.1.2.2).

Painful peripheral sensory neuropathies

In its broadest sense, it is possible to consider painful peripheral sensory neuropathies (PPSN) affecting the body to be either primary or secondary.[98] If they are primary, they are neuropathic pain prior to any active intervention or identifiable disorder; in the trigeminal system, this would include conditions previously known as primary *persistent dentoalveolar pain disorder* (PDAP), now known in the new ICOP system as *persistent idiopathic dentoalveolar pain disorder* (PIDAP, 6.3), and persistent idiopathic facial pain (6.2) This type of primary PPSN can be difficult to diagnose because it is poorly understood and, as ICOP now acknowledges, may present with somatosensory changes that mean it mimics neuropathic pain but without any identifiable active intervention prior to its occurrence.

Secondary PPSNs may be due to a variety of disorders, including hereditary sensory neuropathies (eg, Fabry disease), multifocal lesions of the peripheral nervous system (eg, polyarteritis nodosa causing mononeuritis multiplex), and generalized lesions of the peripheral nervous system (eg, polyneuropathies such as diabetes mellitus). Lesions of the CNS (eg, spinal cord injury) and complex neuropathic disorders (eg, complex regional pain syndrome [CRPS] types 1 and 2) may also give rise to neuropathic pain. The most common conditions causing secondary painful trigeminal neuropathies include the following:

- Painful posttraumatic trigeminal neuropathy (PPTTN, ICHD 13.1.2.3) now known as *posttraumatic trigeminal neuropathic pain* in ICOP (4.1.2.3)
- Trigeminal neuropathy attributed to (acute) herpes zoster (ICHD 13.1.2.1 Painful trigeminal neuropathy attributed to herpes zoster)
- Trigeminal postherpetic neuropathy (ICHD 13.3.2.2 Postherpetic neuralgia of nervus intermedius)
- Trigeminal neuropathic pain attributed to other disorder (includes that caused by MS)

Painful posttraumatic trigeminal neuropathy (PPTTN, ICHD 13.1.2.3, No *ICD* reference currently) and posttraumatic trigeminal neuropathic pain (ICOP 4.1.2.3)

Following the reclassification by ICOP, PPTTN/PTTNP is now a very broad group of disorders including conditions such as those previously known as anesthesia dolorosa, atypical odontalgia and secondary persistent dentoalveolar pain disorder, and postsurgical neuropathy/nerve injury. This section covers each of these conditions in turn, but it is to be noted that they all fall under one diagnostic heading of PPTTN/PTTNP, with the key variable to finally determine the diagnosis being advanced diagnostic testing to detect a lesion of the peripheral trigeminal nerve as detailed later. Without this testing, the diagnosis should be stated as *probable* PPTTN/PTTNP.

Anesthesia dolorosa in the second edition of the ICHD (13.18.1) was a painful area of anesthesia or dysesthesia in the trigeminal nerve distribution. It can arise following peripheral or central (neurosurgical) damage to the trigeminal nerve, ganglion, or nuclear complex, such as that occurring in some neurosurgical management strategies for TN. As a type of deafferentation pain, PPTTN/PTTNP is feared most with rhizotomies, but a review revealed a low incidence rate of PPTTN/PTTNP (< 2%) after radiofrequency thermocoagulation and glycerol injections.[68] Balloon microcompression, MVD, and gamma knife surgery have not typically been associated with the development of PPTTN/PTTNP.[77,99–101] In addition to the characteristic pain, a feature of this condition is decreased sensitivity to pain and temperature in one or more divisions of the trigeminal nerve. Accordingly, central pain results from lesions that affect the trigeminothalamic pathways. Very few studies are available regarding the treatment of anesthesia dolorosa. Therefore, treatment remains anecdotal and usually consists of tricyclic antidepressants and anticonvulsants. Microsurgical repair has shown to be effective in only one out of seven patients.[102] Dorsal root entry zone lesioning has shown some promise in the treatment of anesthesia dolorosa, as has sensory thalamic neurostimulation.[103]

What was previously known as *atypical odontalgia and phantom tooth pain* has been subsumed into PPTTN/PTTNP because of the emerging opinion that atypical odontalgia and phantom tooth pain is likely, at least in part, to be neuropathic in origin.[104] This means that if the pain is present in a plausible dermatome with somatosensory changes (negative "loss" or positive "gain") and it began within 6 months of a nerve injury (eg, extirpation or extraction), the pain can be classified as probable PTTNP (ICOP 4.1.2.3.1), and it can be confirmed as PTTNP/PPTTN (ICOP 4.1.2.3) through imaging or surgical exploration demonstrating nerve lesion or with neurophysiologic diagnostic tests such as blink reflex and laser evoked potentials. In essence, the disorders previously grouped under atypical odontalgia are likely to be characterized by the following[104–107]:

- Persistent pain in a defined area of the dentoalveolus for more than 3 months, which can oscillate in intensity
- Pain characteristics that may include dull aching or burning, worsening pain with changes in barometric pressure, pain or pressure feeling deep within the bone, prickly or itching feelings, and difficulty in communicating the nature or character of pain
- Potentially presenting more frequently in females than in males (proposed 3:1)
- Usually following a deafferentation injury (eg, extraction or extirpation)
- Equivocal response to local anesthesia
- More frequent presentations in anterior teeth and in the maxilla

This group of conditions produces a colloquial "phantom tooth pain." This pain may occur in situations of extirpation and root canal treatment of the tooth that is still in situ despite no demonstrable failure of the root canal treatment or through extraction of the tooth and ongoing pain despite demonstrable clinical and radiographic healing. Given the neuropathic nature of PPTTN/PTTNP, management of a diagnosed deafferentation phantom tooth pain follows the same principles of either topical or systemic neuromodulation covered later in this section.

Recent advances in phantom tooth pain diagnosis include the use of quantitative sensory testing (QST) and/or qualitative sensory testing (QualST) as well as the development of a self-report screening instrument.[108–110] QST has shown to be reliable intraorally and highlighted by objective somatosensory differences between patients suffering from atypical odontalgia and control groups.[111,112] QST is, however, a time-consuming and equipment-dependent process, given its uses. There are 13 tests to examine Aδ, Aβ, and C-fiber function and temporal summation (wind-up); therefore, it is not suited for routine everyday clinical practice. QualST is an abbreviated form of QST that achieves results comparable to QST using simpler equipment available in all clinical facilities: cotton wool, an ice-cold spatula, and a dental probe or explorer.[108,109] The ipsilateral affected side is tested for sensory loss or gain compared to the contralateral side. Sensory loss

1. This pain never stops; it seems to always be there.

   STRONGLY DISAGREE | DISAGREE | NEITHER AGREE NOR DISAGREE | AGREE | STRONGLY AGREE

2. This pain moves around, sometimes it seems to be mainly in one area and at other times it seems to be in other areas.

   STRONGLY DISAGREE | DISAGREE | NEITHER AGREE NOR DISAGREE | AGREE | STRONGLY AGREE

3. This pain is a throbbing type of pain.

   STRONGLY DISAGREE | DISAGREE | NEITHER AGREE NOR DISAGREE | AGREE | STRONGLY AGREE

4. This pain wakes me up at night.

   STRONGLY DISAGREE | DISAGREE | NEITHER AGREE NOR DISAGREE | AGREE | STRONGLY AGREE

5. This pain is best described as sharp, stabbing, or electrical bouts of pain that are intense and brief in duration (lasting for seconds or less).

   STRONGLY DISAGREE | DISAGREE | NEITHER AGREE NOR DISAGREE | AGREE | STRONGLY AGREE

6. This pain gets worse with changes of atmospheric pressure, for example during bad weather, scuba diving, airplane travel.

   STRONGLY DISAGREE | DISAGREE | NEITHER AGREE NOR DISAGREE | AGREE | STRONGLY AGREE

7. This pain feels like it is deep within the tooth or jaw bone.

   STRONGLY DISAGREE | DISAGREE | NEITHER AGREE NOR DISAGREE | AGREE | STRONGLY AGREE

8. This pain feels like a pressure within the tooth or jaw bone.

   STRONGLY DISAGREE | DISAGREE | NEITHER AGREE NOR DISAGREE | AGREE | STRONGLY AGREE

9. This pain is difficult for me to describe to others.

   STRONGLY DISAGREE | DISAGREE | NEITHER AGREE NOR DISAGREE | AGREE | STRONGLY AGREE

10. Some words that might help describe my pain include peculiar, itchy, tingling, or prickling feelings.

   STRONGLY DISAGREE | DISAGREE | NEITHER AGREE NOR DISAGREE | AGREE | STRONGLY AGREE

There are NO more questions to answer in this booklet, thank you.

Fig 6-1 Screening instrument for phantom tooth pain/atypical odontalgia (now classified in ICOP under PTTNP and PIDAP and in ICHD under PPTTN) and scoring instructions.[110]

or gain on the ipsilateral side is one indication that PPTTN/PTTNP may be present. It is also possible to examine wind-up using QualST, and a good description of both QST and QualST has been previously reported.[113] A self-report screening instrument consisting of 10 questions (Fig 6-1) has also demonstrated preliminary promise during pilot testing.[110] This screening instrument concentrates on the key features of PPTTN/PTTNP (the phenomenon that was

FOR OFFICE USE (REMOVE THIS TEXT PRIOR TO ISSUING THE INSTRUMENT TO PATIENTS):

Scoring instructions:

–2 to 2 for strongly disagree to strongly agree for all items except for 3, 4, and 5, where reverse scoring is used (ie, strongly agree is –2 and strongly disagree is 2).

To calculate the total score for the screening instrument, we recommend the simple sum method whereby the response scores of all items are summed. The threshold for a positive screen is ≥ 1.

The interpretation of the screening instrument's threshold score being met or exceeded is that it is not likely that the pain is from an odontogenic or TMD cause. Therefore, neuropathic or idiopathic etiologies may be present and further investigation is warranted.

Below is a scored example of the screening instrument (* indicates reverse scoring item):

Item	Response given	Score
1	Strongly agree	2
2	Agree	1
3*	Neither agree nor disagree	0
4*	Disagree	1
5*	Strongly disagree	2
6	Neither agree nor disagree	0
7	Strongly disagree	–2
8	Strongly agree	2
9	Neither agree nor disagree	0
10	Strongly agree	2
	Total score (sum)	**8**

Interpretation of score: Exceeds threshold of 1 and therefore patient's pain is not likely to be of odontogenic or TMD etiology.

previously described as "atypical odontalgia") within the patient's complaint as described earlier.

Risk factors for any postsurgical neuropathy

Prevention of chronic postsurgical pain with or without neuropathy may be possible. Risk factors evident in diseases and disorders affecting other areas of the body may translate to the orofacial region. Considerations for identification of risk factors may include some of the following[114,115]:

1. Operative risk factors
   - Non-minimal access surgery
   - Lack of use of local anesthetic
   - Poor perioperative pain management
2. Patient factors
   - Fear of pain and surgery, psychologic factors including catastrophizing, anxiety, depression, and other factors
   - Chronic widespread pain or fibromyalgia

Elective surgery should be avoided in patients who may be vulnerable to, or already suffering from, neuropathic pain. Suspicion of neuropathic pain may be heightened by preoperative screening for unusual presentations of pain before and after previous surgery. Neuropathic pain can develop slowly over time, so clinicians should always be cognizant of its potential to emerge over the months following surgery. Diagnosis requires clinical and psychologic assessment and quantitative and or qualitative sensory assessment (see above). ICOP has incorporated the recent suggestions from Finnerup et al[116] and Devine et al[117] to ensure that the label of probable PPTTN/PTTNP is applied rather than PPTTN/PTTNP if imaging, surgical exploration, or neurophysiologic diagnostic testing for nerve lesions/injury is not confirmatory.

There are validated diagnostic screening tools available to help identify any neuropathic pain pre- or postoperatively, although to date the sensitivity and specificity of these instruments are deemed low when used with trigeminal neuropathies.[118,119] The screening tools include the following:

- Leeds Assessment of Neuropathic Symptoms and Signs (LANSS) or its self-reported version (S-LANSS)
- Neuropathic Pain Questionnaire (NPQ)
- Douleur Neuropathique en 4 (DN4)
- painDETECT
- ID-Pain

Performing preoperative screening for patient-specific factors such as the following prior to surgery may also help predict the risk of postsurgical neuropathy:

- *Genetics:* Haplotype for catechol-O-methyltransferase is the most studied single nucleotide polymorphism implicated in postsurgical pain, but others include SCN90A, GCH1, IL10, IL1R2, KCNS1, OPRM1, and P2RX7.[120]
- *Preceding pain:* Intensity and chronicity
- *Psychosocial factors:* Anxiety, depression, fear avoidance, self-efficacy, work, levels of physical activity, somatization, anxiety, and catastrophizing
- *Younger age:* Increased risk of neuropathic pain following breast surgery and herniorrhaphy
- *Older age:* Increased risk of neuropathic pain following other surgery
- *Female sex:* Increased risk of neuropathic pain[114]

Preoperative medication may play a role in minimizing the development of posttraumatic neuropathic pain, but the evidence is limited. In a systematic review of prevention and management of chronic postsurgical (neuropathic) pain, the authors found that while some studies have shown the benefit of perioperative pregabalin in reduction of chronic pain development at 6 and 12 months, others have demonstrated no difference.[121,122] Martinez et al in a more recent systematic review[123] identified no difference in the development of chronic postsurgical pain when comparing treatment with pregabalin or a placebo. Gabapentinoids may have an impact on reducing the development of chronic postsurgical (neuropathic) pain. However, more comprehensive studies are required.

Surgical risk factors may be potentially modifiable. They include the duration and extent of surgical procedure and technique (eg, tension due to retraction of tissues) and level of reported perioperative pain intensity. Modifications to account for these risk factors may include the following:

- Multimodal management of severe acute postsurgical pain
- Minimal access surgery
- Intraoperative use of local anesthesia when patient is undergoing general anesthetic

Assessment

As is commonplace in assessing orofacial pain, the clinician must conduct a holistic evaluation of the patient's pain history, the functional impact, and the psychologic consequences of the pain. The area of neuropathy must be qualified and mapped out within the dermatome distribution of the damaged sensory nerve (Fig 6-2).[124] The ipsilateral and contralateral unaffected dermatome should be subject to at least the following basic mechanosensory examination whether there is sensory gain or loss: Assess the patient's response to light touch (eg, cotton wool), painful stimuli (eg, sharp probe or explorer), and thermal challenge (eg, cold spatula). Visual inspection and palpation should be used to examine for any autonomic changes in color, temperature, sweating, and swelling. Elicited mechanical and thermal allodynia and/or hyperalgesia will reinforce diagnosis of neuropathic pain when there is hyperesthesia rather than a hypoesthetic nerve injury (anesthesia or paresthesia).

There is a role for judicious use of investigations as determined by the presenting patient, their history, and the examination findings. These investigations may include the following:

- Hematologic tests to exclude systemic causes of neuropathy, including CBC, thyroid function tests, C-reactive protein, autoantibody screen, erythrocyte sedimentation rate, creatinine, alanine transaminase, vitamin B_{12}, ferritin, folate, and serum protein immunoelectrophoresis
- HbA1c to assess for risk of diabetes or level of glycemic control in patients known to have diabetes

Imaging of varying forms, such as plain films, computed tomography (CT), or MRI, may be used. Most often, local imaging (eg, cone beam CT) or plain films are indicated if there is a definite history of local damage (eg, mandibular third molar removal or implant placement), but an MRI scan may be indicated if centrally mediated sensory neuropathy is suspected. The recent development of MR neurography may have an emerging role over the next few years in early postsurgical assessment of nerve injuries.[125]

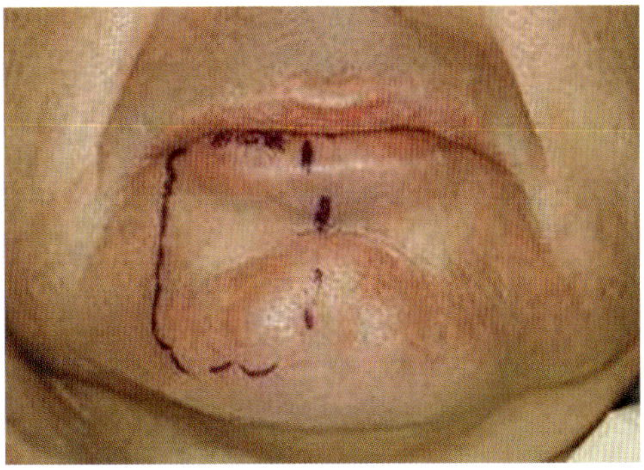

Fig 6-2 Photograph of delineated area of neuropathy at time of initial examination.

Management of PPTTN/PTTNP

A recent Cochrane review[126] concluded that there is a lack of high-quality trials to investigate the effectiveness of all forms of management for iatrogenic inferior alveolar and lingual nerve injuries. Thus, management of PPTTN/PTTNP is mainly extrapolated from other types of neuropathy affecting other areas of the body.

Most patients suffering from iatrogenic inferior alveolar and lingual nerve injuries present with PPTTN/PTTNP mixed with numbness and altered sensation.[124] The pain the patient is experiencing must be assessed, including the related functional and psychologic impact.[127] These aspects must then be managed alongside the pain using psychologic interventions if the patient accepts the important role that psychologic therapies have in managing neuropathic pain. For most patients, it is necessary to use multiple strategies that are tailored to the individual patient's complaint.[128]

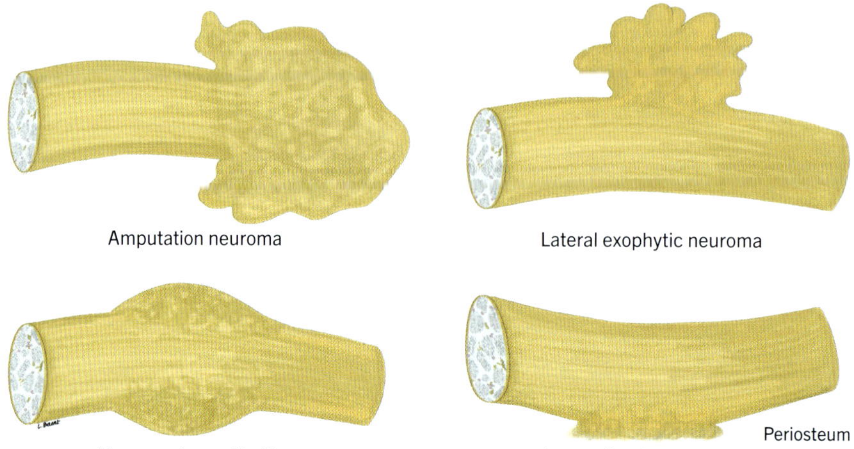

Fig 6-3 Different types of neuromata following macroscopic injury to peripheral branches of trigeminal nerve.

The mechanism of injury drives decision-making and timing of the management of trigeminal nerve injuries. Surgery is urgently indicated for inferior alveolar and lingual nerve injuries related to third molar, implant, or endodontic surgery within 30 hours and rarely up to 3 months but not later.[128] Broad principles for surgical approaches are to immediately repair if a nerve section is identified (by the operator) and to remove an implant within 24 hours of placement if compression by an implant is thought to be the cause. Surgery is not indicated to explore inferior alveolar nerve injuries older than 4 weeks. Exploratory surgery for lingual nerve injuries should occur within 1 to 3 months of injury, but recent data also show that if delayed, positive outcomes can still result.[129–132] A recent case series using cadaveric nerve grafts also demonstrates promise in lingual and inferior alveolar nerve repair where direct anastomoses of nerve stumps is either impossible or inappropriate, eg, due to quality of neural tissue or extrinsic contamination.[133]

Immediate pharmacologic therapy may be indicated alongside surgery for acute sensory nerve injuries. Early management with a corticosteroid taper for 5 to 7 days followed or replaced by 3 weeks of NSAIDs may help reduce the chance of neuropathy following injury.[134–136] If a painful trigeminal nerve injury has been delayed in its presentation to the consulting clinician, or is not associated with a clear-cut macroscopic trauma amenable to surgery, then there may be indications for different pharmacologic therapy.

Tooth extraction or explantation (ie, removal of implant) should be urgently considered in postendodontic and implant-related nerve injuries presenting with neuropathic pain. Earlier surgical exploration may be indicated for lingual nerve injury related to third molar surgery when a CBCT confirms breech of the lingual plates by bur (or chisel). It is crucial, however, to appreciate that surgery is extremely unlikely to resolve neuropathic pain,[137] but for patients with hypoesthetic nerve injuries, early intervention surgery using human cadaver–treated nerve grafts may hold promise for (some) resolution of the hypoaesthesia.[138] Surgical exploration will likely define the type of neuromata and nerve damage (Fig 6-3), but these are not directly correlated with clinical features.[133] As stated earlier, there is an emerging role for MR neurography in the early postsurgical evaluation of suitability for early surgical repair.[125]

Considerations in the case of delayed painful presentations include topical and/or systemic pharmacotherapeutic agents:

TOPICAL AGENTS FOR PAIN. Topical lidocaine 4% or 5% (12 hours on and 12 hours off) patches should be applied to facial skin away from mucous membranes and eyes.[139] Capsaicin either as a cream (0.025%, 0.033%, 0.075%, or 0.10%) or as an 8% patch can be used on the skin to help manage neuropathic pain through its substance P–depleting effects, although the 8% patch is not yet licensed for use in the facial region and the effects of capsaicin in general can be limited by poor tolerance of the burning effect when applied over the first 2 to 4 weeks.[140]

Other compounded off-label topical uses of systemic neuromodulatory agents are also available.[141] Practitioners should be aware of recent concerns about the lack of preclinical safety studies for such topical medications.[142]

BOTULINUM TOXIN. There are a number of recent case reports using botulinum toxin for PPTTN/PTTNP.[143–147] The therapeutic mechanisms of action of botulinum toxin in these cases likely remain similar to those detailed under its use for the management of TN earlier in this chapter.

SYSTEMIC AGENTS FOR PAIN. There are guidelines for the medical management of neuropathic pain in adults.[148–151] The medications used may include selective serotonin-norepinephrine reuptake inhibitors (SSNRIs; venlafaxine, duloxetine, or milnacipran), tricyclic antidepressants (amitriptyline or nortriptyline), or anticonvulsants (pregabalin or gabapentin).

Postsurgical neuropathic pain is rare and not well recognized in the field of dentistry. Current management strategies are extrapolated from evidence from other neuropathic conditions. Thus, research is needed to provide sufficient evidence regarding assessment and management of posttraumatic trigeminal nerve injuries.[152]

Trigeminal neuropathy attributed to (acute) herpes zoster (ICHD 13.1.2.1; ICOP 4.1.2.1)

Chicken pox is caused by the varicella zoster virus (VZV). Following the initial infection with the VZV, the virus remains dormant in the cell bodies of sensory nerves and may reactivate many years later. This type of reactivation is known as *herpes zoster* (or *shingles* in layperson's terms). The incidence rate of herpes zoster is an estimated 0.03% to 0.05%. Herpes zoster largely affects elderly patients or those with impaired immunity. Symptoms of herpes zoster generally include itching, numbness, or a tingly sensation in the affected dermatome, followed by blisters and pain. Most people heal without sequela in about 3 to 4 weeks, but in a small number of people (28.2 to 42 out of 100,000), persistent sensory disturbances or pain may occur.[153] There are now vaccines available to help decrease or prevent herpes zoster in people over the age of 50 years.

Management of the acute pain of painful trigeminal neuropathy attributed to acute herpes zoster will be determined by consideration of a number of factors: degree of symptoms, presence of lesions on the face or eyes, age and immunologic status of the host, and other comorbidities. Antiviral, corticosteroid, and tricyclic antidepressant medications have all been suggested to try to help manage the acute pain and reduce the risk of postherpetic neuropathy.[154] Cochrane reviews, however, cast doubt on the roles of both antiviral and corticosteroid medications in helping prevent postherpetic neuropathy, but they are thought to be beneficial in the management of the acute pain of painful trigeminal neuropathy attributed to acute herpes zoster.[155,156] Because of the immunosuppressive effect of corticosteroids, they should not be given without antivirals.

Trigeminal postherpetic neuropathy (ICHD 13.1.2.2; *ICD-10* B02.22; ICOP 4.1.2.2)

Most people heal completely from an episode of herpes zoster within 3 to 4 weeks without any persisting sequelae. However, some people may have irreversible damage to the skin and sensory disturbances. Whereas persisting or recurrent pain is infrequent in the general population, postherpetic trigeminal neuropathy (previously known as *postherpetic neuralgia*) may affect 50% to 75% of the older population who have had herpes zoster, and its incidence varies from 28.2 per 100,000 persons to 42 per 100,000 persons, depending on the country of study.[153,157] The ICHD describes postherpetic trigeminal neuropathy as unilateral pain developing in temporal relationship to an acute herpes zoster infection that affected one or more branches of the trigeminal nerve and lasting for 3 months or more. The pain usually has a burning character, but there may be superimposed brief, stabbing exacerbations of pain. Postherpetic trigeminal neuropathy may be accompanied by hyperalgesia and allodynia or by profound sensory loss and anesthesia dolorosa. Risk factors for developing postherpetic trigeminal neuropathy include female sex, older age, experience of a prodrome, severe rash, and severe pain.[158]

The pathophysiology of postherpetic trigeminal neuropathic pain is still largely unknown, but peripheral and central mechanisms have been suggested. Cell destruction at the level of the dorsal horn and loss of cutaneous nerve endings have been implicated.[159,160] Baron[161] proposed three different types of postherpetic trigeminal neuropathies: one based on peripheral and central sensitization, one based on predominant degeneration of nociceptive neurons, and one mainly based on skin deafferentation. Depending on the type of underlying mechanism, different symptoms may prevail, and different treatment modalities might be more successful. The existence, value, and implications of this differentiation must be further evaluated.

According to a recent systematic review, the anticonvulsants gabapentin (1,800 mg and 3,600 mg per day) and pregabalin (150 to 600 mg per day) show satisfactory pain relief, as does the tricyclic antidepressant amitriptyline (25 to 150 mg per day).[149] Topical lidocaine has also been advocated for treatment of postherpetic trigeminal neuropathy. To date, there are not enough data to support the use of the newer antidepressants in postherpetic trigeminal neuropathy, but if the conventional medications fail or produce too many side effects, a trial of these medications may be indicated. The efficacy of opioids in postherpetic trigeminal neuropathy is as yet uncertain.[162]

Trigeminal neuropathic pain attributed to another disorder (ICHD 13.1.2.4; ICOP 4.1.2.4)

There are a number of potential causes for this presentation, including space-occupying lesions or disease. The only difference between secondary TN and this category are the clinical characteristics of this category:

- Quality/character and duration of pain is different to neuralgia: continuous or near continuous burning, squeezing, aching, or "pins and needles." Brief paroxysms may occur but are not predominant.
- Evoked pain may or may not be present.
- Somatosensory changes (gain/loss, negative/positive) may be present.

In MS particularly, pain is a common and sometimes multifactorial problem with its pathophysiology being due to either central or peripheral pathology and often dependent on plaque location.

Migraine-type headaches can develop as a consequence of MS or its treatment (ie, interferon).[163] MS is known for its association with the development of TN, and this is likely to be due to the long-term damage to the trigeminal nerve root entry zone.

MS increases the risk of developing TN by a factor of 20.[164] The nature of TN in MS does not usually differ from classical TN other than being more frequently bilateral. Bilateral TN (14% to 31% in MS) or TN in a young patient may be indicative of underlying MS.[165] TN will precede MS in only 0.3% of patients.[166] Interestingly, only a minority of patients with MS show vascular compression of the trigeminal nerve root. Decompression procedures on these few specific patients often relieve the neuralgia-like symptoms.[167] Management of this type of pain is the same as that of TN.

Central Neuropathic Pain (ICHD 13.13)

This new category in the ICHD is subdivided into central neuropathic pain attributed to MS and central poststroke pain (CPSP).

Central neuropathic pain attributed to MS (ICHD 13.13.1)

Pain is a frequent symptom in MS and may have a variety of potential mechanisms, including pain resulting from the disease process, but also pain as a result of the disability. Any lesion from the spinal dorsal horn or spinal trigeminal nucleus to the cerebral cortex can cause central neuropathic pain attributed to MS.

Neuropathic pain in MS shares the generic features of neuropathic pain as previously described. This pain may be episodic or constant, although constant pain is more typical. With the exception of some of the stereotyped manifestations (such as TN, optic neuritis, or painful tonic spasms), the clinical features of the neuropathic pain in MS are often not specific for the site of the lesion or the underlying pathology. Anecdotally, central neuropathic pain affecting the face and head attributed to MS is much less frequent than TN. Diagnostic pointers for central neuropathic pain attributed to MS include evidence of CNS disease, distribution of pain (sometimes regional or cranial nerve or occasionally root), and the presence of other neurologic symptoms or signs (mostly sensory).

Central poststroke pain (ICHD 13.13.2; *ICD-10* G89.0, *ICD-11* MG30.50)

Central poststroke pain (CPSP) is characterized by unilateral facial or head pain, dysesthesia, and impaired sensation to pinprick and temperature that occurs within 6 months of a stroke and is not due to a lesion of the trigeminal nerve (with imaging demonstrating a lesion in an appropriate site). CPSP is attributed to a lesion somewhere along the spinothalamic pathway and by definition is the result of a vascular lesion (eg, ischemic or hemorrhagic infarction). The pain is not limited to the facial and cranial area; similar symptoms may be experienced in the entire half of the body contralateral to the infarction (such as after a thalamic stroke). Similar pain can be produced by lesions that involve the ascending pain pathways elsewhere in the CNS, and the term *central pain* is used to indicate such involvement.

Few RCTs investigating treatment modalities for CPSP have been performed. A 2006 systematic review identified amitriptyline and lamotrigine as the most effective medications, followed by mexiletine and phenytoin.[168] Carbamazepine did not appear effective, whereas gabapentin, although promising, was not studied sufficiently. This review also indicated that intravenous ketamine, propofol, and lidocaine might be helpful for short-term treatment. Invasive procedures may have a place when pharmacologic management fails. The available data are mostly anecdotal but suggest that deep brain stimulation and cortical stimulation may be helpful.[169]

Neurodegenerative Diseases as Causes for Central Pain

There is a growing awareness that neuropathic pain can be an important feature of neurodegenerative conditions.[170] This has been perhaps best defined in Parkinson disease, a degenerative neurologic disorder with motor and nonmotor features. Pain is a common symptom in patients with Parkinson disease.[171] This includes primary pain (ie, central pain arising from the CNS) and secondary pain (eg, pain arising from the musculoskeletal system). Central pain in Parkinson disease is estimated to have a prevalence of 10% to 12%.[171] Central pain is recognized in a number of different areas, including the mouth, rectum, vagina, abdomen, chest, and testes. Fil et al[171] have reviewed pain in Parkinson disease and propose that it might result from pathologic changes in structures involved in the nociceptive system. In some patients, this pain might respond to dopaminergic therapy, but conventional analgesics and tricyclic antidepressants are recommended otherwise.

Tolosa-Hunt syndrome (ICHD 13.8; *ICD-10* H51.9)

Tolosa-Hunt syndrome is characterized by episodes of orbital pain accompanied by paralysis of one or more of cranial nerves III, IV, or VI. One or more of these nerves will contain lesions caused by granulomatous inflammation of superior orbital fissure, cavernous sinus, or orbit as demonstrated by MRI or biopsy. More specific differential diagnoses should be considered, including vasculitis or vascular, neurologic, inflammatory, infiltrative, or space-occupying processes, such as pseudotumor of the orbit, temporal arteritis, and ophthalmoplegic migraine. Episodes are said to have a duration of 8 weeks in untreated patients; patients experience relief of pain within 72 hours of initiation of corticosteroid therapy. If suspected, referral to a neurologist is recommended.

Complex regional pain syndrome (CRPS) (no ICHD category; *ICD-10* G90.50, *ICD-11* 8D8A)

Complex regional pain syndrome (CRPS) is a term that has been coined to replace two different disorders of the autonomic nervous system. CRPS 1 has been proposed to replace the term *reflex sympathetic dystrophy* (*ICD-10* G90.59, *ICD-11* 8D8A.00), and CRPS 2 has been proposed to replace the term *causalgia*, also described as *mononeuritis* (*ICD-10* G58.9, *ICD-11* 8D8A.01). The replacements have not been widely accepted, and the older terms are still frequently used.

According to the IASP, CRPS is characterized by persistent, often burning pain accompanied by allodynia and hyperalgesia and at some point accompanied by swelling, changes in blood flow, and/or abnormal sudomotor activity. In CRPS 1, the symptoms occur after a mild injury and are disproportionate to the initiating event, whereas in CRPS 2, there is evidence of nerve damage preceding the persistent pain. A 2007 revision to the IASP criteria has been proposed.[172] The criteria include four symptom categories, of which at least three must be reported and at least two must be present at the time of evaluation. The four categories consist of sensory, vasomotor, sudomotor/edema, and motor/trophic changes. The distinction between CRPS 1 and CRPS 2 was maintained, and a third diagnosis, *CRPS not otherwise specified* (*ICD-10* G90.50, *ICD-11* 8D8A.0Z), was added for patients not fully meeting the criteria.

The pathophysiology of CRPS remains unclear, and it may be peripherally or centrally mediated and of neuropathic, inflammatory, or immunologic origin.[173] Estimates of the incidence of CRPS range between 5 and 26 cases per 100,000 persons.[174,175] Women are afflicted about three times more often than men.[174] CRPS is typically found in the upper or lower extremities, with the upper extremities more often involved than the lower extremities, and it is not generally described as occurring in the head and neck. A review of the available literature between 1947 and 2000 identified only 13 cases with head and neck involvement.[176] The typical features, such as loss of function and skin atrophy, were rarely seen, and therefore, the diagnoses in most of these cases were debatable.

In some cases of CRPS, the peripheral nociceptors become sensitive to adrenergic stimulation. In those cases, any increase in activity of the sympathetic nervous system is likely to increase the pain experience. Increased levels of emotional stress and even visual or auditory stimuli can markedly increase the pain intensity. Typically, this pain is responsive to sympathetic blockade, and in such cases, the term *sympathetically maintained pain* is appropriate. Studies trying to resolve which features (eg, mechanical allodynia, cold allodynia) might predict a favorable response to sympathetic blockade have shown contrasting results.[177–179] High anxiety levels, litigation, and disability may be related to poor treatment response to a sympathetic blockade.[178]

Treatment of CRPS generally includes physical rehabilitation, psychologic interventions, and pharmacologic management.[173,180] Few RCTs with adequate sample sizes are available with regard to the treatment of CRPS, and no particular pharmacologic or intervention strategy appears to stand out. Therefore, at this time, pharmacologic treatment should follow the treatment paradigms for neuropathic pain. In the case of sympathetically maintained pain, a series of sympathetic blocks is indicated.[181]

Other Conditions Potentially Associated with Some Elements or Signs and Symptoms of Neuropathy

Through both ongoing research and the creation of ICOP, some disorders now sit between neuropathy and idiopathic etiologies and are included in this chapter because it is the most appropriate situation for them. These include the following:

- Burning mouth syndrome (ICOP 6.1)
- Persistent idiopathic facial pain (ICOP 6.2)
- Persistent idiopathic dentoalveolar pain disorder (ICOP 6.3)
- Occlusal dysesthesia or phantom bite syndrome (unclassified in ICHD and ICOP, as it does not cause pain)
- Numb chin syndrome (unclassified as a distinct entity in ICHD and ICOP, as it does not cause pain)
- Red ear syndrome
- First bite syndrome

Burning mouth syndrome (ICHD 13.11; *ICD-10* K14.6, *ICD-11* DA0F.0; ICOP 6.1)

Burning mouth syndrome (BMS) is "characterized by unremitting oral burning or similar pain for more than two hours per day over three months in the absence of detectable oral mucosal changes."[5,182] If BMS has been present for less than 3 months, it should be defined as probable BMS until the pain has remained for more than 3 months. Within ICOP, BMS is defined as having a purely idiopathic etiology with or without somatosensory changes detectable with qualitative or quantitative sensory testing. According to ICOP definition, BMS is a primary pain condition and all systemic and local causes must be excluded (Box 6-2[183,184]). ICOP also states that if there are secondary conditions, they should be

Box 6-2 Local and systemic factors thought to be potentially causative for secondary burning symptoms in the mouth[183,184]

Local factors
- Alcohol-based mouthwash
- Allergy (serum IgE and patch test for dental materials patient is exposed to)
- Chewing tobacco use
- Ciguatera neurotoxin exposure
- Dehydration, mouth breathing, or nasal obstruction
- Gastric reflux
- Infection (bacterial, fungal, viral)
- Mechanical (trauma or reduced tongue space from poorly fitting prostheses)
- Oral lesions: erosive lichen planus; geographic tongue; leukoplakia, neoplasia, pemphigoid; pemphigus; vesiculobullous conditions
- Parafunctional habits
- Stomatitis: allergy-induced, aphthous,radiation-induced
- Xerostomia (salivary flow rate)

Systemic factors
- Autoimmune conditions (Sjögren syndrome)
- Endocrine: diabetes mellitus (HbA1c), hypothyroidism (thyroid function tests), menopause
- *Helicobacter pylori* (antibodies to *H pylori*)
- Medication (eg, angiotensin-converting enzyme inhibitors, angiotensin II receptor blockers, antiretrovirals, psychotropic, anticholinergic, clonazepam, chemotherapeutic agents)
- Neuropathy: nutritional neuropathy (check serum ferritin, vitamins B1, B6, B12, folate, and zinc); peripheral neuropathy due to systemic disease (eg, HIV, sarcoidosis, MS)

Ig, immunoglobulin.

Examinations should reflect those undertaken for peripheral neuropathies and conditions listed earlier in the chapter. If any of the factors listed above are discovered to contribute to the burning mouth symptoms, then a diagnosis of 1.2.1, oral mucosal pain, according to ICOP, should be made.

coded within section 1.2.1 "Oral mucosal pain." Recent efforts have been made alongside ICOP to provide a more comprehensive set of research diagnostic criteria to help ensure homogeneity and comparability of sample cohorts in future studies.[185]

BMS is a poorly understood pain condition that most probably has elements of neuropathy with both peripheral and central components. Reported prevalence rates of burning mouth symptoms in general populations vary from 0.7% to 15%, with variation likely based on whether a study was a survey or a clinical assessment, the population assessed, and the geographic location under study.[186–188] Burning mouth symptoms appear most commonly in postmenopausal women—12.2% in the 50–69-year age group—and are extremely rare in both men and women under the age of 30 years.[186]

The burning pain of BMS commonly presents with a bilateral symmetric distribution, with the most frequently affected areas including the anterior two-thirds, dorsum, and lateral borders of the tongue; the anterior hard palate; and the mucosa of the lower lip; it often occurs in more than one oral site.[189,190] Onset often appears to be spontaneous in around 50% of patients; however, 17% to 33% of patients may attribute the onset of pain to an upper respiratory tract infection, a previous dental procedure, or medication use (including antibiotics). Others report that onset of symptoms occurred following traumatic life stressors.[188,189] Symptoms may be continuously present for significant periods of time (months to years) without cessation or remission, and only a small number (3% of patients within 5 years of onset) demonstrate complete remission.[191] Burning is usually a constant daily phenomenon, and around one-third of patients experience symptoms both day and night.[186,189] Most patients report minimal symptoms on awakening, after which the symptoms crescendo through the day toward the evening. A large proportion of patients experience intensification of the burning related to presence of personal stressors and fatigue or eating acidic, hot, or spicy foods. Equally, however, a proportion of patients report reduction or alleviation of burning through oral intake or stimulation and distraction.[192]

BMS is associated with many possible factors, including anxiety, depression, and personality disorders, particularly in postmenopausal women, but it is unclear if pain initiates the psychologic disorder or vice versa.[184,186,193,194] Approximately 21% of BMS patients present with significant psychologic distress, but BMS patients show no evidence of significant clinical depression, anxiety, and somatization. Moreover, BMS patients report less interference in their daily activities than other chronic pain patients.[195]

There are various regional and local phenomena that have been associated with BMS. These include altered parotid gland function and salivary composition.[196,197] BMS patients generally exhibit greater vasoreactivity, suggesting involvement of the autonomic nervous system.[198] Evidence supports two theories for etiology, but conclusive data are still unavailable, hence BMS sits within the idiopathic categorization of ICOP: *(1)* a neuropathic imbalance between the gustatory and sensory systems; or *(2)* a peripheral and/or central sensory neuropathy. A role for some form of neuropathy in BMS seems likely given that varying somatosensory changes (gain or loss) have repeatedly been identified in some patients with BMS.[199,200]

It is thought that inhibitory influences between the gustatory and sensory systems help to maintain a sensory balance in the tongue. Hypothetically, therefore, disruption in this equilibrium through altered chorda tympani dysfunction could then lead to lingual nerve hyperfunction and a neuropathic-based burning sensation. The role of an imbalance between the gustatory (chorda tympani or glossopharyngeal) and sensory systems (lingual or glossopharyngeal) is uncertain, especially given that gray matter changes are present in the pain matrix of those with BMS as opposed to dysgeusia, but there are data supporting interplay between sensory and gustatory trigeminal pathways.[201–203] Further studies are needed to elucidate this complex and putative relationship.

BMS may result not only from hyperactivity of the sensory component of the trigeminal nerve following loss of central inhibition but also from damage to the chorda tympani.[204–206] This damage results in reduced inhibition of the trigeminal nerve that in turn leads to an intensified response to oral irritants and eventually to neuropathic pain. The exact mechanisms and interactions, however, are obscure, and the evidence is unclear.

A sensory neuropathy is suggested by findings that the sensory threshold in the tongue was significantly higher in BMS patients than in controls.[207,208] BMS patients have a significantly lower density of epithelial nerve fibers in the anterior two-thirds of the tongue, with some correlation to symptom duration.[209,210] Experimental evidence suggests the existence of several diagnostic BMS-neuropathy subgroups, including peripheral neuropathy and centrally mediated pain.[203,211–215] Studies examining the identification of a predominantly peripherally driven BMS as opposed to a predominantly centrally driven BMS have used a lingual block to make this determination. They have demonstrated that topical medication, specifically clonazepam, is more effective in those with a peripherally driven BMS and that its therapeutic effect may be mediated by γ-aminobutyric acid A (GABA-A) receptors present on peripheral afferents in the tongue.[216,217]

Management options for BMS are limited because of the incomplete understanding of the etiology and pathophysiologic processes for this disorder. Current treatment approaches include the following, which can be combined[140]:

- Cognitive behavioral approaches
- Topical management using analgesics, anxiolytics, artificial sweeteners, and low-level laser therapy
- Systemic management using antidepressants, anticonvulsants, and atypical analgesics or antipsychotics

One of the most intensively investigated pharmacologic agents for BMS is clonazepam, for which there are meta-analysis data supporting its efficacy both systemically and topically.[218] A recent clinical evidence update suggests that cognitive behavioral therapy is likely to be beneficial and that there is a trade-off between risks and benefits with the use of clonazepam, given its potential for dependency.[219] The same review suggests that α-lipoic acid, benzydamine hydrochloride, selective serotonin reuptake inhibitors (SSRIs), and tricyclic antidepressants are of unknown effectiveness.

Persistent idiopathic facial pain (ICHD 13.12; *ICD-10* G50.9, *ICD-11* 8A85; ICOP 6.2)

This category has historically been referred to as *atypical facial pain*. It is a term that when applied essentially means that no absolute mechanism or characteristics can be determined that allow the presenting pain to be assigned to any other diagnostic category. It may or may not belong in a neuropathic pain classification given the wide variation in its presentation as only some of this continuum represents potential neuropathy.[181] The incidence of persistent idiopathic facial pain is estimated at 4.4 per 100,000 person-years, and lifetime prevalence is estimated at 0.03% with a predilection for presenting in middle-aged to older women.[199,220,221]

The current ICHD and ICOP suggests that persistent idiopathic facial pain can be diagnosed only when pain is present for more than 3 months, occurring daily with episodes of pain lasting for greater than 2 hours, in a poorly localized manner, and following an unrecognized dermatome pattern. ICOP goes further, allowing classification with and without somatosensory changes on use of qualitative or quantitative sensory testing. The character of persistent idiopathic facial pain can be described in a variety of ways, including a dull aching, nagging quality. It is also prone to acute exacerbations, with one of the aggravators being stress. It may present with psychiatric comorbidity and significant psychosocial disability. Prior to the diagnosis, all other local or systemic causes and intracranial causes (eg, intracranial mass lesions) must be excluded. This may require additional assessment by an otorhinolaryngologist and/or a neurologist. In the process of evaluating potential other types of underlying pathology, hematologic and imaging investigations may be necessary, including an MRI of the head and/or face to exclude intra- and extracranial causes of the pain. QST may also be of benefit to determine if there are any neuropathic elements contributing to the overall pain picture of persistent idiopathic facial pain.[199]

As there are no RCTs that include large samples of patients with persistent idiopathic facial pain, treatment typically relies on therapies proven successful in studies for other persistent orofacial pains, predominantly cognitive behavioral therapy and/or any of the following therapeutic agents: tricyclic antidepressants, SSNRIs, gabapentin, and pregabalin.[222,223]

Persistent idiopathic dentoalveolar pain disorder (unclassified in ICHD; ICOP 6.3)

This diagnostic grouping in ICOP accounts for those pains well-localized intraorally to a dentoalveolar segment or site when there has not been a potentially causative dental/surgical intervention in that region recently, ie, > 6 months since last intervention, as otherwise it would be categorized under 4.1.2.3 under PTTNP. Previous names for this new grouping include primary persistent dentoalveolar pain disorder, and atypical odontalgia that was not closely temporally associated with a deafferentation injury.

The pain is usually well-localized and rarely occurs in multiple sites. Its character is variable, but it is included in the self-report screener in Fig 6-1 on pages 138–139. It can be described as dull, deep, and pressure-like and may be prone to exacerbations.[105] To make the diagnosis, pain should be present for more than 2 hours per day for more than 3 months without a causative event being closely temporally related. If pain is present for less than 3 months, a "probable" diagnosis can be made until the 3-month threshold is surpassed. Local causes must have been excluded, and appropriate imaging should also have been completed to formalize the diagnosis. Rarely, somatosensory changes that are not confined to a neuroanatomically defined region are present, and therefore, ICOP allows for this diagnosis with and without somatosensory changes as determined by qualitative or quantitative sensory testing. Management of this condition is ill-defined and follows that of persistent idiopathic facial pain.

Occlusal dysesthesia, also known as phantom bite syndrome/occlusion (unclassified in ICHD and ICOP)

Patients with occlusal dysesthesia (OD) present with a primary complaint of an uncomfortable and/or incorrect occlusion, usually accompanied by emotional distress.[224,225] Even though this is largely unverifiable, OD patients are convinced of the validity of their complaints and the belief that mechanical and/or surgical dental interventions will accomplish correction.[224] Repeated and failed treatments by clinicians serve to reinforce the patient's potentially hypervigilant state in respect to the occlusion and/or that something is seriously wrong with the occlusion.[226–230] Clinicians often pursue a course of multiple occlusal readjustment appointments, which usually results in increasingly distressing symptomatology reported by the patient. Reassurances that the patient suffers from no occlusal problems usually induce further distress.

The onset of OD can occur at any stage of dental treatment. However, patients typically associate the origin of phantom bite syndrome with the construction of extensive dental prostheses.[231] OD is observed in all age groups with no clear sex predilection; adolescents undergoing orthodontic treatment may also experience OD.[224,232] OD is usually painless; when pain accompanies OD in patients with a history of extractions or multiple surgical interventions, an additional diagnosis of peripheral painful traumatic trigeminal neuropathy should be considered. Patients with OD may describe the need for repositioning of the mandible (often protrusion) to obtain some relief. Further complaints may include the feeling that the tongue is too big or disturbed sensations in the gingiva.[225]

Whether OD is a neuropathic disorder is debatable. Originally, patients with OD were considered to be suffering from a form of monosymptomatic hypochondriacal psychosis, which is an uncommon psychiatric disorder characterized by a single delusion as the sole symptom.[224,233] Although OD cases are often characterized by a number of psychosocial disorders, current thinking links the initiating pathophysiology to physical components.[231,234,235] The first possibility is occlusal hyperawareness or iatrogenic dysproprioception.[236] Following changes in the dental occlusion, it is necessary to adapt to or relearn new jaw movements and proprioception. Patients with OD suffer because they are unable to adapt to even small changes in the dental occlusion. Additionally, patients with OD may become distressed by the lack of familiarity of their own bite. This is based on the theory that the sensation derived through tooth contact acts as a self-identifier.[225,233] In other words, when placing one's teeth together, one confirms the "self." A further possibility is that when tissue damage (apicoectomies, extractions, implants) has formed part of the initiation of OD, the pathophysiology may be due to neuropathic mechanisms, as occurs in traumatic neuropathy.[225] Peripheral painful traumatic neuropathy may present with disturbed proprioception, allodynia, and pain, explaining the symptomatology of OD.[15] In many ways, it is similar to the "phantom pain" described by amputees—hence the original term *phantom bite*.

Pain in OD may arise from comorbid traumatic neuropathy, and this should be treated accordingly. Comorbidity of OD with TMDs has been reported, and although successful therapy of the TMD does not alleviate symptoms of OD, it improves the patient's quality of life.[231,237] Treatment of OD itself is difficult—any further attempts to "equilibrate" the occlusion or grind down specific areas that bother the patient will usually lead to no improvement or worsening of symptoms.[238] Based on case reports, the use of acrylic guards does not relieve OD symptoms.[231] In a small case series, the use of milnacipran, an SSNRI, improved OD symptoms in five out of six patients.[239] A psychiatric consultation or a psychologic assessment is a specific consideration. A combined approach beginning with a behavioral medicine consultation and initiation of SSNRI therapy is recommended. A serious attempt must be made to demonstrate the futility of any further interventions, and patients should be encouraged to adopt a coping approach incorporating relaxation and cognitive behavioral therapy.[230,240]

Numb chin syndrome

Having outlined the various subtypes of painful trigeminal neuropathies present, it is pertinent to mention and clarify a predominantly non-painful condition whose definition and use seems to have gained favor in recent years. This increase in use is presumably, and understandably, because of its desirable facilitatory function in teaching as a simple heuristic, but its use has no real taxonomic or ontologic basis. The condition is *numb chin syndrome*, which is essentially a form of mental or inferior alveolar nerve (partial) sensory loss. The features of this syndrome are anesthesia, paresthesia, and—very occasionally—dysesthesia in the mental dermatome.[241] It is likely that those with dysesthesia were misdiagnosed with this "syndrome" and should have been classified under ICOP 4.1.2 ("Other trigeminal neuropathic pain").

Sensory disturbance in the mental dermatome can be caused by a variety of events, disorders, or diseases, including dental procedures (eg, local anesthesia, implants, surgical endodontics) and pathologies (eg, odontogenic infection or neoplasia in close proximity to the nerve).

The presence of signs and symptoms of numb chin syndrome should not be dismissed in the absence of odontogenic causes, because they can be related to (occult) local or systemic malignant neoplastic conditions.[242–244] In recent years, numerous case reports have been published indicating a wide variety of underlying causes, including but not limited to MS, use of antiresorptive medications (bisphosphonates), vagal and hypoglossal paralysis, leukemic vasculitis, non-Hodgkin lymphoma, B-cell lymphoma, and other metastatic cancers. Under these circumstances, immediate referral to the relevant medical practitioner is paramount. Signs and symptoms of numbness should not be dismissed, because they play an important part in ensuring health professionals are aware of its potential red flag status. It does not, however, constitute a diagnosis, and because it is rarely painful, it does not fit well into the current ICHD or ICOP unless it is painful and/or is due to either a systemic or traumatic cause.

Red ear syndrome (unclassified in ICHD and ICOP)[245]

As the name suggests, this rare and painful condition affects the auricle/pinna of the ear. There is a burning pain and an erythema that affects the auricle for 30 to 60 minutes in the majority of cases described in the literature, although some individuals have experienced the symptoms for up to 4 hours. The attacks occur daily, and individuals may experience up to 20 attacks in a day. Attacks may be triggered (heat, touch, physical exercise, neck movement) or occur spontaneously.

The maximum intensity is sometimes felt in the ear lobe, and pain may radiate to the cheek, mandible, and occiput. It can present bilaterally or unilaterally and may or may not be side-locked. There is only a very slight female preponderance of 1.25:1 female to male, and the condition usually presents in the fourth and fifth decades.

It is an exceedingly rare condition with around 100 cases described in the literature since first being described by Lance in 1994.[246] Its etiology and pathophysiology therefore remain enigmatic, and hence it remains unclassified in ICHD.

Red ear syndrome has been reported secondary to TMD, upper cervical spine pathology, and thalamic lesions, and therefore, MRIs of brain and C-spine are warranted. In the primary variant of the syndrome, there has been a focus on trigemino-autonomic dysregulation. As Lambru et al[245] point out though, the parasympathetic facial outflow is not known to be capable of initiating vasodilation in the ear because this is controlled by the sympathetic nervous system. However, it may be similar to trigeminal autonomic cephalalgias, where there is a sympathetic deficit at the same time as increased parasympathetic outflow to the ear thereby resulting in erythema.

Management is somewhat empirical, and the following have been helpful in limited cases reported in the literature: ice packs, greater auricular nerve block, NSAIDs, tricyclic antidepressants, serotonergic agonists and antagonists, beta-blockers, calcium channel blockers, and anticonvulsants, of which gabapentin has been the most tried medication while providing benefit.

First bite syndrome (unclassified in ICHD and ICOP)[247,248]

This syndrome was first described in 1986 and is now accepted as presenting as a sudden and intense pain in the parotid region associated with the first bite of some food. The pain intensity usually is extreme, then decreases slowly with each subsequent bite, but this feature can substantially vary between individuals. In the majority (~95%) of cases, the syndrome generally occurs either days or months after a variety of upper neck surgery, such as lymph node dissection, parapharyngeal* and infratemporal* space surgery, (deep lobe*) parotid surgery, cervical sympathetic chain surgery,* carotid artery surgery, and styloid process resection (* indicates greater probability with this type of surgery). It may also occur following radiosurgery in the trigeminal region.[249]

In a small number of cases, the condition arises spontaneously without surgery, and in these cases, appropriate imaging of the ipsilateral parapharyngeal space as well as the parotid and submandibular glands is crucial to exclude occult malignancy because this is the most frequent cause of spontaneous onset of first bite syndrome. Clinicians should also consider repeat imaging if the condition continues without abatement in the event that the first imaging is negative, because there are cases within the literature where pathology has developed over time.

The pathophysiology of the condition is thought to relate to an imbalance between the parasympathetic and sympathetic supply to the parotid gland's myoepithelial cells, resulting in an intense contraction of these cells with first bite. This imbalance is purported to be brought about through surgical trauma or malignant tumor (in cases without surgical intervention) affecting parts of those neural systems. Although this somewhat simplistic explanation is attractive, it is likely that the mechanisms are more multifactorial and yet to be fully understood.

Management of this syndrome that has been reported to be effective in the literature includes time itself in helping to resolve symptoms over the space of 12 months, intraparotid injection of botulinum toxin, and anticonvulsants alone or in combination with tricyclic antidepressants. There are, however, no trial data on the definitive management of this condition.

References

1. Costigan M, Scholz J, Woolf CJ. Neuropathic pain: A maladaptive response of the nervous system to damage. Annu Rev Neurosci 2009;32:1–32.
2. International Association for the Study of Pain. Terminology. 2017. https://www.iasp-pain.org/resources/terminology/. Accessed 16 Aug 2022.
3. Jensen TS. Mechanisms of neuropathic pain. In: Pain 1996: An Updated Review: Refresher Course Syllabus. Seattle: IASP, 1996:77–86.
4. The International Classification of Headache Disorders, 3rd edition. Cephalalgia 2018;38:1–211.
5. International Classification of Orofacial Pain, 1st edition (ICOP). Cephalalgia 2020;40:129–221.
6. Di Stefano G, Maarbjerg S, Nurmikko T, Truini A, Cruccu G. Triggering trigeminal neuralgia. Cephalalgia 2018;38:1049–1056.
7. Cheshire WP. Trigeminal neuralgia: Diagnosis and treatment. Curr Neurol Neurosci Rep 2005;5:79–85.
8. Truini A, Galeotti F, Cruccu G. New insight into trigeminal neuralgia. J Headache Pain 2005;6:237–239.
9. Devor M, Wood I, Sharav Y, Zakrzewska JM. Trigeminal neuralgia during sleep. Pain Pract 2008;8:263–268.
10. Haviv Y, Khan J, Zini A, Almoznino G, Sharav Y, Benoliel R. Trigeminal neuralgia (part I): Revisiting the clinical phenotype. Cephalalgia 2016;36:730–746.
11. Neto HS, Camilli JA, Marques MJ. Trigeminal neuralgia is caused by maxillary and mandibular nerve entrapment: Greater incidence of right-sided facial symptoms is due to the foramen rotundum and foramen ovale being narrower on the right side of the cranium. Med Hypotheses 2005;65:1179–1182.
12. Bendtsen L, Zakrzewska JM, Heinskou TB, et al. Advances in diagnosis, classification, pathophysiology, and management of trigeminal neuralgia. Lancet Neurol 2020;19:784–796.
13. Reinard K, Nerenz DR, Basheer A, et al. Racial disparities in the diagnosis and management of trigeminal neuralgia. J Neurosurg 2017;126:368–374.
14. Benoliel R, Zini A, Khan J, Almoznino G, Sharav Y, Haviv Y. Trigeminal neuralgia (part II): Factors affecting early pharmacotherapeutic outcome. Cephalalgia 2016;36:747–759.
15. Benoliel R, Zadik Y, Eliav E, Sharav Y. Peripheral painful traumatic trigeminal neuropathy: Clinical features in 91 cases and proposal of novel diagnostic criteria. J Orofac Pain 2012;26:49–58.
16. Di Stefano G, La Cesa S, Truini A, Cruccu G. Natural history and outcome of 200 outpatients with classical trigeminal neuralgia treated with carbamazepine or oxcarbazepine in a tertiary centre for neuropathic pain. J Headache Pain 2014;15:34.
17. Cruccu G, Di Stefano G, Truini A. Trigeminal neuralgia. N Engl J Med 2020;383:754–762.
18. Jannetta PJ. Arterial compression of the trigeminal nerve at the pons in patients with trigeminal neuralgia. J Neurosurg 1967;26:159–162.
19. Love S, Coakham HB. Trigeminal neuralgia: Pathology and pathogenesis. Brain 2001;124:2347–2360.
20. Coffey RJ, Fromm GH. Familial trigeminal neuralgia and Charcot-Marie-Tooth neuropathy. Surg Neurol 1991;35:49–53.
21. Devor M, Amir R, Rappaport ZH. Pathophysiology of trigeminal neuralgia: The ignition hypothesis. Clin J Pain 2002;18:4–13.
22. Rappaport HZ, Devor M. Trigeminal neuralgia: The role of self-sustaining discharge in the trigeminal ganglion. Pain 1994;56:127–138.
23. Lisney SJW, Devor M. Afterdischarge and interactions among fibers in damaged peripheral nerve in the rat. Brain Res 1987;415:122–136.
24. Beaver DL. Electron microscopy of the gasserian ganglion in trigeminal neuralgia. J Neurosurg 1967;26:138–150.

25. Di Stefano G, Yuan JH, Cruccu G, Waxman SG, Dib-Hajj SD, Truini A. Familial trigeminal neuralgia—Asystematic clinical study with a genomic screen of the neuronal electrogenisome. Cephalalgia 2020;40:767–777.
26. Wiffen PJ, Derry S, Moore RA, Kalso EA. Carbamazepine for chronic neuropathic pain and fibromyalgia in adults. Cochrane Database Syst Rev 2014;4: CD005451.
27. Taylor JC, Brauer S, Espir ML. Long-term treatment of trigeminal neuralgia with carbamazepine. Postgrad Med J 1981;57:16–18.
28. Reisner L, Pettengill CA. The use of anticonvulsants in orofacial pain. Oral Surg Oral Med Oral Pathol Oral Radiol Endod 2001;91:2–7.
29. Chen Z, Liew D, Kwan P. Real-world efficiency of pharmacogenetic screening for carbamazepine-induced severe cutaneous adverse reactions. PLoS One 2014;9:e96990.
30. Locharernkul C, Shotelersuk V, Hirankarn N. Pharmacogenetic screening of carbamazepine-induced severe cutaneous allergic reactions. J Clin Neurosci 2011;18:1289–1294.
31. Oomens MA, Forouzanfar T. Pharmaceutical management of trigeminal neuralgia in the elderly. Drugs Aging 2015;32:717–726.
32. Mushiroda T, Takahashi Y, Onuma T, et al. Association of HLA-A*31:01 screening with the incidence of carbamazepine-induced cutaneous adverse reactions in a Japanese population. JAMA Neurol 2018;75: 842–849.
33. Ferrell PB, McLeod HL. Carbamazepine, HLA-B*1502 and risk of Stevens-Johnson syndrome and toxic epidermal necrolysis: US FDA recommendations. Pharmacogenomics 2008;9:1543–1546.
34. Royal M, Wienecke G, Movva V, et al. Open label trial of oxcarbazepine in neuropathic pain. Pain Med 2001;2:250–251.
35. Zakrzewska JM, Patsalos PN. Oxcarbazepine: A new drug in the management of intractable trigeminal neuralgia. J Neurol Neurosurg Psychiatry 1989;52: 472–476.
36. Zakrzewska JM, Linskey ME. Trigeminal neuralgia. BMJ 2014;348:g474–g474.
37. Jorns TP, Zakrzewska JM. Evidence-based approach to the medical management of trigeminal neuralgia. Br J Neurosurg 2007;21:253–261.
38. Leandri M, Lundardi G, Inglese M, et al. Lamotrigine in trigeminal neuralgia secondary to multiple sclerosis. J Neurol 2000;247:556–558.
39. Zakrzewska JM, Chaudhry Z, Nurmikko TJ, Patton DW, Mullens LE. Lamotrigine (Lamictal) in refractory trigeminal neuralgia: Results from a double-blind placebo controlled crossover trial. Pain 1997;73:223–230.
40. Fromm GH, Terrence CF, Chattha AS. Baclofen in the treatment of trigeminal neuralgia: Double-blind study and long-term follow-up. Ann Neurol 1984;15:240–244.
41. Cheshire WP Jr. Defining the role for gabapentin in the treatment of trigeminal neuralgia: A retrospective study. J Pain 2002;3:137–142.
42. Birse F, Derry S, Moore RA. Phenytoin for neuropathic pain and fibromyalgia in adults. Cochrane Database Syst Rev 2012;2012:CD009485.
43. Wiffen PJ, Derry S, Bell RF, et al. Gabapentin for chronic neuropathic pain in adults. Cochrane Database Syst Rev 2017;6:CD007938.
44. Obermann M, Yoon MS, Sensen K, Maschke M, Diener HC, Katsarava Z. Efficacy of pregabalin in the treatment of trigeminal neuralgia. Cephalalgia 2008;28: 174–181.
45. Pérez C, Navarro A, Saldaña MT, Martínez S, Rejas J. Patient-reported outcomes in subjects with painful trigeminal neuralgia receiving pregabalin: Evidence from medical practice in primary care settings. Cephalalgia 2009;29:781–790.
46. Gilron I, Booher SL, Rowan JS, Max MB. Topiramate in trigeminal neuralgia: A randomized, placebo-controlled multiple crossover pilot study. Clin Neuropharmacol 2001;24:109–112.
47. Solaro C, Uccelli MM, Brichetto G, Gaspperini C, Mancardi G. Topiramate relieves idiopathic and symptomatic trigeminal neuralgia. J Pain Symptom Manage 2001;21:367–368.
48. Wang Q-P, Bai M. Topiramate versus carbamazepine for the treatment of classical trigeminal neuralgia. CNS Drugs 2011;25:847–857.
49. Zhang J, Yang M, Zhou M, He L, Chen N, Zakrzewska JM. Non-antiepileptic drugs for trigeminal neuralgia. Cochrane Database Syst Rev 2013;12:CD004029.
50. Mittal SO, Safarpour D, Jabbari B. Botulinum toxin treatment of neuropathic pain. Semin Neurol 2016; 36:73–83.
51. Shackleton T, Ram S, Black M, Ryder J, Clark GT, Enciso R. The efficacy of botulinum toxin for the treatment of trigeminal and postherpetic neuralgia: A systematic review with meta-analyses. Oral Surg Oral Med Oral Pathol Oral Radiol 2016;122:61–71.
52. Hu Y, Guan X, Fan L, et al. Therapeutic efficacy and safety of botulinum toxin type A in trigeminal neuralgia: A systematic review. J Headache Pain 2013;14:72.
53. Bendtsen L, Zakrzewska JM, Abbott J, et al. European Academy of Neurology guideline on trigeminal neuralgia. Eur J Neurol 2019;26:831–849.
54. Zakrzewska JM, Palmer J, Morisset V, et al. Safety and efficacy of a Nav1.7 selective sodium channel blocker in patients with trigeminal neuralgia: A double-blind, placebo-controlled, randomised withdrawal phase 2a trial. Lancet Neurol 2017;16:291–300.

55. Kotecha M, Cheshire WP, Finnigan H, et al. Design of phase 3 studies evaluating vixotrigine for treatment of trigeminal neuralgia. J Pain Res 2020;13:1601–1609.
56. Mechtler L, Hart P, Bargnes V, Saikali N. Medical cannabis treatment in patients with trigeminal euralgia (P5.10-020). Neurol 2019;92:P5.10-020.
57. Gajofatto A. Refractory trigeminal neuralgia responsive to nabiximols in a patient with multiple sclerosis. Mult Scler Relat Disord 2016;8:64–65.
58. WHO. WHO expert committee on drug dependence. World Health Organ Tech Rep Ser 2012;(973):1–26.
59. Freo U, Romualdi P, Kress HG. Tapentadol for neuropathic pain: A review of clinical studies. J Pain Res 2019;12:1537.
60. Goodman CW, Brett AS. Gabapentinoids for pain: Potential unintended consequences. Am Fam Physician 2019;100:672–675.
61. Kapil V, Green JL, Le Lait MC, Wood DM, Dargan PI. Misuse of the γ-aminobutyric acid analogues baclofen, gabapentin and pregabalin in the UK.[letter]. Br J Clin Pharmacol 2014;78:190–191.
62. Hägg S, Jönsson AK, Ahlner J. Current evidence on abuse and misuse of gabapentinoids. Drug Saf 2020;43:1235–1254.
63. Peters G, Nurmikko TJ. Peripheral and gasserian ganglion-level procedures for the treatment of trigeminal neuralgia. Clin J Pain 2002;18:28–34.
64. Murali R, Rovit RL. Are peripheral neurectomies of value in the treatment of trigeminal neuralgia? An analysis of new cases and cases involving previous radiofrequency gasserian thermocoagulation. J Neurosurg 1996;85:435–437.
65. Oturai AB, Jensen K, Eriksen J, Madsen F. Neurosurgery for trigeminal neuralgia: Comparison of alcohol block, neurectomy, and radiofrequency coagulation. Clin J Pain 1996;12:311–315.
66. Pradel W, Hlawitschka M, Eckelt U, Herzog R, Koch K. Cryosurgical treatment of genuine trigeminal neuralgia. Br J Oral Maxillofac Surg 2002;40:244–247.
67. Zakrzewska JM, Thomas DGT. Patient's assessment of outcome after three surgical procedures for the management of trigeminal neuralgia. Acta Neurochir (Wien) 1993;122:225–230.
68. Lopez BC, Hamlyn PJ, Zakrzewska JM. Systematic review of ablative neurosurgical techniques for the treatment of trigeminal neuralgia. Neurosurg 2004;54:973–983.
69. Lee S-T, Chen J-F. Percutaneous trigeminal ganglion balloon compression for treatment of trigeminal neuralgia, part II: Results related to compression duration. Surg Neurol 2003;60:149–153.
70. Skirving DJ, Dan NG. A 20-year review of percutaneous balloon compression of the trigeminal ganglion. J Neurosurg 2001;94:913–917.
71. Taarnhøj P. Decompression of the trigeminal root and the posterior part of the ganglion as treatment in trigeminal neuralgia. J Neurosurg 1952;9:288–290.
72. Love JG. Decompression of the gasserian ganglion and its posterior root for trigeminal neuralgia. Postgrad Med 1954;15:1–4.
73. Jannetta PJ. Treatment of trigeminal neuralgia by suboccipital and transtentorial cranial operations. Neurosurg 1977;24:538–549.
74. Kalkanis SN, Eskandar EN, Carter BS, Barker FG. Microvascular decompression surgery in the United States, 1996 to 2000: Mortality rates, morbidity rates, and the effects of hospital and surgeon volumes. Neurosurg 2003;52:1251–1262.
75. Maarbjerg S, Wolfram F, Gozalov A, Olesen J, Bendtsen L. Significance of neurovascular contact in classical trigeminal neuralgia. Brain 2015;138:311–319.
76. Henson CF, Goldman HW, Rosenwasser RH, et al. Glycerol rhizotomy versus gamma knife radiosurgery for the treatment of trigeminal neuralgia: An analysis of patients treated at one institution. Int J Radiat Oncol Biol Phys 2005;63:82–90.
77. Kondziolka D, Perez B, Flickinger JC, Habeck M, Lunsford LD. Gamma Knife radiosurgery for trigeminal neuralgia. Arch Neurol 1998;55:1524.
78. McNatt SA, Yu C, Giannotta SL, Zee C–H, Apuzzo ML, Petrovich Z. Gamma Knife radiosurgery for trigeminal neuralgia. Neurosurg 2005;56:1295–1303.
79. Sheehan J, Pan H-C, Stroila M, Steiner L. Gamma Knife surgery for trigeminal neuralgia: Outcomes and prognostic factors. J Neurosurg 2005;102:434–441.
80. Dvorak T, Finn A, Price LL, et al. Retreatment of trigeminal neuralgia with Gamma Knife radiosurgery: Is there an appropriate cumulative dose. J Neurosurg 2009;111:359–364.
81. Huang C-F, Chiou S-Y, Wu M-F, Tu H-T, Liu W-S. Gamma Knife surgery for recurrent or residual trigeminal neuralgia after a failed initial procedure. J Neurosurg 2010;113:172–177.
82. Kimball BY, Sorenson JM, Cunningham D. Repeat Gamma Knife surgery for trigeminal neuralgia: Long-term results. J Neurosurg 2010;113:178–183.
83. Park KJ, Kondziolka D, Berkowitz O, et al. Repeat gamma knife radiosurgery for trigeminal neuralgia. Neurosurg 2012;70:295–305; discussion 305.
84. Aubuchon AC, Chan MD, Lovato JF, et al. Repeat Gamma Knife radiosurgery for trigeminal neuralgia. Int J Radiat Oncol Biol Phys 2011;81:1059–1065.
85. Helis CA, Lucas JT Jr, Bourland JD, Chan MD, Tatter SB, Laxton AW. Repeat radiosurgery for trigeminal neuralgia. Neurosurg 2015;77:755–761.

86. Tuleasca C, Carron R, Resseguier N, et al. Repeat Gamma Knife surgery for recurrent trigeminal neuralgia: Long-term outcomes and systematic review. J Neurosurg 2014;121(suppl):210–221.
87. Park SC, Kwon DH, Lee DH, Lee JK. Repeat Gamma-Knife radiosurgery for refractory or recurrent trigeminal neuralgia with consideration about the optimal second dose. World Neurosurg 2016;86:371–383.
88. Spatz AL, Zakrzewska JM, Kay EJ. Decision analysis of medical and surgical treatments for trigeminal neuralgia: How patient evaluations of benefits and risks affect the utility of treatment decisions. Pain 2007;131:302–310.
89. Zakrzewska JM, Akram H. Neurosurgical interventions for the treatment of classical trigeminal neuralgia. Cochrane Database Syst Rev 2011;2011:CD007312.
90. Cruccu G, Gronseth G, Alksne J, et al. AAN-EFNS guidelines on trigeminal neuralgia management. Eur J Neurol 2008;15:1013–1028.
91. Dworkin RH, O'Connor AB, Kent J, et al. Interventional management of neuropathic pain: NeuPSIG recommendations. Pain 2013;154:2249–2261.
92. Manzoni GC, Torelli P. Epidemiology of typical and atypical craniofacial neuralgias. Neurol Sci 2005;26 (suppl 2):s65–s67.
93. Rushton JG, Stevens JC, Miller RH. Glossopharyngeal (vagoglossopharyngeal) neuralgia: A study of 217 cases. Arch Neurol 1981;38:201–205.
94. Rozen TD. Trigeminal neuralgia and glossopharyngeal neuralgia. Neurol Clin 2004;22:185–206.
95. Kondo A. Follow-up results of using microvascular decompression for treatment of glossopharyngeal neuralgia. J Neurosurg 1998;88:221–225.
96. Stieber VW, Bourland JD, Ellis TL. Glossopharyngeal neuralgia treated with Gamma Knife surgery: Treatment outcome and failure analysis. J Neurosurg 2005;102:155–157.
97. Aguggia M. Typical facial neuralgias. Neurol Sci 2005;26:s68–s70.
98. Baron R. Mechanisms of disease: Aeuropathic pain—A clinical perspective. Nat Clin Pract Neurol 2006;2:95–106.
99. Brown JA, Pilitsis JG. Percutaneous balloon compression for the treatment of trigeminal neuralgia: Results in 56 patients based on balloon compression pressure monitoring. Neurosurg Focus 2005;18:1–5.
100. Chang JW, Chang JH, Park YG, Chung SS. Microvascular decompression in trigeminal neuralgia: A correlation of three-dimensional time-of-flight magnetic resonance angiography and surgical findings. Stereotact Funct Neurosurg 2000;74:167–174.
101. Gorgulho A, De Salles AA, McArthur D, et al. Brainstem and trigeminal nerve changes after radiosurgery for trigeminal pain. Surg Neurol 2006;66:127–135.
102. Gregg JM. Studies of traumatic neuralgia in the maxillofacial region: Symptom complexes and response to microsurgery. J Oral Maxillofac Surg 1990;48:135–140
103. Nashold BS, el-Naggar A, Mawaffak Abdulhak M, Ovelmen-Levitt J, Cosman E. Trigeminal nucleus caudalis dorsal root entry zone: A new surgical approach. Stereotact Funct Neurosurg 1992;59:45–51.
104. Baad-Hansen L. Atypical odontalgia – Pathophysiology and clinical management. J Oral Rehabil 2008; 35:1–11.
105. Durham J, Exley C, John MT, Nixdorf DR. Persistent dentoalveolar pain: The patient's experience. J Orofac Pain 2013;27:6–13.
106. Graff-Radford SB, Solberg WK. Atypical odontalgia. J Craniomandib Disord 1992;6:260–265.
107. Melis M, Lobo SL, Ceneviz C, et al. Atypical odontalgia: A review of the literature. Headache 2003;43:1060–1074.
108. Baad-Hansen L, Pigg M, Ivanovic SE, et al. Chairside intraoral qualitative somatosensory testing: Reliability and comparison between patients with atypical odontalgia and healthy controls. J Orofac Pain 2013;27: 165–170.
109. Baad-Hansen L, Pigg M, Ivanovic SE, et al. Intraoral somatosensory abnormalities in patients with atypical odontalgia—A controlled multicenter quantitative sensory testing study. Pain 2013;154:1287–1294.
110. Durham J, Stone SJ, Robinson LJ, Ohrbach R, Nixdorf DR. Development and preliminary evaluation of a new screening instrument for atypical odontalgia and persistent dentoalveolar pain disorder. Int Endod J 2019;52:279–287.
111. Baad-Hansen L, Pigg M, Yang G, List T, Svensson P, Drangsholt M. Reliability of intra-oral quantitative sensory testing (QST) in patients with atypical odontalgia and healthy controls – a multicentre study. J Oral Rehabil. 2015;42:127–135.
112. Pigg M, Baad-Hansen L, Svensson P, Drangsholt M, List T. Reliability of intraoral quantitative sensory testing (QST). Pain 2010;148:220–226.
113. Svensson P, Baad-Hansen L, Pigg M, et al. Guidelines and recommendations for assessment of somatosensory function in oro-facial pain conditions—A taskforce report. J Oral Rehabil 2011;38:366–394.
114. Kehlet H, Jensen TS, Woolf CJ. Persistent postsurgical pain: Risk factors and prevention. Lancet 2006;367:1618–1625.
115. Schreiber KL, Kehlet H, Belfer I, Edwards RR. Predicting, preventing and managing persistent pain after breast cancer surgery: The importance of psychosocial factors. Pain Manag 2014;4:445–459.

116. Finnerup NB, Haroutounian S, Kamerman P, et al. Neuropathic pain: An updated grading system for research and clinical practice. Pain 2016;157:1599–1606.
117. Devine M, Hirani M, Durham J, Nixdorf DR, Renton T. Identifying criteria for diagnosis of post-traumatic pain and altered sensation of the maxillary and mandibular branches of the trigeminal nerve: A systematic review. Oral Surg Oral Med Oral Pathol Oral Radiol 2018;125:526–540.
118. Elias LA, Yilmaz Z, Smith JG, et al. PainDETECT: A suitable screening tool for neuropathic pain in patients with painful post-traumatic trigeminal nerve injuries. Int J Oral Maxillofac Surg 2014;43:120–126.
119. Herrero Babiloni A, Nixdorf DR, Law AS, et al. Initial accuracy assessment of the modified S-LANSS for the detection of neuropathic orofacial pain conditions. Quintessence Int 2017;48:419–429.
120. James SK. Chronic postsurgical pain: Is there a possible genetic link. Br J Pain 2017;11:178–185.
121. Mishriky BM, Waldron NH, Habib AS. Impact of pregabalin on acute and persistent postoperative pain: A systematic review and meta-analysis. Br J Anaesth 2015;114:10–31.
122. Thapa P, Euasobhon P. Chronic postsurgical pain: Current evidence for prevention and management. Korean J Pain 2018;31:155–173.
123. Martinez V, Pichard X, Fletcher D. Perioperative pregabalin administration does not prevent chronic postoperative pain: Systematic review with a meta-analysis of randomized trials. Pain 2017; 158:775–783.
124. Renton T, Yilmaz Z. Profiling of patients presenting with posttraumatic neuropathy of the trigeminal nerve. J Orofac Pain 2011;25:333–344.
125. Van der Cruyssen F, Peeters F, Croonenborghs TM, et al. A systematic review on diagnostic test accuracy of magnetic resonance neurography versus clinical neurosensory assessment for post-traumatic trigeminal neuropathy in patients reporting neurosensory disturbance. Dentomaxillofac Radiol 2021;50: 20200103.
126. Coulthard P, Kushnerev E, Yates JM, et al. Interventions for iatrogenic inferior alveolar and lingual nerve injury. Cochrane Database Syst Rev 2014:CD005293.
127. Smith JG, Elias LA, Yilmaz Z, et al. The psychosocial and affective burden of posttraumatic neuropathy following injuries to the trigeminal nerve. J Orofac Pain 2013;27:293–303.
128. Renton T, Yilmaz Z. Managing iatrogenic trigeminal nerve injury: A case series and review of the literature. Int J Oral Maxillofac Surg 2012;41:629–637.
129. Atkins S, Kyriakidou E. Clinical outcomes of lingual nerve repair. Br J Oral Maxillofac Surg 2021;59:39–45.
130. Strauss ER, Ziccardi VB, Janal MN. Outcome assessment of inferior alveolar nerve microsurgery: A retrospective review. J Oral Maxillofac Surg 2006;64: 1767–1770.
131. Susarla SM, Kaban LB, Donoff RB, Dodson TB. Does early repair of lingual nerve injuries improve functional sensory recovery? J Oral Maxillofac Surg 2007;65: 1070–1076.
132. Susarla SM, Kaban LB, Donoff RB, Dodson TB. Functional sensory recovery after trigeminal nerve repair. J Oral Maxillofac Surg 2007;65:60–65.
133. Zuniga JR. Sensory outcomes after reconstruction of lingual and inferior alveolar nerve discontinuities using processed nerve allograft—A case series. J Oral Maxillofac Surg 2015;73:734–744.
134. Galloway EB, Jensen RL, Dailey AT, Thompson BG, Shelton C. Role of topical steroids in reducing dysfunction after nerve injury. Laryngoscope 2000; 110:1907–1910.
135. Jancso G, Kiraly E, Jancso-Gabor A. Pharmacologically induced selective degeneration of chemosensitive primary sensory neurones. Nature 1977;270: 741–743.
136. Kraut RA, Chahal O. Management of patients with trigeminal nerve injuries after mandibular implant placement. J Am Dent Assoc 2002;133:1351–1354.
137. Zuniga JR, Yates DM, Phillips CL. The presence of neuropathic pain predicts postoperative neuropathic pain following trigeminal nerve repair. J Oral Maxillofac Surg 2014;72:2422–2427.
138. Zuniga JR, Yates DM. Factors determining outcome after trigeminal nerve surgery for neuropathic pain. J Oral Maxillofac Surg 2016;74:1323–1329.
139. Khawaja N, Yilmaz Z, Renton T. Case studies illustrating the management of trigeminal neuropathic pain using topical 5% lidocaine plasters. Br J Pain 2013;7:107–113.
140. Christoforou J, Balasubramaniam R, Klasser GD. Neuropathic orofacial pain. Current Oral Health Reports. 2015;2:148–157.
141. Nasri-Heir C, Khan J, Heir GM. Topical medications as treatment of neuropathic orofacial pain. Dent Clin North Am 2013;57:541–553.
142. Al-Musawi M, Durham J, Whitworth JM, Stone SJ, Nixdorf DR, Valentine RA. Effect of topical neuromodulatory medications on oral and skin keratinocytes. J Oral Pathol Med 2017;46:134–141.
143. Devine M, Taylor S, Renton T. Chronic post-surgical pain following the placement of dental implants in the maxilla: A case series. Eur J Oral Implantol 2016;9 (suppl 1):179–186.

144. García-Sáez R, Gutiérrez-Viedma Á, González-García N, Gómez-Mayordomo V, Porta-Etessam J, Cuadrado ML. OnabotulinumtoxinA injections for atypical odontalgia: An open-label study on nine patients. J Pain Res 2018;11:1583–1588.
145. Herrero Babiloni A, Kapos FP, Nixdorf DR. Intraoral administration of botulinum toxin for trigeminal neuropathic pain. Oral Surg Oral Med Oral Pathol Oral Radiol 2016;121:e148–e153.
146. Kim SY, Kim YK, Yun PY, Bae JH. Treatment of non-odontogenic orofacial pain using botulinum toxin-A: A retrospective case series study. Maxillofac Plast Reconstr Surg 2018;40:21.
147. Moreno-Hay I, Mishra P, Okeson JP. Intraoral administration of botulinum toxin for continuous dentoalveolar neuropathic pain: A case series. J Oral Facial Pain Headache 2019;33:160–164.
148. Dworkin RH, O'Connor AB, Audette J, et al. Recommendations for the pharmacological management of neuropathic pain: An overview and literature update. Mayo Clin Proc 2010;85:S3–S14.
149. Finnerup NB, Attal N, Haroutounian S, et al. Pharmacotherapy for neuropathic pain in adults: A systematic review and meta-analysis. Lancet Neurol 2015; 14:162–173.
150. National Institute for Health and Care Excellence. Neuropathic pain in adults: Pharmacological management in non-specialist settings. 2013.
151. van Seventer R, Bach FW, Toth CC, et al. Pregabalin in the treatment of post-traumatic peripheral neuropathic pain: A randomized double-blind trial. Eur J Neurol 2010;17:1082–1089.
152. Veitz-Keenan A, Keenan JR. Trials needed to identify best management of iatrogenic inferior alveolar and lingual nerve injuries. Evid Based Dent 2015;16:29.
153. van Hecke O, Austin SK, Khan RA, Smith BH, Torrance N. Neuropathic pain in the general population: A systematic review of epidemiological studies. Pain 2014;155:654–662.
154. Cohen JI. Clinical practice: Herpes zoster. N Engl J Med 2013;369:255–263.
155. Chen N, Li Q, Yang J, Zhou M, Zhou D, He L. Antiviral treatment for preventing postherpetic neuralgia. Cochrane Database Syst Rev 2014:CD006866.
156. Han Y, Zhang J, Chen N, He L, Zhou M, Zhu C. Corticosteroids for preventing postherpetic neuralgia. Cochrane Database Syst Rev 2013:CD005582.
157. Wiffen PJ, Derry S, Moore RA, et al. Antiepileptic drugs for neuropathic pain and fibromyalgia—An overview of Cochrane reviews. Cochrane Database Syst Rev 2013;11:CD010567.
158. Jung BF, Johnson RW, Griffin DR, Dworkin RH. Risk factors for postherpetic neuralgia in patients with herpes zoster. Neurol 2004;62:1545–1551.
159. Oaklander AL. The density of remaining nerve endings in human skin with and without postherpetic neuralgia after shingles. Pain 2001;92:139–145.
160. Wree A, Schmitt O, Usunoff K. Neuroanatomy of pain and neuropathology of herpes zoster and postherpetic neuralgia. In: Gross G, Doerr H (eds). Herpes Zoster: Recent Aspects of Diagnosis and Control. Basel, Switzerland: Karger, 2006:58–68.
161. Baron R. Postherpetic neuralgia and other neurologic complications. In: Gross G, Doerr H (eds). Herpes Zoster: Recent Aspects of Diagnosis and Control. Basel, Switzerland: Karger, 2006:69–80.
162. McNicol ED, Midbari A, Eisenberg E. Opioids for neuropathic pain. Cochrane Database Syst Rev 2013;8:CD006146.
163. Kenner M, Menon U, Elliott DG. Multiple sclerosis as a painful disease. Int Rev Neurobiol 2007;79:303–321.
164. Katusic S, Beard CM, Bergstralh E, Kurland LT. Incidence and clinical features of trigeminal neuralgia, Rochester, Minnesota, 1945-1984. Ann Neurol 1990;27:89–95.
165. De Simone R, Marano E, Brescia Morra V, et al. A clinical comparison of trigeminal neuralgic pain in patients with and without underlying multiple sclerosis. Neurol Sci 2005;26 (suppl 2):s150–s151.
166. Hooge JP, Redekop WK. Trigeminal neuralgia in multiple sclerosis. Neurol 1995;45:1294–1296.
167. Broggi G, Ferroli P, Franzini A, Servello D, Dones I. Microvascular decompression for trigeminal neuralgia: Comments on a series of 250 cases, including 10 patients with multiple sclerosis. J Neurol Neurosurg Psychiatry 2000;68:59–64.
168. Frese A, Husstedt IW, Ringelstein EB, Evers S. Pharmacologic treatment of central post-stroke pain. Clin J Pain 2006;22:252–260.
169. Nicholson BD. Evaluation and treatment of central pain syndromes. Neurol 2004;62:S30–6.
170. de Tommaso M, Arendt-Nielsen L, Defrin R, Kunz M, Pickering G, Valeriani M. Pain in neurodegenerative disease: Current knowledge and future perspectives. Behav Neurol 2016;b:7576292.
171. Fil A, Cano-de-la-Cuerda R, Muñoz-Hellín E, Vela L, Ramiro-González M, Fernández-de-Las-Peñas C. Pain in Parkinson disease: A review of the literature. Parkinsonism Relat Disord 2013;19:285–294.
172. Harden RN, Bruehl S, Stanton-Hicks M, Wilson PR. Proposed new diagnostic criteria for complex regional pain syndrome. Pain Med 2007;8:326–331.
173. Stanton-Hicks MD, Burton AW, Bruehl SP et al. An updated interdisciplinary clinical pathway for CRPS: Report of an expert panel. Pain Pract 2002;2:1–16.

174. de Mos M, de Bruijn AG, Huygen FJ, Dieleman JP, Stricker BH, Sturkenboom MC. The incidence of complex regional pain syndrome: A population-based study. Pain 2007;129:12–20.
175. Sandroni P, Benrud-Larson LM, McClelland RL, Low PA. Complex regional pain syndrome type I: Incidence and prevalence in Olmsted county, a population-based study. Pain 2003;103:199–207.
176. Melis M, Zawawi K, al-Badawi E, Lobo Lobo S, Mehta N. Complex regional pain syndrome in the head and neck: A review of the literature. J Orofac Pain 2002;16:93–104.
177. Dellemijn PL, Fields HL, Allen RR, McKay WR, Rowbotham MC. The interpretation of pain relief and sensory changes following sympathetic blockade. Brain 1994;117:1475–1487.
178. Hartrick CT, Kovan JP, Naismith P. Outcome prediction following sympathetic block for complex regional pain syndrome. Pain Pract 2004;4:222–228.
179. Rommel O, Malin JP, Zenz M, Jänig W. Quantitative sensory testing, neurophysiological and psychological examination in patients with complex regional pain syndrome and hemisensory deficits. Pain 2001; 93:279–293.
180. Perez RS, Zollinger PE, Dijkstra PU, et al. Evidence based guidelines for complex regional pain syndrome type 1. BMC Neurol 2010;10:20.
181. Tran DQ, Duong S, Bertini P, Finlayson RJ. Treatment of complex regional pain syndrome: A review of the evidence. Can J Anaesth 2010;57:149–166.
182. Scala A, Checchi L, Montevecchi M, Marini I, Giamberardino MA. Update on burning mouth syndrome: Overview and patient management. Crit Rev Oral Biol Med 2003;14:275–291.
183. Crow HC, Gonzalez Y. Burning mouth syndrome. Oral Maxillofac Surg Clin North Am 2013;25:67–76, vi.
184. Renton T. Burning Mouth Syndrome. Rev Pain 2011;5:12–17.
185. Currie CC, Ohrbach R, De Leeuw R, et al. Developing a research diagnostic criteria for burning mouth syndrome: Results from an international Delphi process. J Oral Rehabil 2021;48:308–331.
186. Bergdahl M, Bergdahl J. Burning mouth syndrome: Prevalence and associated factors. J Oral Pathol Med 1999;28:350–354.
187. Lipton JA, Ship JA, Larach-Robinson D. Estimated prevalence and distribution of reported orofacial pain in the United States. J Am Dent Assoc 1993;124:115–121.
188. Tammiala-Salonen T, Hiidenkari T, Parvinen T. Burning mouth in a Finnish adult population. Community Dent Oral Epidemiol 1993;21:67–71.
189. Grushka M, Sessle BJ. Burning mouth syndrome. Dent Clin North Am 1991;35:171–184.
190. van der Ploeg HM, van der Wal N, Eijkman MA, van der Waal I. Psychological aspects of patients with burning mouth syndrome. Oral Surg Oral Med Oral Pathol 1987;63:664–668.
191. Sardella A, Lodi G, Demarosi F, Bez C, Cassano S, Carrassi A. Burning mouth syndrome: A retrospective study investigating spontaneous remission and response to treatments. Oral Dis 2006;12:152–155.
192. Suarez P, Clark GT. Burning mouth syndrome: An update on diagnosis and treatment methods. J Calif Dent Assoc 2006;34:611–622.
193. Al Quran FA. Psychological profile in burning mouth syndrome. Oral Surg Oral Med Oral Pathol Oral Radiol Endod 2004;97:339–344.
194. Maina G, Albert U, Gandolfo S, Vitalucci A, Bogetto F. Personality disorders in patients with burning mouth syndrome. J Pers Disord 2005;19:84–93.
195. Carlson CR, Miller CS, Reid KI. Psychosocial profiles of patients with burning mouth syndrome. J Orofac Pain 2000;14:59–64.
196. Granot M, Nagler RM. Association between regional idiopathic neuropathy and salivary involvement as the possible mechanism for oral sensory complaints. J Pain 2005;6:581–587.
197. Lamey PJ, Murray BM, Eddie SA, Freeman RE. The secretion of parotid saliva as stimulated by 10% citric acid is not related to precipitating factors in burning mouth syndrome. J Oral Pathol Med 2001;30:121–124.
198. Heckmann SM, Heckmann JG, Hilz MJ et al. Oral mucosal blood flow in patients with burning mouth syndrome. Pain 2001;90:281–286.
199. Forssell H, Jääskeläinen S, List T, Svensson P, Baad-Hansen L. An update on pathophysiological mechanisms related to idiopathic oro-facial pain conditions with implications for management. J Oral Rehabil 2015;42:300–322.
200. Mo X, Zhang J, Fan Y, Svensson P, Wang K. Thermal and mechanical quantitative sensory testing in Chinese patients with burning mouth syndrome—A probable neuropathic pain condition. J Headache Pain 2015;16:84d.
201. Boucher Y, Simons CT, Carstens MI, Carstens E. Effects of gustatory nerve transection and/or ovariectomy on oral capsaicin avoidance in rats. Pain 2014;155:814–820.
202. Cruz A, Green BG. Thermal stimulation of taste. Nature 2000;403:889–892.
203. Sinding C, Gransjøen AM, Schlumberger G, Grushka M, Frasnelli J, Singh PB. Grey matter changes of the pain matrix in patients with burning mouth syndrome. Eur J Neurosci 2016;43:997–1005.

204. Bartoshuk LM, Snyder DJ, Grushka M, Berger AM, Duffy VB, Kveton JF. Taste damage: Previously unsuspected consequences. Chem Senses 2005;30(suppl 1):i218–219.
205. Eliav E, Kamran B, Schaham R, Czerninski R, Gracely RH, Benoliel R. Evidence of chorda tympani dysfunction in patients with burning mouth syndrome. J Am Dent Assoc 2007;138:628–633.
206. Femiano F. Damage to taste system and oral pain: Burning mouth syndrome. Minerva Stomatol 2004;53:471–478.
207. Grushka M, Sessle BJ, Howley TP. Psychophysical assessment of tactile, pain and thermal sensory functions in burning mouth syndrome. Pain 1987;28:169–184.
208. Svensson P, Bjerring P, Arendt-Nielsen L, Kaaber S. Sensory and pain thresholds to orofacial argon laser stimulation in patients with chronic burning mouth syndrome. Clin J Pain 1993;9:207–215.
209. Lauria G, Majorana A, Borgna M, et al. Trigeminal small-fiber sensory neuropathy causes burning mouth syndrome. Pain 2005;115:332–337.
210. Puhakka A, Forssell H, Soinila S, et al. Peripheral nervous system involvement in primary burning mouth syndrome-results of a pilot study. Oral Dis 2016;22:338–344.
211. Albuquerque RJC, de Leeuw R, Carlson CR, Okeson JP, Miller CS, Andersen AH. Cerebral activation during thermal stimulation of patients who have burning mouth disorder: An fMRI study. Pain 2006;122:223–234.
212. Borelli V, Marchioli A, Di Taranto R, et al. Neuropeptides in saliva of subjects with burning mouth syndrome: A pilot study. Oral Dis 2010;16:365–374.
213. Forssell H, Jääskeläinen S, Tenovuo O, Hinkka S. Sensory dysfunction in burning mouth syndrome. Pain 2002;99:41–47.
214. Hagelberg N, Forssell H, Rinne JO, et al. Striatal dopamine D1 and D2 receptors in burning mouth syndrome. Pain 2003;101:149–154.
215. Jääskeläinen SK. Pathophysiology of primary burning mouth syndrome. Clin Neurophysiol 2012;123:71–77.
216. Grémeau-Richard C, Dubray C, Aublet-Cuvelier B, Ughetto S, Woda A. Effect of lingual nerve block on burning mouth syndrome (stomatodynia): A randomized crossover trial. Pain 2010;149:27–32.
217. Tan SN, Song E, Dong XD, Somvanshi RK, Cairns BE. Peripheral GABAA receptor activation modulates rat tongue afferent mechanical sensitivity. Arch Oral Biol 2014;59:251–257.
218. Cui Y, Xu H, Chen F, et al. Efficacy evaluation of clonazepam for symptom remission in burning mouth syndrome: A meta-analysis. Oral Dis 2015;22:503–511.
219. Zakrzewska J, Buchanan JA. Burning mouth syndrome. BMJ Clin Evid 2016;2016:1301.
220. Koopman JS, Dieleman JP, Huygen FJ, de Mos M, Martin CG, Sturkenboom MC. Incidence of facial pain in the general population. Pain 2009;147:122–127.
221. Mueller D, Obermann M, Yoon MS, et al. Prevalence of trigeminal neuralgia and persistent idiopathic facial pain: A population-based study. Cephalalgia 2011;31:1542–1548.
222. Forssell H, Tasmuth T, Tenovuo O, Hampf G, Kalso E. Venlafaxine in the treatment of atypical facial pain: A randomized controlled trial. J Orofac Pain 2004;18:131–137.
223. List T, Axelsson S, Leijon G. Pharmacologic interventions in the treatment of temporomandibular disorders, atypical facial pain, and burning mouth syndrome. A qualitative systematic review. J Orofac Pain 2003;17:301–310.
224. Marbach JJ. Phantom bite. Am J Orthod 1976;70:190–199.
225. Marbach JJ. Orofacial phantom pain: Theory and phenomenology. J Am Dent Assoc 1996;127:221–229.
226. Hollins M, Walters S. Experimental hypervigilance changes the intensity/unpleasantness ratio of pressure sensations: Evidence for the generalized hypervigilance hypothesis. Exp Brain Res 2016;234:1377–1384.
227. McDermid AJ, Rollman GB, McCain GA. Generalized hypervigilance in fibromyalgia: Evidence of perceptual amplification. Pain 1996;66:133–144.
228. Michelotti A, Iodice G. The role of orthodontics in temporomandibular disorders. J Oral Rehabil 2010;37:411–429.
229. Raphael KG, Marbach JJ, Gallagher RM. Somatosensory amplification and affective inhibition are elevated in myofascial face pain. Pain Med 2000;1:247–253.
230. Reeves JL, Merrill RL. Diagnostic and treatment challenges in occlusal dysesthesia. J Calif Dent Assoc 2007;35:198–207.
231. Jagger RG, Korszun A. Phantom bite revisited. Br Dent J 2004;197:241–243.
232. Clark GT, Minakuchi H, Lotaif AC. Orofacial pain and sensory disorders in the elderly. Dent Clin North Am 2005;49:343–362.
233. Marbach JJ. Phantom bite syndrome. Am J Psychiatry 1978;135:476–479.
234. Marbach JJ, Varoscak JR, Blank RT, Lund P. "Phantom bite": Classification and treatment. J Prosthet Dent 1983;49:556–559.
235. Marbach JJ. Psychosocial factors for failure to adapt to dental prostheses. Dent Clin North Am 1985;29:215–233.
236. Klineberg I. Occlusion: Principles and Assessment. Oxford: John Wright, 1991.

237. Clark GT, Simmons M. Occlusal dysesthesia and temporomandibular disorders: Is there a link. Alpha Omegan 2003;96:33–39.
238. Leon-Salazar V, Morrow L, Schiffman EL. Pain and persistent occlusal awareness: What should dentists do. J Am Dent Assoc 2012;143:989–991.
239. Toyofuku A, Kikuta T. Treatment of phantom bite syndrome with milnacipran—A case series. Neuropsychiatr Dis Treat 2006;2:387–390.
240. Hara ES, Matsuka Y, Minakuchi H, Clark GT, Kuboki T. Occlusal dysesthesia: A qualitative systematic review of the epidemiology, aetiology and management. J Oral Rehabil 2012;39:630–638.
241. Kalladka M, Proter N, Benoliel R, Czerninski R, Eliav E. Mental nerve neuropathy: Patient characteristics and neurosensory changes. Oral Surg Oral Med Oral Pathol Oral Radiol Endodod 2008;106:364–370.
242. Baskaran RK, Krishnamoorthy, Smith M. Numb Chin Syndrome—A reflection of systemic malignancy. World J Surgl Oncol 2006;4:52.
243. Halachmi S, Madeb R, Madjar S, Wald M, River Y, Nativ O. Numb chin syndrome as the presenting symptom of metastatic prostate carcinoma. Urology 2000;55:286.
244. Lossos A, Siegal T. Numb chin syndrome in cancer patients: Etiology, response to treatment, and prognostic significance. Neurol 1992;42:1181–1184.
245. Lambru G, Miller S, Matharu MS. The red ear syndrome. J Headache Pain 2013;14:83.
246. Lance JW. The mystery of one red ear. Clin Exp Neurol 1994;31:13–18.
247. Laccourreye O, Werner A, Garcia D, Malinvaud D, Tran Ba Huy P, Bonfils P. First bite syndrome. Eur Ann Otorhinolaryngol Head Neck Dis 2013;130:269–273.
248. Linkov G, Morris LG, Shah JP, Kraus DH. First bite syndrome: Incidence, risk factors, treatment, and outcomes. Laryngoscope. 2012;122:1773–1778.
249. Redon S, Graillon N, Régis J, Donnet A. First bite syndrome after trigeminal radiosurgery: Case report and pathophysiology. Headache 2018;58:1680–1681.

7

Intraoral Pain Disorders

Key Points

- Intraoral pain disorders (both acute and chronic) are a common complaint in both healthy and medically complex patients.
- Diagnosis of oral pain can be complicated by referred or radiating pain and by proximity of multiple afferent nerve fibers.
- Even though painful conditions of various etiologies may overlap, there are typically distinguishing features that will direct the clinician to the correct diagnosis.
- Dental and periodontal pains generally have an infectious or inflammatory etiology but in rare instances may have systemic or extraoral causes.
- Periodontal disease is associated with increased risk of multiple systemic disorders, such as cardiovascular disease, cerebrovascular disease, and irritable bowel syndrome.
- Mucosal (soft tissue) oral pain has a more varied etiology, with traumatic, viral, fungal, autoimmune, and iatrogenic causes predominating.

Odontogenic Pain

Pain described by the patient as "toothache" may occasionally confound the clinician during the diagnostic process because perception of tooth sensitivity can be experienced due to dental disease, or it can arise in other tissues, either adjacent to the tooth or anatomically distant (ie, referred pain). For example, regional pain from adjacent structures, other orofacial pain disorders, and distant disease such as central nervous system (CNS) lesions (eg, tumors) may refer pain to teeth and mimic the symptoms of toothache. Similarly challenging is the fact that dental pathology may refer pain to other teeth or distant locations in the maxillofacial area or the neck, which can mimic other types of facial pain. Although the origin of most dental and acute orofacial pain can be easily located, the clinician must be aware of these other possibilities, which become more likely with chronic, intractable symptoms.

As a first step in the diagnosis process, the clinician must determine if the pain is truly odontogenic in origin. If it can be attributed to dental disease, it is then necessary to determine if the pain is of pulpal or periodontal origin (or both). These odontogenic disorders, and their corresponding *The International Classification of Diseases, Eleventh Revision* (*ICD*-11) codes, are presented below. The *ICD-10* codes are also provided for reference. Furthermore, the International Classification of Orofacial Pain, 1st edition (ICOP), also provides descriptions and diagnostic criteria of these intraoral pain disorders.[1] Nonodontogenic sources of pain that may mimic toothache, as well as mucosal pains, are reviewed later in this chapter.

Pulpal pain (*ICD-11* DA09.0, *ICD-10* K04.0)

The dental pulp is a visceral tissue that is richly innervated and vascularized. Pain that originates in the pulp has characteristics similar to other types of visceral pain, which tend to be deep, dull, or aching and may sometimes be difficult to localize.[2–5] Pulpitis, which may be reversible or irreversible, is caused by inflammation of the pulpal tissue.[6]

Reversible pulpitis

Reversible pulpitis is characterized by a short, sharp, hyperalgesic response that subsides soon (ie, seconds) after the stimulus is removed. The pain must be provoked and typically does not occur spontaneously. Irritants such as hypertonic solutions (eg, sugary food) or thermal extremes may cause focal stimulation, which produces a brief pain.[7] It is worth noting that pain from reversible pulpitis is a symptom, not a disease process.

Irreversible pulpitis

Irreversible pulpitis is characterized by prolonged pain, either spontaneous or provoked by a stimulus. This type of pain tends to be variable and may be intermittent or continuous, moderate or severe, sharp or dull, localized or diffuse, and affected by the time of day or body position. The intensity of the pain may also vary over time, and the tooth may go through asymptomatic periods. Pulpal inflammation is typically more severe and more widespread than in reversible pulpitis, and it may progress to pulpal necrosis.[7]

Nonvital tooth pain

Pulpal necrosis (*ICD-11* DA09.1, *ICD-10* K04.1) results from untreated pulpitis, exposure of the pulp to oral bacteria, traumatic injury, or other events that cause long-term interruption of the blood supply to the tissue. Pulpal necrosis may be partial or total. Partial necrosis may have some of the symptoms associated with irreversible pulpitis, which is common in multirooted teeth. Total necrosis is asymptomatic as long as no other disease process (ie, infection) affects the adjacent innervated tissues.[7] If pulpal disease extends beyond the apex of the tooth, pain becomes both spontaneous and continuous and can be exacerbated by percussion but not by temperature changes.

Etiology of pulpal pain

Tooth hypersensitivity may occur when dentinal tubules are exposed to the oral environment, causing fluid movement that affects the pulp.[8,9] Attrition (*ICD-11* DA08.10, *ICD-10* K03.0), abrasion (*ICD11* DA08.11, *ICD-10* K03.1), abfraction, erosion (*ICD-11* DA08.12, *ICD-10* K03.2), dental caries (*ICD-11* DA08.0, *ICD-10* K02.9), gingival recession (*ICD-11* DA0D.0, *ICD-10* K06.0), toothbrush trauma, periodontal diseases (*ICD-11* DA0C.Y, *ICD-10* K05.30), or periodontal surgery may expose coronal and/or radicular dentin. The factors leading to acute pulpal pain can be grouped into three general categories: bacterial, traumatic, and iatrogenic.

BACTERIAL. Bacteria or their metabolic byproducts are introduced into the pulp as a result of dental caries, inadequate restorations, enamel and/or dentin fractures, or anomalous tracts from the periodontium or from the systemic blood supply (bacteremia and retrograde infection).[10–13]

TRAUMATIC (*ICD-11* DA08.Y, *ICD-10* K03.8). Direct trauma to a tooth can cause pulpitis, acute pulpalgia, incomplete fracture, or complete fracture with exposure of dentin or the pulp. Trauma may subluxate or completely avulse a tooth, with consequent disruption of the apical blood supply and subsequent pulpitis or necrosis.[14]

IATROGENIC. The process of restoring teeth may cause pulpitis and acute pulpalgia. Heat and vibration from dental procedures, depth of preparation, dehydration of dentin, insertion of pin-retained restorations, and accidental pulp exposure have been well documented. Pulpal changes have also been reported following impressions in which bacteria were forced through the dentinal tubules. Furthermore, many dental materials and chemicals have the potential to irritate or injure the pulp.

Pathophysiology of pulpal pain

Myelinated (Aδ) and unmyelinated (C) afferent nerve fibers innervate the dental pulp. The Aδ fibers arborize in the coronal part of the tooth, just below the odontoblasts, where they lose their myelin sheath and form the plexus of Raschkow.[4,9,15] This plexus sends free nerve endings onto and through the odontoblastic cell layer, where they contact the odontoblastic processes at the pulpal end of the dentinal tubule.[16] The intimate association of Aδ fibers with the odontoblast is referred to as the *pulpodentinal complex*.[17] If the cellular or fluid contents of the dentinal tubules are sufficiently disturbed to involve the odontoblastic cell layer, the Aδ fibers become excited.[18–20] These nociceptive signals are perceived as sharp (bright), momentary pain that resolves when the stimulus is removed.[7] If an external irritant is of significant magnitude to cause pulpal inflammation, a vascular response (hyperemia) can lead to an increase in tissue pressure (perceived as pain), which increases as inflammation increases.[21]

A tooth with localized inflammation can also produce Aδ fiber pain with other types of excitation. Inflammatory mediators such as bradykinin, 5-hydroxytryptamine (5-HT, also known as *serotonin*), and prostaglandin E2 can sensitize the Aδ fibers, heightening their response to stimulants. As exaggerated Aδ fiber pain subsides, a dull, throbbing ache remains, associated with inflammatory involvement of nociceptive C-fibers.[7] This type of pain occurs with more severe tissue injury and is modulated by chronic inflammatory mediators, vascular changes in blood volume and blood flow, and increases in intrapulpal pressure. When C-fiber pain dominates over Aδ fiber pain, the symptom is more diffuse and poorly localized and may be referred to other sites. C-fiber pain typically signifies irreversible tissue damage as the inflammation increases.[7] Pain may begin as a short, lingering discomfort, which can escalate to intense, prolonged episodes or constant, throbbing pain. When a caries lesion contacts the pulp, the cellular inflammatory response changes from mostly mononuclear to polymorphonuclear leukocytes (neutrophils), resulting in microabscesses within the inflammatory lesion, at which point pulpitis typically becomes irreversible.[22,23] Complete necrosis of the pulp may occur rapidly, or it may take years to develop; symptomatology covers the spectrum from severe pain to complete analgesia.

Clinical characteristics of pulpal pain

Pulpal pain usually presents as a visceral, deep, dull, aching sensation.[5] This pain may be superimposed with pulsing and throbbing, or it may be sharp, burning, and lancinating due to local nerve sensitization rather than to vascular or neuropathic mechanisms. Clinical symptoms correlate poorly with the histologic status of the pulp.[24–26] Severe pain may be associated with early histopathologic changes, while a tooth that is asymptomatic may be necrotic. Pulpal pain can be modified by many factors, including heat and cold, pressure from occlusal contacts, head position, and the intensity of the offending stimulus. In addition, pain perception is complex and is affected by pain signaling, emotional state, and sociocultural background.[9]

When the pain is referred, it tends to follow a laminated segmental pattern within the trigeminal system. Maxillary teeth commonly refer pain to maxillary and mandibular teeth on the same side and to cutaneous locations on the face, superior to the maxillary teeth. Mandibular teeth tend to refer pain to maxillary and mandibular teeth on the same side. Anterior teeth may refer pain to both sides of the face.[27] Cutaneous referral patterns start at the level of the ear and project to locations on the face inferior to the ear.[28]

Differential diagnosis of pulpal pain

The first step in the diagnostic process is to determine whether the patient with a toothache is experiencing pain from an odontogenic or a nonodontogenic source. The tooth causing the odontogenic pain is usually identified by the presence of pathology to explain the pain (eg, caries or large restoration, combined with historic, clinical, and radiographic findings).[7] When a suspicious tooth is located, diagnosis may be confirmed by increased pain on application of a noxious stimulation (chemical, thermal, mechanical, or electric sources). If the pain can be influenced by local irritation, the tooth should be anesthetized to determine if the pain is blocked. If local anesthesia has no effect, pain from a nonodontogenic source should be considered. If administration of anesthesia decreases but does not eliminate the pain, there may be a nonanesthetized source contributing to the pain.

Once a conclusion regarding the source has been reached, the next step is to determine if the pain is of pulpal or periodontal origin. Pain of pulpal origin tends to respond to a stimulus at a given threshold and may be difficult to localize. Teeth that have only pulpal involvement are generally not sensitive to percussion. Teeth that have periodontal and/or periapical involvement typically respond to percussion or pressure on a graduated basis, and the pain is more likely to be localized.[7] Reversible pulpitis is characterized by stimulated pain of brief duration that ceases seconds after removal of the stimulus. Cold and electric stimulation provoke a brief response, and sensitivity to percussion is uncommon.[7] Irreversible pulpitis is characterized by stimulated pain of prolonged duration and/or by spontaneous pain. There may be no sensitivity to percussion until the inflammatory process extends to the periapex.[7] A necrotic pulp is asymptomatic until it becomes infected and inflammation extends to periapical tissues. The tooth is not responsive to either cold or electric pulp testing; however, there may be extreme sensitivity to percussion if the periapex is inflamed.[7]

Management considerations for pulpal pain

Optimal treatment for dentin hypersensitivity is still being debated, but overall it can include the following management modalities based on the patient presentation: *(1)* oral hygiene education; *(2)* diet and behavioral modification to eliminate predisposing factors; *(3)* application of noninvasive desensitizing to occlude the dentin tubules; *(4)* restoration with a composite resin, veneer, or crown; or *(5)* application of dentin bonding agents to seal the tubules.[29]

Treatment for reversible pulpitis targets removal of the pain-causing stimulus, such as caries, and restoration of lost tooth structures. Treatment of irreversible pulpitis or a necrotic pulp requires root canal therapy or extraction of the tooth. Systemic antibiotics are contraindicated when disease is localized to the pulp. A necrotic pulp is devoid of blood circulation, so no systemic medication will penetrate the space.

Acute periodontal pain (*ICD-11* DA0C.0, *ICD-10* K05.6)

The periodontium (ie, periodontal ligament and alveolar bone) is of mesenchymal origin. Therefore, periodontal pain tends to be more localized in comparison to visceral pain of pulpal origin. Localization of the source of pain is attributed to the proprioceptive and mechanoreceptive sensation of the periodontium.[30] Periodontal pain is generally dull and aching. Inflammatory fluid may cause displacement of the tooth in the socket with a resulting acute malocclusion and typical localization of the pain with biting or chewing. The diseased site readily responds to provocation proportionate to the stimulus.[5] At minimal levels of stimulation, the patient may describe an innocuous sensation such as itching or moderate dull aching; at severe levels, the patient may describe unrelenting, aching, and throbbing pain. Factors that may increase periodontal pain include occlusal contact, head position, the intensity of the stimulus, and CNS modulation. Periodontal pain, like pulpal pain, may stimulate secondary central excitatory activity, resulting in regional pain referral around the head and neck, to muscle overload with the potential to develop myalgia, myofascial trigger points, and autonomic effects such as sinus congestion, conjunctival injection, lacrimation, nasal drainage, and eyelid edema or drooping. Sites of prior pain are more likely to be sites of referred pain. Periodontal pain localized to a single tooth is usually associated with a gingival or periodontal abscess or a combined periodontal-endodontic lesion.[31]

Gingival abscess (*ICD-11* DA0C.4, *ICD-10* K0.500)

CLINICAL CHARACTERISTICS. The gingival abscess is a relatively rare entity. It usually arises as a result of foreign body impaction or trauma to previously healthy tissue and is confined to the marginal gingiva. It presents as a painful, possibly fluctuant swelling. The surface may be erythematous, smooth, and shiny associated with spontaneous drainage.[32]

ETIOLOGY. The precipitating cause of a gingival abscess is usually an impacted foreign object (eg, popcorn kernel) or trauma followed by infection.

PATHOPHYSIOLOGY. The gingival abscess consists of a purulent focus in the connective tissue surrounded by an inflammatory infiltrate.

MANAGEMENT CONSIDERATIONS. Treatment is by incision and drainage, followed by oral rinses with warm salt water, and may require removal of the causative agent. On rare occasions, irrigation and gentle debridement of the soft tissue lesion may be required.[33,34]

Periodontal abscess (*ICD-11* DA0C.4, *ICD-10* K05.20)

CLINICAL CHARACTERISTICS. Periodontal abscesses arise as acute or recurrent inflammatory swellings in periodontally diseased dental sites. The classic periodontal abscess is a localized swelling of the gingiva and/or the alveolar mucosa. These lesions often have an erythematous, violaceous, or cyanotic appearance and may be fluctuant. Pain is variable and can range from a deep ache of low intensity to severe discomfort. The pain is often exacerbated by chewing and percussion. The affected tooth may be mobile and may be slightly extruded. Fever and malaise may occur in cases of a severe abscess.[32,34–37] Suppuration may be noted from the pocket orifice. The tooth is usually vital.[32,34]

ETIOLOGY. The infectious cause of the lesion is the periodontal microbial flora, which is usually composed of pathogens such as *Porphyromonas gingivalis*, *Prevotella intermedia*, *Fusobacterium nucleatum*, *Peptostreptococcus micros*, and *Tannerella forsythia*.[38–40] It may arise from chronic periodontitis that cannot drain into the periodontal pocket or from trauma or extension of pulpal inflammation into the periapical tissues.[33,34,41] A lateral pulp canal may also cause an abscess in the periodontal space, which technically is not a periodontal abscess and requires root canal therapy.

PATHOPHYSIOLOGY. A periodontal abscess is usually an exacerbation of a preexisting chronic periodontal condition. More than 300 species of microorganisms have been isolated from periodontal pockets, but only a small number are considered pathogenic.[42,43] Most of the tissue destruction found in established periodontal lesions is a result of the mobilization of the host immunity via activation of monocytes, lymphocytes, fibroblasts, and other host cells. Engagement of these cellular elements by bacterial factors, in particular bacterial lipopolysaccharide, is thought to stimulate production of both catabolic cytokines and inflammatory mediators including arachidonic acid metabolites such as prostaglandin E2. Cytokines stimulate inflammatory responses that cause tissue destruction via activation of tissue metalloproteinases, a major pathway for connective tissue attachment loss and bone loss in most forms of periodontitis.[44,45]

MANAGEMENT CONSIDERATIONS. Treatment consists of establishing drainage (usually through the pocket orifice) and gentle debridement of the root surface and pocket wall under local anesthesia, accompanied by copious irrigation. Occlusal adjustment is sometimes indicated. Unless the tooth is beyond salvage, it is usually prudent to resolve the symptoms and then reassess the periodontal status. The endodontic status (ie, vitality) of the tooth should also be determined.

Periradicular (periapical) abscess (*ICD-11* DA09.6Z, *ICD-10* K04.7)

CLINICAL CHARACTERISTICS. Pulpal infection may induce an inflammatory reaction that may lead to periradicular abscess formation. Clinical characteristics include rapid onset, spontaneous pain, and acute response to percussion, purulence, and swelling. It must be distinguished from the periodontal abscess, although both processes may be operant in the case of a combined periodontal-endodontic lesion. One helpful element for differentiation is that the periodontal abscess occurs in a setting of periodontal attachment loss and pocket formation. The initial pain associated with a radicular abscess is intense when confined to bone, and it subsides following formation of a sinus tract (drainage) into the soft tissues. The infection may drain in the oral cavity or spread along fascial planes and result in cellulitis. In addition, bacteremia may occur, resulting in systemic infection. If the infection localizes, it may progress to a fluctuant swelling that may eventually drain.

ETIOLOGY. A periradicular abscess usually develops from a necrotic pulp that becomes infected, with spread of infection into the periradicular tissues. Occasionally, it may develop from exacerbation of chronic periodontitis located near the tooth apex (called *phoenix abscess*).

PATHOPHYSIOLOGY. The periradicular abscess is initiated by infiltration of bacteria into the apical periodontal ligament from an infection in the pulp, causing an acute inflammatory reaction.

MANAGEMENT CONSIDERATIONS. Management involves treating the cause of the abscess, which is endodontic (root canal therapy), or extraction of the offending tooth. Spread of the infection may require drainage of exudates and/or systemic antibiotics. Signs and symptoms such as fever, swelling of the infraorbital region or other masticatory or cervical spaces due to extension along fascial planes, trismus, stridor, or elevation of the floor of the mouth may indicate significant danger and typically require urgent intervention. In such cases, oral antibiotics are insufficient, and the patient should be immediately referred to a hospital.[7]

Pericoronitis (*ICD-11* DA0B.6, *ICD-10* K05.20)

CLINICAL CHARACTERISTICS. Pericoronitis is a localized infection within the soft tissue that surrounds the crown of an impacted or partially erupted tooth, most commonly a third molar. Clinical features may include an erythematous, swollen, suppurating gingival lesion that is tender and may cause radiating pain to the ear, throat, and floor of the mouth. The patient may experience a foul taste and inability to open or fully close the jaws. Swelling of the cheek in the region of the angle of the mandible is common, as is lymphadenopathy. The patient may also experience signs and symptoms of systemic complications such as fever, leukocytosis, and malaise.

ETIOLOGY. The typical process involves bacterial colonization of the pericoronal space, which triggers inflammation. Food debris or foreign objects may also become trapped under the gingival tissue covering the crown, thereby contributing to the inflammatory process.

PATHOPHYSIOLOGY. A diverse microflora of several facultative and obligate anaerobic bacteria, similar to that of a diseased periodontal pocket, exist in pericoronitis.[46] The byproducts of these bacteria may lead to cellulitis, which may follow the spread of the infection posteriorly into the oropharyngeal area and medially to the base of the tongue, making it difficult for the patient to swallow. Depending on the severity of the infection, lymph node involvement of the submandibular, posterior cervical, deep cervical, and retropharyngeal regions may occur.

MANAGEMENT CONSIDERATIONS. An irrigating syringe should be used to perform lavage under the gingiva with sterile saline or chlorhexidine solution, as well as the potential addition of hydrogen peroxide.[47] Removal of the tooth is generally indicated when the acute episode has resolved. Removal of the operculum is sometimes advocated in lieu of extraction; however, the soft tissue frequently regrows, resulting in the same local conditions that lead to infection. Abscess formation is common and leads to the need for surgical drainage and appropriate antibiotic therapy. Patients presenting with trismus, fever greater than 101°F, and facial swelling are candidates for referral to an oral and maxillofacial surgeon. Cellulitis that extends along fascial planes to involve other anatomical spaces requires aggressive treatment due to the potential for morbidity and—rarely—mortality.[48]

Combined periodontal-endodontic lesions (*ICD-11* DA0C.Y, *ICD-10* K05.5)

These lesions may be of primary pulpal origin or of periodontal origin. They may occur in a patient with preexisting periodontitis or in a setting of relatively good periodontal health. If the lesion is primarily endodontic in origin, root canal treatment alone may lead to resolution; however, this can only occur if the lesion is of recent onset.[49]

CLINICAL CHARACTERISTICS. The clinical presentation includes pain upon pressure and percussion, increased tooth mobility, probing depth and attachment loss, and swelling of the marginal gingiva, simulating a periodontal abscess. The suppurative process may cause the formation of a narrow, deep pocket that may be traced to the apex with a gutta-percha cone or a periodontal probe. Pulp testing is negative, or in a multirooted tooth it may show an abnormal response. All these signs, including radiographic findings, are somewhat variable.[7]

ETIOLOGY AND PATHOPHYSIOLOGY. The etiology and pathophysiologic processes are detailed in the preceding sections on periodontal and periradicular abscess.

MANAGEMENT CONSIDERATIONS. The periodontal component of the combined lesion may resolve subsequent to root canal therapy, and therefore it is preferable to perform this treatment first and allow for a suitable period of healing. If the periodontal lesion persists, further treatment will be required.[49] Of note is that vertical root fracture may show similar signs and symptoms, and is often associated with a previously endodontically treated tooth. Electric pulp testing may help separate these two lesions.

Pulpal and periodontal pain secondary to fractured teeth (*ICD-11* NA02.6, *ICD-10* K03.81)

Tooth fractures occur in approximately 5% of adults annually.[50] In most cases, the fracture of a cusp or a split tooth are readily diagnosed. Surface cracks, or *craze lines*, are considered incomplete tooth fractures. These incomplete fractures are usually asymptomatic but when painful, they may be due to "cracked tooth syndrome," which can be difficult to diagnose.[7]

CLINICAL CHARACTERISTICS. Patients with a cracked tooth may have complaints of sporadic, sharp, momentary pain on biting or releasing, along with occasional pain from cold stimuli. Sometimes, patients may indicate the pain occurs minutes after chewing.[7] In contrast with other tooth-related pains, the pain of a cracked tooth is usually easily located.[51]

ETIOLOGY. A fracture rarely occurs in teeth that are without caries or have no or small restorations. Predisposing factors include loss of support due to caries or large restorations, inadequate cusp protection by restorations, developmental weaknesses of the tooth, a history of local trauma, and clenching or bruxing habits.[52,53]

PATHOPHYSIOLOGY. The pain associated with a cracked tooth occurs when occlusal forces spread portions of the crown, exposing the underlying dentin. Momentary hydrostatic movement of fluid within the dentinal tubules causes pain.

DIFFERENTIAL DIAGNOSIS. The diagnosis of a cracked tooth is usually made from history and clinical tests. Generally, percussion, palpation, mobility, and probing are within normal limits if the crack is confined to the crown. The most useful test is biting on successive cusps with a firm object such as a wood stick or Tooth Slooth (Professional Results) until the pain is reproduced. Staining and transillumination may also disclose subtle fractures. In addition, the use of a microscope greatly facilitates the observation of fractures.[54] Electric pulp testing will produce normal responses unless the pulp is involved. Cold testing may be productive, whereas heat may not be helpful. Fracture lines are not visible on radiographs when they run mesiodistally and are not in the plane of the x-ray beam. While CBCT imaging may be useful in detecting certain types of cracks, this is inconsistent and cannot be relied upon as a sole diagnostic test.[55,56] If the fracture extends into the root, a periodontal defect may be observed adjacent to the fracture. At this point, the pulp may have become necrotic. Sharp pain and cold sensitivity are not common. Typically, a dull ache on biting might be present when the periodontal ligament is inflamed, resulting in tenderness on percussion.[51–53]

MANAGEMENT CONSIDERATIONS. Early detection of cracked teeth is essential, and therapy depends on the severity of symptoms, location and extent of the crack.[51,53,57,58] Temporary stabilization can be achieved with an orthodontic stainless-steel band or a provisional crown until an overlay or full crown can be fabricated. Root canal therapy with or without stabilization has been advocated. In cases with extensive cracks, extraction may be necessary.[7]

Systemic factors and dental disease

Systemic conditions may modify host response to oral infection and increase risk for cariogenic, periodontal, or other infectious processes where oral pain is a prominent feature. These conditions include diabetes mellitus, anemia, diseases causing altered neutrophil count and function, immunosuppression (pathologic or medically induced), tobacco use, nutrient and caloric deficiencies, hormone abnormalities, and emotional stress.[59–64] Additionally, pathologic conditions and/or medications that affect exocrine secretions may influence oral homeostasis through effects on saliva. Rheumatic diseases such as arthritis, Sjögren syndrome, systemic lupus, and systemic sclerosis (scleroderma) are counted among the most common inducers of pathologic changes in salivary glands. Dehydration, alcoholism, and a large variety of medications induce hyposalivation without significant change in glandular tissues. In addition, genetic diseases that affect calcification may interfere in mineralization of teeth. Most common among these are osteogenesis imperfecta and the related dentinogenesis and amelogenesis imperfecta. Diagnosis and treatment of these patients involve unusual complexity.

Dental disease, most notably periodontal disease, is associated with and potentially causative of multiple systemic disorders with high morbidity and mortality rates. These disorders include cardiovascular disease (CVD), cerebrovascular disease, irritable bowel syndrome (IBS), Alzheimer disease, diabetes mellitus, respiratory tract infections, and adverse pregnancy outcomes.[59–64] While the exact mechanism(s) of association is not known, proposed mechanisms include the induction of systemic inflammation resulting from the local inflammatory response as well as from translocated oral microbiota into the bloodstream.[61] Additionally, translocated oral bacteria may lead to gut dysbiosis and altered gut epithelial cell barrier function in genetically vulnerable individuals under challenging environmental conditions, further contributing to chronic low-grade systemic inflammation.[65–67] Therapeutically, recent evidence has shown that periodontal therapy may reduce the incidence of adverse cardiovascular events, although further studies are needed to confirm whether this is clinically significant.[61]

Nonodontogenic Toothache

When the patient reports "toothache," the clinician must determine if the pain has its origin in dental structures or if pain is referred from other sites.[68] Effective treatment can only be provided following a correct diagnosis. Because dental pain is so commonly treated in the dental office and nonodontogenic tooth pain is uncommon, these latter cases are often inappropriately treated with dental therapy before appropriate diagnosis of the cause. The appropriate diagnosis is often only determined after multiple treatment failures that may include invasive and irreversible procedures such as root canal therapy and tooth extractions have been trialed.[69–71]

Nonodontogenic toothache may be differentiated from odontogenic toothache by local provocation. Pulpal and periodontal pains are increased by local stimulation such as percussion, heat, cold, or bite forces. When the pain is not increased by provocation, the clinician should be suspicious of a nondental etiology. Local anesthetic may be helpful in differentiating true dental pain from pain referred to the teeth. Local anesthetic placed at the site of the nonodontogenic toothache often will be ineffective because the site of pain report is not the true source. Pain can be referred to the teeth from multiple sources including myofascial trigger points in the masseter (most common muscle source), temporalis, temporal tendon, medial pterygoid, lateral pterygoid, and anterior digastric muscles.[72,73] Maxillary sinusitis or a regional tumor may be a source of maxillary tooth pain. Nonodontogenic toothache may also result from continuous neuropathic pain (ie, deafferentation, neuritis, neuroma, persistent dentoalveolar pain), episodic neuropathic pain disorders (ie, neuralgias), and other neoplastic or neurovascular disorders. CNS disease and cardiac pain may also be experienced as toothache.[74,75] In some instances, psychiatric comorbidities may also contribute to tooth pain.[76] Knowing the pain characteristics and referral patterns for each of these sources is essential for accurate differential diagnosis and appropriate treatment.

Potential identifiers of nonodontogenic toothache include the following:

- Spontaneous multiple-tooth pain
- Migrating tooth pain
- Stimulating, burning, electric/lancinating pain, nonpulsatile toothaches
- Constant/persistent, unremitting toothaches
- Persistent, recurrent toothaches
- Pain referral to region of tooth from muscle trigger points
- Associated autonomic symptoms such as tearing, conjunctival injection, regional sweating, and other vascular phenomena
- Regional pain and paresthesia
- Severe headache
- Associated migrainous symptoms such as nausea, photophobia, phonophobia, or both photophobia and phonophobia
- Recent cold, allergy, stuffiness, and coughing with pain in maxillary teeth
- Inadequate clinical or radiographic dental cause for the pain
- Failure of local anesthesia to significantly reduce pain
- Failure of the toothache to respond to reasonable dental therapy

Oral Mucosal Pain

Local mucogingival and glossal pains

Localized mucosal pain is often associated with a detectable lesion resulting from physical, chemical, or thermal trauma; infection; inflammation; neoplasia; immune dysfunction; or other origin. The pain experienced is typically localized to the site of mucosal change. A response to stimulation (eg, eating spicy or acidic foods or contact with toothpaste) is representative in intensity and location, and topical anesthetic at the site modulates the pain. By contrast, for diffuse mucosal pain, it may be difficult to identify the specific cause unless widespread lesions are obvious. This type of pain may result from a direct insult to the tissues due to local or CNS lesions that require special studies or bacterial, viral, or fungal infection, which can be identified by the characteristic appearance of the oral mucosa and confirmed with diagnostic testing.

Diffuse pain may also be due to radiation therapy and cytotoxic or targeted chemotherapy, which may result in acute mucositis with severe generalized pain that may persist past healing of the lesions as chronic mucosal pain. Burning sensation of the oral mucosa, particularly the tongue, may result from neuropathy/neuralgia, hyposalivation, use of certain medications, and in some cases, nutrient deficiency diseases. Generalized diffuse pain with a symmetric distribution in the oral mucosa, with a burning quality that may be accompanied by a change in taste, may represent burning mouth disorder (see chapter 6).[37]

Necrotizing disease (necrotizing gingivitis *ICD-11* 1C1H.Z; necrotizing periodontitis *ICD-11* DA0C.30; medication-related osteonecrosis of the jaw *ICD-11* FB81.2)

Necrotizing mucosal conditions are generally characterized by severe pain, and they often hemorrhage on slight provocation. The term *necrotizing periodontal diseases* includes the somewhat arbitrary terms *necrotizing gingivitis* (NG) and *necrotizing periodontitis* (NP), which have been used to distinguish necrotizing conditions that present with or without attachment loss.[77] Tissue necrosis of gingiva or periodontium may run a short course or may become chronic; therefore, the term *acute* has been deleted. Likewise, the preferred terminology no longer includes *ulcerative*, as the ulcerations are secondary to the occurrence of the necrotic tissue.[78]

Spontaneous or, more commonly, trauma- and/or extraction-associated soft tissue and jawbone necrosis has been described in association with antiresorptive bone medications or osteolytic inhibitors such as bisphosphonates and receptor activator of nuclear factor κB ligand inhibitors and antiangiogenic medications. Cases related to other biologic therapies have also been reported.[79] *Medication-related osteonecrosis of the jaw (MRONJ)* may be a consideration if these conditions are met: *(1)* history of current or previous use of antiresorptive or antiangiogenic drugs; *(2)* bone exposure in the mandible or maxilla of more than 8 weeks' duration through an intraoral or extraoral fistula(e); and *(3)* no history of radiation to jaws or metastatic disease of the jaws.[80] Of note, MRONJ is often painless.

CLINICAL CHARACTERISTICS. NG/NP is characterized by painful, hyperemic, fiery erythematous gingiva and punched-out ulceration of the interdental papilla. The lesions bleed easily and are often covered with a gray necrotic pseudomembrane. The patient may complain of bad breath and inability to eat. Occasionally, systemic symptoms are seen, such as malaise and low-grade fever. The lesions may occasionally involve other areas of the oral mucosa (necrotizing ulcerative stomatitis), which is usually seen in debilitated or immunocompromised individuals (also known as *noma*, *gangrenous stomatitis*, and *cancrum oris*).[34,81] When the condition occurs in immunocompetent individuals, which is usually the case, the patient is often a young adult with poor hygiene who is also a heavy frequent smoker. Patients who do not fit this profile should be evaluated for potential predisposing immunosuppressive conditions, including blood dyscrasia and HIV/AIDS.

ETIOLOGY. Vascular changes associated with emotional stress, tobacco use, poor oral hygiene, local trauma, fatigue, and impaired host defense predispose the individual to infection and tissue necrosis.[81]

PATHOPHYSIOLOGY. NG was originally referred to as a *fusospirochetal disease*. More recently, *P intermedia* has been implicated, along with various *Treponema spp*, *Fusobacterium spp*, and *Selenomonas spp*.[82]

MANAGEMENT CONSIDERATIONS. Treatment of NG/NP consists of gentle mechanical debridement; systemic antibiotic therapy with metronidazole, tetracycline, or doxycycline; and 0.12% chlorhexidine mouth rinse.

Aphthous stomatitis (*ICD-11* DA01.10, *ICD-10* K12.0)

Aphthous stomatitis is the most common oral mucosal disease affecting the general population. Aphthae may present in three clinical forms: minor, major, and herpetiform. Aphthous minor is the most widespread form, with a prevalence of 17.7% of the general population (80% of the cases of aphthous stomatitis). The prevalence of the major form ranges from 10% to 15%.[83] Herpetiform cases comprise 7% to 10%.[84–88] As there is a tendency for recurrence, the condition may be referred to as *recurrent aphthous stomatitis* (RAS). In lay terms it is referred to as *canker sores*.

CLINICAL CHARACTERISTICS. Pain is the most characteristic symptom of RAS. Aphthous minor appears as discrete, painful, shallow, recurrent ulcers, covered by a yellowish-gray pseudomembrane, that are surrounded by an erythematous halo. Ulcers typically number one to five at any one time and measure < 2 to 8 mm in diameter. These lesions are painful and usually heal within 10 to 14 days without scar formation.[83] Aphthous major produces ulcers that are usually > 10 mm in diameter, may persist for weeks, and may be recurrent or present continuously for extended periods. They appear as very painful, large, deep-based ulcers containing a yellow-gray necrotic center, and they may develop raised, rolled borders with a predilection for the lips, soft palate, posterior aspect of the tongue, and tonsillar fauces. These lesions may heal with scarring. Herpetiform aphthae occur as pinpoint crops of small ulcers that sometimes coalesce, creating a look reminiscent of a herpetic infection and typically there are 10 or more ulcers with this subtype.[83,89,90] In all types of aphthae, ulcers predominantly involve nonkeratinized mucosa of the mouth: the labial and buccal mucosae, maxillary and mandibular sulci, nonattached gingiva, floor of the mouth, ventral surface of the tongue, soft palate, and tonsillar fauces. Ulcers of this type typically spare the keratinized mucosa of the dorsum of the tongue, the attached gingiva, and the hard palate. While patients may develop submandibular lymphadenopathy, fever is rare.[89]

ETIOLOGY. The underlying cause(s) of RAS are unclear and is in all likelihood multifactorial. Proposed factors that play a role in triggering the development of RAS include hormonal changes, trauma, stress, food allergies, systemic diseases (Crohn disease, celiac disease, ulcerative colitis), and genetically acquired immune disturbances.[90] Foods associated with aphthous stomatitis include bovine milk protein, glutens, chocolate, nuts, cinnamon, spices, and preservatives.[89,90] A number of medications are known to cause aphthous-like lesions, including nonsteroidal anti-inflammatory drugs (NSAIDs) and "targeted" cancer therapies (eg, mammalian target of rapamycin [mTOR] inhibitors).[91] Deficiencies of ferritin and vitamin B_{12} have also been associated with this condition.[92] Nevertheless, the complete etiology remains unknown.

PATHOPHYSIOLOGY. The development of aphthous ulcers within the oral mucosa is considered to be a result of an immune response to a yet to be identified factor(s) in the oral mucosa from one or more of the triggers mentioned above.[90] Genetic polymorphisms of interleukins (IL) such as IL-1β and IL-6 are robust predictors of RAS, while polymorphisms for IL-10 and IL-12 were not.[92–94] Overexpression of polymorphisms of tumor necrosis factor (TNF) are found in some studies but not others.[92,93] In summary, most evidence indicates an imbalance between pro-inflammatory (TNF, IL-15, interferon-g) and anti-inflammatory (TGF-B, IL-10) cytokines, particularly of the Th1-type immune response, while T helper cell regulatory components are diminished.[95,96] This scenario provides a predisposition toward autoimmune cellular responses in RAS.

MANAGEMENT CONSIDERATIONS. The management of RAS aims to reduce pain and morbidity as well as lesion size and duration. In cases where stress or nutritional or systemic diseases are identified, the underlying condition should be managed. RAS responds quickly to the administration of low-, medium-, or high-potency corticosteroids. These products are available as topicals, elixirs, and systemic medications.[97] Medication potency should match disease severity. For example, RAS minor may be managed with topical triamcinolone. Minor ulcers or those in favorable locations spared from mastication, such as the posterior vestibule, may not need any treatment. Herpetiform RAS, due to its multiple lesions in a variety of intraoral sites, can be practically managed with dexamethasone or prednisolone elixirs. RAS major may be treated with more potent topicals such as fluocinonide or clobetasol. More severe cases may be managed with a 7–10-day burst of prednisone.[97] Recalcitrant major apthae can be managed via intralesional corticosteroid injection. While corticosteroids are the mainstay in RAS management, there are alternatives if steroid therapy fails or is contraindicated.[98] Colchicine, levamisole, dapsone, zinc, azathioprine, pentoxifylline, and cautery have been studied in RAS and have shown some efficacy.[98–102]

Infections

Viral infection (*ICD-11* primary herpetic gingivostomatitis 1F00.02, recurrent herpes labialis 1F00.01, other specified herpes simplex virus infection of skin or mucous membrane 1F00.0Y, herpes zoster 1E91.Z, postherpetic neuralgia 1E91.5)

Herpes family viruses often cause oral mucosal and salivary gland infection in either primary or reactivated form. The most common pathogens affecting the oral mucosa are the herpes simplex virus (HSV) members (HSV 1 and 2, primarily the former). Research has identified a relatively high prevalence of human herpes virus (HHV) 6, 7, and 8 in the oral mucosa.[103] The varicella zoster virus (VZV) is present in all patients with a history of chicken pox, whereas cytomegalovirus (CMV) or Epstein-Barr virus (EBV) may be latent within salivary gland tissue lymphocytes. Common to all herpes viruses is the fact that after primary exposure (which may or may not produce overt disease), the virus achieves a dormant state and is subject to episodic reactivation.

PRIMARY HERPETIC GINGIVOSTOMATITIS. Primary herpetic gingivostomatitis occurs in individuals without prior exposure to the virus. These infections are seen mostly in children and young adults. When symptomatic, the clinical manifestations include diffuse oral lesions and possible systemic involvement. The initial presentation has rapid onset of generalized prodromal signs and symptoms, including erythema, pruritus, fever, malaise, headache, irritability, and regional lymphadenopathy, followed by the development of frank oral lesions that consist of severe generalized inflammation and vesicles primarily involving keratinized mucosa of the lips, gingiva, tongue, and palate. The vesicles rupture rapidly, forming shallow, ragged, painful ulcerations with a yellowish center and erythematous borders. The lesions begin as clustered, punctate (1–2-mm rounded) ulcerations that may coalesce to form irregular lesions that usually heal within 2 weeks.[104] In some cases, extraoral ulcerations develop on the skin and vermillion borders of the lips, with resultant crusting and oozing. Severe pain, foul odor, and increased salivation may accompany the oral lesions. Diagnosis is most often based on the history and clinical presentation. Laboratory diagnosis is not usually necessary except in the setting of immunosuppression or atypical presentation. However, if required, a Tzanck test involves light microscopic examination of cells smeared from the ulcer.[105]

Active herpetic lesions should be considered infectious until complete re-epithelialization. Patients should be warned of the possibility of transmission to others, especially infants and the immunocompromised. Autoinoculation of the virus into other receptive mucosal sites (eg, the eye) is also possible. For dental professionals, herpetic whitlow and herpetic conjunctivitis is a professional risk.

RECURRENT INTRAORAL HERPES (RIH). Recurrent infections are caused by reactivation of the virus, which is latent in the trigeminal ganglion. The clinical characteristic of RIH is unilateral vesicular eruptions surrounded by erythema, followed by crusting and healing. The eruptions are often preceded by a prodromal tingling sensation. Oral mucosal lesions are usually restricted to small clusters of vesicles (1–3 mm in size) that rupture, resulting in punctate ulcers, typically on the palatal gingiva (occasionally elsewhere on the gingiva) unilaterally.[104] The lesions may be triggered by ultraviolet light exposure, stress, immunosuppression, or dental procedures. The lesions are usually self-limiting, resolving within several days.[105] Extraoral lesions may appear on the skin, genitalia, anal and perianal areas, eyes (keratitis, keratoconjunctivitis), and nervous system (encephalitis, meningitis) in those undergoing cancer chemotherapy, taking immunosuppressant medications during organ transplant, or in advanced cases of AIDS.[103,106,107]

RECURRENT HERPES LABIALIS (RHL). RHL is a common, painful, and unsightly perioral lesion affecting about a quarter of the general population. In lay terms, it is referred to as a *fever blister* or *cold sore*. Stress and sun exposure are known triggers. Prior to lesions appearing on the upper or lower lip (unilateral), there is an itchy, tingly prodrome the day before. A cluster of vesicles appear and rapidly ulcerate, and the lesions coalesce. The entire course runs 10 to 14 days without intervention. The lesion is contagious the first 5 days. Treatment is directed at controlling pain, lesion size, and to a limited extent, lesion duration. Topical treatment includes acyclovir 5%, penciclovir 1%, and OTC N-Docosanol 1% creams applied every 2 hours while awake for the first 4 to 5 days of the lesion.[97,103] The systemic antiviral valacyclovir 1000 mg twice a day for just the first day can accomplish the same goal.[97] If RHL recurrences are too frequent throughout the year, daily prophylactic suppression treatment with valacyclovir or famciclovir is recommended.[103]

ETIOLOGY. The typical route of HSV transmission is physical contact with an infected individual by someone who has not been previously exposed to the virus. During the primary infection, only about 50% of individuals show clinical signs and symptoms, while most experience a subclinical course. This latter group becomes seropositive and can be identified through laboratory evaluation of circulating antibodies to HSV.[108] Approximately 90% of adults are seropositive for HSV 1 and about 35% for HSV 2, which are the most common agents for mucosal lesions.

PATHOPHYSIOLOGY. The incubation period for primary infection ranges from several days to 2 weeks after exposure to the virus. The clinical picture consists of a vesiculo-ulcerative eruption on the mucosal tissues at the site of inoculation. Following resolution of primary herpetic gingivostomatitis, the virus becomes latent in the trigeminal ganglia. Reactivation of the virus is not fully understood but may follow exposure to ultraviolet light, trauma and stress, or immunosuppression, causing a secondary or recurrent infection. Virions assemble and migrate along the nerve and enter epidermal cells, causing vesicles that ulcerate at the epithelial surface. Because the humoral and cell-mediated arms of the immune system have been sensitized to HSV antigens, the lesions typically remain localized, and systemic symptoms are rare. As the secondary lesion resolves, the virus returns to its latent state.[108] It is worth noting that viral shedding occurs commonly in infected individuals, from oral and genital sites without clinical symptoms or overt lesions. Hence, contagion can occur even in the absence of clinical lesions. In immunosuppressed patients, recurrent lesions may spread, persist for longer periods, and present atypical appearances including ulceration of attached and unattached mucosa in contrast to those of non-immunosuppressed patients.

VARICELLA ZOSTER INFECTION. Primary infection with VZV (chicken pox) is also a disease with recurrent episodes termed *shingles* or *herpes zoster* (HZ). It is estimated that in the United States, more than 90% of adults are susceptible to VZV reactivation.[109] With an estimated 30% chance of reactivation over the lifetime, about one million cases of HZ occur in the United States annually. Common causes of reactivation include age above 60 years, immunosuppression, or trauma. Reactivation of VZV has a typical onset with pain that can be severe, followed by segmental distribution of lesions that may involve the head, neck, and oral cavity. HZ may run its course, and the virus becomes latent in immunocompetent patients but may spread locoregionally or cause systemic infection in immunosuppressed individuals.

The clinical characteristics of HZ include the development of a unilateral rash, typically within affected dermatomes of the trunk, but it can occur on the face. Nasal involvement requires an ophthalmology consult because the infection can then involve the eye via the nasociliary nerve. The rash scabs after 7 to 10 days and resolves in 2 to 4 weeks. In addition to facial lesions and exanthem, lesions may occur intraorally as well as on the palate, characteristically and abruptly stopping at the midline. The pain is burning, and the affected area exhibits allodynia. When the lesions of HZ involve the external auditory canal in the presence of ipsilateral facial paralysis, hearing deficits, and other auditory symptoms, it is classified as Ramsay Hunt syndrome. Postherpetic neuralgia (PHN) is quite common after HZ and may result in persisting chronic neuropathic pain following resolution of active infection. PHN may last 120 days or more post rash.[110]

Management of HZ includes the use of antivirals early in its course, preferably starting within 72 hours, with agents such as acyclovir 800 mg five times a day, valacyclovir 1000 mg three times a day, or famciclovir 500 mg three times a day for 7 to 10 days.[110] The use of corticosteroids in conjunction with antivirals is controversial; the thought is that it decreases perineural inflammation. There are two vaccines available for shingles prevention in older adults: the earlier Zostavax vaccine and the newer Shingrix vaccine. The US Centers for Disease Control and Prevention's Advisory Committee on Immunization Practices (ACIP) recommends adults above age 50 receive the preferred Shingrix vaccine, as it reduces HZ by 90% in immunocompetent individuals.[111,112]

The management of PHN is important because the pain is severe and adversely affects quality of life, sleep, and activities of daily living. The risk of PHN increases with age.[112] PHN management is similar to that of other neuropathic pains. Topical treatment can include lidocaine patches, capsaicin, and compounded pain creams. Systemic medications include the gabapentinoids, tricyclic antidepressants, serotonin-norepinephrine reuptake inhibitors, tramadol, and possibly opioids.[110,113] A nonpharmacologic intervention that has shown some success is transcutaneous electric nerve stimulation (TENS), which may be used by itself or as an adjunct with other treatments.[114] Cognitive behavioral therapy should be considered because patients with neuropathic pain diagnoses have a higher degree of pain catastrophizing relative to other orofacial pain diagnoses.[115]

OTHER HERPES VIRUSES. Occasionally, oral lesions may be induced by CMV and HHV 8, which are responsible for ulcerations in immunocompromised patients and in Kaposi sarcoma. Acute infection by CMV and the EBV may cause mononucleosis-like symptoms.

Candidiasis (*ICD-11* 1F23.0, *ICD-10* B37.0)

Candidiasis encompasses a group of mucosal and cutaneous conditions most commonly caused by the yeast *Candida albicans*. Other members of the *Candida* genus such as *C tropicalis*, *C krusel*, *C parapsilosis*, *C guilliermondi*, and *C dubliniensis* are rarely the cause of disease; however, continuing overuse of antifungals has led to an increase in the prevalence of strains that are resistant to common drugs, particularly in immunosuppressed individuals.[116,117] *Candida* species are opportunistic pathogens that may lead to clinical overgrowth and frank, local, and—rarely—systemic infection due to changes in oral conditions, oral flora, and systemic status of the host.[118]

PSEUDOMEMBRANOUS CANDIDIASIS. The pseudomembranous form occurs most commonly in infants, elderly patients, and those with white cell or immune deficiencies. The lesions present as superficial, curd-like white plaques that wipe off, leaving an erythematous, eroded, or ulcerated surface. Plaques are composed of fungal organisms, keratotic debris, inflammatory cells, desquamated epithelial cells, bacteria, and fibrin. The lesions commonly affect the palate, buccal mucosa and mucobuccal folds, lateral and dorsal aspects of the tongue, and oropharynx. Patients may have no symptoms or may complain of tenderness, mucosal burning, taste change, and odynophagia. Predisposing factors include a history of medication with broad-spectrum antibiotics or corticosteroids, hyposalivation, wearing of removable dentures, tobacco use, nutritional deficiency, diabetes, malignancy, chemotherapy, radiation therapy, and cell-mediated immune dysfunction, including that induced by HIV.

ERYTHEMATOUS (ATROPHIC) CANDIDIASIS. Erythematous lesions are most often seen on the middorsal tongue (median rhomboid glossitis or glossal central papillary atrophy) and on denture-bearing areas of the palate. Oral tenderness, burning, taste change, and odynophagia are common. Predisposing factors are the same as those listed above. Erythematous candidiasis may also occur under dentures, presenting with erythema and edema on a velvety or pebbly surface (ie, papillary hyperplasia). Chronic candida infections are also capable of producing a hyperplastic tissue response with inter- and intracellular invasion of the epithelium. White lesions may include palpable thickness and irregular surface texture with or without erythema. These lesions are mostly asymptomatic. Predisposing factors include inherited or acquired altered cellular immunity and general local risk factors for candidiasis. Angular cheilitis presents as localized erythema and/or ulcerations, unilaterally or bilaterally at the commissures of the lips. The lesions may be painful, eroded, and crusted when extending onto the skin surface. Angular cheilitis is often associated with intraoral forms of candidiasis. Predisposing factors include loss of vertical dimension of occlusion, drooling at the corners of the mouth, lip-licking and/or thumb- or digit-sucking habits, and risk factors common to all other forms of candidiasis. Angular cheilitis is often a mixed infection of *Candida* and salivary species of streptococci and staphylococci. The diagnosis of candidiasis may be made from the patient history and the clinical appearance and distribution of the mucosal lesions. When necessary, especially in an immunocompromised individual, identification of the organism is made in a culture or smear from the lesion. For hyperplastic lesions, biopsy followed by microscopy with fungal stain is necessary.[119]

MANAGEMENT CONSIDERATIONS. The underlying risk factors for candidiasis should be identified and managed when possible, or recolonization and recurrence of infection is likely, as the yeast can rarely be completely eliminated. Oral candidiasis is most often treated with antifungal agents such as topical polyenes (nystatin) and azoles (clotrimazole, miconazole). Oral preparations in the form of troches or adherent patches provide the advantage of prolonged contact of the medication with the lesions.[100] The angular cheilitis lesions respond well to broad-spectrum antimicrobials or combination therapy containing an antifungal and a topical steroid (miconazole with betamethasone dipropionate or nystatin with triamcinolone acetonide). Persistent lesions may require addition of antibacterial creams, such as mupirocin (Bactroban) and treatment of oral infection/colonization. Recurrence is common if the underlying risk factors are not managed. In cases of refractory candidiasis and for chronic mucocutaneous candidiasis, a 2-week course of a systemic antifungal such as fluconazole, ketoconazole, or itraconazole is a common choice.[120] For persisting cases, amphotericin B or next-generation antifungals are available.

Mucosal trauma

Trauma is a common cause of irritation and ulceration of the oral mucosa. Traumatic oral lesions may be accidental, factitial, or iatrogenic and may result from physical, chemical, or thermal insults to the tissue.[121] Hyposalivation may predispose a patient to traumatic lesions of the mucosa due to inadequate lubrication. Chemical and thermal burns are rare because the oral mucosa is quite resistant to heat and acid or alkaline compounds. Thermal burns usually affect the hard palate and are most commonly caused by ingestion of hot liquids or hot melted cheese ("pizza palate"). Electrical burns are almost exclusively seen in children who may bite electric cords. Mucositis due to cancer therapies, including radiation and/or chemotherapy for head and neck cancer or other solid tumors, and hematopoietic malignancies, are common significant and treatment-limiting complications (see below). Chemical burns can be a consequence of deliberate or accidental ingestion of caustic agents; prolonged contact with aspirin or vitamin C tablets; use of undiluted oral antiseptics; contamination of prosthesis with denture cleaners; or accidental contact with phosphoric, chromic, or trichloroacetic acid during dental treatment. As the offending cause or agent is usually quickly discontinued or deleted, most traumatic injuries to the oral mucous membranes are acute in nature. Management includes identification of the cause, discontinuation of the offending agent, management of risk factors (eg, hyposalivation), and symptomatic care.[121]

Cancer pain (chronic cancer pain *ICD-11* MG30.10, *ICD-10* G89.3; oral mucositis *ICD-11* DA01.11; *ICD-10* K12.30)

Approximately 3% of all malignancies in the United States are oral and oropharyngeal, with 90% of these being oral squamous cell carcinomas (OSCCs). Annually in the United States, there are nearly 45,000 new cases and more than 9,000 deaths due to head and neck cancers. Improved survival rates have been reported in recent years, reflecting change in cancer etiology involving human papilloma virus (HPV) and changes in cancer therapy. Unfortunately, the improvement does not appear related to early detection, as approximately two-thirds of OSCCs are diagnosed in advanced stages.[122,123] Discomfort is common at diagnosis, and management remains difficult both because the neural mechanisms underlying cancer pain are poorly understood and because there is a lack of adequate pharmacologic management options.[124] Oral involvement by hematologic cancers and orofacial spread of metastatic cancer frequently cause oral pain. Pain from cancer may be due to the malignant disease itself or to anticancer therapy. Pain from

OSCCs may be due to ulceration; pressure on nerves; invasion of nerves, vessels, muscle, and periosteum; or secondary infection. When intraoral neoplasms become large, patients may complain of paresthesia or hypoesthesia that may be accompanied by loose teeth; mass or swelling; and/or restriction of tongue, lip, or jaw movement.[125] Also, as with other painful conditions involving the orofacial structures, pain from cancer may be felt at the primary site, may be referred to another site, or both.

Symptoms from metastatic lesions of the jaw may be the first indication of a distant tumor or may occur during the course of the disease—most commonly breast, prostate, colon, or lung cancer—frequently causing unilateral pain, paresthesia, or anesthesia. Hematologic cancers may involve gingival tissues directly and may be associated with intraoral infection (eg, pericoronitis). Lymphoma commonly involves lymphatic tissues of the head and neck and can present with cervical adenopathy and/or infiltration of gingival tissues with or without discomfort. Cancers and cancer treatments may both produce inflammatory cytokines and release nociceptive and sensitizing molecules that stimulate nerve pain, such as bradykinin, substance P, and endothelin-1.[126]

Pain due to cancer treatment

Head and neck cancer treatment may include surgery, radiation therapy, chemotherapy, targeted agents, and immunotherapy. Treatment-induced acute pain occurs due to surgery or due to mucositis induced by radiation or chemotherapy. The most distressing side effect of head and neck cancer therapy is pain due to oral mucositis (OM). In radiation therapy, OM develops following release of reactive oxygen species, pro-inflammatory cytokines, and sensitizing and nociceptive molecules (eg, bradykinin, 5-HT, prostaglandins, substance P). When ulcerative mucositis is present, the condition is aggravated by secondary microbial irritation, resulting in further upregulation of pro-inflammatory cytokines and nociceptive molecules. In cycled chemotherapy, OM and associated pain may occur in up to 25% of patients; it is more common in patients with mucositis in prior courses of chemotherapy and is more common in later cycles. In hematopoietic stem cell transplant (HSCT), symptomatic OM occurs in more than half of patients, and as in radiation therapy, it may be the most significant acute symptom these patients experience.

In radiation therapy, OM may persist for a few weeks following completion of therapy; with chemotherapy alone, OM may persist for 1 to 2 weeks; and in combined chemotherapy and radiation therapy, it may continue for 1 to 2 months or even longer periods. Other mucosal pain-inducing mechanisms may be present in patients undergoing cancer therapy. In immunosuppressed and myelosuppressed patients, herpes viruses are common causes of mucosal lesions and pain. Following HSCT, oral graft versus host disease (GVHD) may be a cause of symptomatic mucosal lesions (see immune-mediated mucosal lesions). Lastly, many cytotoxic agents (eg, platinum and taxane agents) may affect nerve cells, producing neurogenic pain that can manifest in the orofacial region. All of these mechanisms can induce mucosal pain and changes to taste that can affect oral function, nutrient and energy intake, and quality of life. Post–cancer treatment muscle fibrosis can occur with surgical intervention and radiation therapy and may be increased in patients with chemotherapy. Head and neck cancer patients may experience fibrosis, limiting movement of the tongue, lips, and jaw. Neuropathy following head and neck cancer treatment and radiation therapy– and/or chemotherapy-induced neuropathy is common and may result in orofacial pain.

Management of cancer-related oral pain is dependent on its cause and presentation. Tumor-induced symptoms will regress with anticancer treatment. Postsurgical pain is managed with acute pain medication. Oral pain from cancer or cancer treatment often may present with neuropathic descriptors and may be treated with antidepressants, anticonvulsants, and possibly in combination with opioid analgesics.[126] In 2020, the International Society of Oral Oncology updated its clinical practice guidelines for the management of OM.[127] The recommendations endorsed treatments based on levels of evidence in treating and/or preventing OM. Basic oral care was recommended via patient education, professional dental hygiene, and sodium bicarbonate and chlorhexidine rinses. Additional recommended therapies were cryotherapy/ice chips, benzydamine mouthwash, and photobiomodulation (low-level laser therapy). Keratinocyte growth factor 1 was recommended with autologous HSCT cases.

Geographic tongue (benign migratory glossitis, erythema migrans) (*ICD-11* DA03.1, *ICD-10* K14.1)

CLINICAL CHARACTERISTICS. Geographic tongue is a benign inflammatory disorder that is characterized by multiple well-demarcated zones of erythema (resembling a map, hence "geographic") located on the dorsum and lateral borders of the tongue. Lesions may be present in the buccal mucosa and lip (stomatitis areata migrans) and rarely other oral surfaces.[128–130] The condition is not usually symptomatic but may occasionally present with a burning sensation, often related to the consumption of food (particularly spicy, hot foods, or food and drink high in acid content), likely related to tissue inflammation. Fissured tongue is frequently observed. Lesions vary in size and shape and may have episodic occurrence.[108]

ETIOLOGY. The etiology of geographic tongue remains unclear. The lesion has not been linked to stress and/or infection. It has been suggested that it may represent a manifestation of psoriasis.[108,128]

PATHOPHYSIOLOGY. Loss of adhesion molecules may underlie the clinical findings of red areas (atrophic tongue) surrounded by a white border of less attached epithelium.

MANAGEMENT CONSIDERATIONS. Reassurance and education are generally the only treatments indicated. When symptomatic, topical steroids and/or analgesics may be helpful.[129,130]

Immune-mediated inflammatory conditions

Painful oral conditions may occur due to drug-induced reactions or subsequent to hyposalivation induced by many medications, including tricyclic antidepressants, antipsychotics, muscle relaxants, antihistamines, anticonvulsants, diuretics, anxiolytics, opioid analgesics, and antihypertensive agents. A number of inflammatory/immune disorders may present only in the oral cavity or associated with clinical extraoral manifestations, including lichen planus, aphthous stomatitis, erythema multiforme, mucous membrane (cicatricial or bullous) pemphigoid, pemphigus vulgaris, and lupus erythematosus. Pain is common with these lesions. Oral lichen planus is the most common immune-mediated condition and can cause pain due to inflammation, including neurogenic inflammation/sensitization and mucosal ulceration. Pain is commonly aggravated by spicy, acidic, and highly flavored foods or oral care products. A number of other systemic diseases are known to present with erythematous, erosive, ulcerative, or hemorrhagic—and generally painful—lesions in the oral cavity. These include discoid and systemic lupus erythematosus, uncontrolled diabetes mellitus, uremia, Crohn disease, and blood dyscrasias, such as leukemia and pancytopenia, agranulocytosis, cyclic neutropenia, and sickle cell anemia. GVHD is an inflammatory condition that may follow allogeneic bone marrow (hematopoietic) stem cell transplant that may affect oral tissues, resulting in lichenoid or lupus-like lesions.

Clinical signs and symptoms are rarely pathognomonic, so diagnosis of systemic and/or immune-mediated oral lesions requires laboratory testing, including specific blood components and biopsy specimen immunofluorescence studies. Therefore, these lesions should be referred to specialists or hospital practices for appropriate evaluation. Management of diagnosed immune-mediated lesions requires therapy that involves local and/or systemic immune modulation, with initial treatment often consisting of corticosteroids. Pain relief is typically rapid after inception of appropriate therapy and can be further managed with topical anesthetics or systemic analgesics. Lack of response to immunoactive drugs should increase suspicion of primary or secondary infection of the lesions. Complete remission of the disease is a rare outcome, and these conditions generally require chronic treatment and frequent follow-ups.

Mucosal pain secondary to HIV

The number of oral lesions in HIV-infected individuals has decreased considerably since the introduction of effective antiretroviral therapy. Nevertheless, painful lesions persist in this population and are directly related to immune incompetence.[131] Orofacial pain may be due either directly to HIV infection or to comorbid conditions, including mucosal infection and necrotizing diseases.[132] Causes of oral pain in this population may include herpetic gingivostomatitis, recurrent zoster, candidiasis, progressive gingival and periodontal disease, necrotizing gingivitis or periodontitis, or Kaposi sarcoma or other malignant disease (eg, OSCC, lymphoma), among others.[133] Pain may also be due to HIV-associated peripheral neuropathy.[134] As with all conditions, a proper diagnostic evaluation and identification of disease processes must precede treatment (other than palliation). Painful oral ulcerative conditions are often seen and may be caused by a variety of pathogens, including fungi, viruses, parasites, and bacteria, or they could represent aphthous lesions or tumor.[135–140] The treatment of oral pain in the patient with HIV/AIDS will depend on the specific diagnosis. Symptom management employing analgesics including NSAIDs or acetaminophen to control mild to moderate pain is generally indicated. If the pain is not adequately controlled, an opioid may be prescribed. Various chemotherapeutic or analgesic mouth rinses or topical agents may also be useful in some cases.

Newer Trends

Electronic cigarettes/vaping (vaping-related disorder *ICD-11* RA0.00, *ICD-10* U07.0)

The advent and popularity of electronic cigarettes (e-cigarettes) has gained much traction in the past 10 years, particularly among younger people. Unlike traditional cigarettes where one would inhale smoke, with e-cigarettes one inhales vapor. Hence, this practice is called "vaping," and e-cigarettes are also called "vapes." A basic vape device consists of an atomizer, a power source (battery), and a cartridge containing solution. The solution contains nicotine, flavors, and numerous particles, some of which are toxic and carcinogenic. The user inserts the end of the device into the mouth. Activating a switch manually, or automatically upon inspiration, vaporizes the liquid.

There are two general kinds of vaping techniques and devices. With mouth-to-lung (MTL) vapes, such as the popular brand Juul, the user inhales the vapor from the device into the mouth and subsequently into the lungs. The second technique is called a "lung hit," in which the user simply takes a longer "drag" directly into the lungs. This second technique produces much more vapor by virtue of the fact that lung volume is greater than mouth volume, and thus much more vapor is inhaled and released on exhalation. This plume of vapor coming from the mouth gives vaping its characteristic look.

The prevalence of US adults who use e-cigarettes is 3.2%, but use is an astonishing 20.8% among high school students.[141] Vaping remains controversial. Proponents extol the lower nicotine and carcinogen levels, and vaping may serve as a viable nicotine replacement alternative among smokers who are unable or unwilling to quit. Opponents point out that vaping may be a gateway to smoking and the flavors associated with vaping target younger users. Both traditional smokers and vapers are at risk for the carcinogenic effects of these habits. Periodontal bone loss, attachment loss, peri-implantitis, and inflammatory cytokine production is higher in smokers and vapers compared to those who do not use nicotine products. The most common oral lesions associating with vaping is nicotinic stomatitis, hairy tongue, and angular cheilitis.[142] The oral health professional must remain vigilant and conduct appropriate, periodic oral cancer screening exams.

COVID-19 considerations (COVID-19 virus identified *ICD-11* RA0.10, *ICD-10* U07.1)

From the end of 2019 and through the time of this writing, coronavirus disease 2019 (COVID-19) has been a deadly worldwide pandemic caused by severe acute respiratory syndrome coronavirus 2 (SARS-CoV-2) and its variants. The symptoms that were first described in the literature of 41 patients were fever (98%,) cough (76%), dyspnea (55%), and myalgia or fatigue (44%).[143] SARS-CoV-2 can be present in saliva in up to 92% of symptomatic patients and declines over time.[144] The most common oral symptom is dysgeusia, often comorbid with a loss of the sense of smell.[145] To date, there are no pathognomonic oral lesions of COVID-19. Reports in the literature have described lesions on the vesiculo-erosive spectrum, papules, depapillated tongue, erythema, edema, and petechiae. The diagnoses for these findings included aphthous stomatitis, candidiasis, herpetiform lesions, or generalized mucositis. Site involvement, in descending order, was tongue (38%), labial mucosa (26%), and palate (22%), with 68% of the lesions being painful.[146] There have also been recent reports of parotitis as a presenting finding in emergency departments among patients who tested positive for COVID-19.[147] Currently, it is unknown if these reported lesions represent a sign of COVID-19 disease and whether the pathogenesis involves mucosal tissues. On the other hand, these lesions may be secondary representations of the patient's overall systemic condition during a viral attack and the body's immunologic response to it.

References

1. International Classification of Orofacial Pain, 1st edition (ICOP). Cephalalgia 2020;40:129–221.
2. McCarthy PJ, McClanahan S, Hodges J, Bowles WR. Frequency of localization of the painful tooth by patients presenting for an endodontic emergency. J Endod 2010;36:801–805.
3. Kayaoglu G, Ekici M, Altunkaynak B. Mechanical Allodynia in Healthy Teeth Adjacent and Contralateral to Endodontically Diseased Teeth: A Clinical Study. J Endod 2020;46:611–618.
4. Jain N, Gupta A, Meena N. An insight into neurophysiology of pulpal pain: Facts and hypotheses. Korean J Pain 2013;26:347–355.
5. Okeson J. Bell's Oral and Facial Pain, ed 7. Chicago: Quintessence, 2014.
6. Dabuleanu M. Pulpitis (reversible/irreversible). J Can Dent Assoc 2013;79:d90.
7. Berman L HK. Cohen's Pathways of the Pulp, ed 12. St Louis: Elsevier, 2020.
8. Addy M. Etiology and clinical implications of dentine hypersensitivity. Dent Clin North Am 1990;34:503–514.
9. Abd-Elmeguid A, Yu DC. Dental pulp neurophysiology: Part 1. Clinical and diagnostic implications. J Can Dent Assoc 2009;75:55–59.
10. Fouad AF. Microbiological Aspects of Traumatic Injuries. J Endod 2019;45:S39–S48.

11. Adachi T, Nakanishi T, Yumoto H, et al. Caries-related bacteria and cytokines induce CXCL10 in dental pulp. J Dent Res 2007;86:1217–1222.
12. Ricucci D, Siqueira JF Jr, Li Y, Tay FR. Vital pulp therapy: Histopathology and histobacteriology-based guidelines to treat teeth with deep caries and pulp exposure. J Dent 2019;86:41–52.
13. Gutmann JL, Manjarrés V. Historical and contemporary perspectives on the microbiological aspects of endodontics. Dent J (Basel) 2018;6:49.
14. Lima TFR, Dos Santos SL, da Silva Fidalgo TK, Silva EJNL. Vitality tests for pulp diagnosis of traumatized teeth: A systematic review. J Endod 2019;45:490–499.
15. Kim S. Neurovascular interactions in the dental pulp in health and inflammation. J Endod 1990;16:48–53.
16. Holland GR. The odontoblast process: Form and function. J Dent Res 1985;64 (special issue):499–514.
17. Goldberg M, Lasfargues JJ. Pulpo-dentinal complex revisited. J Dent 1995;23:15–20.
18. Trowbridge HO. Intradental sensory units: Physiological and clinical aspects. J Endod 1985;11:489–498.
19. Brännström M, Aström A. The hydrodynamics of the dentine; Its possible relationship to dentinal pain. Int Dent J 1972;22:219–227.
20. Brännström M, Lindén LA, Aström A. The hydrodynamics of the dental tubule and of pulp fluid. A discussion of its significance in relation to dentinal sensitivity. Caries Res 1967;1:310–317.
21. Van Hassel HJ. Physiology of the human dental pulp. Oral Surg Oral Med Oral Pathol 1971;32:126–134.
22. Lin L, Langeland K. Light and electron microscopic study of teeth with carious pulp exposures. Oral Surg Oral Med Oral Pathol 1981;51:292–316.
23. Torneck CD. Changes in the fine structure of the dental pulp in human caries pulpitis. 1. Nerves and blood vessels. J Oral Pathol 1974;3:71–82.
24. Garfunkel A, Sela J, Ulmansky M. Dental pulp pathosis. Clinicopathologic correlations based on 109 cases. Oral Surg Oral Med Oral Pathol 1973;35:110–117.
25. Seltzer S. Classification of pulpal pathosis. Oral Surg Oral Med Oral Pathol 1972;34:269–287.
26. Seltzer S, Bender IB, Ziontz M. The dynamics of pulp inflammation: Correlations between diagnostic data and actual histologic findings in the pulp. Oral Surg Oral Med Oral Pathol 1963;16:969–977.
27. Wright EF, Gullickson DC. Dental pulpalgia contributing to bilateral preauricular pain and tinnitus. J Orofac Pain 1996;10:166–168.
28. Wright EF. Pulpalgia contributing to temporomandibular disorder-like pain: A literature review and case report. J Am Dent Assoc 2008;139:436–440.
29. Liu XX, Tenenbaum HC, Wilder RS, Quock R, Hewlett ER, Ren YF. Pathogenesis, diagnosis and management of dentin hypersensitivity: An evidence-based overview for dental practitioners. BMC Oral Health 2020;20:220.
30. van Steenberghe D. The structure and function of periodontal innervation. A review of the literature. J Periodontal Res 1979;14:185–203.
31. Armitage GC. Development of a classification system for periodontal diseases and conditions. Ann Periodontol 1999;4:1–6.
32. Meng HX. Periodontal abscess. Ann Periodontol 1999;4:79–83.
33. Herrera D, Roldán S, Sanz M. The periodontal abscess: A review. J Clin Periodontol 2000;27:377–386.
34. Herrera D, Alonso B, de Arriba L, Santa Cruz I, Serrano C, Sanz M. Acute periodontal lesions. Periodontol 2000 2014;65:149–177.
35. Laudenbach JM, Kumar SS. Common dental and periodontal diseases. Dermatol Clin 2020;38:413–420.
36. de Leeuw R, Klasser G. Orofacial Pain: Guidelines for Assessment, Diagnosis, and Management, ed 6. Chicago: Quintessence, 2018.
37. Silva GL, Soares RV, Zenóbio EG. Periodontal abscess during supportive periodontal therapy: A review of the literature. J Contemp Dent Pract 2008;9:82–91.
38. Jaramillo A, Arce RM, Herrera D, Betancourth M, Botero JE, Contreras A. Clinical and microbiological characterization of periodontal abscesses. J Clin Periodontol 2005;32:1213–1218.
39. Topoll HH, Lange DE, Müller RF. Multiple periodontal abscesses after systemic antibiotic therapy. J Clin Periodontol 1990;17:268–272.
40. Herrera D, Roldán S, González I, Sanz M. The periodontal abscess (I). Clinical and microbiological findings. J Clin Periodontol 2000;27:387–394.
41. O'Brien TJ. Diagnosis and treatment of periodontal and gingival abscesses. J Ont Dent Assoc 1970;47:16–18.
42. Rafiei M, Kiani F, Sayehmiri K, et al. Prevalence of anaerobic bacteria (P.gingivalis) as major microbial agent in the incidence periodontal diseases by meta-analysis. J Dent (Shiraz) 2018;19:232–242.
43. Moore WE, Moore LV. The bacteria of periodontal diseases. Periodontol 2000 1994;5:66–77.
44. Offenbacher S. Periodontal diseases: Pathogenesis. Ann Periodontol 1996;1:821–878.
45. Birkedal-Hansen H. Role of cytokines and inflammatory mediators in tissue destruction. J Periodontal Res 1993;28:500–510.
46. Leung WK, Theilade E, Comfort MB, Lim PL. Microbiology of the pericoronal pouch in mandibular third molar pericoronitis. Oral Microbiol Immunol 1993;8:306–312.

47. Lone PA, Jamwal R, Suden A, Lone BA. Comparison of two different irrigating solutions i.e. 3% hydrogen peroxide and 0.12 % chlorhexidine in pericoronitis of partially erupted mandibular third molars, without antibiotics. Int J Contemp Med Res 2015;3:3353–3356.
48. Haggerty CJ, Laughlin RM (eds). Atlas of Operative Oral and Maxillofacial Surgery. Hoboken: Wiley-Blackwell, 2015.
49. Newman MG, Takei H, Klokkevold P, Carranza F. Newman and Carranza's Clinical Periodontology. St Louis: Elsevier, 2019.
50. Bader JD, Martin JA, Shugars DA. Preliminary estimates of the incidence and consequences of tooth fracture. J Am Dent Assoc 1995;126:1650–1654.
51. Wright EF, Bartoloni JA. Diagnosing, managing, and preventing cracked tooth syndrome. Gen Dent 2012; 60:e302–e307.
52. Banerji S, Mehta SB, Millar BJ. Cracked tooth syndrome. Part 1: Aetiology and diagnosis. Br Dent J 2010;208: 459–463.
53. Gill T, Pollard AJ, Baker J, Tredwin C. Cracked tooth syndrome: Assessment, prognosis and predictable management strategies. Eur J Prosthodont Restor Dent 2021;29:209–217.
54. Mamoun JS, Napoletano D. Cracked tooth diagnosis and treatment: An alternative paradigm. Eur J Dent 2015;9:293–303.
55. Gao A, Cao D, Lin Z. Diagnosis of cracked teeth using cone-beam computed tomography: Literature review and clinical experience. Dentomaxillofac Radiol 2021;50:20200407.
56. PradeepKumar AR, Shemesh H, Nivedhitha MS, et al. Diagnosis of vertical root fractures by cone-beam computed tomography in root-filled teeth with confirmation by direct visualization: A systematic review and meta-analysis. J Endod 2021;47:1198–1214.
57. Banerji S, Mehta SB, Millar BJ. Cracked tooth syndrome. Part 2: Restorative options for the management of cracked tooth syndrome. Br Dent J 2010; 208:503–514.
58. Banerji S, Mehta SB, Millar BJ. The management of cracked tooth syndrome in dental practice. Br Dent J 2017;222:659–666.
59. Albandar JM, Susin C, Hughes FJ. Manifestations of systemic diseases and conditions that affect the periodontal attachment apparatus: Case definitions and diagnostic considerations. J Clin Periodontol 2018;45 (suppl 20):S171–S189.
60. Jepsen S, Caton JG, Albandar JM, et al. Periodontal manifestations of systemic diseases and developmental and acquired conditions: Consensus report of workgroup 3 of the 2017 World Workshop on the Classification of Periodontal and Peri-Implant Diseases and Conditions. J Clin Periodontol 2018;45 (suppl 20):S219–S229.
61. Sanz M, Del Castillo AM, Jepsen S, et al. Periodontitis and cardiovascular diseases. Consensus report. Glob Heart 2020;15:1.
62. Romandini M, Baima G, Antonoglou G, Bueno J, Figuero E, Sanz M. Periodontitis, edentulism, and risk of mortality: A systematic review with meta-analyses. J Dent Res 2021;100:37–49.
63. Chandan JS, Thomas T. The impact of inflammatory bowel disease on oral health. Br Dent J 2017;222:549–553.
64. Bui FQ, Almeida-da-Silva CLC, Huynh B, et al. Association between periodontal pathogens and systemic disease. Biomed J 2019;42:27–35.
65. Lira-Junior R, Figueredo CM. Periodontal and inflammatory bowel diseases: Is there evidence of complex pathogenic interactions? World J Gastroenterol 2016;22:7963–7972.
66. She YY, Kong XB, Ge YP, et al. Periodontitis and inflammatory bowel disease: A meta-analysis. BMC Oral Health 2020;20:67.
67. Inaba H, Amano A. Roles of oral bacteria in cardiovascular diseases--from molecular mechanisms to clinical cases: Implication of periodontal diseases in development of systemic diseases. J Pharmacol Sci 2010;113:103–109.
68. De Laat A. Differential diagnosis of toothache to prevent erroneous and unnecessary dental treatment. J Oral Rehabil 2020;47:775–781.
69. Greene CS, Manfredini D. Mismanagement of dentoalveolar pain: What are the clinical consequences? J Am Dent Assoc 2022;153:79–85.
70. Yatani H, Komiyama O, Matsuka Y, et al. Systematic review and recommendations for nonodontogenic toothache. J Oral Rehabil 2014;41:843–852.
71. Renton T. Tooth-related pain or not? Headache 2020;60:235–246.
72. Wright EF. Referred craniofacial pain patterns in patients with temporomandibular disorder. J Am Dent Assoc 2000;131:1307–1315.
73. Duffin PS, Smith A, Hawkins JM. Nonodontogenic odontalgia referred from the temporal tendon: A case report. J Endod 2020;46:1530–1534.
74. Kreiner M, Okeson J, Tanco V, Waldenström A, Isberg A. Orofacial pain and toothache as the sole symptom of an acute myocardial infarction entails a major risk of misdiagnosis and death. J Oral Facial Pain Headache 2020;34:53–60.
75. Sexton C, Lalloo R, Stormon N, et al. Oral health and behaviours of people living with Multiple Sclerosis in Australia. Community Dent Oral Epidemiol 2019;47: 201–209.
76. Miura A, Tu TTH, Shinohara Y, et al. Psychiatric comorbidities in patients with Atypical Odontalgia. J Psychosom Res 2018;104:35–40.

77. Rowland RW. Necrotizing ulcerative gingivitis. Ann Periodontol 1999;4:65–73.
78. Herrera D, Retamal-Valdes B, Alonso B, Feres M. Acute periodontal lesions (periodontal abscesses and necrotizing periodontal diseases) and endo-periodontal lesions. J Clin Periodontol 2018;45(suppl 20):S78–S94.
79. Bouganim N, Dranitsaris G, Amir E, Clemons M. Optimising the use of bone-targeted agents in patients with metastatic cancers: A practical guide for medical oncologists. Support Care Cancer 2011;19:1687–1696.
80. Ruggiero SL, Dodson TB, Fantasia J, et al. American Association of Oral and Maxillofacial Surgeons position paper on medication-related osteonecrosis of the jaw--2014 update. J Oral Maxillofac Surg 2014;72:1938–1956.
81. Laskaris G. Oral manifestations of infectious diseases. Dent Clin North Am 1996;40:395–423.
82. Loesche WJ, Syed SA, Laughon BE, Stoll J. The bacteriology of acute necrotizing ulcerative gingivitis. J Periodontol 1982;53:223–230.
83. Chattopadhyay A, Shetty KV. Recurrent aphthous stomatitis. Otolaryngol Clin North Am 2011;44:79–88, v.
84. Axéll T, Henricsson V. Association between recurrent aphthous ulcers and tobacco habits. Scand J Dent Res 1985;93:239–242.
85. Natah SS, Konttinen YT, Enattah NS, Ashammakhi N, Sharkey KA, Häyrinen-Immonen R. Recurrent aphthous ulcers today: A review of the growing knowledge. Int J Oral Maxillofac Surg 2004;33:221–234.
86. Bagán JV, Sanchis JM, Milián MA, Peñarrocha M, Silvestre FJ. Recurrent aphthous stomatitis. A study of the clinical characteristics of lesions in 93 cases. J Oral Pathol Med 1991;20:395–397.
87. Wray D, Vlagopoulos TP, Siraganian RP. Food allergens and basophil histamine release in recurrent aphthous stomatitis. Oral Surg Oral Med Oral Pathol 1982;54:388–395.
88. Jurge S, Kuffer R, Scully C, Porter SR. Mucosal disease series. Number VI. Recurrent aphthous stomatitis. Oral Dis 2006;12:1–21.
89. Woo SB, Sonis ST. Recurrent aphthous ulcers: A review of diagnosis and treatment. J Am Dent Assoc 1996;127:1202–1213.
90. Slebioda Z, Szponar E, Kowalska A. Etiopathogenesis of recurrent aphthous stomatitis and the role of immunologic aspects: Literature review. Arch Immunol Ther Exp (Warsz) 2014;62:205–215.
91. Siegel MA, Balciunas BA. Medication can induce severe ulcerations. J Am Dent Assoc 1991;122:75–77.
92. Bazrafshani MR, Hajeer AH, Ollier WE, Thornhill MH. IL-1B and IL-6 gene polymorphisms encode significant risk for the development of recurrent aphthous stomatitis (RAS). Genes Immun 2002;3:302–305.
93. Guimarães AL, Correia-Silva Jde F, Sá AR, et al. Investigation of functional gene polymorphisms IL-1beta, IL-6, IL-10 and TNF-alpha in individuals with recurrent aphthous stomatitis. Arch Oral Biol 2007;52:268–272.
94. Bazrafshani MR, Hajeer AH, Ollier WE, Thornhill MH. Polymorphisms in the IL-10 and IL-12 gene cluster and risk of developing recurrent aphthous stomatitis. Oral Dis 2003;9:287–291.
95. Lewkowicz N, Kur B, Kurnatowska A, Tchorzewski H, Lewkowicz P. Expression of Th1/Th2/Th3/Th17-related genes in recurrent aphthous ulcers. Arch Immunol Ther Exp (Warsz) 2011;59:399–406.
96. Lewkowicz N, Lewkowicz P, Banasik M, Kurnatowska A, Tchórzewski H. Predominance of Type 1 cytokines and decreased number of CD4(+)CD25(+high) T regulatory cells in peripheral blood of patients with recurrent aphthous ulcerations. Immunol Lett 2005;99:57–62.
97. Hargitai IA. Painful Oral Lesions. Dent Clin North Am 2018;62:597–609.
98. Akintoye SO, Greenberg MS. Recurrent aphthous stomatitis. Dent Clin North Am 2014;58:281–297.
99. Cabras M, Carrozzo M, Gambino A, et al. Value of colchicine as treatment for recurrent oral ulcers: A systematic review. J Oral Pathol Med 2020;49:731–740.
100. Sharda N, Shashikanth MC, Kant P, Jain M. Levamisole and low-dose prednisolone in the treatment of reccurent aphthous stomatitis. J Oral Pathol Med 2014;43:309–316.
101. Sharquie KE, Najim RA, Al-Hayani RK, Al-Nuaimy AA, Maroof DM. The therapeutic and prophylactic role of oral zinc sulfate in management of recurrent aphthous stomatitis (ras) in comparison with dapsone. Saudi Med J 2008;29:734–738.
102. Olson JA, Silverman S Jr. Double-blind study of levamisole therapy in recurrent aphthous stomatitis. J Oral Pathol 1978;7:393–399.
103. Stoopler ET. Oral herpetic infections (HSV 1-8). Dent Clin North Am 2005;49:15–29, vii.
104. Sapp JP, Eversole LR, Wysocki GP. Contemporary Oral and Maxillofacial Pathology. St Louis: Mosby, 1997.
105. Chauvin PJ, Ajar AH. Acute herpetic gingivostomatitis in adults. A review of 13 cases, including diagnosis and management. J Can Dent Assoc 2002;68:247–251.
106. Corey L, Spear PG. Infections with herpes simplex viruses (2). N Engl J Med 1986;314:749–757.

107. Scully C. Ulcerative stomatitis, gingivitis, and skin lesions. An unusual case of primary herpes simplex infection. Oral Surg Oral Med Oral Pathol 1985;59: 261–263.
108. Regezi JA, Sciubba JJ, Pogrel MA. Atlas of Oral and Maxillofacial Pathology. London: Saunders, 2000.
109. Weaver BA. Herpes zoster overview: Natural history and incidence. J Am Osteopath Assoc 2009;109(suppl 2):S2–S6.
110. Thakur R, Philip AG. Chronic pain perspectives: Treating herpes zoster and postherpetic neuralgia: An evidence-based approach. J Fam Pract 2012;61(9 suppl):S9–S15.
111. James SF, Chahine EB, Sucher AJ, Hanna C. Shingrix: The new adjuvanted recombinant herpes zoster vaccine. Ann Pharmacother 2018;52:673–680.
112. Dooling KL, Guo A, Patel M, et al. Recommendations of the Advisory Committee on Immunization Practices for Use of Herpes Zoster Vaccines. MMWR Morb Mortal Wkly Rep 2018;67:103–108.
113. Lin CS, Lin YC, Lao HC, Chen CC. Interventional treatments for postherpetic neuralgia: A systematic review. Pain Physician 2019;22:209–228.
114. Kolšek M. TENS—An alternative to antiviral drugs for acute herpes zoster treatment and postherpetic neuralgia prevention. Swiss Med Wkly 2012;141: w13229.
115. Dinan JE, Hargitai IA, Watson N, Smith A, Schmidt JE. Pain catastrophising in the oro-facial pain population. J Oral Rehabil 2021;48:643–653.
116. Appleton SS. Candidiasis: Pathogenesis, clinical characteristics, and treatment. J Calif Dent Assoc 2000; 28:942–948.
117. Staab JF, Bradway SD, Fidel PL, Sundstrom P. Adhesive and mammalian transglutaminase substrate properties of Candida albicans Hwp1. Science 1999;283:1535–1538.
118. Farah CS, Ashman RB, Challacombe SJ. Oral candidosis. Clin Dermatol 2000;18:553–562.
119. Neville BW DD, Allen CM, Bouquot J. Oral & Maxillofacial Pathology, ed 2. Philadelphia: Saunders, 2002.
120. Muzyka BC, Epifanio RN. Update on oral fungal infections. Dent Clin North Am 2013;57:561–581.
121. Cifuentes M, Davari P, Rogers RS, 3rd. Contact stomatitis. Clin Dermatol 2017;35:435–440.
122. Vokes EE. Head and neck cancer. In: Kasper D, Fauci A, Hauser S, Longo D, Jameson JL, Loscalzo J (eds). Harrison's Principles of Internal Medicine, ed 19. New York: McGraw-Hill, 2015:502–505.
123. Barasch A, Safford M, Eisenberg E. Oral cancer and oral effects of anticancer therapy. Mt Sinai J Med 1998;65:370–377.
124. Viet CT, Schmidt BL. Biologic mechanisms of oral cancer pain and implications for clinical therapy. J Dent Res 2012;91:447–453.
125. Sarkar R. Pathological and clinical features of primary osseous tumours of the jaw. J Bone Oncol 2014;3:90–95.
126. Epstein JB, Miaskowski C. Oral pain in the cancer patient. J Natl Cancer Inst Monogr 2019;2019:lgz003.
127. Elad S, Cheng KKF, Lalla RV, et al. MASCC/ISOO clinical practice guidelines for the management of mucositis secondary to cancer therapy. Cancer 2020;126:4423–4431.
128. Assimakopoulos D, Patrikakos G, Fotika C, Elisaf M. Benign migratory glossitis or geographic tongue: An enigmatic oral lesion. Am J Med 2002;113:751–755.
129. Scully C, Felix DH. Oral medicine—Update for the dental practitioner: Red and pigmented lesions. Br Dent J 2005;199:639–645.
130. Pass B, Brown RS, Childers EL. Geographic tongue: Literature review and case reports. Dent Today 2005; 24:54,56–57.
131. Schofferman J. Care of the terminally ill person with AIDS. Int Ophthalmol Clin 1989;29:127–130.
132. Dios PD, Ocampo A, Miralles C, Limeres J, Tomás I. Changing prevalence of human immunodeficiency virus-associated oral lesions. Oral Surg Oral Med Oral Pathol Oral Radiol Endod 2000;90:403–404.
133. Gennaro S, Naidoo S, Berthold P. Oral health & HIV/AIDS. MCN Am J Matern Child Nurs 2008;33:50–57.
134. Kaku M, Simpson DM. HIV neuropathy. Curr Opin HIV AIDS 2014;9:521–526.
135. Bruce AJ, Rogers RS 3rd. Oral manifestations of sexually transmitted diseases. Clin Dermatol 2004;22: 520–527.
136. Campisi G, Pizzo G, Mancuso S, Margiotta V. Gender differences in human immunodeficiency virus-related oral lesions: An Italian study. Oral Surg Oral Med Oral Pathol Oral Radiol Endod 2001;91:546–551.
137. Cannon M, Cesarman E. Kaposi's sarcoma-associated herpes virus and acquired immunodeficiency syndrome-related malignancy. Semin Oncol 2000; 27:409–419.
138. Depaola LG. Human immunodeficiency virus disease: natural history and management. Oral Surg Oral Med Oral Pathol Oral Radiol Endod 2000;90:266–270.
139. Detels R, Tarwater P, Phair JP, Margolick J, Riddler SA, Muñoz A. Effectiveness of potent antiretroviral therapies on the incidence of opportunistic infections before and after AIDS diagnosis. Aids 2001;15:347–355.
140. Clarkson E, Mashkoor F, Abdulateef S. Oral viral infections: Diagnosis and management. Dent Clin North Am 2017;61:351–363.
141. Creamer MR, Wang TW, Babb S, et al. Tobacco product use and cessation indicators among adults—United States, 2018. MMWR Morb Mortal Wkly Rep 2019;68:1013–1019.

142. Ralho A, Coelho A, Ribeiro M, et al. Effects of electronic cigarettes on oral cavity: A systematic review. J Evid Based Dent Pract 2019;19:101318.
143. Huang C, Wang Y, Li X, et al. Clinical features of patients infected with 2019 novel coronavirus in Wuhan, China. Lancet 2020;395:497–506.
144. To KK, Tsang OT, Yip CC, et al. Consistent detection of 2019 novel coronavirus in saliva. Clin Infect Dis 2020;71:841–843.
145. Thomas DC, Baddireddy SM, Kohli D. Anosmia: A review in the context of coronavirus disease 2019 and orofacial pain. J Am Dent Assoc 2020;151:696–702.
146. Iranmanesh B, Khalili M, Amiri R, Zartab H, Aflatoonian M. Oral manifestations of COVID-19 disease: A review article. Dermatol Ther 2021;34:e14578.
147. Lechien JR, Chetrit A, Chekkoury-Idrissi Y, et al. Parotitis-like symptoms associated with COVID-19, France, March–April 2020. Emerg Infect Dis 2020;26:2270–2271.

8

Differential Diagnosis and Management of TMDs

Key Points

- Temporomandibular disorders (TMDs) rarely result in disabling conditions.
- There is no single cause for all TMDs. Benign TMD signs and symptoms are very common among the general population and are generally self-limiting.
- Only 3.6% to 7% of the general population have TMDs severe enough that they seek treatment. Patients with pain-free temporomandibular joint (TMJ) clicking generally do not need treatment; reassurance and education about this benign condition usually suffices.
- Management of TMDs should include the identification and addressing the effect of contributing factors such as parafunctional oral habits.
- Smoking habits and certain disorders may influence TMD symptoms and prognosis, so these factors should be addressed.
- Management of TMDs may include self-management instructions, oral appliances, pharmacotherapy, and physical therapy.
- Generally, invasive surgical management is indicated only after reasonable nonsurgical efforts have failed and when the patient's quality of life is significantly affected.
- Radiographic structural changes consistent with degenerative joint disease (DJD) should not be used as the sole guide for treatment decisions.

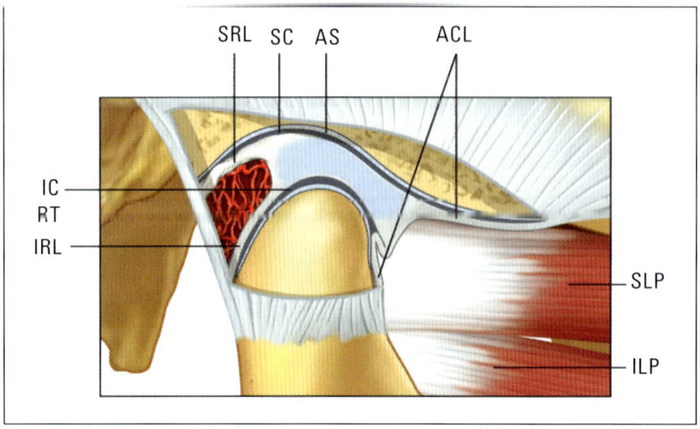

Fig 8-1 Normal anatomy of the TMJ. ACL, anterior capsular ligament (collagenous); AS, articular surface; IRL, inferior retrodiscal lamina (collagenous); RT, retrodiscal tissues; SC and IC, superior and inferior joint cavities; SLP and ILP, superior and inferior lateral pterygoid muscles; SRL, superior retrodiscal lamina (elastic). (Reproduced with permission from Okeson.[1])

Anatomy of the Masticatory Structures

Temporomandibular articulation occurs in the TMJs, two of the most complex joints of the body. The TMJ is technically considered a ginglymoarthrodial joint because each TMJ provides for both hinging or rotation movements in one plane (a criterion for a ginglymoid joint) and for gliding or translation movements (a criterion for an arthrodial joint).[1] The TMJ is formed by the mandibular condyle fitting into the mandibular (glenoid) fossa of the temporal bone (Fig 8-1).[1] Separating these two bones from direct contact is the interposed articular disc (sometimes inappropriately called a *meniscus*). The articular portion of the healthy disc is composed of dense fibrous connective tissue, devoid of any nerves or vessels; conversely, the posterior attachment of the disc is richly vascularized and innervated.[2–4] Collateral ligaments attach the disc to the condyle both medially and laterally. These ligaments permit rotational movement of the disc on the condyle during opening and closing of the mouth.

This so-called "condyle-disc complex" translates out of the fossa during extended mouth opening (Fig 8-2).[1] Therefore, in the normal joint, rotational movement occurs between the condyle and the inferior surface of the disc during early opening (the inferior joint space), and translation takes place in the space between the superior surface of the disc and the fossa (the superior joint space) during later opening. Movement of the joint is lubricated by synovial fluid, which also acts as a medium for transporting nutrients and waste products to and from the articular surfaces. Unlike most synovial joints, the articulating surfaces of the TMJs are lined with dense fibrocartilage instead of hyaline cartilage.[5] This is an important feature because fibrocartilage has a greater ability to repair itself than does hyaline cartilage. This implies that the management of arthritic conditions of the TMJ may be different from that of other synovial joints.[6]

Movement of the TMJs is achieved by a group of skeletal muscles called the *muscles of mastication*. These muscles are comparable to other skeletal muscles in physiology and ergonomics.[7] Although the muscles of mastication are the primary muscles that provide mandibular movement, other associated muscles of the head and neck provide secondary support during mastication. The masticatory muscles include the masseter, medial pterygoid, and temporalis muscles, which predominantly elevate the mandible (mouth closing); the digastric

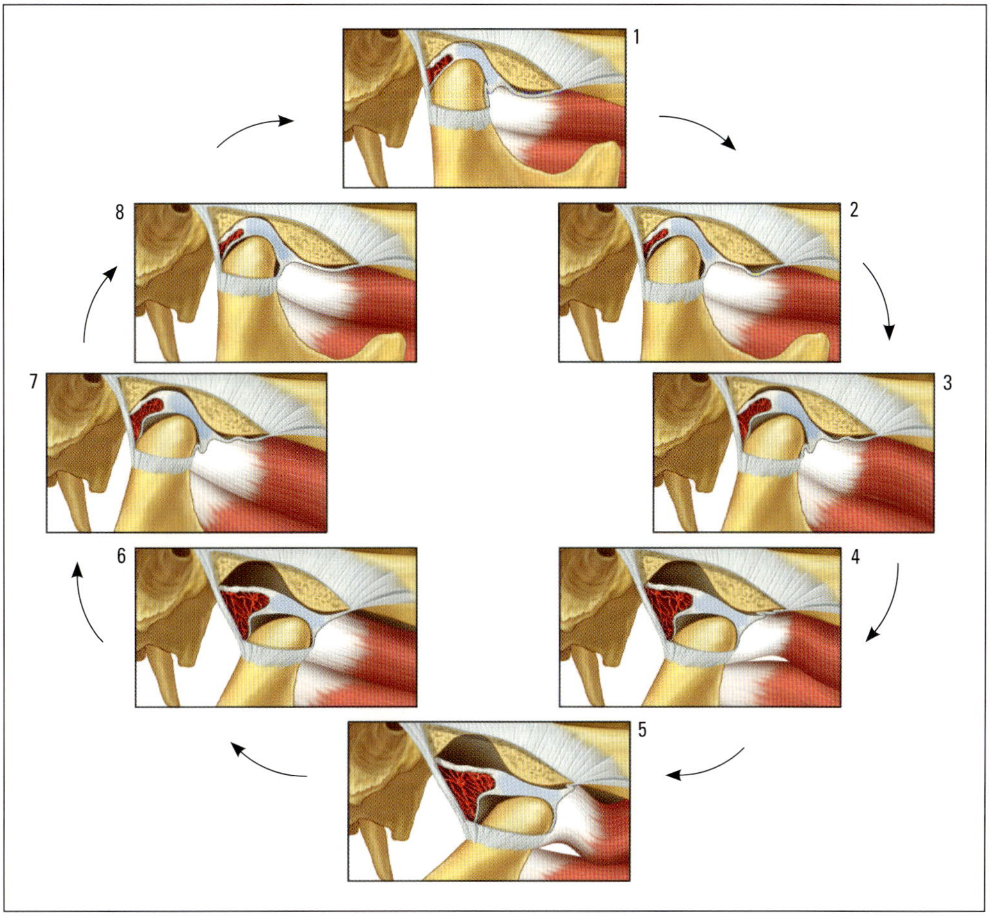

Fig 8-2 Normal functional movement of the condyle and disc during the full range of opening and closing. Note that the disc is rotated posteriorly on the condyle as the condyle is translated out of the fossa. The closing movement is the exact opposite of opening. (Reproduced with permission from Okeson.[1])

muscles, which assist in mandibular depression (mouth opening); the inferior lateral pterygoid muscles, which assist in protruding and lateral movements of the mandible; and the superior lateral pterygoid muscles, which provide stabilization for the condyle and disc during function.[8–11] The masticatory muscles are involved in various orofacial functions, including talking, chewing, and swallowing. A number of muscle behaviors are nonfunctional (ie, parafunctional) and are categorized under the broad term of *bruxism,* which currently is defined as repetitive masticatory activity characterized by clenching or grinding of the teeth and/or bracing or thrusting of the mandible and specified as either sleep or awake.[12]

Defining TMDs

TMDs encompass a group of musculoskeletal and neuromuscular conditions that involve the

TMJs, the masticatory muscles, and all associated tissues.[13] Most recently, *TMDs* were defined as a set of diseases and disorders that are related to alteration in the structure, function, or physiology of the masticatory system and that may be associated with other systemic and comorbid medical conditions. TMDs are the most prevalent type of chronic orofacial pain.[14] TMDs represent clusters of related disorders in the masticatory system with many common symptoms. The most frequent presenting symptom is pain, usually localized in the muscles of mastication or the preauricular area. Chewing or other mandibular activities usually aggravate the pain. In addition to complaints of pain, patients with these disorders frequently have limited mandibular movements and TMJ sounds that are most frequently described as clicking, popping, grating, or crepitus.

Common patient complaints include jaw ache, earache, headache, and facial pain. Nonpainful masticatory muscle hypertrophy and abnormal occlusal wear associated with oral parafunction, such as bruxism (eg, clenching and grinding), may be related problems. Pain or dysfunction due to nonmusculoskeletal causes such as otolaryngologic, neurologic, vascular, neoplastic, or infectious disease in the orofacial region is not considered to be a primary TMD even though secondary musculoskeletal pain may be present.

Epidemiology of TMDs

Reports on the prevalence of TMDs from cross-sectional epidemiologic studies vary considerably from study to study because of differences in terminology, operational definitions, data collection, analytic approaches (eg, single-factor versus multiple factor analysis), and bias. A systematic review including only studies adopting the Research Diagnostic Criteria for TMDs[15,16] reported a prevalence of up to 13% for masticatory muscle pain, up to 16% for disc derangement disorders, and up to 9% for TMJ pain disorders in the general population.[17] While the prevalence of the different diagnoses in TMDs within patient populations varied widely, the results of a meta-analysis showed a prevalence of 45%, 41%, and 30% for muscle disorders, disc derangement disorders, and joint pain disorders, respectively.[17] Data from the National Health Interview Survey from 2009 show that 5% of the U.S. adult population (11.5 million people) had self-reported jaw or face pain in the preceding 3 months.[18] Consistently, based on population data from 2017 to 2018, it was estimated that 4.8% of US adults had pain in the region of the TMJ that could be related to TMD.[14,19] Moreover, using a random sample of adult women in the US, the examiner confirmed that prevalence of TMD was estimated at 10%.[20]

Other studies show that TMDs are primarily a condition of young and middle-aged adults, rather than of children or the elderly, and are approximately twice more common in women than in men.[18,21,22] Data on the association between race and TMD are not consistent. TMD prevalence has been reported higher in African American people and Hispanic women compared to white women,[20] but longitudinal data show that both the rate of TMD symptoms and the rate of first-onset TMD were greater in African American people, although the persistency of the symptoms is higher in white people. [23] In addition, TMDs are often remitting, self-limiting, or fluctuating over time; the progression to a potentially more serious nonreducing disc status or chronic and disabling intracapsular TMJ disease is relatively uncommon.[24–28] In fact, recent data demonstrated that 76% and 71% of soft and hard tissue diagnoses, respectively, remained stable after an 8-year follow-up.[29]

Only 3.6% to 7% of individuals with TMDs have been estimated to require treatment, and the annual incidence rate is estimated to be 2%.[30–35] For painful TMDs specifically, the most recent estimate for first onset was 3.9%, with 50% of the cases maintaining the condition after 6 months.[23] Because joint sounds are common, often pain free, not progressive, and with poor sensitivity to identify most intracapsular conditions,[15] it is important to avoid overtreatment of benign chronic reducing and nonreducing disc displacement in the absence of pain and impaired function.[28] According to magnetic resonance imaging (MRI) studies, it is estimated that up to 35% of asymptomatic individuals appear to have disc displacements.[36]

Painful TMD conditions such as myofascial pain and arthralgia have been associated with facial trauma, third molar removal, clenching, physical symptoms (somatization), and the female sex.[37] Cigarette smoking has been associated with an increased risk of TMDs in young adults, and higher levels of pain, psychosocial distress, and sleep disturbances are reported among TMD patients.[38,39]

Specifically, several longitudinal studies have supported that poor sleep quality and sleep deficiency are risk factors for the development of chronic pain.[40] The mechanisms involved influence nociceptive processing by deactivating systems and mediators with analgesic properties and activating those with hyperalgesia properties.[41]

The framework of sleep disorders and hyperalgesia, the association of self-reported sleep disorders (sleep disturbance and obstructive sleep apnea symptoms), atopic conditions, and multiple painful conditions were also evaluated. Findings support elevated odds of TMD incidence among individuals with various sleep-related markers and atopy disorders.[42]

The relationship between painful TMDs and comorbid conditions has been evaluated by several investigators. Myofascial pain patients self-report more severe headaches, fainting and dizzy spells, gastric acid reflux, fibromyalgia, anxiety, depression, psychiatric treatments, phobias, and frequent sore throats compared with arthralgia patients (both diagnoses based on the RDC/TMD).[43] Individuals developing TMDs are also more likely to describe comorbidities such as headaches, muscle soreness, and other body pains.[44]

In fact, headaches have been identified as a risk factor for TMD onset. The TMD incidence rate was 8.4% per year among individuals with mixed headaches and 6.0% among individuals who reported four headaches per month. A dose response effect was observed that aligned with the number of headaches.[45] Moreover, the assessment of chronic overlapping conditions has been intensely evaluated by the Orofacial Pain: Prospective Evaluation and Risk (OPPERA) group. Greater evidence of syndromic presentation was noted among musculoskeletal conditions such as fibromyalgia, TMDs, and low back pain, in contrast to that seen in headache and irritable bowel syndrome. Among TMD cases, 78% had one or more comorbid conditions, with headaches being the dominant tendency.[46]

In a more integrated model, the presence of comorbid conditions was investigated to see if it further modified the phenotype of individuals with TMDs. This relationship was evaluated by implementing a Multisystem Dysregulation Index that included sensory, autonomic, inflammatory, and psychologic domains due to their contribution in pain amplification.[47] Among individuals without comorbid persistent pain (only 8% among cases of the study population), the predominant dysregulation was in the sensory domain, which represented the presence of generalized somatic sensitization. Among those with one persistent painful comorbid condition (49%), the psychologic dysregulation was the only domain associated with the increased risk of having a TMD. For those individuals with two or more comorbid conditions (42%), a multisystem dysregulation was observed that included sensory, psychologic, and autonomic domains, indicating that multisystem dysregulation is associated with common persistent pain conditions.[47]

A relevant contribution of the OPPERA study has been the integration of clinical characteristics, autonomic function, psychophysical response to experimental pain, psychosocial characteristics, and environmental exposures to identify three major clusters of individuals. These clusters were identified as "Adaptive," "Pain Sensitive," and "Global Symptoms." The lowest proportion of TMD cases (8.5%), which had lower pain sensitivity and lower psychologic distress, were assigned to the Adaptive cluster.[48] The Pain Sensitivity cluster made up 52.5% of the cases, which had more sensitivity to pain-evoking pressure stimuli (PPT), higher levels of psychologic distress, and a slightly greater response to experimental pain sensitivity compared to the Adaptive group.[48] The Global Symptoms group, which comprised 39% of the cases, had the highest pain sensitivity and psychologic distress, a vastly increased risk of pain severity, physical and mental dysfunction, greater TMD pain intensity, and the greatest burden of comorbid pain, with an overall higher risk of TMD onset.[48]

International comparisons of comorbid pain conditions among women with TMD pain were evaluated among women from Italy, Sweden, and Saudi Arabia. Using a case-control design that was age-matched in the respective centers, it was found that comorbid pain prevalence, intensity, and disability differ among women from these cultures. The comorbid conditions studied were head, chest, back, and abdominal pain, and all comorbid conditions were consistently higher among the cases than the controls. The prevalence of back pain was higher among women from Saudi Arabia. Saudi Arabian women experienced more interference from the back pain than women from Sweden and Italy. Headache did not differ among the groups, but the intensity was lower among the women from Sweden.[49]

Consistent results have been presented among adolescents from Canada, France, and Brazil, and the most common comorbidities among short- and long-term painful TMDs were headaches, back pain, and allergies.[50]

Overall, as presented in a recent systematic review, individuals with TMDs have a higher prevalence of comorbid chronic pain conditions, including back pain, myofascial syndrome, stomach pain, migraines, irritable bowel syndrome, and fibromyalgia.[51]

Etiology of TMDs

No unambiguous universal cause of TMDs has been identified because determining causation requires more than just phenotyping the conditions under study and/or describing their distribution based on observational studies. Nevertheless, the methodologic quality of such observational studies is key to determining their internal and external validity and to then transfer such knowledge to clinical care. For this reason, most of the factors discussed in this section are not proven causal, but are instead associated with TMDs. Factors that may cause the onset of TMDs are called *initiating or precipitating factors*, factors that increase the risk of TMDs are called *predisposing factors*, and factors that interfere with healing or enhance the progression of TMDs are called *perpetuating* or *maintaining factors*. Under varying circumstances, individual factors may serve any or all of these roles. There is not a single etiologic factor or a unique theoretical model that can explain the onset of TMDs.

Bone and TMJ soft tissue remodeling and muscle tone regulation are all adaptive physiologic responses to injury or change. Loss of structural integrity, altered function, or biomechanical stresses in the system can compromise adaptability and increase the likelihood of dysfunction, dysregulation, or pathology.[52] Current data support that in vivo mechanobehavioral quantification linked to computer models of strain-regulated biochemical events may elucidate the mechanisms responsible for growth, maintenance, and deterioration of TMJ tissues.[53]

Direct extrinsic trauma to any component of the masticatory system can spontaneously initiate loss of structural integrity and concomitantly alter function, thereby reducing the adaptive capacity in the system. In addition, there are other contributing anatomical, systemic, pathophysiologic, and psychosocial factors that may sufficiently reduce the adaptive capacity of the masticatory system and result in TMDs.

Trauma

Trauma is described as any force applied to the mastication structures that exceeds that of normal functional loading. Most trauma can be divided into three types: *(1)* the result of a sudden and usually isolated blow to the structures (*direct trauma*), *(2)* that associated with a sudden blow but without direct contact to the affected structures (*indirect trauma*), and *(3)* the result of prolonged, repeated force over time (*microtrauma*).

Direct trauma

There is general agreement that direct trauma (ie, macrotrauma) to the mandible or the TMJ produces injury via impact and is accompanied in close temporal proximity with signs and symptoms of inflammation. If the forces lead to structural failure, loss of function may quickly follow. Direct trauma resulting in mandibular fracture in adults has been associated with increased signs and symptoms of TMDs; however, these may not result in patients seeking treatment.[54] In children, condylar and subcondylar fractures in girls—but not boys—were associated with increased TMD symptoms over time.[55] More significant fractures may result in disc displacement.[56] Patients with TMDs report physical trauma more often than non-TMD patients.[57] The accuracy of recall of TMD symptoms associated with a traumatic event may be compromised, making it difficult to clearly link the traumatic event with the symptom onset.[58] Other forms of trauma such as wide or prolonged mouth opening, third molar extraction, and intubation have been reported as associated with TMDs.[59,60] Self-reported jaw injury due to yawning or prolonged opening is significantly higher in patients with TMDs.[57] Transient and permanent dysfunction of the TMJ after upper airway management procedures has been reported, but controlled trials and longitudinal studies are not available in the English-language literature.[61,62]

More recently, it was reported that both perceived single injury events and multiple events predicted a greater incidence of painful TMD.[63] Such increased incidence is amplified in individuals with enhanced laboratory-tested heat-pain sensitivity evaluated on the forearm.[64] Analysis of the nested case-control-designed OPPERA data showed a significant association between self-reported jaw injuries attributed to sustained mouth opening, injuries due to yawning, and extrinsic injuries. Overall, jaw injury predicted a 5-fold increase in the odds of painful TMD, illustrating a pronounced influence of jaw injury on painful TMD incidence.[63]

In the OPPERA data, intrinsic injuries related to yawning were reported by 15.5% of the cases compared to 8.0% of the controls. These were related to sustained mouth opening in 17.2% of the cases in contrast to 6.3% in the controls, while extrinsic injuries were reported by 5.2 % of the incident cases versus 1.1% of the controls. Among those who reported injury from sustained mouth opening, only 3% associated it to dental treatment, and no reports were linked to oral intubation.[63]

Indirect trauma

Acceleration-deceleration (flexion-extension) injury (ie, whiplash) with no direct blow to the face may cause symptoms consistent with TMDs, but significant controversy persists as to whether there could be a direct causal relationship. Prospective controlled studies both link and show limited risk for the development of TMD symptoms after whiplash.[65,66] Review of the literature has highlighted these controversies; however, there is some evidence that post-whiplash TMDs can have a different and potentially more protracted clinical course than non-trauma-associated TMDs.[67–69] There is some indication that increased severity of symptoms and structural changes in the lateral pterygoid muscle based on MRI studies may occur in individuals diagnosed with TMD and immediate history of whiplash.[70] Although symptoms in the mandible may be referred from injured cervical structures, a direct causal relationship between mandibular symptoms and indirect trauma has yet to be established.[66,71,72] However, reports seem to indicate increased risk for developing orofacial pain, especially with increased for severity of the indirect trauma.[73]

Computer simulation suggests that low-velocity rear-end impact does not cause mandibular movement or stresses beyond the physiologic range.[74] In support of this finding, human volunteers in simulated rear-end crash tests failed to demonstrate mandibular movement beyond physiologic limits.[75] Thus, while evidence is lacking for a mandibular strain without a direct blow to the mandible following a low-velocity motor vehicle accident, there are recognized pathways of heterotopic pain from the cervical area to the trigeminal area.[76] It is therefore not uncommon to observe symptoms of TMDs following acceleration-deceleration injury to the neck without direct trauma to the face or jaw. The etiologic significance of non-impact injuries is uncertain, and much misinformation is being provided to patients without scientific studies to support the claims.

Microtrauma

Microtrauma has been hypothesized to originate from sustained and repetitious adverse loading of the masticatory system through postural imbalances or from parafunctional behaviors (ie, habits). It has been suggested that postural habits such as forward head position or phone-bracing may create muscle and joint strain and lead to musculoskeletal pain—including headache—in TMD patients.[77]

Parafunctional habits have been most frequently assessed by indirect means such as self-report, questionnaires, reports by a bedroom partner, or tooth wear. These indirect measures of parafunctional habits have resulted in conflicting reports as to the relationship between TMD symptoms and the presence of parafunctional habits. When myofascial TMD patients were compared with controls using polysomnography, the tests did not confirm the patients' self-reports of sleep bruxism more than the controls.[78] Parafunctional habits such as teeth clenching, tooth grinding, lip biting, and abnormal posturing of the mandible are common and usually do not result in TMD symptoms, but they have been suggested as initiating or perpetuating factors in certain subgroups of TMD patients.[79–83] Although the available research and clinical observations generally support this contention, the exact role of parafunctional habits in TMDs remains unclear because few studies have directly assessed these behaviors. Attrition severity secondary to bruxism cannot distinguish TMD patients from asymptomatic individuals, and muscle hyperactivity has not been shown to be associated with arthrogenous TMJ disorders.[84–86] Furthermore, clenching does not cause neuromuscular fatigue because muscles compensate for sustained muscle activity by derecruitment of motor neurons or through slower firing rates.[87]

Despite the lack of evidence that nonexperimentally induced parafunction or clenching can cause TMDs, some studies have shown that experimentally induced parafunction can result in transient pain similar to that reported by patients with TMDs.[81,88–90] The impact of these studies is limited by their small sample sizes. The intensity and frequency of oral parafunctional activity may be exacerbated by stress and anxiety, sleep disorders, and medications (eg, neuroleptics, alcohol, and other substances), although the relationship between sleep bruxism and psychologic factors has been questioned.[91,92] Some forms of masticatory muscle hyperactivity have been associated with emotional behavior and may be mediated via the cortex through the hypothalamus.[93] Intense and persistent parafunction can also occur in patients with neurologic disorders (eg, cerebral palsy) and extrapyramidal disorders (eg, orofacial dyskinesia and epilepsy).[94]

The most commonly believed indication of past sleep bruxism severity is dental attrition.[95] However, dental attrition can also be partly explained by overbite and overjet changes that correlate with age and sex, protrusive guidance schemes, dentofacial morphology, erosive diets, bite force ability, and environmental factors.[96–104] Recent evidence suggests that sleep bruxism may be associated with increased salivation during sleep, resulting in lubrication of oropharyngeal structures, or with increasing the space of the upper airways to aid with airway patency, or both.[105–108] Furthermore, it has been suggested that sleep bruxism plays a protective role as a compensatory mechanism to protect the airway during sleep-related breathing disorders.[109] Therefore, the issue of whether or not sleep bruxism requires management without the presentation of significant problems is debatable. A more pragmatic approach may be to view this as an issue regarding "consequence management," taking into account risk or side effect/benefit ratio.[110] Another problem arises when attrition is used to suggest current bruxism levels. Attrition appears to be episodic in nature and occurs in bursts caused by as yet unspecified factors, and thus any noted attrition may not necessarily represent ongoing or current habits.[111] Moreover, it is not clear whether sleep bruxism is a pathogenic disorder or a normal physiologic process. Recently, it has been proposed that the terms *normo-bruxism* and *patho-bruxism* should be implemented, avoiding attempts to "cure bruxism" but restoring system homeostasis.[112]

Anatomical factors

Skeletal factors

Skeletal factors include adverse biomechanical relationships that can be genetic, developmental, or iatrogenic in origin. Severe skeletal malformations, inter-arch and intra-arch discrepancies, and past injuries to the teeth may play a role in TMDs, but this role may be weaker than previously believed. For example, while it is known that disc displacement is common in children with facial skeletal abnormalities such as retrognathia, it cannot be said that these anatomical anomalies are etiologic.[113] Furthermore, TMD patients with disc displacement generally do not have an increased prevalence of forward head posture.[114] A steep articular eminence has also been proposed as an etiologic factor in internal derangement of the TMJ. In asymptomatic individuals, a steeper eminence was associated with an increased posterior rotation of the disc, posing a potential anatomical risk factor.[115] However, several studies have shown that in TMJs with disc displacement without reduction and TMJs with osseous changes, the eminence was less steep than in TMJs with disc displacement with reduction or TMJs without osseous changes, indicating adaptive remodeling.[116–118] In addition, unilateral joint sounds were associated with the side with the less steep condylar movement path. [119]

Occlusal relationships

Historically, the dental profession has viewed occlusal parameters as a primary etiologic factor for TMDs; nevertheless, such clinical views supported by case reports and anecdotal publications have been challenged and dismantled.[120] Occlusal features such as working and nonworking posterior contacts and discrepancies between the retruded contact position (RCP) and intercuspal position (ICP) have commonly been identified as predisposing, initiating, and perpetuating factors. The evidence suggests that the influence of the occlusion on the onset and development of TMDs is low.[121,122] Among the occlusal factors evaluated, loss of posterior support and unilateral crossbite show some association across studies.[121]

Several occlusal factors (eg, large overjet, minimal anterior overlap and anterior skeletal open bite, unilateral posterior crossbite, occlusal slides > 2 mm, and lack of firm posterior tooth contact) were found to be more prevalent in patients than in convenience samples. However, this is possibly due to condylar positional changes following intracapsular alterations associated with the disease process itself. Therefore, these occlusal factors may be the result rather than the cause of the disease.[121,123] Previous studies have lacked reliable occlusal measurement techniques and data collection methods, which may explain the diversity of some findings. Nevertheless, little evidence is available to implicate occlusal factors in TMD etiology.

Despite the historic views, findings support the absence of a disease-specific association to support the hypothesis of dental occlusion as an etiologic parameter in the pathophysiology of TMD. Furthermore, clinicians are encouraged to abandon the historical gnathologic paradigm in TMD practice.[124] Moreover, it is time for the dental profession and the orofacial pain specialty to endorse the robust 21st century literature, supported by solid scientific methodology, which provides evidence-based knowledge on the nonexisting etiologic role of occlusion.[120]

Pathophysiologic factors

Systemic factors

Systemic pathophysiologic conditions may influence local TMDs and should generally be managed in cooperation with the patient's primary care physician or other medical specialists. These conditions can include degenerative, endocrine, infectious, metabolic, neoplastic, neurologic, rheumatologic, and vascular disorders. Systemic factors can act simultaneously at a central and local (peripheral) level.[125,126]

Generalized joint laxity (hypermobility) has been cited as a possible contributing factor to TMDs and has proven to be significantly more prevalent in patients with internal derangements than with other types of TMDs or in normal controls.[26,127–131] Altered collagen metabolism may also play a role in joint laxity, and the collagen composition in TMJs with painful disc displacement compared with asymptomatic joints has been found to differ in the total value and ratio of collagen types, fibroblasts density, dimension of arterial lumens, and distribution of elastic fibers.[129,132]

Nevertheless, there is only a weak correlation between the mobility of peripheral joints or the trunk and mandibular mobility, and research has yet to demonstrate that joint laxity can predict the potential for developing TMDs.[127]

Local (peripheral) factors

Local pathophysiologic factors of TMDs such as masticatory efficiency appear to be multifactorial and involve such a large span of individual variation that it is difficult to establish norms.[133] In addition, chewing force is also influenced by sex, age, and pain levels.[134–140] Masticatory muscle tenderness is not always related to variation in muscle activity or the site or side of reported tenderness. Muscle tenderness does not appear to be the result of inflammation but is probably related to prolonged central hyperexcitability and altered CNS processing following peripheral tissue injury.[141] Cervical muscle activity has been shown to influence masticatory muscle activity, probably involving a primary afferent reflex response.[142–144] Thus, a primary cervical or TMJ disorder may precipitate a secondary masticatory muscle condition. Muscle hyperalgesia can also result from TMJ inflammation.[145]

Of great concern to the clinician is the distinction between pathologic and adaptive responses to disease in the TMJ. Histologic studies suggest that cartilage thickness and composition adapt to shearing stresses during functional loading.[146] Maintenance of an intact articular surface is to be expected, even in the face of osteoarthritic changes, allowing for both stable morphologic relationships and histologic compatibility between the articulating components.[147–149] Therefore, even though morphologic change is mostly irreversible, it usually achieves and maintains stability and should be considered adaptive.[150] In this light, the goal of treating osteoarthritic changes should not be to restore earlier morphology but to encourage the body's adaptive response to pathophysiologic processes.

In early disc derangements, signs of osteoarthritis are not apparent. Disc derangements with reduction may persist for many years without development of radiographically visible changes or symptoms.[151] Disc derangements in later stages with osteoarthritic changes occur possibly in parallel but may also represent independent processes, and 50% will show some active cellular osteoblastic or osteoclastic activity.[152,153] Osteoarthritic changes, alterations in synovial fluid viscosity, and inadequate or altered lubrication may initiate derangement of the TMJ articular disc.[154,155] Synovial fluid analyses attempting to correlate biochemical signs of inflammation with pain reveal abnormal concentrations of plasma proteins or neurotransmitters and inflammatory cytokines.[156–161] While still controversial, cytokine profiles of patients with intracapsular TMDs do appear to be different from controls.[162]

In addition, basic research has presented substantial data to support the role of the calcitonin gene-related peptide (CGRP) in the underlying pathologic mechanisms of TMDs due to its involvement in the development of peripheral and central sensitization[163] independent of inflammatory mechanisms.[164] In more detail, CGRP upregulated expression in both trigeminal neurons and satellite glia cells suggest its participation in the complex modulation of orofacial pain.[165] Additional research in this area, including clinical trials, could elucidate the role of targeted neuropeptides as therapeutic interventions in a subset of individuals with TMDs and comorbid pain conditions.

Frictional "sticking" of the disc has been proposed to cause internal derangement of the TMJ with the forces dependent on the type of clenching task, with the greater impact at ICP and during a unilateral molar clench.[166–168] According to experimental models and animal studies, the forces are also increased by reduced congruity between the opposing surfaces and by flat, unrounded surfaces.[168–171] The forces are affected by disc thickness and area and by mandibular deformation during clenching.[170,172] Interestingly, nonworking tooth contacts have been hypothesized to reduce loads within the joint and act as a stress breaker for the clenching forces.[168] Intracapsular pressure may also affect TMDs.[173] With joint movement, the alternating pressure acts as a pump for joint lubrication, nutrition, blood supply, drug delivery, waste removal, and even condylar growth. Thus, any interruption through immobilization or prolonged clenching might have the potential to initiate or advance TMD signs and symptoms.

Female hormones might play a role in TMJ disc disease compromise, but this has not been proven because the presence of both estrogen and progesterone receptors within the articular disc has been both confirmed and denied.[174,175] However, data from an experimental animal model study suggest there is an additive effect of estrogen deficiency and mechanical stress in structural changes of the TMJ.[176] Clinical randomized controlled trials (RCTs) indicate that estrogen does not play a role in the etiology of TMDs, whereas cohort studies and case-control studies show contrasting results.[177–181] The etiologic explanations for progression from disc displacement to osteoarthritis and osteoarthritic changes are multifactorial and include failure of the reparative articular chondrocyte response due to metabolic dysfunction and relative or absolute overloading due to excessive mechanical forces leading to articular cartilage biochemical failure.[52,182] Remodeling, in contrast, is a physiologic response to accommodate an altered disc position.[147] Thus, it is probable that a mechanical breakdown in the articular disc (eg, a perforation) rather than an unusual disc position leads to osteoarthritis and/or osteoarthritic changes following disc displacement.[183] It is not certain, however, that all gross abnormalities of disc morphology will lead to osteoarthritis because one experimental animal study suggests that the TMJ may be capable of healing disc perforations within a relatively short time.[184] Mechanical stress may also lead to the accumulation of damaging free radicals in affected articular tissues of susceptible individuals. This condition is called *oxidative stress*.[185] It has been proposed that free radicals may be responsible for the formation of adhesions in the TMJ by cross-linking of proteins.[186]

Genetic factors

While the body of literature regarding genetic susceptibility for TMDs is an expanding field, genetic association studies have been limited. The relationship between catechol-O-methyltransferase (*COMT*) polymorphism, pain sensitivity, and the risk of TMD development has been evaluated, and three genetic variants (haplotypes) of the gene encoding *COMT* were identified and designated as "low pain sensitivity," "average pain sensitivity," and "high pain sensitivity."[187] The haplotypes were associated with experimental pain sensitivity, and the presence of even a single "low pain sensitivity" haplotype was shown to reduce the risk of developing myogenous TMDs. Furthermore, the gene-environment interaction was illustrated by the significant role of stress, which doubles the rate of TMDs among those with low-activity *COMT* haplotypes.[23] Current data from OPPERA did not demonstrate significant variation in TMD incidence by genetic polymorphisms from a panel of candidates' putative genes but found evidence for genetic associations in several pronociceptive intermediate phenotypes and their contributing role.[188] Single-nucleotide polymorphisms (SNPs) representing 358 genes involved in biologic systems associated with pain perception were identified. Specifically, SNPs had stronger associations with nonspecific orofacial symptoms, global psychologic symptoms, stress, negative affect, and heat and temporal summation. These included the following:

- The glucocorticoid receptor gene, which suggests a role of the hypothalamic-pituitary-adrenal system in chronic TMDs
- The serotonin receptor gene, indicating the influence of nociceptive and affective pathways
- The gene encoding the α subunit of the voltage-gated sodium channel NaV 1.1, which is involved in the generation and propagation of action potentials in sensory nerves
- A variation in a gene encoding angiotensin I-converting enzyme implicated in hypertension
- The prostaglandin-endoperoxide synthase 1 gene, a regulator of nociception and inflammatory response
- A variation in the gene encoding amyloid β (A4) precursor protein, which influences synapse formation and neuronal plasticity
- Multiple PDZ domain protein gene, influencing G-protein-coupled receptors involved in nociception and analgesia

These most extensive panel-related candidate genes support the strong indication that multiple genetic and biologic pathways contribute to the risk for TMDs.[188] Extending beyond previous candidate gene investigations, genotype effects within sex were examined to identify variants and pathways potentially underlying sex-specific mechanisms responsible for a higher prevalence of TMD among females. Genome-wide significant associations with chronic TMD were found for three loci, including a single-nucleotide polymorphism on chromosome 3 in males only, suggesting that males and females may develop TMD through different pathophysiologic pathways.[189] Enrichment of genetic associations in a serotonergic signaling pathway among cases suggest that activation of peripheral serotonin receptors elicited local hyperalgesia among individuals with TMD without widespread pain.[23]

Psychosocial factors

Psychosocial factors include individual, interpersonal, and situational variables that impact the patient's capacity to function adaptively. General distress is the most salient single factor across most individuals with chronic TMD pain.[190] General distress is readily assessed (see chapters 2 and 12), and certainly other factors may contribute actively to the measured distress, such as personality characteristics, enduring stressors, a physical response style to stress, or limited coping skills.[191–196]

There is evidence that some patients with TMDs experience more anxiety than healthy control groups and that TMD and orofacial pain symptoms may be only one of several somatic manifestations of emotional distress.[197–200] Some muscle pain may in fact be caused by excessive sympathetic nervous system activity as an overresponse to life stressors, and the attention focused on the pain can adversely affect the intensity of the pain.[201–204] Patients with such complaints often have a history of other stress-related disorders.[200] Depression and anxiety related to other major life events may alter the patient's perception of and tolerance of physical symptoms, causing them to seek more care for what is presented as a problem of the body.[205] Patients with chronic TMDs have been found to have psychosocial and behavioral characteristics similar to patients with lower back pain and headache.[206,207]

Environmental contingencies can greatly complicate treatment by affecting an individual's perception of and responses to pain and disease. Some patients may experience a lessening of distress to the extent that psychogenic symptoms decrease or resolve preexisting psychologic and interpersonal conflicts. This primary gain of symptom formation is distinguished from the secondary gain of social benefits experienced by patients once a disorder is established.[208–210] Secondary gain includes being exempt from ordinary daily responsibilities; being compensated monetarily from insurance or litigation; using the rationalization of "being ill" to avoid unpleasant tasks; and receiving attention from family, friends, or health care workers.[210,211] What the clinician interprets as pain (eg, in response to a clinical examination procedure designed to evoke pain) may be less related to any local nociceptive mechanisms and more a function of pain behavior: how the individual presents his or her distress as motivated by factors beyond the stated complaint.

From the psychosocial domain, the OPPERA study group evaluated 26 psychosocial measures; among them, the frequency of somatic symptoms was the strongest predictor for TMD onset. Other contributors to a lesser degree were psychologic stress, anxiety, obsessive-compulsive feelings, and pain coping strategies.[212] Using a case-control analytical approach as a foundation for their research, the investigators reported that TMD cases are different than controls across multiple phenotypic domains including sociodemographic factors, clinical variables, psychologic functioning, pain sensitivity, autonomic responses, and genetic associations. All these elements are providing leading-edge information to the biologic pathways that may elucidate TMD pathophysiology.[213]

More recently, an analysis from the OPPERA study found that there was a strong association between negative mood, perceived stress, pain catastrophizing, and overlapping conditions. The strongest independent predictor of case status for TMD, fibromyalgia, and lower back pain was the measure of somatic symptoms, thereby emphasizing the relevance of psychologic functioning characterization in the management of individuals with chronic pain conditions.[214]

Diagnostic Classification of TMDs

The classification of TMDs is hampered by limited knowledge of the etiology and the natural progression of these disorders, and yet, advancement in our knowledge is dependent upon an accepted taxonomy and corresponding diagnostic criteria.[16] Diagnostic criteria allow comparisons of patient populations in different studies and provide a common language for developing a conceptual framework to use in the clinic.[215] Any classification scheme or taxonomy must be considered as an evolving framework that will be modified by new findings and with an increased level of understanding. The following outlines are based on the Diagnostic Criteria for Temporomandibular Disorders (DC-TMD), which include the most common TMDs with sensitivity and specificity values, and the expanded taxonomy, which includes less common TMDs without validity estimates (Box 8-1 and Table 8-1).[15,216] In addition, a summary of a newly published tool, the International Classification of Orofacial Pain (ICOP),[217] limited to TMD diagnoses, is presented in Figs 8-3 and 8-4.

This new tool is a comprehensive research and diagnostic manual that amalgamates the International Classification of Headache Disorders, 3rd edition (ICHD-3),[218] *The International Classification of Disease, Eleventh Revision* (*ICD-11*),[219] and the International Association for the Study of Pain (IASP)[220] structure and terminology in a hierarchical presentation of diagnoses and respective criterion, while incorporating some elements of the DC-TMD.[15]

Other disorders and conditions with limited literature are also included.

Box 8-1 **Expanded TMD taxonomy**

Temporomandibular joint disorders

1. Joint pain (*ICD-10* M26.62)
   A. Arthralgia
   B. Arthritis
2. Joint disorders
   A. Disc-condyle complex disorders (*ICD-10* M26.62)
      i. Disc displacement with reduction
      ii. Disc displacement with reduction with intermittent locking
      iii. Disc displacement without reduction with limited opening
      iv. Disc displacement without reduction without limited opening
   B. Other hypomobility disorders (*ICD-10* M26.61)
      i. Adhesions/adherence
      ii. Ankylosis
         a. Fibrous ankylosis
         b. Osseous ankylosis
   C. Hypermobility disorders
      i. Subluxation (*ICD-10* S03.0XXA)
      ii. Luxation (*ICD-10* S03.0XXA)
         a. Closed dislocation (*ICD-10* S03.0XXA)
         b. Recurrent dislocation (*ICD-10* M26.69)
         c. Ligamentous laxity (*ICD-10* M24.20)
3. Joint diseases
   A. Degenerative joint diseases (*ICD-10* M19.91)
      i. Osteoarthrosis
      ii. Osteoarthritis
   B. Condylysis (*ICD-10* M26.69)
   C. Osteochondritis dissecans (*ICD-10* M93.20)
   D. Osteonecrosis (*ICD-10* M87.08)
   E. Systemic arthritides (rheumatoid arthritis: *ICD-10* M06.9)
   F. Neoplasm (benign: *ICD-10* D16.5; malignant: *ICD-10* C41.1)
   G. Synovial chondromatosis (*ICD-10* D48.0)
4. Fractures
   A. Closed fracture of condylar process (*ICD-10* S02.61XA)
   B. Closed fracture of subcondylar process (*ICD-10* S02.62XA)
   C. Open fracture of condylar process (*ICD-10* S02.61XB)
   D. Open fracture of subcondylar process (*ICD-10* S02.62XB)
5. Congenital/developmental disorders
   A. Aplasia (*ICD-10* Q67.4)
   B. Hypoplasia (*ICD-10* M27.8)
   C. Hyperplasia (*ICD-10* M27.8)

Masticatory muscle disorders

1. Muscle pain limited to the orofacial region
   A. Myalgia (*ICD-10* M79.1)
      i. Local myalgia
      ii. Myofascial pain
      iii. Myofascial pain with referral
   B. Tendonitis (*ICD-10* M67.90)
   C. Myositis
      i. Noninfective (*ICD-10* M60.9)
      ii. Infective (*ICD-10* M60.009)
   D. Spasm (*ICD-10* M62.838)
2. Contracture
   A. Muscle (*ICD-10* M62.40)
   B. Tendon
3. Hypertrophy (*ICD-10* M62.9)
4. Neoplasms
   A. Jaw
      i. Malignant (*ICD-10* C41.1)
      ii. Benign (*ICD-10* D16.5)
   B. Soft tissues of head, face, and neck
      i. Malignant (*ICD-10* C49.0)
      ii. Benign (*ICD-10* D21.0)
5. Movement disorders
   A. Orofacial dyskinesia
      i. Abnormal involuntary movements (*ICD-10* R25.1 [tremor unspecified]; R25.2 [cramp and spasm]; R25.3 [fasciculations])
      ii. Ataxia, unspecified (*ICD-10* R27.0); muscular incoordination (*ICD-10* R27.9)
      iii. Subacute, due to drugs; oral tardive dyskinesia (*ICD-10* G24.01)
   B. Oromandibular dystonia
      i. Acute, due to drugs (*ICD-10* G24.02)
      ii. Deformans, familial, idiopathic, and torsion dystonia (*ICD-10* G24.1)
6. Masticatory muscle pain attributed to systemic/central disorders
   A. Fibromyalgia (*ICD-10* M79.7)
   B. Centrally mediated myalgia (*ICD-10* M79.1)

Headache disorders

1. Headache attributed to TMDs (*ICD-10* G44.89 or *ICD-10* R51)

Associated structures

1. Coronoid hyperplasia (*ICD-10* M27.8)

Table 8-1 *ICD-10* to *ICD-11* mapping

General: Temporomandibular joint disorders (*ICD-10* M26.6; *ICD-11* DA0E.8)				
	ICD-10	***ICD-10* definition**	***ICD-11***	***ICD-11* definition**
Joint disorders				
Joint pain	M26.62	Arthralgia of the TMJ	DA0E.8	Temporomandibular joint disorders
Arthralgia	M26.62	Arthralgia of the TMJ	DA0E.8	Temporomandibular joint disorders
Disc-condyle complex disorders	M26.63	Articular disc disorder TMJ	DA0E.8	Temporomandibular joint disorders
Other hypomobility disorders	M26.61	Adhesions and ankylosis TMJ	FA34.4	Ankylosis of joint
Adhesions/ adherence	M26.61	Adhesions and ankylosis TMJ	FA37.Y	Other specified certain joint disorders, not elsewhere classified
Ankylosis	M26.61	Adhesions and ankylosis TMJ	FA34.4	Ankylosis of joint
Fibrous ankylosis	M26.61	Adhesions and ankylosis TMJ	FA34.4	Ankylosis of joint
Osseous ankylosis	M26.61	Adhesions and ankylosis TMJ	FA34.4	Ankylosis of joint
Hypermobility disorders				
Subluxation	S03.00	Dislocation of jaw	NA03.0	Dislocation of jaw
Luxation	S03.00	Dislocation of jaw	NA03.0	Dislocation of jaw
Closed dislocation	S03.00	Dislocation of jaw	NA03.0	Dislocation of jaw
Recurrent dislocation	M26.69	Other specified disorders TMJ	NA03.0	Dislocation of jaw
Ligamentous laxity	M24.20	Disorder of ligament unspecified site	FA34.1	Disorder of ligament
Joint diseases				
Degenerative joint diseases	M19.91	Primary osteoarthritis unspecified site	FA03.0	Primary osteoarthritis of other specified joint
Osteoarthrosis	M19.91	Primary osteoarthritis unspecified site	FA03.0	Primary osteoarthritis of other specified joint
Osteoarthritis	M19.91	Primary osteoarthritis unspecified site	FA03.0	Primary osteoarthritis of other specified joint
Condylysis	M26.69	Other specified disorders of TMJ	NA	

Table 8-1 *(cont) ICD-10* to *ICD-11* mapping

General: Temporomandibular joint disorders (*ICD-10* M26.6; *ICD-11* DA0E.8)				
	ICD-10	***ICD-10* definition**	***ICD-11***	***ICD-11* definition**
Osteochondritis dissecans	M93.20	Osteochondritis dissecans	FB82.1	Osteochondrosis or osteochondritis dissecans
Osteonecrosis	M87.08	Idiopathic aseptic necrosis of bone	FB81.0	Idiopathic aseptic osteonecrosis
Systemic arthritides (rheumatoid arthritis)	M06.9	Rheumatoid arthritis, unspecified	FA20.Z	Rheumatoid arthritis, serology unspecified
Neoplasm (benign)	D16.5	Benign neoplasm of lower jaw bone	2E83.1	Benign osteogenic tumors of bone or articular cartilage of lower jaw
Neoplasm (malignant)	C41.1	Malignant neoplasm of mandible	2D4Z	Malignant neoplasm, primary site unspecified
Synovial chondromatosis	D48.0	Neoplasm of uncertain behavior of bone and articular cartilage	2F7B	Neoplasms of uncertain behavior of bone or articular cartilage
Fractures				
Closed fracture of condylar process	S02.61	Fracture of condylar process of mandible	NA02.70	Fracture of condylar process of mandible
Closed fracture of subcondylar process	S02.62	Fracture of subcondylar process of mandible	NA02.71	Fracture of subcondylar process of mandible
Congenital/developmental disorders				
Aplasia	Q67.4	Other congenital deformities of skull, face, and jaw	LD0Z	Structural developmental anomalies primarily affecting one body system, unspecified
Hypoplasia	M27.8	Other specified diseases of jaws	DA0E.0Y	Other specified major anomalies of jaw size
Hyperplasia	M27.8	Other specified diseases of jaws	DA0E.0Y	Other specified major anomalies of jaw size
Masticatory muscle disorders				
Muscle pain limited to the orofacial region				
Myalgia	M79.1	Myalgia	FB56.2	Myalgia
Tendonitis	M67.90	Disorder of synovium and tendon, unspecified	FB42	Certain specified disorders of synovium or tendon

Table 8-1 *(cont) ICD-10* to *ICD-11* mapping

General: Temporomandibular joint disorders (*ICD-10* M26.6; *ICD-11* DA0E.8)				
	ICD-10	***ICD-10* definition**	***ICD-11***	***ICD-11* definition**
Myositis noninfective	M60.9	Myositis, unspecified	FB32	Certain specified disorders of muscle
Myositis infective	M60.009	Infective myositis, unspecified site	FB30	Infectious myositis
Spasm	M62.838	Other muscle spasm	MB47.3	Spasm
Contracture (muscle)	M62.40	Contracture of muscle	FB32.4	Contracture of muscle
Hypertrophy	M62.9	Disorder of muscle, unspecified	DA0E.7	Dentofacial parafunctional disorders (includes hypertrophy of chewing muscles)
Neoplasms				
Jaw malignant	C41.1	Malignant neoplasm of mandible	2D4Z	Malignant neoplasm, primary site unspecified
Jaw benign	D16.5	Benign neoplasm of lower jaw bone	2F5Z	Benign neoplasm
Soft tissue of head, face, and neck				
Malignant	C49.0	Malignant neoplasm: Connective and soft tissue of head, face, and neck	2B5K	Unspecified malignant soft tissue tumors or sarcomas of bone or articular cartilage of other or unspecified sites
Benign	D21.0	Other benign neoplasms of connective and other soft tissue	2E8Z	Benign mesenchymal neoplasms, unspecified
Movement disorders				
Orofacial dyskinesia				
Abnormal involuntary movements				
Tremor unspecified	R25.1	Tremor, unspecified	8A04.Y	Other specified disorders associated with tremor
Cramp and spasm	R25.2	Cramp and spasm	MB47.3	Spasm
Fasciculations	R25.3	Fasciculation	MB47.5	Fasciculation
Ataxia, unspecified	R27.0	Ataxia, unspecified	MB45.0	Ataxia, unspecified
Muscular incoordination	R27.9	Unspecified lack of coordination	MB45.Y	Other specified lack of coordination

Table 8-1 *(cont)* ***ICD-10*** **to** ***ICD-11*** **mapping**

General: Temporomandibular joint disorders (*ICD-10* M26.6; *ICD-11* DA0E.8)				
	ICD-10	***ICD-10* definition**	***ICD-11***	***ICD-11* definition**
Subacute, due to drugs; oral tardive dyskinesia	G24.01	Drug-induced subacute dyskinesia	8A02.10	Drug-induced dystonia
Oromandibular dystonia				
Acute due to drugs	G24.02	Drug-induced acute dystonia	8A02.10	Drug-induced dystonia
Deformans, familiar, ideopathic and torsion dystonia	G24.1	Idiopathic familial dystonia	8A02.0Y	Other specified primary dystonia
Masticatory muscle pain attributed to systemic/central disorders				
Fibromyalgia	M79.7	Fibromyalgia	MG30.01	Chronic widespread pain
Centrally mediated myalgia	M79.1	Myalgia	FB56.2	Myalgia
Headache disorders	G44.89	Other headache syndrome	8A84.Y	Other specified secondary headache
Headache attributed to TMD	G44.89 & R51 (headache)		MG30.63	Headache or orofacial pain associated with chronic secondary temporomandibular disorders
Associated structures				
Coronoid hyperplasia	M27.8	Other specified diseases of jaws	DA0E.0Y	Other specified major anomalies of jaw size

Note: In most cases, modifiers (eg, right or left) or subclasses are not included in codes.
Data from https://icd.who.int/en/. Accessed 20 Sept 2022.

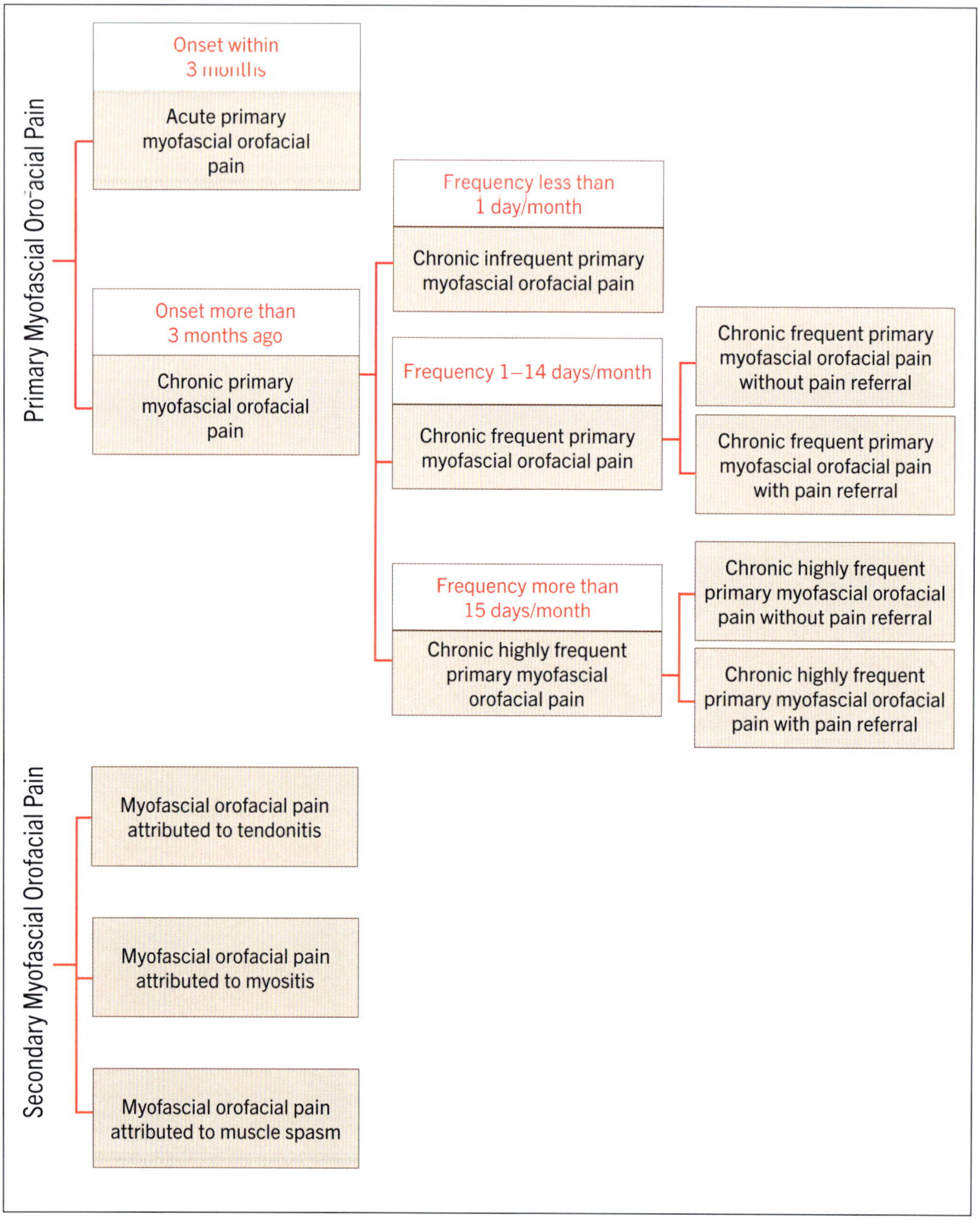

Fig 8-3 Classification of myofascial orofacial pain based on the ICOP.[217]

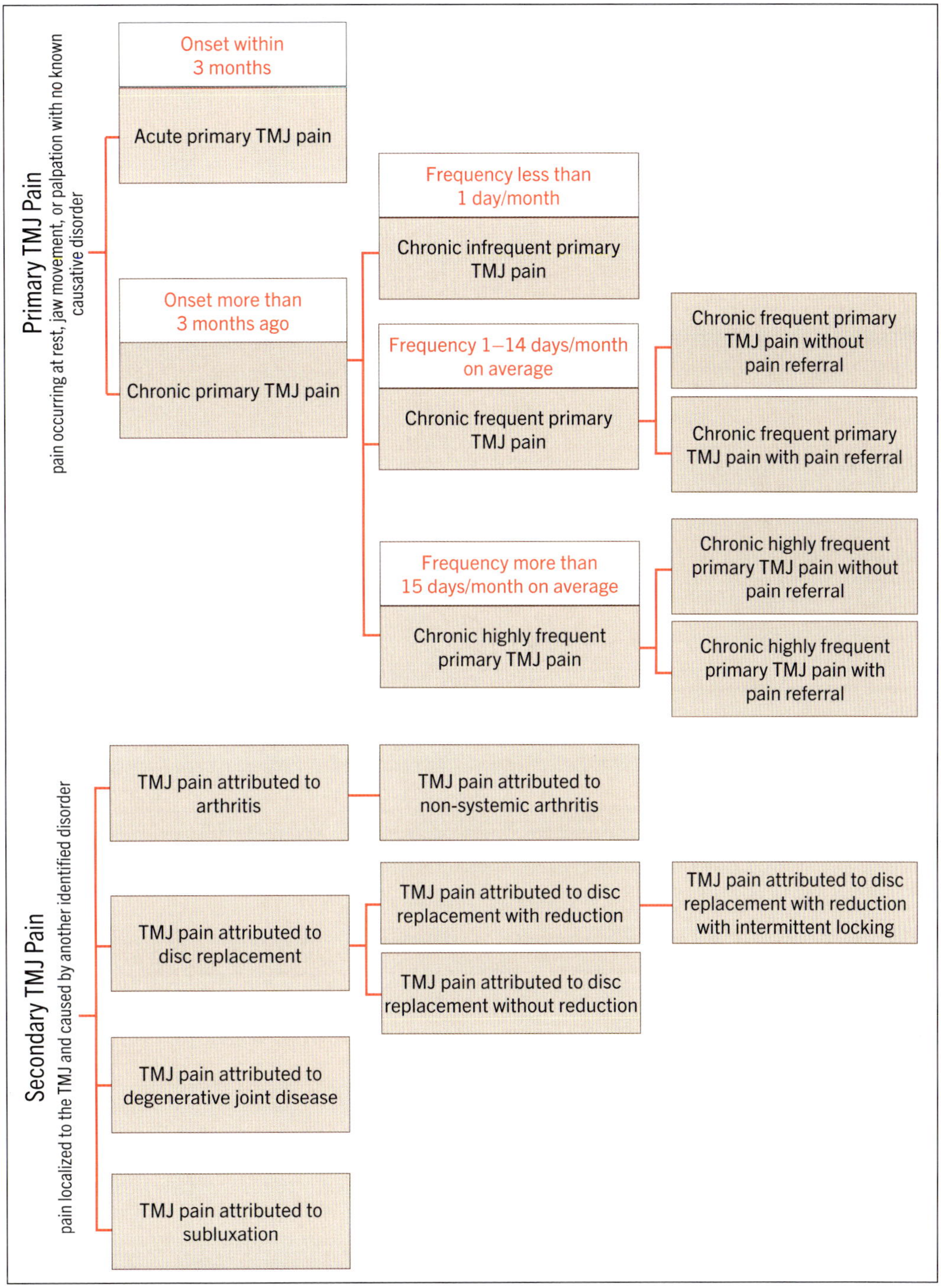

Fig 8-4 Classification of TMJ pain based on the ICOP.[217]

TMJ disorders

Joint pain

Previously described as synovitis, capsulitis, and retrodiscitis, joint pain has been explained in the biomedical model as an inflammatory process of the synovial lining of the TMJ that can be due to infection, an immunologic condition secondary to cartilage degeneration, or trauma. Joint pain is characterized by localized pain that is exacerbated by function and parafunction. On occasion, there may be a fluctuating swelling that decreases the ability to occlude on the ipsilateral posterior teeth.

ARTHRALGIA. This is pain of joint origin affected by jaw movement, function, or parafunction and replication of this pain with provocation testing, either during mandibular movement or palpation of the TMJs. Sensitivity is 0.89, and specificity is 0.98.

History is positive for both of the following:

- In the past 30 days, pain in the jaw, in the temple, in front of the ear, or in the ear with examiner confirmation of pain location in a masticatory structure
- Pain altered with jaw movement, function, or parafunction

Confirmation of the pain location in the TMJ area includes at least one of the following tests:

- Palpation of the lateral pole (0.5 kg pressure) or around the lateral pole (1.0 kg pressure)
- Maximum unassisted or assisted opening, right or left lateral movements, or protrusive movements

Examination of the TMJ elicits a report of *familiar pain* (defined as similar or like the pain the patient has experienced in the masticatory area palpated during the last 30 days).

ARTHRITIS. This is pain of joint origin with clinical characteristics of inflammation or infection: edema, erythema, and/or increased temperature. It may arise in association with trauma. Associated symptoms can include occlusal changes such as ipsilateral posterior open bite if intra-articular swelling is present unilaterally. This disorder has also been referred to as *synovitis* or *capsulitis*; however, these terms limit the sites of nociception. With this localized condition, there should be no history of systemic inflammatory disease. Sensitivity and specificity have not been established.

History is positive for arthralgia as defined above as well as one of the following:

- Swelling, redness, and/or increased temperature in front of the ear
- Dental occlusal changes resulting from articular inflammatory exudate (eg, posterior open bite)

Examination is positive for arthralgia as defined above as well as one of the following:

- Presence of edema, erythema, and/or increased temperature over the TMJs
- Reduction in dental occlusal contacts noted between two consecutive measurements

Unilateral or bilateral posterior open bite must not be attributable to other causes. The patient is negative for rheumatologic disease, including those in systemic arthritides. The pain is not better accounted for by another pain diagnosis.

Joint disorders

Articular disc displacement is the most common TMJ arthropathy and is characterized by several stages of clinical dysfunction that involve the condyle-disc relationship. It is characterized by an abnormal relation or misalignment of the articular disc relative to the condyle. Although posterior and mediolateral displacements of the articular disc have been described,[221,222] the usual direction for displacement is in an anterior or anteromedial direction.[223–227] Nevertheless, pain or mandibular movement symptoms are not specific for disc derangement disorders, and the disc position is not related to any presenting symptoms.[228,229]

The causes of disc displacement are not agreed upon; however, it is postulated that in the majority of cases, elongated or torn ligaments binding the disc to the condyle permit the disc to displace.[230] Lubrication impairment is also suggested as a possible etiologic factor of disc displacement.[155,166] Disc displacement is subdivided into disc displacement with reduction and disc displacement without reduction.

DISC-CONDYLE COMPLEX DISORDERS

Disc displacement with reduction. This is an intracapsular biomechanical disorder involving the condyle-disc complex. In the closed mouth position, the disc is in an anterior position relative to the condyle, and the disc reduces upon opening of the mouth. Medial and lateral displacement of the disc may also be present. Clicking, popping, or snapping noises may occur with disc reduction. Using MRI as the reference standard, sensitivity is 0.34, and specificity is 0.92. Although not required for this diagnosis and without diagnostic validity, elimination of the opening and closing noise, if present, with protrusion can help corroborate this diagnosis.

History is positive for the following:

- In the last 30 days, any noise(s) present with jaw movement or function, or patient report of joint sounds during the examination

Examination is positive for at least one of the following:

- Both an opening and closing clicking, popping, or snapping noise detected with palpation during at least one of three repetitions of jaw opening and closing
- Either an opening or closing clicking, popping, or snapping noise detected with palpation during at least one of three repetitions of opening and closing and a clicking, popping, and/or snapping noise detected with palpation during at least one of three repetitions of left lateral, right lateral, or protrusive movements

When this diagnosis needs to be confirmed, the imaging analyses criteria—using TMJ MRI—are positive for both of the following:

- In the maximum intercuspal position, the posterior band of the disc is located anterior to the 11:30 position, and the intermediate zone of the disc is anterior to the condyle and the articular eminence
- On full opening, the intermediate zone of the disc is positioned between the condyle and the articular eminence

Disc displacement with reduction with intermittent locking. This is an intracapsular biomechanical disorder involving the condyle-disc complex. In the closed mouth position, the disc is in an anterior position relative to the condyle, and the disc intermittently reduces with opening of the mouth. When the disc does not reduce with opening of the mouth, intermittent limited mandibular opening occurs. When the limited opening occurs, a maneuver may be needed to unlock the TMJ. Medial and lateral displacement of the disc may also be present. Clicking, popping, or snapping noises may occur with disc reduction. Although not required for this diagnosis, occurrence of intermittent closed lock during the clinical examination can help corroborate this diagnosis. Using MRI as the reference standard, sensitivity is 0.38, and specificity is 0.98.

History is positive for both of the following:

- In the last 30 days or during the examination itself, any noises present with jaw movement or function
- In the last 30 days, report of intermittent locking with limited opening or evidence of intermittent locking during clinical examination

Examination is positive for the following:

- Disc displacement with reduction as defined previously

When this diagnosis needs to be confirmed, the imaging analysis criteria are the same as for disc displacement with reduction. If locking occurs during imaging, then an imaging-based diagnosis of disc displacement without reduction will be rendered, and clinical confirmation of reversion to intermittent locking is needed.

Disc displacement without reduction with limited opening. This is an intracapsular biomechanical disorder involving the condyle-disc complex. In the closed mouth position, the disc is in an anterior position relative to the condyle and the disc does not reduce with opening of the mouth. Medial and lateral displacement of the disc may also be present. This disorder is associated with limited mandibular opening that does not reduce with the clinician or patient performing a manipulative maneuver. This is also referred to as *closed lock*. Using MRI as the reference standard, sensitivity is 0.80, and specificity is 0.97.

History is positive for both of the following:

- Jaw lock or catch so that it will not open all the way
- Limitation in jaw opening severe enough to interfere with the ability to eat

Examination is positive for the following:

- Maximum assisted opening (passive stretch) < 40 mm including vertical incisal overlap

When this diagnosis needs to be confirmed, the imaging analysis criteria—using TMJ MRI—are positive for both of the following:

- In the maximum intercuspal position, the posterior band of the disc is located anterior to the 11:30 position, and the intermediate zone of the disc is anterior to the condyle and the articular eminence
- On full opening, the intermediate zone of the disc is positioned anterior to the condyle

Disc displacement without reduction without limited opening. This is an intracapsular biomechanical disorder involving the condyle-disc complex. In the closed mouth position, the disc is anterior relative to the condyle, and the disc does not reduce with opening of the mouth. Medial and lateral displacement of the disc may also be present. This disorder is not associated with limited mandibular opening. Using MRI as the reference standard, sensitivity is 0.54, and specificity is 0.79.

History is the same as defined for disc displacement without reduction with limited opening.

Examination is positive for the following:

- Maximum assisted opening (passive stretch) > 40 mm including vertical incisal overlap
- When this diagnosis needs to be confirmed, the imaging analysis criteria are the same as for disc displacement without reduction with limited opening

OTHER HYPOMOBILITY DISORDERS. Intra-articular fibrous adhesions and ankyloses are characterized by restricted mandibular movement with deflection to the affected side on opening that may occur as a long-term sequela of trauma, including mandibular fracture. In case of bilateral involvement, asymmetries in mandibular movements during clinical examination will be less pronounced or absent. The diagnostic criteria of mandibular movement asymmetries are for unilateral causes of hypomobility. Hypomobility is firm and unyielding because of intra-articular fibrous adhesions, more widespread fibrotic changes in the capsular ligaments (fibrous ankylosis), and/or, less frequently, the formation of a bony mass that results in fusion of the joint components (bony ankylosis). The condition is usually not associated with pain. The most frequent cause of TMJ ankylosis is macrotrauma; less frequent causes are infection of the mastoid or middle ear, systemic disease, and inadequate surgical treatment of the condylar area.

Adhesions and adherence. Fibrous adhesions within the TMJ are thought to occur mainly in the superior compartment of the TMJ. They produce decreased movement of the disc-condyle complex. Adhesions may occur secondary to joint inflammation that results from direct trauma, excessive loading, or systemic conditions such as a polyarthritic disease. They are typically associated with disc-condyle complex disorders.

History is positive for both of the following:

- No history of TMJ clicking (historically to differentiate from disc displacement without reduction with limited opening)
- History of loss of jaw mobility

Examination is positive for all of the following:

- Limited range of motion on opening
- Uncorrected deviation of the jaw to the affected side on opening if present unilaterally
- Marked limited laterotrusion to the contralateral side if unilateral

When this diagnosis needs to be confirmed, arthrography, MRI, or arthroscopy may show the presence of adhesions. Sensitivity and specificity have not been established.

Ankylosis. TMJ ankyloses are differentiated by the type of tissues that are causing them: fibrous or bony. In fibrous ankylosis, there are no gross bony changes and no radiographic findings other than absence of ipsilateral condylar translation on opening. Bony ankylosis is characterized by the union of the bones of the TMJ as a result of bone cell proliferation; this may cause complete immobility of that joint. It is characterized by radiographic evidence of bone proliferation with marked deflection to the affected side and marked limited laterotrusion to the contralateral side. Sensitivity and specificity have not been established for these disorders.

Fibrous ankylosis. History is positive for the following:

- History of progressive loss of jaw mobility

Examination is positive for all of the following:

- Severe limited range of motion on opening
- Uncorrected jaw deviation to the affected side
- Marked limited laterotrusion to the contralateral side

Computed tomography or cone beam CT (CBCT) is positive for both of the following:

- Imaging findings of decreased ipsilateral condylar translation on opening
- Imaging findings of a joint space between ipsilateral condyle and eminence

Bony ankylosis. History is positive for the following:

- History of progressive loss of jaw mobility
  Examination is positive for the following:
- Absence of or severely limited jaw mobility with all movements

CT/CBCT is positive for the following:

- Imaging-based evidence of bone proliferation with obliteration of part or all of the joint space

HYPERMOBILITY DISORDERS. Hypermobility disorders include two types of TMJ dislocations in which the disc-condyle complex is positioned anterior to the articular eminence and is unable to return to a closed position without a specific maneuver by the patient (ie, subluxation or partial dislocation) or by the clinician (ie, luxation or dislocation). The latter disorder is also referred to as *open lock*. Note that the condyle is frequently anterior to the eminence at full mouth opening and thus by itself is not a predictor of hypermobility disorders. The duration of dislocation may be momentary or prolonged. Pain may occur at the time of dislocation with residual pain following the episode.

Subluxation. This is a condition involving the disc-condyle complex and the articular eminence. In the open mouth position, the disc-condyle complex is positioned anterior to the articular eminence and is unable to return to normal closed mouth position without a manipulative maneuver by the patient. When the patient needs the assistance of the clinician to reduce the dislocation and normalize the jaw position, it is called *luxation* or *open lock*. Using history only, sensitivity is 0.98, and specificity is 1.00.

History is positive for both of the following:

- In the last 30 days, jaw locking or catching in a wide-open mouth position, even for a moment, so the patient could not close from the wide-open position
- Inability to close the mouth from wide opening without a self-maneuver

No examination findings are required. If the patient presents with this disorder, he or she is then found clinically positive for inability to return to a normal closed mouth position without manipulative patient maneuver.

Luxation. This is a condition in which the disc-condyle complex is positioned anterior to the articular eminence and is unable to return to the fossa without a specific manipulative maneuver by a clinician. This is also referred to as *open lock*. Sensitivity and specificity have not been established.

History is positive for both of the following:

- Report of inability to close from wide opening
- Report that mouth closing can be achieved only with a specific mandibular maneuver by the clinician

Examination is positive for one of the following persistent presentations:

- Wide open mouth
- Protruded jaw position
- Lateral position to the contralateral side if unilateral

When this diagnosis needs to be confirmed, CT/CBCT or MRI scans are positive for the following:

- The condyle is anterior to the articular eminence with the patient attempting to close the mouth

Joint diseases

Osteoarthritis (ie, osteoarthrosis or degenerative joint disease [DJD]) is defined as a degenerative condition of the joint characterized by deterioration and abrasion of articular tissue and concomitant remodeling of the underlying subchondral bone due to overload of the remodeling mechanism. The progressive loss of articular cartilage in the osteoarthritic TMJ results from an imbalance between predominantly chondrocyte-controlled reparative and degradative processes.[231] The process accelerates as proteoglycan depletion, collagen fiber network disintegration, and fatty degeneration weaken the functional capacity of the articular cartilage. Different kinds of biochemical markers have been determined in the synovial fluid of TMJs with osteoarthritis. These include interleukin-6 (IL-6), tissue inhibitor metalloproteinase-1 (TIMP-1), matrix metalloproteinases, heat shock protein (HSP), transforming growth factor β 1 (TGF-β1), bone morphogenetic protein 2 (BMP-2), chondroitin-4-sulfate (C4S) and chondroitin-6-sulfate (C6S), keratan sulfate (KS), and human leukocyte antigen D related (HLA-DR).[232–242] The clinical and diagnostic value of these markers remains to be evaluated because similar markers have also been present in other joint diseases. Radiographic evidence typically lags behind articular tissue changes.[243] The early changes in the synovial membrane, such as synovial intima hyperplasia, cell hypertrophy with subsequent loss of fibrous material in the intima matrix, and articular cartilage, are only detectable with biopsy and arthroscopy.[182,244,245] Thus, osteoarthrosis frequently escapes early clinical detection.[246]

DEGENERATIVE JOINT DISEASE (DJD). Degenerative disorders involving the joint are characterized by deterioration of articular tissue with concomitant osseous changes in the condyle and articular eminence. Using CT/CBCT as the reference standard, sensitivity is 0.55, and specificity is 0.61.

History is positive for one of the following:

- In the past month, any joint noises present with jaw movement or function
- Patient report of any noises during the examination

Examination is positive for the following:

- Crepitus detected with palpation during at least one of the following: maximum unassisted opening, maximum assisted opening, right or left lateral movements, or protrusive movements

CT/CBCT is positive for at least one of the following:

- Subchondral cyst
- Erosion
- Generalized sclerosis
- Osteophyte

Flattening and/or cortical sclerosis are considered indeterminate findings for DJD and may represent normal variation, aging, remodeling, or a precursor to frank DJD.

CONDYLYSIS/IDIOPATHIC CONDYLAR RESORPTION. This is an idiopathic degenerative condition leading to the loss of condylar height and a progressive anterior open bite. The condition occurs spontaneously, is mainly bilateral, and occurs primarily in adolescent and young adult females.[216] The presence of pain or joint sounds is variable. In early stages, dental occlusal changes may not be evident, but imaging findings would be positive. It has been suggested that it may be a severe form of DJD and that low estrogen levels may be implicated.[247] Sensitivity and specificity have not been established.

History is positive for the following:

- Progressive dental occlusal changes

Examination is positive for both of the following:

- Anterior open bite
- Evidence of progressive dental occlusal changes with either occlusal facets that cannot be approximated or change in sequential occlusal measurement over time based on overbite, overjet, or intercuspal contacts

Imaging includes CT/CBCT evidence of partial or total condylar resorption or change with sequential imaging over time from lateral cephalometric images, which may include clockwise mandibular rotation, increase in mandibular plane angle, or increased A point–nasion–B point. Serologic tests for rheumatologic disease, including systemic arthritides, must be negative.

OSTEOCHONDRITIS DISSECANS. This is a joint condition in which a piece of cartilage and a small bone fragment break loose from the end of the bone and result in loose osteochondral fragments within the joint. The pathophysiology is unclear. It usually occurs in the knee and elbow and is often related to sports. Case reports describe the condition in the TMJ, but little is known about signs and symptoms. Sensitivity and specificity have not been established.

History is positive for any of the following:

- Arthralgia as previously defined
- Joint noises with mandibular movement or swelling

Examination is positive for one of the following:

- Same clinical findings as operationalized for arthralgia
- Crepitus detected by the examiner during palpation or reported by patient during mandibular movements
- Maximum assisted opening plus vertical overlap < 40 mm
- Swelling around the affected joint

CT/CBCT will provide positive findings for loose osteochondral fragments within the joint. Serologic tests for rheumatologic disease, including systemic arthritides, must be negative.

OSTEONECROSIS. Osteonecrosis is a painful condition most commonly affecting the ends of long bones such as the femur. Other common sites include the humerus and the knees. The condition is found in the mandibular condyle on MRI as decreased signal in T1 weighted or proton density images and on T2-weighted images (sclerosis pattern) and can be combined with increased signal on T2 images (edema). The cause, clinical significance, and need for treatment are unknown.

To diagnose osteonecrosis, the patient must fulfill criteria for arthralgia as previously defined, and imaging must show a decreased signal in T1-weighted or proton-density MR images and can be combined with an increased signal on T2-weighted images. Additionally, laboratory testing will confirm negative serologic results for rheumatologic disease. Sensitivity and specificity have not been established.

SYSTEMIC ARTHRITIDES. This is joint inflammation resulting in pain or structural changes caused by a generalized systemic inflammatory disease, including rheumatoid arthritis, juvenile idiopathic arthritis, spondyloarthropathies (eg, ankylosing spondylitis, psoriatic arthritis, infectious arthritis, Reiter syndrome), and crystal-induced disease (eg, gout, chondrocalcinosis). Other rheumatologically related diseases that may affect the TMJ include autoimmune disorders and other mixed connective tissue diseases (eg, scleroderma, Sjögren syndrome, lupus erythematosus). This group of arthritides therefore comprises multiple diagnostic categories that are best diagnosed and managed by rheumatologists regarding the general or systemic therapy. Clinical signs and symptoms of an ongoing chronic TMJ inflammation are variable between patients and within a patient over time. They can vary from no signs or symptoms to only pain to only swelling and exudate to only tissue degradation to only growth disturbance. Resorption of condylar structures may be associated with malocclusion such as a progressive anterior open bite. A diagnostic instrument should aim to identify patients with chronic inflammation early and accurately, should not exclude patients with chronic arthritis of long duration, and should not only cover rheumatoid arthritis but the whole range of chronic inflammatory states. Imaging in early stages may not demonstrate osseous findings. Sensitivity and specificity have not been established.

History is positive for both of the following:

- Rheumatologic diagnosis of a systemic inflammatory joint disease
- TMJ pain or noises present in the past month or TMJ pain that worsens with the episodes and exacerbations of the systemic inflammatory joint disease

Examination is positive for both of the following:

- Rheumatologic diagnosis of a systemic joint disease
- Arthritis signs and symptoms as defined previously or crepitus detected with palpation during maximum unassisted and assisted opening, lateral, and protrusive movements

Imaging criteria are the same as for DJD; CT/CBCT is positive for at least one of the following:

- Subchondral cyst
- Erosion
- Generalized sclerosis
- Osteophyte

NEOPLASM (TMJ). A *neoplasm* is new, often uncontrolled growth of abnormal tissue, in this case arising or involving the TMJ or supporting structures. Neoplasms in this area may be benign, malignant, or metastatic. Although neoplasia as an underlying cause of TMJ dysfunction is rare, it is well known in the literature.[248] Approximately 3% of malignant neoplasia metastasizes to the jaws.[249,250] Neoplasia most frequently extending to the TMJ region causing pain and dysfunction are squamous cell carcinomas of the maxillofacial region and primary nasopharyngeal tumors.[251–258] Neoplasia arising in the parotid gland, such as adenoid cystic carcinomas and mucoepidermoid carcinomas, may produce TMJ pain and dysfunction.[259–261] The most common signs and symptoms are reduced opening, crepitation, occlusal changes, pain with function, and swelling.[262] If the condyle is involved, there is frequently development of a facial asymmetry with a midline shift as that seen in condylar hyperplasia.[263] The most common treatment is surgery. Diagnostic imaging and biopsy are essential when a neoplasm is suspected. Sensitivity and specificity have not been established.

SYNOVIAL CHONDROMATOSIS. *Synovial chondromatosis* is a cartilaginous metaplasia of the mesenchymal remnants of the synovial tissue of the joint. Its main characteristic is the formation of cartilaginous nodules that may be pedunculated and/or detached from the synovial membrane, becoming loose bodies within the joint space. Calcification of the cartilage can occur (ie, osteochondromatosis). The disease may be associated with malocclusion, such as a progressive ipsilateral posterior open bite. Imaging is needed to establish the diagnosis. Sensitivity and specificity have not been established.

History must be positive for at least one of the following:

- Report of preauricular swelling
- Arthralgia as previously defined
- Progressive limitation in mouth opening
- Presence of joint noises in the last month

Examination must confirm at least one of the following:

- Preauricular swelling
- Arthralgia as previously defined
- Maximum assisted opening (passive stretch) < 40 mm including the vertical incisal overlap
- Crepitus as per DJD

MRI or CT/CBCT of the TMJ must be positive for at least one of the following:

- MRI: multiple chondroid nodules, joint effusion, and amorphous iso-intensity signal tissues within the joint space and capsule
- CT/CBCT: loose calcified bodies in the soft tissues of the TMJ

Histologic examination confirms cartilaginous metaplasia.

Fractures

Direct traumatic force can injure all related bony components of the masticatory system (ie, temporal bone, maxilla, zygoma, sphenoid bone, and mandible). This trauma can be related to the following conditions: fracture, dislocation, contusion, or laceration of articular surfaces, ligaments, and disc, with or without intraarticular hemarthrosis. Sequelae could include adhesions, ankylosis, occlusal abnormalities, or joint degeneration.[264] Patients with nonsurgical treated dislocated fractures may be prone to symptoms of TMDs, functional disorders, and occlusal disorders.[264] Fractures of the condylar process may result in facial asymmetry; in general, there are greater skeletal changes when the fracture occurs earlier in life. Closed treatments have reportedly also resulted in facial asymmetries, even in adults.[265] Sensitivity and specificity have not been established.

Examples of fractures are the following:

- Closed fracture of condylar process
- Closed fracture of subcondylar process
- Open fracture of condylar process
- Open fracture of subcondylar process

History must be positive for both of the following:

- Trauma to the orofacial region
- A preauricular swelling, arthralgia as previously defined, or limited mouth opening

Examination is positive for at least one of the following:

- Preauricular swelling
- Arthralgia as previously defined
- Maximum assisted opening (passive stretch) < 40 mm including vertical incisal overlap

Imaging is positive for evidence of fracture.

Congenital/developmental disorders

APLASIA. *Aplasia* is defined as a typically unilateral absence of the condyle and incomplete development of the articular fossa and eminence, resulting in facial asymmetries. It is commonly associated with other congenital anomalies (eg, oculo-auriculo-vertebral spectrum [Goldenhar syndrome], hemifacial microsomia, and mandibulofacial dysostosis [Treacher Collins syndrome]).[266,267] It is occasionally bilateral, and in such cases, asymmetry is not present, but micrognathia is the dominant clinical manifestation. The condition may be associated with malocclusion, which may include open bite. Sensitivity and specificity have not been established.

History must be positive for both of the following:

- Progressive development of mandibular asymmetry or micrognathia from birth or early childhood
- Development of malocclusion, which may include posterior open bite

Examination is positive for both of the following:

- Confirmation of mandibular asymmetry, with deviation of the chin to the affected side or micrognathia
- Inability to detect the condyle upon palpation during mandibular movements

Imaging will show both of the following:

- Severe hypoplasia of the fossa and eminence
- Aplasia of the condyle

HYPOPLASIA. *Hypoplasia* is defined as incomplete development or underdevelopment of the cranial bones or the mandible. Growth is proportionately reduced and less severe than in aplasia. This condition bridges the continuum from aplasia to normal condylar size. Condylar hypoplasia can be secondary to facial trauma. The condition may be associated with malocclusion, which may include open bite. Sensitivity and specificity have not been established.

History must be positive for both of the following:

- Progressive development of mandibular asymmetry or micrognathia from birth or early childhood
- Development of malocclusion, which may include posterior open bite

Examination must confirm this history.

Imaging using CT/CBCT will show at least one of the following:

- Hypoplasia of the fossa
- Hypoplasia of the condyle
- Shortened mandibular ramus height

HYPERPLASIA. *Hyperplasia* is an overdevelopment of the cranial bones or mandible. It is a nonneoplastic increase in the number of normal cells. It can occur unilaterally or bilaterally as a localized enlargement such as condylar hyperplasia, or as an overdevelopment of the entire mandible or side of the face. Sensitivity and specificity have not been established.

To diagnose hyperplasia, the history must be positive for progressive development of mandibular or facial asymmetry, and the examination must confirm this history. Imaging using panoramic radiography and/or CT/CBCT and single-photon emission CT are positive for the following:

- Asymmetry in mandibular ramus height
- Increased uptake of technetium-99m hydroxy diphosphonate on bone scintigraphy scan (nuclear imaging)

Masticatory muscle disorders

The mechanisms that produce pain in skeletal muscles are still not well understood. Overuse of a normally perfused muscle or ischemia of a normally working muscle may cause pain.[268–271] Sympathetic and fusimotor reflexes can produce changes in the blood supply and muscle tone.[272,273] Furthermore, different psychologic or emotional states can alter muscle tone.[201,274] Neurons that mediate pain from skeletal muscles are subject to strong modulatory influences. Endogenous substances (eg, bradykinin, serotonin, prostaglandins, neuropeptides, and substance P) can sensitize the nociceptive endings very easily. Painful muscle conditions not only lead to increased sensitivity of peripheral nociceptors but also produce hyperexcitability in the central nervous system, resulting in central sensitization presenting with localized hyperalgesia and allodynia.[275–277]

Some systemic conditions that produce muscle pain are polymyalgia rheumatica, polymyositis, dermatomyositis, lupus erythematosus, and fibromyalgia (ie, chronic widespread pain). Fibromyalgia is of particular interest because it may easily be confused with a regional masticatory muscle disorder. When fibromyalgia is suspected, a referral to a rheumatologist is necessary.

Muscle pain limited to the orofacial region

MYALGIA. Pain of muscle origin is modified by jaw movement, function, or parafunction, and replication of this pain is elicited with provocation testing of the temporalis or masseter muscles, which are the muscles involved with highest prevalence. Although not required in the criteria, a positive finding with the specified provocation tests when examining the other masticatory muscles can help to corroborate this diagnosis if the location of the pain associated with the chief complaint is in these muscles; limited mandibular range of motion may also be present. Hypothetically, based on the work by the validation research group and later on by the DC/TMD international community, three subtypes of myalgia can be identified, but only myalgia and myofascial pain with referral are the clinical diagnoses with diagnostic validity values; the other two diagnoses—local myalgia and myofascial pain with spreading—do not have sensitivity and specificity estimates, and therefore, they are not validated.

History must be positive for both of the following:

- Pain in the jaw, temple, ear, or in front of the ear in the last 30 days
- Pain modified by jaw function or parafunction

In addition, the clinical examination will reveal confirmation of the localization of the pain in the masticatory muscle structure, confirmed by the examiner, and report of familiar pain during vertical mandibular movements or palpation of the masticatory muscles. The sensitivity and specificity estimates are 0.90 and 0.99, respectively.

Local myalgia. This involves pain of muscle origin plus a report of pain localized only to the site of palpation (immediate site to stimulation). Limitation of mandibular movements secondary to pain may be present. Sensitivity and specificity have not been established. The criterion for this diagnostic group limits the familiar pain to be provoked only with palpation and not with mandibular movement.

Myofascial pain with spreading. This involves pain of muscle origin plus a report of pain spreading beyond the location of the palpating fingers but within the boundary of the masticatory muscle being examined. Limitation of mandibular movements secondary to pain may be present. Sensitivity and specificity have not been established.

To diagnose myofascial pain with spreading, the patient must have local myalgia, and the examination of the temporalis or masseter muscle must confirm both of the following:

- Familiar muscle pain with palpation
- Pain with muscle palpation with spreading of the pain beyond the location of palpation but within the boundary of the palpated muscle

Note: Other masticatory muscles may be examined as required.

Myofascial pain with referral. This involves pain of muscle origin as defined for myalgia plus a referral of pain beyond the boundary of the masticatory muscles being palpated, for example, to the ear, tooth, or eye; spreading may be present. The sensitivity and specificity values are 0.86 and 0.98, respectively.

To diagnose myofascial pain with referral, the patient must have myalgia, and the examination of the temporalis or masseter muscle must confirm both of the following:

- Familiar muscle pain with palpation
- Pain with muscle palpation beyond the boundary of the muscle

Other masticatory muscles may be examined as required.

TENDONITIS. Tendonitis involves pain of tendon origin affected by jaw movement, function, or parafunction and replication of this pain with provocation testing of the masticatory tendon. Limitation of mandibular movements secondary to pain may be present. The temporalis tendon is a common site of tendonitis with referred pain to the teeth or other structures. Sensitivity and specificity have not been established.

To diagnose tendonitis, the patient must have myalgia as previously defined, and the examination must confirm the diagnosis of myalgia but restricted to the temporalis tendon. This condition could also apply to other masticatory muscle tendons.

MYOSITIS. This involves pain of muscle origin with clinical characteristics of inflammation or infection: edema, erythema, and/or increased temperature. It generally arises acutely following direct trauma of the muscle or from infection or chronically with autoimmune disease. Limitation of unassisted mandibular movements secondary to pain is often present. Calcification of the muscle can occur (ie, myositis ossificans). Sensitivity and specificity have not been established.

To diagnose myositis, the patient must have local myalgia, and the examination of the temporalis or masseter muscle must confirm both of the following:

- Local myalgia
- Presence of edema, erythema, and/or increased temperature over the muscle

In addition, serologic tests may reveal elevated enzyme levels (eg, creatine kinase), markers of inflammation, and the presence of autoimmune diseases. Other masticatory muscles may be examined as required.

SPASM. This is a sudden, involuntary, reversible tonic contraction of a muscle. Acute malocclusion may be present. Sensitivity and specificity have not been established.

To diagnose a spasm, the patient must report the following:

- Immediate onset of muscle pain modified by function and parafunction as operationalized in myalgia
- Immediate report of limited range of jaw motion

In addition, the examination must confirm both of the following:

- Myalgia that may include all masticatory muscles
- Limited range of jaw motion in the direction that elongates the affected muscle (eg, for jaw closers, opening will be limited to < 40 mm; for the lateral pterygoid muscle, ipsilateral movement will be limited to < 7 mm)

When this diagnosis needs to be confirmed, laboratory testing will confirm elevated electromyographic activity compared with the contralateral unaffected muscle. Sensitivity and specificity have not been established.

Contracture

Contracture is the shortening of a muscle due to fibrosis of tendons, ligaments, or muscle fibers. It is usually not painful unless the muscle is overextended. A history of radiation therapy, trauma, or infection is often present. Sensitivity and specificity have not been established. To diagnose contracture, the patient must have progressive loss of range of motion, and the examination must confirm that unassisted and assisted jaw movements are limited such that maximum assisted opening is < 40 mm. It must also be associated with a hard end feel that has been operationalized as having unyielding resistance to assisted movements as felt by the clinician.

Hypertrophy

Hypertrophy is enlargement of one or more masticatory muscles. It is usually not associated with pain and can be secondary to overuse and/or chronic tensing of the muscle(s). Some cases are familial or genetic in origin. Sensitivity and specificity have not been established. To diagnose hypertrophy, the patient must have enlargement of one or more masticatory muscles as evidenced from photographs or previous records, and the examination must confirm this enlargement. Diagnosis is based on the clinician's assessment of muscle size and requires consideration of craniofacial morphology and ethnicity.

Neoplasm (soft tissues of head, face, and neck)

Neoplasms of the masticatory muscles result from tissue proliferation with histologic characteristics and may be benign (eg, myoma), malignant (eg, rhabdomyosarcoma), or metastatic. They are uncommon. They may present with swelling, spasm, pain during function, limited mouth opening, and/or sensory-motor changes (eg, paresthesias). Diagnostic imaging (typically using CT/CBCT and/or MRI) and biopsy are essential when a neoplasm is suspected. Sensitivity and specificity have not been established.

Movement disorders

OROFACIAL DYSKINESIA. Orofacial dyskinesia involves involuntary, mainly choreatic (dance-like) movements that may involve the face, lips, tongue, and/or jaw. The disorder may result in traumatic injury to the oral mucosa or tongue. It is more common with advancing age and in patients with a history of using neuroleptic medications and/or associated with traumatic brain injury, psychiatric conditions, or other neurologic disorders (eg, Wilson disease). Reduction or discontinuation of the movement pattern could occur when the mouth or face receives sensory stimulation (*sensory trick*). Sensitivity and specificity have not been established.

To allocate these diagnoses, the patient must provide a positive history of neurologic diagnosis of dyskinesia in the orofacial region and history components of myalgia and/ or arthralgia (diagnostic criteria as previously described) that worsens with episodes of dyskinesia.

Examination will be positive for all of the following:

- Sensory and/or motor nerve conduction deficit
- Central and/or peripheral myopathic disease
- Muscular hyperactivity confirmed by intramuscular electromyography (EMG)
- Myalgia and/or arthralgia

OROMANDIBULAR DYSTONIA. Oromandibular dystonia involves excessive, involuntary, and sustained muscle contractions that may involve the face, lips, tongue, and/or jaw. They could be components of a number of central nervous systems disorders, including Parkinson disease and Meige syndrome, and could be an adverse event related to medication usage, notably neuroleptics. Trauma to the brain, head, and neck can trigger the onset of transient or permanent dystonia of the masticatory muscles. The disorder can also be genetically determined. Normally, the dystonia disappears during sleep. The affected muscles are often painful. The condition can make opening and closing the mouth difficult and impair speech, swallowing, and chewing. Sensitivity and specificity have not been established.

To allocate these diagnoses, the patient must provide a positive history of neurologic diagnosis of dystonia in the orofacial region and history components of myalgia and/or arthralgia (diagnostic criteria as previously described) that worsens with episodes of dystonia.

Examination will be positive for all of the following:

- Sensory and/or motor nerve conduction deficit
- Central and/or peripheral myopathic disease
- Dystonia confirmed by intramuscular EMG
- Myalgia and/or arthralgia

Masticatory muscle pain attributed to systemic/central disorders

FIBROMYALGIA. Fibromyalgia involves widespread pain with concurrent masticatory muscle pain (see chapter 10). History and examination are positive for both a rheumatologic-based diagnosis of fibromyalgia and myalgia as previously defined. Sensitivity and specificity have not been established. Historically, in diagnosing fibromyalgia, there needed to be tenderness in at least 11 of 18 specified sites and the presence of widespread pain denoted as axial pain, right and left pain, and upper and lower segment pain. Current criteria eliminate the tender points and focus on a widespread pain index and symptom severity scale.[278,279]

CENTRALLY MEDIATED MYALGIA. *Centrally mediated myalgia* is defined as chronic, continuous muscle pain that is aggravated by function. Intermittent muscle pain conditions may not produce centrally mediated myalgia, while a prolonged and constant period of muscle pain is likely to lead to the condition. Sensitivity and specificity have not been established.

History must be positive for all of the following:

- Prolonged and continuous pain in the jaw, in the temple, in front of the ear, or in the ear in the past 30 days
- Regional dull, aching pain at rest
- Pain is aggravated by function of the affected muscles
- Presence of at least three nonspecific somatic symptoms, such as sensation of muscle stiffness, weakness, and/or fatigue
- Sensation of acute dental occlusal changes not verified clinically
- Ear symptoms (eg, tinnitus, feeling of fullness, blocked ear), vertigo, dental pain symptoms not attributed to another diagnosis, or headache symptoms not otherwise classifiable by the ICHD-3 (beta version)
- Limited mouth opening (due to pain or myofibrotic contracture)

In addition, the examination must confirm at least two of the following:

- Myalgia
- Evidence of sensory dysfunction (eg, allodynia, paresthesia, dental occlusal awareness)
- Muscular atrophy
- Maximum unassisted opening < 40 mm including vertical incisal overlap

Headache disorders

Headache attributed to TMDs

If the headache is caused by a disorder involving structures in the temporomandibular region, it can be considered a headache attributed to TMDs. According to the International Headache Society, this headache is considered present when there is evidence of a pathologic process affecting the TMJ, muscles of mastication, and/or associated structures, together with evidence of a causal relationship with the headache. Causation is demonstrated when at least two of the following symptoms are present.[274]

- Headache has developed in a temporal relationship to the onset of the TMDs
- Headache has significantly worsened in parallel with progression of the TMDs, and/or headache has significantly improved or resolved in parallel with improvement in or resolution of the TMDs
- Headache is produced or exacerbated by active jaw movements, passive jaw movements, and/or provocative maneuvers applied to temporomandibular structures such as palpation pressure
- When unilateral, headache is ipsilateral to the side of the TMDs

In the DC/TMD, headache attributed to TMDs is included as one of the new diagnostic subtypes.[211] In general, the DC/TMD criteria for this headache closely follow those of the ICHD. An important difference, however, relates to the definition of the TMD subtype that should be present: The DC/TMD specifically links the headache to a pain-related TMD diagnosis like myalgia or arthralgia. Sensitivity and specificity values are 0.89 and 0.98, respectively.

To allocate this diagnosis, both of the following criteria must be met:

- History of headaches of any type localized in the temple region during the last 30 days that are modified by jaw movement in function or parafunction
- During clinical examination, confirmation of the location of the headaches in the temporalis muscle area and report of familiar headache upon palpation of the temporalis muscle or during mandibular movements

Associated structures

Coronoid hyperplasia

Coronoid hyperplasia is progressive enlargement of the coronoid process that impedes mandibular opening when it is obstructed by the zygomatic process of the maxilla. Sensitivity and specificity have not been established.

To diagnose coronoid hyperplasia, the patient must complain of progressive limitation of jaw opening, the examination must confirm the reduction of active and passive maximum jaw opening, and imaging must show an elongated coronoid process that approximates the posterior aspect of the zygomatic process of the maxilla on opening.

Management of TMDs

Management goals for patients with TMDs are similar to those for other orthopedic and/or rheumatologic disorders. They include decreased pain, decreased adverse loading, restoration of function, and resumption of normal daily activities. These management goals are best achieved by a well-defined program designed to treat the physical disorder(s) and to reduce or eliminate the effects of all contributing factors. The treatment options and sequences for TMDs outlined here are consistent with treatment of other musculoskeletal disorders.

As with many musculoskeletal conditions, the signs and symptoms of TMDs over time may be transient and self-limiting, resolving without serious long-term effects.[13] Little is known about which signs and symptoms will progress to more serious conditions in the natural course of TMDs. Therefore, special efforts should be made to avoid early use of aggressive, irreversible treatments. Conservative (ie, reversible), noninvasive treatment such as self-management instructions, behavioral modification, physical therapy, medications, and orthopedic appliances are endorsed for the initial care of nearly all TMDs.[13]

Principles of management

Most patients with TMDs achieve good symptom relief with conservative therapy.[280] More than 85% to 90% of the patients in three longitudinal studies lasting 2 to 10 years had relief of symptoms after conservative treatment.[281–283] Stability was achieved in most cases between 6 and 12 months after the start of treatment.[283] A more recent case series of a 1-year duration demonstrated substantial pain relief and improvement in jaw function utilizing heat, therapeutic exercises, habit management, and a flat plane splint.[284]

In many patients with disc displacement (reducing and nonreducing), painless jaw function is possible with a displaced disc.[285,286] Patients with pain-free clicking TMJs generally do not need treatment except for reassurance and explanation of the condition,[287] whereas patients with nonreducing discs typically respond well to conservative treatment.[286,288,289] Internal derangement of the TMJ often exhibits a natural progression of compensatory adaptation and remodeling.[290,291] Even with progression or with osteoarthritic changes, the outcome is typically benign with adequate masticatory function.[292,293] Myogenous disorders more frequently require recurrent treatment as compared with TMJ articular disorders.[294,295]

Relevant precipitating and perpetuating contributing factors should be identified through the history and clinical examination. Factors such as bruxism and other parafunctional habits, trauma, adverse anatomical relationships, and pathophysiologic and psychosocial conditions may all impact TMDs, but because the majority of these factors are highly prevalent in the general population, their presence in an individual case may be coincidental and not contribute to the TMDs. Therefore, in addition to the physical diagnosis, the goal of each evaluation should be the development of a prioritized problem list of the relevant contributing factors. This has direct implications for the treatment plan and strategic sequencing.

Treatment prognosis can be affected by a number of considerations. Early treatment of acute musculoskeletal pain results in greater patient satisfaction, fewer workdays lost, and reduced chance of development of a chronic pain condition.[296] In cases of chronic TMDs where pain is less frequent and patients engage in greater daily activity, the prognosis is better.[297] The power of nonspecific effects in healing (eg, placebo effect) in the treatment of psychosocial and biologic conditions has been well documented.[298] These effects certainly play a role in the successful treatment of TMDs, and the value of a good doctor–patient relationship should be recognized and used.[299] Despite the documented success of the various forms of conservative care, some patients with TMDs do not improve. Reasons for this vary, but these patients typically fall into two groups: *(1)* patients with an incomplete or incorrect diagnosis or *(2)* patients with unsuccessfully addressed or even unrecognized contributing factors.[285] When multiple contributing factors are present, and especially if the condition is chronic, a pain management program with a multidisciplinary team of clinicians may be needed. It is difficult for an individual clinician to address the multiple contributing factors that may be present in complex chronic pain patients.[300] Treatment options include patient education and self-management, cognitive behavioral therapy (CBT), pharmacotherapy, physical therapy, orthopedic appliances, and possibly surgery. It is important to also remember that Axis II (psychologic) factors need to be considered in the management of all TMDs. These factors are reviewed in chapter 12.

Patient education and self-management

The success of a self-management program depends on patient acceptance, motivation, cooperation, and compliance. The time spent on patient reassurance and education is a significant factor in developing a high level of rapport and treatment compliance. The clinician's explanation of the problem and treatment recommendations should use terminology the patient can understand.

A successful self-management program allows healing and prevents further injury to the musculoskeletal system. This may be enough to control the problem.[301] A self-management routine should include the following: *(1)* education, including explanation, advice, and reassurance; *(2)* self-exercise therapy; *(3)* thermal modalities; *(4)* self-massage therapy; *(5)* diet and nutrition; and *(6)* parafunctional behavior modification.[302] Modification of function (eg, avoidance of heavy mastication, gum chewing, wide yawning, singing, and playing certain musical instruments) as well as parafunctional habit reversal (eg, clenching, bruxing, tongue thrusting, cheek biting, poor sleeping posture, or object biting) should be emphasized.

Offending habits can be modified with habit awareness, motivation to change, and knowledge in how to change. Commitment to conscientious monitoring for the habits can lead to successful habit modification. A simple feedback mechanism, such as visual or audio reminders adapted to the patient's daily activities, should be discussed and implemented (eg, small stickers strategically placed at home, in the patient's vehicle, and at work; alarms sounding from electronic sources; phone apps). Keeping a diary aimed at identifying circumstances and activities that foster the offending habits may also be helpful so that the patient can titrate the need for more or less monitoring during any given day. Progress with habit modification should be discussed at each follow-up appointment with the patient.

A home physiotherapy program has also been proposed for the treatment of TMD pain and dysfunction because it is simple, noninvasive, and cost-effective; allows an easy self-management approach; cultivates good doctor-patient communication; and can be managed by the general practitioner.[303] Emphasis should be placed on patient self-control. A program of heat and/or ice to the affected areas, massage of the affected muscles, and gentle range-of-motion exercises can decrease tenderness and pain and increase range of motion. Heat stimulates muscle relaxation and vascular perfusion. Heat should not be used following an acute injury (ie, < 72 hours) or for acute inflammation or infection. Ice packs are used primarily for local analgesic and anti-inflammatory effects in muscle and joint tissues. Because the temperature differential is greater with cold, a shorter application may produce a greater response. Cold should not be used over areas with poor circulation (eg, as a result of diabetes or radiation) or over open wounds.

Self-management components can be provided to the patient first as essential interventional steps and continued as fundamental for the continuous management with the intent that these elements will be used throughout the patient's life.[302]

Biobehavioral therapy

Behavioral modification for overuse or parafunctional behaviors (habits) remains a central part of the overall treatment program for individuals with TMDs despite the as-yet unclear evidence for their overall role in etiology or in contributing to persistence of the disorder.[304] In general, the clinician should err toward overemphasis on this part of treatment based on the extent by which higher levels of parafunction are observed in individuals with chronic TMDs.[57] International consensus has rated bruxism as a behavior rather than a disorder, where in an otherwise healthy person it could be classified as harmless.[12] In individuals self-reporting bruxism (either by history or with a focused questionnaire) and associating it with adverse consequences, it is logical to consider treatment approaches to reduce the frequency and/or intensity of the behavior.

The success in reducing the frequency and/or intensity of parafunctional behaviors depends on several patient and clinical factors. Patient factors include the level and continuity of awareness of the putative behaviors, long-term motivation and commitment to treatment, and the extent to which other factors (eg, life stress) are uncontrollable triggers for the behaviors.

Clinical factors include curiosity in exploring possible symptom–behavior relationships, persistence in monitoring behavioral patterns and level of patient skills, and ability in effecting behavioral change. Patients whose parafunctional behaviors may seem severe, chronic, and under the control of extensive environmental factors may nevertheless respond quickly to the clinician's initial intervention, while patients whose parafunctional behaviors seem simple may require extensive treatment from a behavioral specialist.[304] Consequently, initiating intervention of parafunctional behaviors is a pragmatic decision for every patient, recognizing that significant modification of their lifestyle is often necessary to alter the contributing factors in the interest of long-term prevention of recurrent TMD pain. If a more structured approach is indicated, strategies for behavior modification such as a habit-reversal program, lifestyle counseling, CBT for stress management, progressive relaxation, hypnosis, and biofeedback should be considered. Treatment should be individualized based on the patient's problems, preferences, and lifestyle.

Biofeedback is a structured therapy based on the theory that when an individual receives information about a desired change and is supported in making the change, the change is more likely to occur.[305,306] In general, biofeedback training uses equipment to measure biologic activity (eg, surface EMG to measure muscle activity). The equipment is designed with a feedback loop so that a patient can receive immediate feedback regarding performance. A number of controlled studies have demonstrated that the use of surface EMG biofeedback can decrease awake tonic muscle activity.[307,308] Most trials evaluating biofeedback for the treatment of TMDs have been undertaken with small sample sizes, and although there is cumulative evidence of effectiveness when biofeedback was compared with controls, there remains a need for large-sample, controlled-outcome trials.[307]

Biofeedback may be less effective in the treatment of sleep bruxism,[309] and is not considered as effective as other modalities.[310] EMG biofeedback to help raise awareness of awake bruxism may help to reduce sleep bruxism, but the evidence is minimal and preliminary.[311] Comprehensive stress management and counseling programs that involve a combination of EMG biofeedback, progressive relaxation, and self-directed lifestyle changes appear to be more effective when used together than any single behavioral treatment. Use of behavioral therapies in conjunction with usual physical medicine and medication therapies also appears to enhance the overall therapeutic effects.[312]

A systematic review evaluating noninvasive interventions for persistent TMD concluded that CBT in addition to standard care yielded better results than standard care alone with regard to life interference and depression as well as pain intensity; however, the latter difference was not deemed to reach clinical importance.[313] Another systematic review on the effect of counseling and self-management for TMDs revealed that these strategies yielded similar positive results in pain reduction and increase in mouth opening compared with the use of interocclusal appliances with no additive effect when used together. The studies included mostly patients with myofascial pain.[314]

Pharmacologic management

Pharmacologic agents may promote patient comfort and rehabilitation when used as part of a comprehensive program. Clinicians who decide to prescribe medications should be familiar with a variety of drugs to realize maximal treatment effect and benefit, avoid unexpected complications, and act in response to adverse drug interactions.

The most widely used pharmacologic agents for the management of TMDs include analgesics, such as nonsteroidal anti-inflammatory drugs (NSAIDs), corticosteroids, and low-dose antidepressants.[315] Pharmacologic agents less often used include gabapentinoids, benzodiazepines, and muscle relaxants. The analgesics, corticosteroids, and benzodiazepines may be indicated for acute TMD pain; NSAIDs and muscle relaxants may be used for both acute and chronic conditions; and the tricyclic antidepressants (TCAs) are primarily indicated for chronic orofacial pain management.

Analgesics

Mild analgesics (nonopiate preparations) are usually the pharmacologic agents of choice to reduce pain associated with TMDs. The nonopioid analgesics are a heterogenous group of compounds that share certain therapeutic actions and side effects. They may be used for mild to moderate pain associated with TMDs. Aspirin, which inhibits prostaglandin synthesis, is the prototype for these compounds. All salicylate drugs are antipyretic, analgesic, and anti-inflammatory, but there are important differences in their effects. Opioid narcotics act on specific opioid receptor sites in the central and peripheral nervous systems. Opioids have central nervous system (CNS) depression qualities and addiction liabilities. They may be considered for short-term use for moderate to severe acute pain.[316]

Drug misuse and abuse are of concern in the pharmacologic management of TMDs. Opioid narcotics produce tolerance and dependence and therefore are most useful in short-term, acute pain conditions. Long-term narcotic analgesic use in patients with chronic TMDs requires careful consideration[316]; adverse effects are common, and with limited evidence of efficacy combined with significant potential for harm, the clinician should be very cautious with their use.[317] Prescribing drugs on a pain-contingent basis to be taken "as needed" for chronic noncancer pain has long been associated with concern that it may lead to abuse for some patients. Recent evidence, however, indicates that time-contingent prescribing of opioids may lead to use of higher amounts and may be associated with more patient concerns regarding their opioid use.[318] Given the continuing controversies and risks associated with long-term opioid use for noncancer pain, all other avenues of treatment should be pursued before relying on narcotic medication for TMD patients.

Nonsteroidal anti-inflammatory drugs

NSAIDs have been reported as effective for mild to moderate inflammatory conditions and acute postoperative pain.[316] Specific for TMDs involving the joint, a systematic review showed some support for use of NSAIDs.[319] There are several chemically dissimilar groups of NSAIDs, which each differ in their antipyretic, analgesic, and anti-inflammatory efficacy.[320] Therefore, if one NSAID fails, another agent may succeed. NSAIDs may have serious side effects, and patients on NSAIDs should therefore be carefully monitored.[321] Gastrointestinal complications form the greatest risk associated with the use of NSAIDs. If gastroprotection is needed, a proton pump inhibitor should be considered in conjunction with NSAID therapy, although these are not without their own set of risks.[322] In adults with asthma, up to 10% may have aspirin-induced asthma. This condition is also precipitated by NSAIDs and can lead to bronchospasm. The classic triad is a history of nasal polyps, aspirin intolerance, and asthma.[323] In addition to increased bleeding risk, there are increased risks associated in patients with cardiovascular or renal disease, however these may be minimized with short courses of therapy.[324] As TMD may become a chronic condition, associated risks with chronic use of NSAIDs increase. Patients should be informed of the risks, especially as they may perceive over-the-counter medication as "safe." Renal effects from the NSAIDs can also cause or increase hypertension as well as lead to acute renal injury.[325] All NSAIDs contain the same black box warning regarding cardiovascular and gastrointestinal toxicity regardless of the route of administration. NSAIDs increase the risk of serious and potentially fatal cardiovascular thrombotic events including myocardial infarction and stroke; risk may occur early in treatment and may increase with the duration of use.

Corticosteroids and sodium hyaluronate

Corticosteroids are potent anti-inflammatory drugs not commonly prescribed for systemic use in the treatment of TMDs due to their side effects. The exception is for acute, severely painful joint inflammation or for joint inflammation associated with the polyarthritides. Intracapsular TMJ injection of corticosteroids (ie, methylprednisolone) has been recommended on a limited basis in cases of acute flare-up of severe joint pain where conservative treatment has been unsuccessful. Although there have been some concerns regarding long-term effects (ie, progression of joint destruction), the 6-month follow-up appears good for alleviating TMJ pain and dysfunction with no or minimal increase of radiographically visible degenerative changes.[326,327]

Sodium hyaluronate is the sodium salt of purified natural sodium hyaluronic acid. Hyaluronic acid is a naturally occurring polysaccharide belonging to the glycosaminoglycan family. In healthy synovial joints, hyaluronic acid maintains viscosity of the synovial fluid and supports the lubricating and shock-absorbing properties of the articular cartilage. Systematic reviews of both corticosteroids and sodium hyaluronate do not show a difference in treatment outcome between the two interventions, and there is currently some support for their use.[319,328,329] Concerns still raised by the reviews involve low enrollment numbers, risk of bias, and short follow-up. Randomized controlled trials (RCTs) are needed to provide evidence of efficacy of corticosteroid or hyaluronate use over standard treatments for TMDs.

There are some studies on injecting platelet-rich plasma (PRP) into intra-articular TMDs. Systematic reviews provide support for the minimally invasive use of PRP as an intra-articular injection for TMJ DJD.[330,331] There is concern, however, on the standardization of preparation, so more RCTs using standardized techniques are recommended.[331] In addition, cost–benefit analyses have not been done comparing these treatments.

BOTULINUM TOXIN. Botulinum toxin has been trialed in the treatment of myofascial trigger points (TPs). An update of a Cochrane review concluded that there is insufficient evidence for botulinum use, highlighting that there is a lot of heterogeneity between the studies, including lack of standardized outcome measurements, treatment modalities, and follow-up.[332] Contrasting results in a more recent systematic review and meta-analysis including only double-blind studies with placebo controls showed that pain intensity was significantly reduced in the botulinum-A groups compared with placebo groups at a relatively long term of 6 months, although the cost-effectiveness is questioned.[333,334]

Benzodiazepines

Benzodiazepines are antianxiety agents that have been administered to patients with chronic pain. These drugs are potentially habit forming, and there is a concern that they may worsen depression in chronic pain patients.[315] A review of studies could not support or refute their use.[335] Benzodiazepines have not shown a superior effect over other medications,[336] and their risk profile is significantly higher than other treatment options.

Muscle relaxants

Muscle relaxants used to reduce skeletal muscle tone are prescribed in an effort to reduce the supposed increased muscle activity associated with TMDs.[337] Experimentally, muscle relaxants depress spinal polysynaptic reflexes preferentially over monosynaptic reflexes. Muscle relaxants affect neuronal activity associated with muscle stretch reflexes, primarily in the lateral reticular area of the brainstem. The oral doses of all of these drugs are well below the levels required to elicit experimental muscle relaxant activity. Therefore, some investigators conclude that their muscle relaxant activity is related only to their sedative effect.[315] Some central skeletal muscle relaxants are available in combination with analgesics.

In TMD patients, cyclobenzaprine was found to be statistically superior to either placebo or clonazepam in reducing jaw pain upon awakening, but neither drug had any effect on sleep improvement.[336] This has been borne out with a systematic review,[319] but as with other pharmacologic treatments, additional RCTs are needed to determine if muscle relaxants are of benefit in treating TMDs. Because there is limited evidence of the efficacy of muscle relaxants in the treatment of TMDs, their use should be limited to a brief trial in conjunction with conservative TMD therapy.

Antidepressants

Antidepressants have been used to manage chronic pain and have demonstrated pain relief that is not associated with depression relief.[338] TCAs, particularly amitriptyline, have analgesic properties independent of antidepressant effect and are prescribed for chronic pain patients with depression and sleep disturbance.[339] The therapeutic effect of these drugs is thought to be related to their ability to increase the availability of the biogenic amines serotonin and norepinephrine at the synaptic junction in the CNS. TCAs are beneficial in dosages as low as 10 mg in the treatment of tension-type headache and musculoskeletal pain.[340] They decrease the number of awakenings, increase slow-wave sleep (δ sleep), and markedly decrease time in rapid eye movement (REM) sleep.[57] For these reasons, it was thought that TCAs might have potential in the treatment of certain types of sleep bruxism; however, double-blind crossover studies reported that amitriptyline did not significantly decrease EMG activity or pain levels but did decrease stress levels associated with sleep bruxism.[341,342] Similarly, a systematic review regarding the use of TCAs in the treatment of TMDs indicated inconsistent or limited quality patient-oriented evidence for the use of this intervention.[343] Amitriptyline has been reported, however, to significantly reduce pain associated with both chronic muscular and TMJ dysfunction, and in combination with CBT showed significant improvement over placebo.[344,345] It has been found to result in an equal amount of pain reduction as occlusal splint therapy, and both were therapeutically more effective than placebo.[346] Some concern has been raised about the likelihood of high placebo effect in the use of amitriptyline,[347] and with all medications, the potential side effects may make the risk greater than the benefit for some patients. The therapeutic doses required to achieve an antidepressant action are significantly larger than those needed to achieve pain control and sleep improvement, so the clinician should be aware that if treatment of depression is a goal, the patient will need to be referred to a practitioner trained and licensed to treat depression. The effect of selective serotonin reuptake inhibitors (SSRIs), selective serotonin-noradrenaline reuptake inhibitors (SSNRIs), and TCAs on pain has been evaluated.[348] In a meta-analysis limited to placebo-controlled trials with an intervention period up to 6 months on a primary depressive disorder population, pain relief was significantly superior in the SSRI and SSNRI groups compared with placebo, but there was no difference between these two drugs. Using a limited number of trials, no significant results were observed with the use of TCAs compared with placebo. Secondary analysis included non-placebo-controlled trials with TCAs showing a trend of improvement but not better than SSRIs and SSNRIs; both analyses with TCAs should be interpreted with caution and are not conclusive. Furthermore, it is important to keep in mind that the transfer of these results to a primary pain population is limited. In a qualitative analysis on the effect of SSRIs in various chronic pain conditions (not specific to TMD), the authors concluded that SSRIs seem to have a positive effect in 70% of the trials.[349] In a Cochrane systematic review, no beneficial effect was found with the use of SSRIs and SNRIs for the prevention of tension-type headaches.[350] In addition to the mixed data on pain control with SSRIs and SNRIs, clinicians should be aware that these drugs have been associated with the development of bruxism within 3 to 4 weeks of initiation or titration.[351] Patients with chronic TMDs are more likely to already be on an antidepressive agent and thus may not be candidates for treatment with these agents.[352]

Gabapentinoids

A well-designed RCT evaluated the effectiveness of gabapentin on the treatment of chronic pain in the masticatory muscles.[352] The authors concluded that this agent was clinically and statistically superior to placebo in reducing pain and hyperalgesia and improving daily function. While this result has not been replicated by other investigators in a randomized clinical trial, promise has been shown for patients who do not respond to TCAs.[353] Most of the trials using this agent focus on neuropathic pain conditions (postherpetic or diabetic) for which pregabalin is cleared by the U.S. Food and Drug Administration (FDA). Gabapentin is FDA cleared for postherpetic neuralgia.

Glucosamine and chondroitin

These nutritional supplements have gained widespread use in the treatment of osteoarthritis with the potential theory that they act as disease-modifying agents not only to reduce the symptoms but also to modify the natural history of osteoarthritis. Although a positive effect with their use has been shown, there are few high-quality trials, specifically in the progression of the disease.[354] In a recent report from a multicenter RCT using these supplements in a knee osteoarthritis model, it was demonstrated that the combination has comparable efficacy to celecoxib in reducing pain and stiffness and increasing function after 3 months, but such effects do not increase at the 6-month follow-up.[355]

The effects of glucosamine hydrochloride (GH) and chondroitin sulfate (CS) have been evaluated in specific TMD populations, first in a pilot study using 1,200 mg of chondroitin and 1,500 mg of glucosamine for 12 weeks. It was reported that participants using GH-CS had improvement in pain, TMJ tenderness, and joint sounds compared to those using over-the-counter medication.[356] In one study, glucosamine sulfate (GS) resulted in a significantly greater decrease in TMJ pain with function compared with ibuprofen, while in another study comparing GS with a placebo, GS seemed to have no superior effect in reducing signs and symptoms of osteoarthritis in the TMJ.[357,358] These conflicting results in the TMD population are consistent with systematic reviews involving other joints.[359] In knee osteoarthritis, the addition of methylsulfonylmethane (MSM) to glucosamine-chondroitin did result in improved pain/stiffness/physical function (measured by the WOMAC scale) over glucosamine-chondroitin alone or placebo. However, the addition of glucosamine-chondroitin-MSM after TMJ arthrocentesis with hyaluronic acid did not demonstrate improvement over the arthrocentesis/hyaluronic acid alone.[360]

Topical medications

Topical NSAIDs are approved to treat osteoarthritis pain (diclofenac formulations), and it is suggested that this formulation has similar effectiveness to oral formulations but with a greater safety profile due to lower serum concentrations.[361] Other formulations have been investigated (eg, ibuprofen, ketoprofen, piroxicam, and indomethacin), and it has been strongly suggested to consider the use of topical diclofenac and ibuprofen in the treatment of acute soft tissue injuries or chronic joint pain–related conditions.[362] A 2012 systematic review failed to show sufficient evidence to support the use of topically applied NSAIDs in painful DJD of the TMJ.[363] A more recent systematic review also concluded there was either limited or insufficient evidence for various topical preparations for TMD.[364]

Other considerations

In a Cochrane systematic review in which only trials comparing active intervention to placebo were included, there was insufficient evidence to either support or refute the use of NSAIDs, benzodiazepines, anticonvulsants, muscle relaxants, propanol, oral GH-CS, and topical capsaicin in the treatment of chronic TMDs.[335] All presented pharmacologic agents have in theory a biologic plausibility, but in general, in the field of TMD as a chronic pain condition, the efficacy and safety of most of them lack evidence due to methodologically compromised data. In addition, this lack of sufficient evidence for pharmacologic interventions may be a result of current limited knowledge of what affects—or does not affect—why certain agents are beneficial for some patients and not others. This can classically be seen in the literature regarding the use of propranolol in TMD. In individuals with comorbid migraine, propranolol has enhanced efficacy in reducing TMD pain.[365] In addition, certain COMT genotypes seem to affect the efficacy of propranolol in TMD patients.[366] We are, however, far from being able to use genotyping to apply the principles of personalized medicine to pharmacotherapy for TMD.

Several other supplements used in pain management have also been suggested for the treatment of primary headaches and osteoarthritis. However, there is a lack of evidence to support their use as primary therapies; therefore, they are mainly suggested as adjuvants. It has been suggested that magnesium provides an analgesic effect in postoperative pain and chronic neuropathic pain as well as increased opioid analgesia, but most of the available data were based on animal studies.[367,368] However, clinical studies have indicated that magnesium supplementation reduces opioid consumption. Vitamins C, D, and E have also been evaluated in the management of pain. Vitamin C exhibits analgesic properties, which may reduce pain and increase quality of life, and has been studied mainly in orthopedic populations.[369] Existing literature does not support vitamin D supplementation as an efficacious independent treatment for pain management.[370] However, there is some suggestion that deficiency in vitamin D is associated with increased risk of TMD.[371,372] It has been suggested that vitamin E plays a role in decreasing the reactive remodeling in osteoarthritis.[373] Nevertheless, no data are specifically available for the management of TMDs with these supplements.

Physical therapy

Physical therapy helps to relieve musculoskeletal pain and to restore normal function by altering sensory input; increasing range of motion; reducing inflammation; decreasing, coordinating, and strengthening muscle activity; and promoting the repair and regeneration of tissues. In most cases, physical therapy is used as an adjunct to other treatments. Systematic reviews have demonstrated that manual physical therapy techniques have support in decreasing pain and increasing range of motion of the jaw.[374] *Manual therapy*, defined as "any hands-on therapy," seems to improve pain, mandibular motion, and pressure pain threshold.[375] This is further evidenced by meta-analysis methodology, which demonstrated that physiotherapy leads to pain reduction and may improve range of motion.[376] While physical therapy has been shown to be better than no treatment, it has not shown superiority to other treatments.[374]

Posture training

The goal of posture training involves the prevention of untoward muscle activity of the head, neck, and shoulder musculature, as well as the masticatory and tongue muscles. The aim should be to maintain orthostatic posture to prevent increased cervical and shoulder muscle activity and possible protrusion of the mandible. The more anterior the head is relative to the spinal column, the greater is its effective weight. Except during function (ie, chewing, swallowing, and speaking), the mandible should be in a relaxed rest position with the teeth separated.[377,378] RCTs of posture training are supportive of using this technique in patients with TMDs.[379] Although posture training is a common physical therapeutic approach, its relationship to TMDs is not well understood and needs further study.[380] A common reversible treatment approach aiming to modify awake parafunctional activity is to monitor and control tongue position, mimicking rest position and reducing muscle activity in principle; nevertheless, available information is controversial because the position of the tongue on the floor of the mouth minimizes muscle activity or has no effect.[377,381,382]

Exercise

Clinical experience suggests that an active exercise program is important for the development and maintenance of normal muscle and joint comfort, function, and stability. One of the objectives of an exercise program is to teach the patient how to avoid activities that are injurious to the involved synovial joints. In addition, exercise has been recommended to stretch and relax the cervical and masticatory muscles, mobilize and stabilize the TMJs, increase muscle strength, and develop normal coordination arthrokinematics (reduce joint clicking).[379] Three types of exercise are generally recommended: *(1)* repetitive exercises to establish coordinated, rhythmic muscle function; *(2)* isotonic exercises to increase range of motion; and *(3)* isometric exercises to increase muscular strength. These exercises are prescribed to achieve specific goals and are modified as the patient progresses. Most patients will not exercise if it increases pain. Therefore, the therapist must initially help the patient achieve some symptom relief with physical agents or modalities. A maintenance level of exercise is recommended to ensure long-term resolution once the patient has reached the goals of treatment. A systematic review and meta-analysis showed that most of the effect sizes for this type of intervention were low to moderate with no clear discrimination of exercises in comparison to other conservative treatments.[383] However, a recent RCT demonstrated that jaw exercises were as effective as an occlusal splint and resulted in lower cost of treatment.[384]

Mobilization

Mobilization techniques are indicated for improving decreased range of motion and pain due to muscle contracture, disc displacement without reduction, and fibrous adhesions in the joint. Muscle relaxation and pain reduction are often required to enhance the effect of mobilization. Thus, a combination of heat, cold, ultrasound, and electric stimulation is often employed before or in conjunction with mobilization. Acute disc displacement without reduction can at times be effectively reduced by manipulation of the mandible.[385] Significantly increased range of motion can be achieved with mobilization compared to splint therapy in individuals with anterior displaced disc without reduction.[386] The mobilization may be accomplished through gripping the mandible firmly with the thumbs on the occlusal surfaces of the posterior teeth. The unaffected side is securely braced, and firm but controlled force is applied to the mandible in a downward, forward, and inward direction.[387,388] Another technique incorporates the patient's voluntary maximal lateral excursive jaw movement to the unaffected side followed by opening through the lateral border path.[388,389] Following mobilization, therapy to maintain joint mobility should be considered, such as orthopedic appliance therapy, relaxation therapy, and exercises.

Physical agents or modalities

Physical agents or modalities used for TMD management include electrotherapy, ultrasound, iontophoresis, anesthetic agents, dry needling, acupuncture, and photobiomodulation (low-level laser therapy).

ELECTROTHERAPY. Electrotherapy devices can produce thermal, histochemical, and physiologic changes in the muscles and joints. These devices include electrogalvanic stimulation (EGS), transcutaneous electrical nerve stimulation (TENS), and microcurrent electric nerve stimulation (MENS). EGS uses a high-voltage, low-amperage, monophasic current of varied frequency. This modality has been applied clinically in an effort to aid in muscle relaxation, reduce inflammation, and increase blood flow to tissues.[379] TENS uses a low-voltage, low-amperage, biphasic current of varied frequency and is designed primarily for sensory counterstimulation in painful disorders.[390] Like EGS, this modality decreases muscle pain and hyperactivity and can aid in muscle reeducation. If significant motor stimulation occurs concurrently, this may impair the analgesic effect and exacerbate acute muscle pain.[391] Although TENS has more traditionally been used outside of the temporomandibular area, application techniques for temporomandibular and cervical pain have been described.

ULTRASOUND. Ultrasound is a frequently used physical treatment modality for musculoskeletal problems. The high-frequency oscillations of the transducer head are converted to heat when transmitted through the tissue. This can heat the tissues to a depth of 5 cm.[392] It has been proposed that ultrasound may be used to produce deep heat in the joints; treat joint contracture by increasing the stretch of the extracapsular soft tissue; decrease chronic pain, muscle contraction, and tendonitis; and facilitate resorption of the calcium deposits of bursitis.[392–394] Ultrasound is also commonly used to carry medication into the tissue through phonophoresis, although the mechanism and efficacy of drug delivery are unknown.[395] A systematic review on the efficacy of ultrasound on the musculoskeletal system revealed that only 2 of 18 placebo-controlled trials showed a statistically and clinically significant benefit of ultrasound. The four trials related to TMDs did not reach the quality standard used in the review. In addition, they did not show any significant benefit of ultrasound.[396] While more recent evidence demonstrated an increase in PPT in the masseter muscle of individuals with myalgia compared to sham ultrasound,[397] there continues to be concerns regarding efficacy and cost-benefit.[398]

IONTOPHORESIS. Iontophoresis is a technique to enhance the transport of drug ions across a tissue barrier. A weak current is used to enhance the transport of drug ions—usually corticosteroids—through the skin into the deeper tissues, where the drug is purported to exert its effect.[399] However, RCTs have not supported the efficacy of this modality to provide pain relief.[400,401]

ANESTHETIC AGENTS. Anesthetic agents have been proposed to be beneficial to TMD therapy. Application of vapocoolant sprays followed by muscle stretching decreases muscle soreness and tightness and is thought to inactivate myofascial TPs.[77,402] To date, there are no RCTs showing efficacy of such therapy, although it has recently been reported to aid in maximum mouth opening.[403]

Local anesthetic injection of myofascial TPs, alone or in conjunction with muscle stretching or mobilization, has been shown to be useful for the management of myofascial pain. Although the anesthetic is useful in pain reduction, it is not the most critical factor in eliminating pain.[404-406] Rather, it appears that the mechanical disruption of the TP by the needle provides the therapeutic effect. TP injections should be used adjunctively with other modalities such as pharmacotherapy, physical therapy, and—in many cases— behavioral medicine techniques.[407] TP injections are usually performed in a series of three to five treatments to an individual muscle group, initially at weekly intervals. Long-acting local anesthetics such as bupivacaine should not be used for muscle injections because of increased myotoxicity, and there is no need to incorporate a vasoconstrictor because the integrated TP physiologic model suggests a localized hypoxic energy associated with sensory and autonomic reflexes.[408,409] In an RCT, the effect of TP injections infiltrating with either saline or anesthetic showed no differences in pain intensity, headache frequency, or intensity between the two intervention groups. It is important to note that the interventions were enhanced with muscle stretching, anti-inflammatory medications, and thermal therapy.[410] More recently, TP injections using saline or lidocaine demonstrated equivalent results, while TP injection using botulinum toxin demonstrated decreased pain.[411]

ACUPUNCTURE. Acupuncture has also been used for the treatment of chronic musculoskeletal pain, but the precise mechanism of action is unknown. Early studies of its application for TMDs suggest that the benefits of acupuncture are comparable with conventional TMD treatments,[297] and continue to be supported.[412] However, one systematic review and meta-analysis of acupuncture demonstrated only limited evidence that acupuncture treatment in TMDs is more effective than sham acupuncture, while others support that conventional acupuncture is effective.[413,414] These contrasting findings suggest there is a need for rigorous clinical trials evaluating acupuncture as an adjunctive therapy before definitive recommendations regarding its application can be made.

PHOTOBIOMODULATION. Photobiomodulation, otherwise known as *low-level laser therapy*, has been used for the treatment of TMDs and is suggested to have bio-stimulating and analgesic effects through direct irradiation without causing a thermal response.[415] Consistent findings support the claim that low-level laser therapy was no better than placebo in reducing chronic TMD pain.[416] Because of the poor methodologic design of the studies and the use of different types, frequencies, and duration of laser radiation in various groups of patients, treatment parameters have not been standardized, and effectiveness cannot be evaluated. Two RCTs published just subsequently to the systematic review time period demonstrated positive effects of the laser therapy compared with controls and positive but equal effects to splint therapy.[417,418] Because of the small sample size of these studies, further research is needed to support the use of low-level laser therapy in TMD treatment. Additional systematic reviews have since shown more promise,[419] however, the protocols have yet to be standardized. One feature yet to be discussed is cost of treatment, as sessions generally occur multiple times throughout the week and continue for a month.

Orthopedic appliance therapy

Orthopedic appliances, such as interocclusal splints, orthotics, orthoses, bite guards, bite planes, night guards, and bruxism appliances, are routinely used in the treatment of TMDs. Based on current theory, removable acrylic resin appliances that cover the teeth have traditionally been used to alter occlusal relationships and to redistribute occlusal forces, to prevent wear and mobility of the teeth, to reduce bruxism and parafunction, to treat masticatory muscle pain and dysfunction, to treat painful TMJs, and to alter structural relationships in the TMJ.[420] Because of heterogenicity in studies regarding TMD diagnosis, splint type, and outcome measures reported, a recent systematic review was unable to support the provision of splints,[421] while other systematic reviews recommend their use in TMD.[422,423]

Historically, studies focusing on appliance therapy have reported a reduction in orofacial pain and other symptoms associated with TMDs.[424] However, most studies have been limited by small sample size, short-term outcome, inadequate control groups, and failure to compare appliance therapy with other forms of treatment. Furthermore, several review papers have concluded that when these appliances were compared with an inactive placebo, they were mildly favorable, performing no better than non-occluding appliances or other types of TMD therapies such as behavioral modification or self-regulation strategies.[425–428] Systematic reviews and meta-analyses have concluded that there is a moderate effect for reduction of pain with the use of splint therapy in TMDs[422,429] and that there is no support for their use from satisfactory scientific evidence.[430] While appliance therapy may not offer a change in pain intensity, a recent systematic review concluded that the efficacy is greater than placebo effect.[431] The three types of orthopedic appliances that are described here include full-coverage stabilizing appliances, partial-coverage appliances, and anterior positioning appliances.

The complications that can occur with the excessive or incorrect use of any appliance include caries, gingival inflammation, mouth odors, speech difficulties, occlusal changes, and psychologic dependence on the appliance. Serious complications can include major, irreversible changes in functional and morphologic occlusal features as a result of long-term, full-time use of these appliances.[432,433] Given that adverse effects are generally not reported,[421] this is an area where more attention needs to be directed. This is a significant concern with partial-arch coverage appliances.

Stabilization appliances

Stabilization appliances cover all the maxillary or mandibular teeth. Stabilization appliances are used as an adjunct for managing symptoms associated with myogenous as well as arthrogenous TMDs.[434–436] Preferably, they are used during sleep only, whereas behavioral modification strategies may be used to increase the patient's awareness and reduce the impact of parafunctional habits on TMDs while awake. Because acrylic is softer than enamel, these appliances have been used to reduce the chance of further tooth attrition in patients with sleep bruxism. Occasionally, they are used to reduce clenching-induced earache and headache,[437–439] although in a RCT the occlusal splint plus usual care did not improve headache outcomes over usual care.[440]

EMG monitoring of the masseter muscle has been used in an attempt to demonstrate a short-term decrease in the level of sleep bruxism activity when an appliance is worn.[441,442] However, studies demonstrated that the response is variable and that sleep bruxism is not eliminated with stabilization appliances.[95,420,443] These studies emphasize the variability of the clinical response to these appliances and the need for careful follow-up. The occlusal surface of the appliance should be adjusted to provide a stable physiologic mandibular posture by creating bilateral, even posterior occlusal contacts for the opposing teeth on closure.[95] Appliances adjusted to a "neuromuscularly determined" jaw position seem to show no advantage over conventional stabilization appliances.[444] Anterior guidance may be provided by acrylic guide ramps in the canine or anterior areas of the appliance to separate the opposing posterior teeth from the appliance in all excursive movements of the mandible. Clinical experience suggests that the occlusal surface of the appliance should be adjusted initially and periodically to compensate for changes in the maxillomandibular relationship as pain, muscle activity, inflammation, edema, or soft tissue structural relations change.

In acute cases, the appliance may be worn full-time for a specified period of time. As symptom reduction occurs, use of the appliance only during sleep is preferred. This is especially true with ongoing sleep bruxism and related morning pain. Patients not showing a positive response within 3 to 4 weeks should be reevaluated. Failure to show an initial positive response does not necessarily indicate a need for more aggressive or prolonged therapy; other factors should be considered, such as chronic pain behavior, noncompliance, misdiagnosis, or degree of TMJ pathology.

Use of a stabilization appliance with adjunctive therapy for pain relief and improved function is also a viable treatment option for TMJ internal derangement.[445–447] Asymptomatic clicks by themselves do not warrant treatment, and studies using TMJ imaging cast doubt on the need for a "correct" or "perfect" disc position.[448]

In the treatment of internal derangement, if improvement is not realized with orthopedic appliance therapy and adjunctive measures, and if significant pain and mechanical symptoms persist, minimally invasive procedures such as arthrocentesis and/or arthroscopy, or more advanced treatments such as open joint surgery may be necessary.

Stabilization appliances fabricated with a soft resilient material appear to have similar results to appliances fabricated from hard acrylic material.[449] Studies comparing soft appliances with hard acrylic appliances have found both to be equally effective in reducing painful symptoms, but they were no more effective than self-management treatment without appliance therapy.[450] Techniques for adjusting soft resilient appliances are available.[388,451] As the material may not last as long as a hard acrylic splint, especially in heavy bruxers, these may be considered "temporary."[452] However, "temporary" use may be all that is needed, especially for acute problems. As soft appliances generally are more affordable for patients,[452] they certainly can be considered as a "first line" approach to treatment. Soft appliances are also best suited for treatment of children with a mixed dentition or incomplete growth as they seem to have minimal effect on dental development.[453]

Partial-coverage appliances

One type of partial-coverage appliance only covers the maxillary central incisors and contacts with only one or two opposing mandibular teeth.[454] The claimed mechanism of action was that occlusal forces applied to a few anterior teeth would be lower than forces applied to a full occlusion, resulting in a decrease in muscle activity and/or diminished loading of the TMJ. While there was a reduction in muscle activity short term (over four nights measured) versus a Michigan splint,[455] there is no evidence for diminished loading of the TMJ. Whereas in a 3-month follow-up study, no differences in improvement were observed between TMD patients wearing this appliance and patients wearing a stabilization appliance, a 6-month follow-up study reported that more patients in the stabilization appliance group improved.[456,457] These results were part of a pilot study, however, so the results were descriptive in nature and self-assessed based on improvement or impairment compared to initial complaints. More recently, it was reported that the use of this type of device as initial therapy did not provide any additional benefit in reducing pain or improving jaw function.[458] A systematic review of this type of appliance indicated that they can be used successfully, but they should only be used in cases where patients will be compliant with their follow-up appointments.[459] Due to its compact size, a less than well-retained appliance worn at night has the potential risk for aspiration. This, combined with the reports of occlusal changes from long-term use,[460] dictate that caution should be used when prescribing this device.

Another partial-coverage oral appliance is one that covers only the posterior teeth. The posterior bite plane is usually fabricated for the mandibular teeth and consists of areas of hard acrylic located over the posterior teeth and connected by a cast metal lingual bar. It has been advocated in cases of loss of vertical dimension or when there is a need to make major changes in anterior positioning of the mandible.[461] The efficacy of this type of appliance has been studied in only one small controlled trial.[462]

Studies supporting the efficacy of partial-coverage appliances in reducing TMD symptoms are limited by number and sample size. In addition, they have the potential to produce a malocclusion and possible internal TMJ changes.[457] There is no evidence that partial-coverage appliances reduce TMD symptoms more effectively than full-arch appliances, and risk–benefit analysis seems to indicate they should be used, if at all, only for the short term and with caution.[463]

Anterior positioning appliances

Anterior positioning appliances, also called *anterior repositioning appliances*, are usually fabricated for the maxillary arch to guide the mandible into a protrusive position. All teeth in the arch are covered, and the opposing teeth are provided with minimal posterior occlusal indentations and a reverse guidance incline in the anterior segment of the appliance.[464] Historically, this design is aimed at providing guidance to a more comfortable therapeutic condyle-disc-fossa relationship. Anterior positioning appliances are used to decrease joint pain, joint noise (clicking), and associated secondary muscle symptoms in TMDs.[465,466] The primary indication for anterior positioning appliance therapy is acute joint pain associated with disc displacement with reduction.[424,467,468] Originally, full-time use of the appliance was suggested with the intent to establish a new jaw position with the disc "recaptured."[469] Although short-term success with full-time wear of anterior positioning appliances was good, long-term success at establishing a new occlusal position with the disc recaptured has not been realized.[27,466,470–472] Therefore, attempts to achieve a new therapeutic mandibular position aimed at restoring the disc-condyle relationship with anterior positioning appliances should be restricted to a few select cases of articular pain that can only be managed by maintained jaw positioning. Given that this may involve substantial time and expense, risk–benefit analysis should be considered prior to initiating treatment, with alternative treatment options discussed with the patient so that adequate informed consent can be obtained. Whether the appliance will be used full-time or part-time, the potential occlusal consequences need to be discussed with the patient prior to treatment because mandibular repositioning can result in irreversible changes in the occlusion (ie, a posterior open bite).[473]

An anterior positioning appliance may be effective in reducing symptoms associated with disc displacement with reduction. Use of the appliance during sleep is also often effective for preventing intermittent disc displacement without reduction on awakening and reducing joint pain. By using the appliance only during sleep, the potential for occlusal changes is greatly reduced. Full-time, short-term wear of the anterior repositioning appliance should be limited to cases of acute disc displacement without reduction (ie, acute closed lock), only if the clinician is able to reduce the disc (ie, unlock the jaw). In such cases, restoring the disc-condyle relationship full time for 5 to 7 days may reduce or prevent additional locking episodes and encourage adaptation. Once joint pain and dysfunction are decreased, appliance use may be gradually reduced to sleep-time wear only, and if needed, eventually converted to (if the design allows it)—or replaced with—a stabilization appliance.

The goal of this treatment is to allow the mandible to approximate the pretreatment occlusal position, as ample evidence has determined that permanent mandibular repositioning as a treatment goal for TMDs does not fall within the standard of medically necessary treatment.[474] This approach is strongly recommended to avoid or minimize the need for unnecessary restorative or orthodontic treatment. The treatment is not intended to correct the disc-condyle relationship but to facilitate control of symptoms similar to other treatments.[475] Clicking is not usually eliminated but may be decreased in intensity. In some instances, returning the patient to the preexisting occlusal condition reinitiates the painful joint symptoms. This is likely due to the lack of adaptation of the retrodiscal tissues. In most instances, immediately returning the patient to the anterior positioning appliance therapy will once again reduce the symptoms. When this occurs, more time should be allowed for tissue adaptation. The need for permanent occlusal therapy is very rare and should not be considered a goal of therapy, but rather necessary due to the potential risks associated with long-term use of repositioning appliances.

Occlusal treatments and TMD therapy

There are valid reasons for occlusal treatment for many dental conditions: lack of inter/intra–arch tooth stability; tooth mobility; fremitus; occlusal-related fracture of a tooth or restoration; tooth sensitivity; altered or compromised masticatory function, swallowing, or speech; and compromised supporting tissues due to adverse loading. Although occlusal-related dental treatment may be necessary for patients with TMDs, it is not necessary for the purpose of treating TMDs.[476] Patients with TMD may still need dental treatment that alters their occlusion (eg, restoring edentulous areas, restoring fractured or carious teeth, or orthodontics) because they desire straighter teeth. However, these treatments are done for dental reasons, not because of TMD problems. It is important to emphasize the lack of evidence for disease-specific associations between TMD and dental occlusion.[124] In addition, it has been well documented that occlusal adjustments and orthodontic therapy are not supported as part of evidence-based treatment for TMD because they do not prevent or treat TMD.[476,477]

The use of anterior positioning appliances in the treatment of TMJ disc displacement to establish a mandibular position with a corrected disc-condyle relationship has led to the concept of two-phase treatment. This treatment approach was especially popular in the late 1970s and the 1980s, well before the emphasis on evidence-based dentistry. Phase 1 involved the use of a splint that altered the occlusion. Phase 2 involved rearticulation of the teeth in the newly acquired jaw position through definitive, irreversible occlusal treatment: occlusal adjustment, restorative or prosthodontic dental treatment, or orthodontic or orthognathic treatment. The scientific literature does not support the need for this two-phase treatment model because definitive occlusal therapy is not required for the effective treatment of TMDs.[121,478] TMDs, especially those involving TMJ pathology, may affect the dental occlusion. In other words, the malocclusion may be a consequence of the TMDs (or their treatment) rather than a cause.[479] The clinician is advised to proceed cautiously, using the least invasive procedures possible, when treating occlusal changes in the TMD patient.[480] The pretreatment intercuspal relationship should be preserved whenever possible.

Orthognathic surgery may be considered in conjunction with orthodontic or restorative or prosthodontic treatment for correction of skeletal malocclusions. However, when orthognathic surgery is considered in TMD patients, it should always follow careful evaluation confirming reasonable symptom resolution and stability of the maxillomandibular relationship. Surgical treatment for skeletal asymmetries and growth anomalies with the specific intent of alleviating pain associated with TMDs is rarely indicated and should only follow careful evaluation and management of any other contributing factors. However, in those TMD patients with severe skeletal malocclusion who desire greater occlusal stability or improved esthetics, orthognathic treatment is often the method of choice.[481–483] A systematic review and meta-analysis from 2017 could not predict which patients might improve or worsen in TMD symptoms after orthognathic surgery.[484] The more recent prospective studies in this review indicated that orthognathic surgery in patients with TMDs may improve the condition; however, there are also reports of exacerbation of TMD signs and symptoms. For TMD patients who desire correction of skeletal malocclusions, orthognathic surgery is an option, but informed consent should emphasize the correction of the malocclusion, not the potential improvement in TMD signs and symptoms.

Surgical therapies

TMJ surgery is an effective treatment for specific articular disorders. However, the complexity of available techniques, potential complications, prevalence of behavioral and psychosocial contributing factors, and the availability of nonsurgical approaches suggest that TMJ surgery should only be used in select cases.

The decision to treat the patient surgically depends on the degree of pathology or anatomical derangement present within the joint, the potential for repair of the condition, the outcome of appropriate nonsurgical treatment, and the degree of impairment the problem creates for the patient. The appropriate duration and complexity of nonsurgical treatment prior to considering surgery are determined by a combination of factors. Factors to be considered include expected prognosis compared with actual improvement realized, the degree of impairment, and the patient's compliance with the program. Patients with complicating factors such as pending litigation, psychologic issues, uncontrolled sleep bruxism, or prior joint surgeries may have a poor surgical prognosis. The clinician must have a full knowledge and appreciation of the potential for surgical failure and potential complications, including neuropathic pain disorders (ie, deafferentation pain). Once this information is available, a realistic discussion of the prognosis, the patient's expectations, and the complicating factors can provide the patient with the information necessary to make an informed decision.

Preoperative and postoperative nonsurgical management must be integrated into the overall surgical treatment plan. This therapy is directed at decreasing the functional load placed on the joint, eliminating or modifying contributing factors such as oral parafunctional habits, and providing appropriate psychologic and medical support. The clinical practice guidelines for TMJ surgery of the American Association of Oral and Maxillofacial Surgeons state that TMJ surgery is only indicated when nonsurgical therapy has been ineffective and is not indicated for asymptomatic or minimally symptomatic cases.[485] In addition, surgery should not be performed for preventive reasons. Indications for surgery include moderate to severe pain or dysfunction that is disabling.[105] Imaging evidence of internal derangement may be indicated. Surgical management may include joint lavage (arthrocentesis), closed surgical procedures (arthroscopy), and open surgical procedures (arthrotomy or arthroplasty), as well as total joint replacement.

Arthrocentesis and arthroscopy

Arthrocentesis involves simple intra-articular irrigation or lavage of the TMJ with or without corticosteroids, hyaluronic acid, or other irrigants. It has been suggested this method may be as effective as arthroscopy when used with joint mobilization in the treatment of intra-articular joint restrictions of mandibular movement such as internal derangement without reduction.[486] However, it also can be used as a palliative procedure for patients with acute episodes of degenerative or rheumatoid arthritis and to relieve pain in patients who have painful clicking in the TMJ that does not respond to medical management.[487,488] Two reviews evaluating outcomes of arthrocentesis performed on patients with different types of internal derangement indicated successful treatment outcomes in about 80% of the cases but noted that most studies could be criticized because of methodologic flaws.[489,490] Other authors, however, report even higher success rates,[486] even long term,[491] and given its lower cost and reduced complications to other surgical therapies, arthrocentesis can be considered an initial surgical therapy if pain or limited function are believed to be a result of an intracapsular disorder.

Arthroscopy allows direct observation and sampling of the joint tissues and shows similar results to arthrocentesis with the advantage of direct visualization.[486] A recent network meta-analysis proposed a hierarchy of recommended treatments that placed arthroscopy, especially combined with intra-articular injections, as recommended for increasing maximum mandibular opening and reducing pain for individuals with arthrogenous TMD.[492] Arthroscopic revision of previous open surgery has been suggested to be helpful in alleviating postoperative pain and intracapsular fibrosis.[493] At this time, arthroscopy is primarily performed in the upper joint space and is used for minor debridement and lavage, removal of minor adhesions, and biopsies. Reduction of symptoms following arthroscopic surgery is not caused by improved disc position; post-arthroscopy MRI scans reveal that a vast majority of patients have persistent anterior disc displacement but increased disc mobility.[494] While the disc can be repositioned arthroscopically with various techniques,[495] there is no reason to expect that this will be any more stable than open joint disc repositioning, and current evidence indicates that there may be no need to reposition the disc.[486] The prognosis of arthroscopy appears comparable to that of discectomy and discoplasty.[496,497] Because arthroscopy is less invasive than open joint surgeries, it should be preferred over them whenever possible. A systematic review published in 2015 reported better pain control and increased maximum opening with arthroscopy over arthrocentesis, but the differences may not be clinically relevant.[498]

Lavage with saline, hyaluronic acid, PRP, or platelet-rich growth factor has been used for both arthrocentesis and arthroscopy. At this time, there has been no clear preference for one over the other.[499]

Arthrotomy and total joint replacement

Open surgical intervention of the TMJ (arthrotomy) is usually required for bony or fibrous ankylosis, neoplasia, severe chronic dislocations, persistent painful disc derangement, and severe osteoarthritis refractory to conservative modalities of treatment.[500] Surgery is less often indicated in displaced condylar fractures, agenesis of the condyle, and severe painful chronic arthritides. Surgery is seldom, if ever, indicated in inflammatory joint disorders, condylysis, and nonpainful degenerative arthritis. Arthrotomy is generally indicated for patients with advanced TMJ disease who meet the surgical criteria and have disease refractory to or not amenable to arthrocentesis or arthroscopic surgical techniques.

Open joint surgical procedures may include discoplasty; disc repositioning or discectomy, with or without replacement; and arthroplasty, which includes high condylectomy and total joint reconstruction or replacements. Discoplasty and disc repositioning with plication have been reported to have an 80% to 90% success rate in reducing joint pain and noise and increasing mouth opening (although mouth opening remains short of normal ranges).[501–504] The discectomy procedure without replacement has the longest history and shows good long-term success (up to 30 years).[505–508] Use of a dermis graft in discectomy does not appear to prevent remodeling, but it may be beneficial in eliminating or preventing joint noises.[509]

The success obtained with less invasive procedures has greatly reduced the need for arthroplasty. Condylectomy (subcondylar osteotomy) and condylotomy are performed infrequently. These procedures have been indicated for more complex diseases or traumatic conditions.[510,511] There can be more postsurgical complications with these procedures, including marked occlusal changes. Modified condylotomy (using an intraoral vertical ramus osteotomy) in the treatment of TMJ internal derangement can reduce related pain and predictably correct disc position.[512–514] Further controlled investigations are needed regarding these applications.

Total joint replacement may be an indicated option due to neoplasm, trauma, ankylosis, or severe deformity developmentally or be caused by disease. Various products are available on the market and, when analyzed, demonstrate postoperative improvement in mouth opening, pain level, and in most cases improvement in diet as defined by lack of dietary restrictions.[515,516] While there continue to be additional replacement systems brought to the market around the world, there is concern about regulatory status and lack of outcome data.[517] As with other joint replacements, patients need to be well educated so they have appropriate expectations. There is a growing body of evidence from other orthopedic areas that psychologic characteristics impact the success of total joint replacement and should be evaluated and addressed prior to surgery.[518]

Conclusion

Despite increasing evidence that TMDs are best managed with conservative reversible treatments, some clinicians continue to choose treatments based on personal biases and belief preferences rather than controlled scientific investigation. There continues to be a need for RCTs regarding nonsurgical and surgical TMD treatment. In addition, studies designed to elucidate the etiology of TMDs are much needed. Practicing clinicians involved in the treatment of TMDs on a daily basis should be knowledgeable in clinical trial methodology and be able to critically appraise the literature upon which they base their treatments. Discriminating readers and clinicians will result, and our patients will benefit.

References

1. Okeson J. Management of Temporomandibular Disorders and Occlusion, ed 7. St Louis: Mosby, 2013.
2. Fried L. Anatomy of the Head, Neck, Face and Jaws, ed 2. Philadelphia: Lea & Febiger, 1980.
3. Scapino RP. The posterior attachment. Its structure, function, and appearance in TMJ imaging studies. Part I. J Craniomandib Disord 1991;5:83–95.
4. Scapino RP. The posterior attachment: Its structure, function, and appearance in TMJ imaging studies. Part 2. J Craniomandib Disord 1991;5:155–166.
5. Du Brul E. The craniomandibular articulation. In: Sicher H, Du Brul E. Sicher's Oral Anatomy, ed 7. St Louis: Mosby, 1980:147–209.
6. Meikle MC. Remodeling. In: Sarnat BG, Laskin DM (eds). The Temporomandibular Joint: A Biological Basis for Clinical Practice, ed 4. Philadelphia: Saunders, 1992:93–107.
7. Waltimo A, Kemppainen P, Könönen M. Maximal contraction force and endurance of human jaw-closing muscles in isometric clenching. Scand J Dent Res 1993;101:416–421.
8. McNamara JA, Jr. The independent functions of the two heads of the lateral pterygoid muscles. Am J Anat 1973;138:197–205.
9. Meyenberg K, Kubik S, Palla S. Relationships of the muscles of mastication to the articular disc of the temporomandibular joint. Helv Odont Acta 1986;30:1–20.
10. Wilkinson TM. The relationship between the disc and the lateral pterygoid muscle in the human temporomandibular joint. J Prosthet Dent 1988;60:715–724.
11. Heylings DJ, Nielsen IL, McNeill C. Lateral pterygoid muscle and the temporomandibular disc. J Orofac Pain 1995;9:9–16.
12. Lobbezoo F, Ahlberg J, Raphael KG, et al. International consensus on the assessment of bruxism: Report of a work in progress. J Oral Rehabil 2018;45:837–844.
13. Greene CS. Managing the Care of Patients with Temporomandibular Disorders: A New Guideline for Care. J Am Dent Assoc 2010;141:1086–1088.
14. Temporomandibular Disorders: Priorities for Research and Care. Washington DC: National Academies of Sciences, Engineering, and Medicine, 2020.
15. Schiffman E, Ohrbach R, Truelove E, et al. Diagnostic Criteria for temporomandibular disorders (DC/TMD) for clinical and research applications: Recommendations of the International RDC/TMD Consortium Network* and Orofacial Pain Special Interest Group†. J Oral Facial Pain Headache 2014;28:6–27.
16. Dworkin SF, LeResche L. Research diagnostic criteria for temporomandibular disorders: Review, criteria, examination and specifications, critique. J Craniomandib Disord 1992;6:301–355.
17. Manfredini D, Guarda-Nardini L, Winocur E, Piccotti F, Ahlberg J, Lobbezoo F. Research diagnostic criteria for temporomandibular disorders: A systematic review of axis I epidemiologic findings. Oral Surg Oral Med Oral Pathol Oral Radiol Endod 2011;112:453–462.
18. Maixner W, Fillingim RB, Williams DA, Smith SB, Slade GD. Overlapping chronic pain conditions: Implications for diagnosis and classification. J Pain 2016;17(9 suppl):T93–T107.

19. Slade G, Durham J. Prevalence, impact and cost of treatment for temporomandibular disorders. Paper commissioned by the Committee on Temporomandibular Disorders (TMDs): From Reserach Discoveries to Clinical Treatment (Appendix C). In: National Academies of Sciences, Engineering, and Medicine. Temporomandibular Disorders: Priorities for Research and Care. Washington, DC: The National Academies Press, 2020.
20. Janal MN, Raphael KG, Nayak S, Klausner J. Prevalence of myofascial temporomandibular disorder in US community women. J Oral Rehabil 2008;35:801–809.
21. LeResche L. Epidemiology of temporomandibular disorders: Implications for the investigation of etiologic factors. Crit Rev Oral Biol Med. 1997;8:291–305.
22. Anastassaki Köhler A, Hugoson A, Magnusson T. Prevalence of symptoms indicative of temporomandibular disorders in adults: Cross-sectional epidemiological investigatons covering two decades. Acta Odontol Scand 2012;70:213–223.
23. Slade GD, Ohrbach R, Greenspan JD, et al. Painful temporomandibular disorder: Decade of discovery from OPPERA studies. J Dent Res 2016;95:1084–1092.
24. Randolph CS, Greene CS, Moretti R, et al. Conservative management of temporomandibular disorders: A posttreatment comparison between patients from a university clinic and from private practice. Am J Orthod Dentofac Orthop 1990;98:77–82.
25. Nickerson JW, Boering G. Natural course of osteoarthrosis as it relates to internal derangement of the temporomandibular joint. Oral Maxillofac Surg Clin North Am 1989;1:1–19.
26. Magnusson T, Carlsson GE, Egermark I. Changes in clinical signs of craniomandibular disorders from the age of 15-25 years. J Orofac Pain 1994;8:207–215.
27. Lundh H, Westesson PL, Kopp S. A three-year follow-up of patients with reciprocal temporomandibular joint clicking. Oral Surg Oral Med Oral Pathol 1987;63:530–533.
28. de Leeuw R, Boering G, Stegenga B, de Bont LG. Temporomandibular joint osteoarthrosis: Clinical and radiographic characteristics 30 years after nonsurgical treatment. A preliminary report. Cranio 1993;11: 15–24.
29. Schiffman EL, Ahmad M, Hollender L, et al. Longitudinal stability of common TMJ structural disorders. J Dent Res 2017;96:270–276.
30. Rugh JD, Solberg WK. Oral health status in the United States: Temporomandibular disorders. J Dent Educ 1985;49:398–406.
31. Dworkin SF, Le Resche L. Temporomandibular disorder pain: Epidemiologic data. APS Bulletin 1993;(April/May):12.
32. Schiffman EL, Fricton JR, Haley DP, Shapiro BL. The prevalence and treatment needs of subjects with temporomandibular disorders. J Am Dent Assoc 1990;120:295–303.
33. Greene CS, Marbach JJ. Epidemiologic studies of mandibular dysfunction: A critical review. J Prosthet Dent 1982;48:184–190.
34. De Kanter RJ, Käyser AF, Battistuzzi PG, Truin GJ, Van 't Hof MA. Demand and need for treatment of craniomandibular dysfunction in the Dutch adult population. J Dent Res 1992;71:1607–1612.
35. Dworkin SF, Huggins KH, LeResche L, et al. Epidemiology of signs and symptoms in temporomandibular disorders: Clinical signs in cases and controls. J Am Dent Assoc 1990;120:273–281.
36. Larheim TA, Westesson P, Sano T. Temporomandibular joint disk displacement: Comparison in asymptomatic volunteers and patients. Radiology 2001;218: 428–432.
37. Huang GJ, LeResche L, Critchlow CW, Martin MD, Drangsholt MT. Risk factors for diagnostic subgroups of painful temporomandibular disorders (TMD). J Dent Res 2002;81:284–288.
38. Sanders AE, Maixner W, Nackley AG, et al. Excess risk of temporomandibular disorders associated with cigarette smoking in young adults. J Pain 2012;13:21–31.
39. de Leeuw R, Eisenlohr-Moul T, Bertrand P. The association of smoking status with sleep disturbance, psychological functioning, and pain severity in patients with temporomandibular disorders. J Orofac Pain 2013;27:32–41.
40. Afolalu EF, Ramlee F, Tang NKY. Effects of sleep changes on pain-related health outcomes in the general population: A systematic review of longitudinal studies with exploratory meta-analysis. Sleep Med Rev 2018;39:82–97.
41. Haack M, Simpson N, Sethna N, Kaur S, Mullington J. Sleep deficiency and chronic pain: Potential underlying mechanisms and clinical implications. Neuropsychopharmacology 2020;45:205–216.
42. Sanders AE, Greenspan JD, Fillingim RB, Rathnayaka N, Ohrback R, Slade GD. Associations of sleep disturbance, atopy, and other health measures with chronic overlapping pain conditions. J Oral Facial Pain Headache 2020;34:s73–s84.
43. Klasser GD, Bassiur J, de Leeuw R. Differences in reported medical conditions between myogenous and arthrogenous TMD patients and its relevance to the general practitioner. Quintessence Int 2014;45:157–167.
44. Bonato LL, Quinelato V, De Felipe Cordeiro PC, De Sousa EB, Tesch R, Casado PL. Association between temporomandibular disorders and pain in other regions of the body. J Oral Rehabil 2017;44:9–15.

45. Tchivileva IE, Ohrbach R, Fillingim RB, Greenspan JD, Maixner W, Slade GD. Temporal change in headache and its contribution to the risk of developing first-onset temporomandibular disorder in the orofacial pain: Prospective evaluation and risk assessment (OPPERA) study. Pain 2017;158:120–129.
46. Slade GD, Greenspan JD, Fillingim RB, Maixner W, Sharma S, Ohrbach R. Overlap of five chronic pain conditions: Temporomandibular disorders, headache, back pain, irritable bowel syndrome, and fibromyalgia. J Oral Facial Pain Headache 2020;34:s15–s28.
47. Chen H, Nackley A, Miller V, Diatchenko L, Maixner W. Multisystem dysregulation in painful temporomandibular disorders. J Pain 2013;14:983–996.
48. Bair E, Gaynor S, Slade GD, et al. Identification of clusters of individuals relevant to temporomandibular disorders and other chronic pain conditions: The OPPERA study. Pain 2016;157:1266–1278.
49. Al-Harthy M, Michelotti A, List T, Ohrbach R. Influence of culture on pain comorbidity in women with and without temporomandibular disorder-pain. J Oral Rehabil 2017;44:415–425.
50. Velly AM, Botros J, Bolla MM, et al. Painful and non-painful comorbidities associated with short- and long-term painful temporomandibular disorders: A cross-sectional study among adolescents from Brazil, Canada and France [epub ahead of print 27 Dec 2021]. J Oral Rehabil doi:10.1111/joor.13280.
51. Kleykamp BA, Ferguson MC, McNicol E, et al. The prevalence of comorbid chronic pain conditions among patients with temporomandibular disorders: A systematic review [epub ahead of print 21 Dec 2021] J Am Dent Assoc doi:10.1016/j.adaj.2021.08.008.
52. Stegenga B. Osteoarthritis of the temporomandibular joint organ and its relationship to disc displacement. J Orofac Pain 2001;15:193–205.
53. Nickel JC, Iwasaki LR, Gonzalez YM, Gallo LM, Yao H. Mechanobehavior and ontogenesis of the temporomandibular joint. J Dent Res 2018;11:1185–1192.
54. Al-Hashmi A, Al-Azri A, Al-Ismaily M, Goss AN. Temporomandibular disorders in patients with mandibular fractures: A preliminary comparative case-control study between South Australia and Oman. Int J Oral Maxillofac Surg 2011;40:1369–1372.
55. Leuin S, Frydendall E, Gao D, Chan KH. Temporomandibular joint dysfunction after mandibular fracture in children: A 10-year review. Arch Otolaryngol Head Neck Surg 2011;137:10–14.
56. Dwivedi AND, Tripathi R, Gupta PK, Tripathi S, Garg S. Magnetic resonance imaging evaluation of temporomandibular joint and associated soft tissue changes following acute condylar injury. J Oral Maxillofac Surg 2012;70:2829–2834.
57. Ohrbach R, Fillingim RB, Mulkey F, et al. Clinical findings and pain symptoms as potential risk factors for chronic TMD: Descriptive data and empirically identified domains from the OPPERA case-control study. J Pain 2011;129(11 suppl):T27–T45.
58. Salé H, Hedman L, Isberg A. Accuracy of patients' recall of temporomandibular joint pain and dysfunction after experiencing whiplash trauma: A prospective study. J Am Dent Assoc 2010;141:879–886.
59. Sahebi S, Moazami F, Afsa M, Zade MRN. Effect of lengthy root canal therapy sessions on temporomandibular joint and masticatory muscles. J Dent Res Dent Clin Dent Prospects 2010;4:95–97.
60. Huang GJ, Rue TC. Third-molar extraction as a risk factor for temporomandibular disorder. J Am Dent Assoc 2006;137:1547–1554.
61. Gould DB, Banes CH. Iatrogenic disruptions of right temporomandibular joints during orotracheal intubation causing permanent closed lock of the jaw. Anesth Analg 1995;81:191–194.
62. Domino KB, Posner KL, Caplan RA, Cheney FW. Airway injury during anesthesia: A closed claims analysis. Anesthesiology 1999;91:1703–1711.
63. Sharma S, Ohrbach R, Fillingim RB, Greenspan JD, Slade G. Pain sensitivity modifies risk of injury-related temporomandibular disorder. J Dent Res 2020;99:530–536.
64. Greenspan JD, Slade GD, Bair E, et al. Pain sensitivity risk factors for chronic TMD: Descriptive data and empirically identified domains from the OPPERA case control study. J Pain 2011;12(11 suppl):T61–T74.
65. Salé H, Isberg A. Delayed temporomandibular joint pain and dysfunction induced by whiplash trauma: A controlled prospective study. J Am Dent Assoc 2007;138:1084–1091 [erratum 2007;138:1426].
66. Kasch H, Hjorth T, Svensson P, Nyhuus L, Jensen TS. Temporomandibular disorders after whiplash injury: A controlled, prospective study. J Orofac Pain 2002; 16:118–128.
67. Fernandez CE, Amiri A, Jaime J, Delaney P. The relationship of whiplash injury and temporomandibular disorders: A narrative literature review. J Chiropr Med 2009;8:171–186.
68. Epstein JB, Klasser GD. Whiplash-associated disorders and temporomandibular symptoms following motor-vehicle collisions. Quintessence Int 2011;42:c1–c14.
69. Häggman-Henrikson B, Rezvani M, List T. Prevalence of whiplash trauma in TMD patients: A systematic review. J Oral Rehabil 2014;41:59–68.
70. Lee YH, Lee KM, Auh QS. MRI-based assessment of masticatory muscle changes in TMD patients after whiplash injury. J Clin Med 2021;10:1404.
71. Goldberg HL. Trauma and the improbable anterior displacement. J Craniomandib Disord 1990;4:131–134.

72. Burgess JA, Kolbinson DA, Lee PT, Epstein JB. Motor vehicle accidents and TMDs: Assessing the relationship. J Am Dent Assoc 1996;127:1767–1772.
73. Häggman-Henrikson B, Lampa E, Marklund S, Wänman A. Pain and disability in the jaw and neck region following whiplash trauma. J Dent Res 2016:95:1155–1160.
74. Pérez del Palomar A, Doblaré M. Dynamic 3D FE modelling of the human temporomandibular joint during whiplash. Med Eng Phys 2008;30:700–709.
75. Hernández IA, Fyfe KR, Heo G, Major PW. Mandibular kinematics associated with simulated low-velocity rear-end impacts. J Oral Rehabil 2006;33:566–575.
76. Wright EF. Referred craniofacial pain patterns in patients with temporomandibular disorders. J Am Dent Assoc 2000;131:1307–1315.
77. Simons DG, Travell JG, Simons LS. Apropos of all muscles. In: Johnson EP (ed). Travell & Simons' Myofascial Pain and Dysfunction: The Trigger Point Manual, ed 2. Baltimore: Lippincott Williams & Wilkins,1999:94–177.
78. Raphael KG, Sirois DA, Janal MN, et al. Sleep bruxism and myofascial temporomandibular disorders: A laboratory-based polysomnographic investigation. J Am Dent Assoc 2012;143:1223–1231.
79. Lobbezoo-Scholte AM, de Leeuw JR, Steenks MH, Bosman F, Buchner R, Olthoff LW. Diagnostic subgroups of craniomandibular disorders. Part I: Self-report data and clinical findings. J Orofac Pain 1995;9:24–36.
80. Dao TT, Lund JP, Lavigne GJ. Comparison of pain and quality of life in bruxers and patients with myofascial pain of the masticatory muscles. J Orofac Pain 1994; 8:350–356.
81. Glaros AG, Forbes D, Shanker J, Glass EG. Effect of parafunctional clenching on temporomandibular disorder pain and proprioceptive awareness. Cranio 2000;18:198–204.
82. Glaros AG, Burton E. Parafunctional clenching, pain, and effort in temporomandibular disorders. J Behav Med 2004;27:91–100.
83. Castelo PM, Gavião MB, Pereira LJ, Bonjardim LR. Relationship between oral parafunctional/nutritive sucking habits and temporomandibular joint dysfunction in primary dentition. Int J Paediatr Dent 2005;15: 29–36.
84. Pullinger AG, Seligman DA. The degree to which attrition characterizes differentiated patient groups of temporomandibular disorders. J Orofac Pain 1993;7: 196–208.
85. Rugh JD. Association between bruxism and TMD. In: McNeill C (ed). Current Controversies in Temporomandibular Disorders. Chicago: Quintessence, 1992:29–31.
86. de Leeuw JR, Steenks MH, Ros WJ, Lobbezoo-Scholte AM, Bosman F, Winnubst JA. Multidimensional evaluation of craniomandibular dysfunction. I: Symptoms and correlates. J Oral Rehabil 1994;21:501–514.
87. Junge D, Clark GT. Electromyographic turns analysis of sustained contraction in human masseter muscles at various isometric force levels. Arch Oral Biol 1993;38:583–588.
88. Kamisaka M, Yatani H, Kuboki T, Matsuka Y, Minakuchi H. Four-year longitudinal course of TMD symptoms in an adult population and the estimation of risk factors in relation to symptoms. J Orofac Pain 2000; 14:224–232.
89. Magnusson T, Egermark I, Carlsson GE. A longitudinal epidemiologic study of signs and symptoms of temporomandibular disorders from 15 to 35 years of age. J Orofac Pain 2000;14:310–319.
90. Arima T, Svensson P, Arendt-Nielsen L. Experimental grinding in healthy subjects: A model for postexercise jaw muscle soreness? J Orofac Pain 1999;13:104–114.
91. Pierce CJ, Chrisman K, Bennett ME, Close JM. Stress, anticipatory stress, and psychologic measures related to sleep bruxism. J Orofac Pain 1995;9:51–56.
92. Lobbezoo F, Naeije M. Bruxism is mainly regulated centrally, not peripherally. J Oral Rehabil 2001;28: 1085–1091.
93. Weiner S, Shaikh MB, Siegel A. Electromyographic activity in the masseter muscle resulting from stimulation of hypothalamic behavioral sites in the cat. J Orofac Pain 1993;7:370–377.
94. Fahn S. The extrapyramidal disorders. In: Wyngaarden JB, Smith LH (eds). Cecil Textbook of Medicine, vol 2, ed 17. Philadelphia: Saunders, 1985:2068–2079.
95. Holmgren K, Sheikholeslam A, Riise C. Effect of a full-arch maxillary occlusal splint on parafunctional activity during sleep in patients with nocturnal bruxism and signs and symptoms of craniomandibular disorders. J Prosthet Dent 1993;69:293–297.
96. Silness J, Johannessen G, Røystrand T. Longitudinal relationship between incisal occlusion and incisal tooth wear. Acta Odontol Scand 1993;51:15–21.
97. Bernhardt O, Gesch D, Splieth C, et al. Risk factors for high occlusal wear scores in a population-based sample: Results of the Study of Health in Pomerania (SHIP). Int J Prosthodont 2004;17:333–339.
98. Johansson A, Fareed K, Omar R. Lateral and protrusive contact schemes and occlusal wear: A correlational study in a young adult Saudi population. J Prosthet Dent 1994;7:159–164.
99. Waltimo A, Nyström M, Könönen M. Bite force and dentofacial morphology in men with severe dental attrition. Scand J Dent Res 1994;102:92–96.

100. Krogstad O, Dahl BL. Dento facial morphology in patients with advanced attrition. Eur J Orthod 1985;7:57–62.
101. Varrela J. Effects of attritive diet on craniofacial morphology: A cephalometric analysis of a Finnish skull sample. Eur J Orthod 1990;12:219–223.
102. Helkimo E, Ingergvall B. Bite force and functional state of the masticatory system in young men. Swed Dent J 1978;2:167–175.
103. Johansson A, Omar R, Fareed K, Haraldson T, Kiliaridis S, Carlsson GE. Comparison of the prevalence, severity and possible causes of occlusal tooth wear in two young adult populations. J Oral Rehabil 1993;20:463–471.
104. Ekfeldt A. Incisal and occlusal tooth wear and wear of some prosthodontic materials. An epidemiological and clinical study. Swed Dent J Suppl 1989;65:1–62.
105. Khoury S, Rouleau GA, Rompré PH, Mayer P, Montplaisir JY, Lavigne JG. A significant increase in breathing amplitude precedes sleep bruxism. Chest 2008;134:332–337.
106. Miyawaki S, Lavigne GJ, Pierre M, Guitard F, Montplaisir JY, Kato T. Association between sleep bruxism, swallowing-related laryngeal movement, and sleep positions. Sleep 2003;26:461–465.
107. Thie NMR, Kato T, Bader G, Montplaisir JY, Lavigne GJ. The significance of saliva during sleep and the relevance of oromotor movements. Sleep Med Rev 2002;6:213–227.
108. Lavigne GJ, Kato T, Kolta A, Sessle BJ. Neurobiological mechanisms involved in sleep bruxism. Crit Rev Oral Biol Med 2003;14:30–46.
109. Simmons JH, Prehn R. Airway protection: The missing link between nocturnal bruxism and obstructive sleep apnea. Sleep 2009;32:(A218).
110. Lobbezoo F, van der Zaag J, van Selms MK, Hamburger HL, Naeije M. Principles for the management of bruxism. J Oral Rehabil 2008;35:509–523.
111. Johansson A, Haraldson T, Omar R, Kiliaridis S, Carlsson GE. A system for assessing the severity and progression of occlusal tooth wear. J Oral Rehabil 1993;20:125–131.
112. Svensson P, Lavigne G. Clinical bruxism semantics beyond academic debates: Normo- and pathobruxism as a new proposal. J Oral Rehabil 2020;47:547–548.
113. Schellhas KP, Pollei SR, Wilkes CH. Pediatric internal derangements of the temporomandibular joint: Effect on facial development. Am J Orthod Dentofacial Orthop 1993;104:51–59.
114. Armijo-Olivo S, Rappoport K, Fuentes J, et al. Head and cervical posture in patients with temporomandibular disorders. J Orofac Pain 2011;25:199–209.
115. Isberg A, Westesson PL. Steepness of articular eminence and movement of the condyle and disk in asymptomatic temporomandibular joints. Oral Surg Oral Med Oral Pathol Oral Radiol Endod 1998;86:152–157.
116. Panmekiate S, Petersson A, Akerman S. Angulation and prominence of the posterior slope of the eminence of the temporomandibular joint in relation to disc position. Dentomaxillofac Radiol 1991;20:205–208.
117. Ren YF, Isberg A, Westesson PL. Steepness of the articular eminence in the temporomandibular joint. Tomographic comparison between asymptomatic volunteers with normal disk position and patients with disk displacement. Oral Surg Oral Med Oral Pathol Oral Radiol Endod 1995;80:258–266.
118. Yamada K, Tsuruta A, Hanada K, Hayashi T. Morphology of the articular eminence in temporomandibular joints and condylar bone change. J Oral Rehabil 2004;31:438–444.
119. Wabeke KB, Spruijt RJ, Habets LL. Spatial and morphologic aspects of temporomandibular joints with sounds. J Oral Rehabil 1995;22:21–27.
120. Greene CS, Manfredini D. Treating temporomandibular disorders in the 21st century: Can we finally eliminate the "third pathway"? J Oral Facial Pain Headache 2020;34:206–216.
121. Türp JC, Schindler H. The dental occlusion as a suspected cause for TMDs: Epidemiological and etiological considerations. J Oral Rehabil 2012;39:502–512.
122. Luther F. TMD and occlusion part II. Damned if we don't? Functional occlusal problems: TMD epidemiology in a wider context. Br Dent J 2007;202:E3.
123. Vanderas AP. Relationship between craniomandibular dysfunction and malocclusion in white children with and without unpleasant life events. J Oral Rehabil 1994;21:177–183.
124. Manfredini D, Lombardo L, Siciliani G. Temporomandibular disorders and dental occlusion. A systematic review of association studies: End of an era? J Oral Rehabil 2017;44:908–923.
125. Byrd KE, Stein ST. Effects of lesions to the trigeminal motor nucleus on temporomandibular disc morphology. J Oral Rehabil 1990;17:529–540.
126. Hagberg C, Hellsing G, Hagberg M. Perception of cutaneous electrical stimulation in patients with craniomandibular disorders. J Craniomandib Disord 1990;4:120–125.
127. Hesse JR, Naeije M, Hansson TL. Craniomandibular stiffness toward maximum mouth opening in healthy subjects: A clinical and experimental investigation. J Craniomandib Disord 1990;4:257–266.

128. Buckingham RB, Braun T, Harinstein DA, et al. Temporomandibular joint dysfunction syndrome: A close association with systemic joint laxity (the hypermobile joint syndrome). Oral Surg Oral Med Oral Pathol 1991;72:514–519.
129. Westling L. Temporomandibular joint dysfunction and systemic joint laxity. Swed Dent J Suppl 1992;81:1–79.
130. De Coster PJ, Van den Berghe LI, Martens LC. Generalized joint hypermobility and temporomandibular disorders: Inherited connective tissue disease as a model with maximum expression. J Orofac Pain 2005; 19:47–57.
131. Kavuncu V, Sahin S, Kamanli A, Karan Ayse, Aksoy C. The role of systemic hypermobility and condylar hypermobility in temporomandibular joint dysfunction syndrome. Rheumatol Int 2006;26:257–260.
132. Pereira FJ, Lundh H, Eriksson L, Westesson PL. Microscopic changes in the retrodiscal tissues of painful temporomandibular joints. J Oral Maxillofac Surg 1996;54:461–468.
133. Akeel R, Nilner M, Nilner K. Masticatory efficiency in individuals with natural dentitions. Swed Dent J 1992;16:191–198.
134. Ahlberg JP, Kovero OA, Hurmerinta KA, Zepa I, Nissinen MJ, Könönen MH. Maximal bite force and its association with signs and symptoms of TMD, occlusion, and body mass index in a cohort of young adults. Cranio 2003;21:248–252.
135. Kohyama K, Mioche L, Bourdiol P. Influence of age and dental status on chewing behavior studied by EMG recordings during consumption of various food samples. Gerodontology 2003;20:15–23.
136. Stegenga B, de Bont LGM, de Leeuw R, Boering G. Assessment of mandibular function impairment associated with temporomandibular joint osteoarthrosis and internal derangement. J Orofac Pain 1993;7:193–195.
137. Wang K, Arima T, Arendt-Nielsen L, Svensson P. EMG-force relationships are influenced by experimental jaw-muscle pain. J Oral Rehabil 2000;27:394–402.
138. Shiau YY, Peng CC, Wen SC, Lin LD, Wang JS, Lou KL. The effects of masseter muscle pain on biting performance. J Oral Rehabil 2003;30:978–984.
139. Mioche L, Bourdiol P, Monier S, Martin JF, Cormier D. Changes in jaw muscles activity with age: Effects on food bolus properties. Physiol Behav 2004;82:621–627.
140. Hansdottir R, Bakke M. Joint tenderness, jaw opening, chewing velocity, and bite force in patients with temporomandibular joint pain and matched healthy control subjects. J Orofac Pain 2004;18:108–113.
141. Reid KI, Gracely RH, Dubner RA. The influence of time, facial side, and location on pain-pressure thresholds in chronic myogenous temporomandibular disorder. J Orofac Pain 1994;8:258–265.
142. Browne PA, Clark GT, Yang Q, Nakano M. Sternocleidomastoid muscle inhibition induced by trigeminal stimulation. J Dent Educ 1993;72:1503–1508.
143. Clark GT, Browne PA, Nakano M, Yang Q. Co-activation of sternocleidomastoid muscles during maximum clenching. J Dent Res 1993;72:1499–1502.
144. Hu JW, Yu XM, Vernon H, Sessle BJ. Excitatory effects on the neck and jaw muscle activity of inflammatory irritant applied to cervical paraspinal tissues. Pain 1993;55:243–250.
145. Okuda-Akabane K. Hyperalgesic change over the craniofacial area following urate crystal injection in the rabbit's temporomandibular joint. J Oral Rehabil 1994;21:311–322.
146. Bibb CA, Pullinger A, Baldioceda R. The relationship of undifferentiated mesenchymal cells to TMJ articular tissue thickness. J Dent Res 1992;71:1816–1821.
147. Juniper RP. The shape of the condyle and position of the meniscus in temporomandibular joint dysfunction. Br J Oral Maxillofac Surg 1994;32:71–76.
148. Pullinger AG, Baldioceda F, Bibb CA. Relationship of TMJ articular soft tissue to underlying bone in young adult condyles. J Dent Res 1990;69:1512–1518.
149. de Bont LG, Boering G, Liem RS, Havinga P. Osteoarthritis of the temporomandibular joint: A light microscopic and scanning electron microscopic study of the articular cartilage of the mandibular condyle. J Oral Maxillofac Surg 1985;43:481–488.
150. Stegenga B, De Bont LGM. TMJ growth, adaptive modeling and remodeling, and compensatory mechanisms. In: Laskin DM, Greene CS, Hylander WL (eds). Temporomandibular Disorders: An evidence-Based Approach to Diagnosis and Treatment. Chicago: Quintessence, 2006:53–64.
151. de Leeuw R, Boering G, Stegenga B, de Bont LG. Radiographic signs of temporomandibular joint osteoarthrosis and internal derangement 30 years after nonsurgical treatment. Oral Surg Oral Med Oral Pathol Oral Radiol Endod 1995;79:382–92.
152. Luder HU. Articular degeneration and remodeling in human temporomandibular joints with normal and abnormal disc position. J Orofac Pain 1993;7:391–402.
153. Bade DM, Lovasko JH, Dimitroff M, Jones TD, Hirsch M. Clinical comparison of temporomandibular joint sound auscultation and emission imaging studies. J Orofac Pain 1994;8:55–60.
154. Toller PA. The synovial apparatus and temporomandibular joint function. Br Dent J 1961;40:347–353.

155. Nitzan DW. The process of lubrication impairment and its involvement in temporomandibular joint disc displacement: A theoretical concept. J Oral Maxillofac Surg 2001;59:36–45.
156. Fujimura K, Segami N, Yoshitake Y, et al. Electrophoretic separation of the synovial fluid proteins in patients with temporomandibular joint disorders. Oral Surg Oral Med Oral Pathol Oral Radiol Endod 2006;101:463–468.
157. Herr MM, Fries KM, Upton LG, Edsberg LE. Potential biomarkers of temporomandibular joint disorders. J Oral Maxillofac Surg 2011;69:41–47.
158. Slade GD, Conrad MS, Diatchenko L, et al. Cytokine biomarkers and chronic pain: Association of genes, transcription, and circulating proteins with temporomandibular disorders and widespread palpation tenderness. Pain 2011;152:2802–2812.
159. Gulen H, Ataoglu H, Haliloglu S, Isik K. Proinflammatory cytokines in temporomandibular joint synovial fluid before and after arthrocentesis. Oral Surg Oral Med Oral Pathol Oral Radiol Endod 2009;107:e1–e4.
160. Kaneyama K, Segami N, Yoshimura H, Honjo M, Demura N. Increased levels of soluble cytokine receptors in the synovial fluid of temporomandibular joint disorders in relation to joint effusion on magnetic resonance images. J Oral Maxillofac Surg 2010;68: 1088–1093.
161. Kim YK, Kim SG, Kim BS, et al. Analysis of the cytokine profiles of the synovial fluid in a normal temporomandibular joint: Preliminary study. J Craniomaxillofac Surg 2012;40:e337–e341.
162. Kellesarian SV, Al-Kheraif AA, Vohra F, et al. Cytokine profile in the synovial fluid of patients with temporomandibular joint disorders: A systematic review. Cytokine 2016;77:98–106.
163. Cady RJ, Glenn JR, Smith KM, Durham PL. Calcitonin gene-related peptide promotes cellular changes in trigeminal neurons and glia implicated in peripheral and central sensitization. Mol Pain 2011;7:94.
164. Romero-Reyes M, Pardi V, Akerman S. A potent and selective calcitonin gene-related peptide (CGRP) receptor antagonist, MK-8825, inhibits responses to nociceptive trigeminal activation: Role of CGRP in orofacial pain. Exp Neurol 2015;271:95–103.
165. Liang H, Hu H, Shan D, et al. CGRP Modulates Orofacial Pain through Mediating Neuron-Glia Crosstalk. J Dent Res 2021;100:98–105.
166. Nitzan DW. 'Friction and adhesive forces'--possible underlying causes for temporomandibular joint internal derangement. Cells Tissues Organs 2003;174:6–16.
167. Erhardson S, Sheikholeslam A, Forsberg CM, Lockowandt P. Vertical forces developed by the jaw elevator muscles during unilateral maximal clenching and their distribution on teeth and condyles. Swed Dent J 1993;17:23–34.
168. Korioth TW, Hannam AG. Mandibular forces during simulated tooth clenching. J Orofac Pain 1994;8:178–189.
169. Nickel JC, McLachlan KR. An analysis of surface congruity in the growing human temporomandibular joint. Arch Oral Biol 1994;39:315–321.
170. Nickel JC, McLachlan KR. In vitro measurement of the stress-distribution properties of the pig temporomandibular joint. Arch Oral Biol 1994;39:439–448.
171. Scapino RP, Canham PB, Finlay HM, Mills DK. The behaviour of collagen fibers in stress relaxation and stress distribution in the jaw-joint disc of rabbits. Arch Oral Biol 1996;41:1039–1052.
172. Korioth TW, Hannam AG. Deformation of the human mandible during simulated tooth clenching. J Dent Res 1994;73:56–66.
173. Nitzan DW. Intraarticular pressure in the functioning human temporomandibular joint and its alteration by uniform elevation of the occlusal plane. J Oral Maxillofac Surg 1994;52:671–679.
174. Abubaker AO, Raslan WF, Sotereanos GC. Estrogen and progesterone receptors in temporomandibular joint discs of symptomatic and asymptomatic persons: A preliminary study. J Oral Maxillofac Surg 1993;51:1096–1100.
175. Campbell JH, Courey MS, Bourne P, Odziemiec C. Estrogen receptor analysis of human temporomandibular disc. J Oral Maxillofac Surg 1993;51:1101–1105.
176. Wu Y, Kadota-Watanabe C, Ogawa T, Moriyama Keiji. Combination of estrogen deficiency and excessive mechanical stress aggravates temporomandibular joint osteoarthritis in vivo. Arch Oral Biol 2019;102: 39–46.
177. Glaros AG, Baharloo L, Glass EG. Effect of parafunctional clenching and estrogen on temporomandibular disorder pain. Cranio 1998;16:78–83.
178. LeResche L, Saunders K, Von Korff MR, Barlow W, Dworkin SF. Use of exogenous hormones and risk of temporomandibular disorder pain. Pain 1997;69: 153–160.
179. Dao TT, Knight K, Ton-That V. Modulation of myofascial pain by the reproductive hormones: A preliminary report. J Prosthet Dent 1998;79:663–670.
180. LeResche L, Sherman JJ, Huggins K, et al. Musculoskeletal orofacial pain and other signs and symptoms of temporomandibular disorders during pregnancy: A prospective study. J Orofac Pain 2005;19:193–201.

181. Ribeiro-Dasilva MC, Fillingim RB, Wallet SM. Estrogen-induced monocytic response correlates with tmd pain: A case control study. J Dent Res 2017;96:285–291.
182. Stegenga B. Temporomandibular Joint Osteoarthrosis and Internal Derangement: Diagnostic and Therapeutic Outcome Assessment [thesis]. Groningen: University of Groningen, 1991.
183. Wonwatana S, Kronman JH, Clark RE, Kabani S, Mehta N. Anatomic basis for disk displacement in temporomandibular joint (TMJ) dysfunction. Am J Orthod Dentofacial Orthop 1994;105:257–264.
184. Lang TC, Zimmy ML, Vijayagopal P. Experimental temporomandibular joint disc perforation in the rabbit: A gross morphological, biochemical, and ultrastructural analysis. J Oral Maxillofac Surg 1993;51: 1115–1128.
185. Milam SB, Zardeneta G, Schmitz JP. Oxidative stress and degenerative temporomandibular joint disease: A proposed hypothesis. J Oral Maxillofac Surg 1998;56:214–223.
186. Dijkgraaf LC, Zardeneta G, Cordewener FW, et al. Crosslinking of fibrinogen and fibronectin by free radicals: A possible initial step in adhesion formation in osteoarthritis of the temporomandibular joint. J Oral Maxillofac Surg 2003;61:101–111.
187. Diatchenko L, Slade GD, Nackley AG, et al. Genetic basis for individual variations in pain perception and the development of a chronic pain condition. Hum Mol Genet 2005;14:135–143.
188. Smith SB, Mir E, Bair E, et al. Genetic variants associated with development of TMD and its intermediate phenotypes: The genetic architecture of TMD in the OPPERA prospective cohort study. J Pain 2013;14(12 suppl):T91–T101.
189. Smith S, Parisien M, Bair E, et al. Genome-wide association reveals contribution of MRAS to painful temporomandibular disorder in males. Pain 2019;160:579-591.
190. Fillingim RB, Ohrbach R, Greenspan JD, et al. Potential psychosocial risk factors for chronic TMD: Descriptive data and empirically identified domains from the OPPERA case-control study. J Pain 2011;12(11 suppl):T46–T60.
191. Rugh JD, Solberg W. Psychological implications in temporomandibular pain and dysfunction. In: Zarb GA, Carlsson GE, (eds). Temporomandibular Joint Function and Dysfunction. Copenhagen: Munksgaard, 1979:239–258.
192. Wänman A, Agerberg G. Etiology of craniomandibular disorders: Evaluation of some occlusal and psychosocial factors in 19-year-olds. J Craniomandib Disord 1991;5:35–44.
193. Eversole LR, Stone CE, Matheson D, Kaplan H. Psychometric profiles and facial pain. Oral Surg Oral Med Oral Pathol 1985;60:269–274.
194. Southwell J, Deary IJ, Geissler P. Personality and anxiety in temporomandibular joint syndrome patients. J Oral Rehabil 1990;17:239–243.
195. Flor H, Birbaumer N, Schulte W, Roos R. Stress-related electromyographic responses in patients with chronic temporomandibular pain. Pain 1991;46:145–152.
196. de Leeuw JR, Steenks MH, Ros WJ, Bosman F, Winnubst JA, Scholte AM. Psychosocial aspects of craniomandibular dysfunction. An assessment of clinical and community findings. J Oral Rehabil 1994;21:127–143.
197. List T, Wahlund K, Larsson B. Psychosocial functioning and dental factors in adolescents with temporomandibular disorders: A case-control study. J Orofac Pain 2001;15:218–227.
198. Wright AR, Gatchel RJ, Wildenstein L, Riggs R, Buschang P, Ellis Edward, 3rd. Biopsychosocial differences between high-risk and low-risk patients with acute TMD-related pain. J Am Dent Assoc 2004; 135:474–483.
199. Manfredini D, Bandettini di Poggio A, Cantini E, Dell'Osso L, Bosco M. Mood and anxiety psychopathology and temporomandibular disorder: A spectrum approach. J Oral Rehabil 2004;31:933–940.
200. De Leeuw R, Bertoli E, Schmidt JE, Carlson CR. Prevalence of post-traumatic stress disorder symptoms in orofacial pain patients. Oral Surg Oral Med Oral Pathol Oral Radiol Endod 2005;99:558–568.
201. Carlson CR, Okeson JP, Falace DA, Nitz AJ, Curran SL, Anderson D. Comparison of psychologic and physiologic functioning between patients with masticatory muscle pain and matched controls. J Orofac Pain 1993;7:15–22.
202. Arntz A, Dreessen L, De Jong P. The influence of anxiety on pain: Attentional and attributional mediators. Pain 1994;56:307–314.
203. Jones DA, Rollman GB, Brooke RI. The cortisol response to psychological stress in temporomandibular dysfunction. Pain 1997;72:171–182.
204. Turner JA, Dworkin SF, Mancl L, Huggins KH, Truelove EL. The roles of beliefs, catastrophizing, and coping in the functioning of patients with temporomandibular disorders. Pain 2001;92:41–51.
205. Magni G, Moreschi C, Rigatti-Luchini S, Merskey H. Prospective study on the relationship between depressive symptoms and chronic musculoskeletal pain. Pain 1994;56:289–297.
206. Turk DC, Rudy TE. The robustness of an empirically derived taxonomy of chronic pain patients. Pain 1990;43:27–35.

207. Aghabeigi B, Feinmann C, Glover V, et al. Tyramine conjugation deficit in patients with chronic idiopathic temporomandibular joint and orofacial pain. Pain 1993;54:159–163.
208. Mechanic D. The concept of illness behavior: Culture, situation and personal predisposition. Psychol Med 1986;16:1–7.
209. Pilowsky I, Smith QP, Katsikitis M. Illness behavior and general practice utilization: A prospective study. J Psychosom Res 1987;31:177–183.
210. Pearce JMS. Psychosocial factors in chronic disability. Med Sci Monit 2002;8:RA275–281.
211. Fordyce WE. Behavioral Methods for Chronic Pain and Illness. St Louis: Mosby, 1976.
212. Fillingim RB, Ohrbach R, Greenspan JD, et al. Psychological factors associated with development of TMD: the OPPERA prospective cohort study. J Pain 2013; 14(12 suppl):T75–T90.
213. Fillingim RB, Slade GD, Diatchenko L, et al. Summary of findings from the OPPERA baseline case-control study: Implications and future directions. J Pain 2011;12(11 suppl):T102–T107.
214. Fillingim RB, Ohrbach R, Greenspan JD, et al. Associations of psychologic factors with multiple chronic overlapping pain conditions. J Oral Facial Pain Headache 2020;34:s85–s100.
215. Fries JF, Hochberg MC, Medsger TA Jr, Hunder GG, Bombardier C. Criteria for rheumatic disease: Different types and different functions. The American College of Rheumatology Diagnostic and Therapeutic Criteria Committee. Arthritis Rheum 1994;37:454–462.
216. Peck CC, Goulet JP, Lobbezoo F, et al. Expanding the taxonomy of the diagnostic criteria for temporomandibular disorders (DC/TMD). J Oral Rehabil 2014; 41:2–23.
217. International classification of orofacial pain, 1st edition (ICOP). Cephalalgia 2020;4:129–221.
218. Headache Classification Committee of the International Headache Society (IHS) the international classification of headache disorders, 3rd edition. Cephalalgia 2018;38:1–211.
219. World Health Organization. International Classification of Diseases 11th Revision. https://icd.who.int/browse11/l-m/en. Accessed 31 May 2021.
220. International Association for the Study of Pain. IASP Terminology. https://www.iasp-pain.org/Education/Content.aspx?ItemNumber=1698. Accessed 31 May 2021.
221. Blankestijn J, Boering G. Posterior dislocation of the temporomandibular joint. Int J Oral Surg 1985;14: 437–443.
222. Westesson PL, Larheim TA, Tanaka H. Posterior disc displacement in the temporomandibular joint. J Oral Maxillofac Surg 1998;56:1266–1273.
223. Khoury MD, Dolan E. Sideways dislocation of the temporomandibular joint meniscus: The edge sign. AJNR AM J Neuroradiol 1986;7:869–872.
224. Westesson PL, Kurita K, Ericksson L, Katzberg RW. Cryosectional observations of functional anatomy of the temporomandibular joint. Oral Surg Oral Med Oral Pathol 1989;68:247–251.
225. Liedberg J, Westesson PL, Kurita K. Sideways and rotational displacement of the temporomandibular joint disc: Diagnosis by arthrography and correlation to cryosectional morphology. Oral Surg Oral Med Oral Pathol 1990;69:757–763.
226. Kurita K, Westesson PL, Tasaki M, Liedberg J. Temporomandibular joint: Diagnosis of medial and lateral disc displacement with anterioposterior arthrography. Correlation with cryosections. Oral Surg Oral Med Oral Pathol Oral Radiol Endod 1992;73:364–368.
227. Isberg-Holm AM, Westesson PL. Movement of disc and condyle in temporomandibular joints with clicking: An arthrographic and cineradiographic study on autopsy specimens. Acta Odontol Scand 1982;40: 151–164.
228. Tallents RH, Hatala M, Katzberg RW, Westesson PL. Temporomandibular joint sounds in asymptomatic volunteers. J Prosthet Dent 1993;69:298–304.
229. Davant TS 6th, Greene CS, Perry HT, Lautenschlager EP. A quantitative computer-assisted analysis of the disc displacement in patients with internal derangement using sagittal view and magnetic resonance imaging. J Oral Maxillofac Surg 1993;51:974–979.
230. Stegenga B, De Bont LG, Boering G, van Willigen JD. Tissue responses to degenerative changes in the temporomandibular joint: A review. J Oral Maxillofac Surg 1991;49:1079–1088.
231. Dijkgraaf LC, de Bont LG, Boering G, Liem RS. The structure, biochemistry, and metabolism of osteoarthritic cartilage: A review of the literature. J Oral Maxillofac Surg 1995;53:1182–1192.
232. 232. Shinoda C, Takaku S. Interleukin-1 beta, interleukin-6, and tissue inhibitor of metalloproteinase-1 in the synovial fluid of the temporomandibular joint with respect to cartilage destruction. Oral Dis 2000;6:383–90.
233. Kubota T, Kubota E, Matsumoto A, et al. Identification of matrix metalloproteinases (MMPs) in synovial fluid from patients with temporomandibular disorder. Eur J Oral Sci 1998;106:992–998.
234. Nordahl S, Alstergren P, Eliasson S, Kopp S. Interleukin-1beta in plasma and synovial fluid in relation to radiographic changes in arthritic temporomandibular joints. Eur J Oral Sci 1998;106:559–563.

235. Tanaka A, Kumagai S, Kawashiri S, et al. Expression of matrix metalloproteinase-2 and -9 in synovial fluid of the temporomandibular joint accompanied by anterior disc displacement. J Oral Pathol Med 2001, 30:59–64.
236. Kanyama M, Kuboki T, Kojima S, et al. Matrix metalloproteinases and tissue inhibitors of metalloproteinases in synovial fluids of patients with temporomandibular joint osteoarthritis. J Orofac Pain 2000;14: 20–30.
237. Suzuki T, Segami N, Nishimura M, Hattori H, Nojima T. Analysis of 70Kd heat shock protein expression in patients with internal derangement of the temporomandibular joint. Int J Oral Maxillofac Surg 2000;29: 301–304.
238. Fang PK, Ma XC, Ma DL, Fu KY. Determination of interleukin-1 receptor antagonist, interleukin-10, and transforming growth factor-beta1 in synovial fluid aspirates of patients with temporomandibular disorders. J Oral Maxillofac Surg 1999;57:922–928.
239. Suzuki T, Bessho K, Segami N, Nojima T, Iizuka T. Bone morphogenetic protein-2 in temporomandibular joints with internal derangement. Oral Surg Oral Med Oral Pathol Oral Radiol Endod 1999;88:670–673.
240. Murakami KI, Shibata T, Kubota E, Maeda H. Intra-articular levels of prostaglandin E2, hyaluronic acid, and chondroitin-4 and -6 sulfates in the temporomandibular joint synovial fluid of patients with internal derangement. J Oral Maxillofac Surg 1998;56:199–203.
241. Ratcliffe A, Israel HA, Saed-Nejad F, Diamond B. Proteoglycans in the synovial fluid of the temporomandibular joint as an indicator of changes in cartilage metabolism during primary and secondary osteoarthritis. J Oral Maxillofac Surg 1998;56:204–208.
242. Fu K, Ma X, Zhang Z, Pang X, Chen W. Interleukin-6 in synovial fluid and HLA-DR expression in synovium from patients with temporomandibular disorders. J Orofac Pain 1995;9:131–137.
243. Carlsson GE. Mandibular dysfunction and temporomandibular joint pathosis. J Prosthet Dent 1980; 43:658–662.
244. Dijkgraaf LC, Liem RS, de Bont LG. Ultrastructural characteristics of the synovial membrane in osteoarthritic temporomandibular joints. J Oral Maxillofac Surg 1997;55:1269–1280.
245. Dijkgraaf LC, Spijkervet FK, de Bont LG. Arthroscopic findings in osteoarthritic temporomandibular joints. J Oral Maxillofac Surg 1999;57:255–268.
246. Israel HA, Diamond B, Saed-Nejad F, Ratcliffe A. Osteoarthritis and synovitis as major pathoses of the temporomandibular joint: Comparison of clinical diagnosis with arthroscopic morphology. J Oral Maxillofac Surg 1998;56:1023–1027.
247. Milam SB. TMJ osteoarthritis. In: Laskin DM, Greene CS, Hylander WL (eds). Temporomandibular Disorders: An Evidence-Based Approach To Diagnosis And Treatment. Chicago: Quintessence, 2006:105 124.
248. Warner BF, Luna MA, Newland TR. Temporomandibular joint neoplasms and pseudotumors. Adv Anat Pathol 2000;7:365–381.
249. Sánchez Aniceto G, García Peñín A, de la Mata Pages R, Montalvo Moreno JJ. Tumors metastatic to the mandible: Analysis of nine cases and review of the literature. J Oral Maxillofac Surg 1990;48:246–251.
250. Nortjé CJ, van Rensburg LJ, Thompson IO. Case report. Magnetic resonance features of metastatic melanoma of the temporomandibular joint and mandible. Dentomaxillofac Radiol 1996;25:292–297.
251. Orlean SL, Robinson NR, Ahern JP, Mallon CF, Blewitt G. Cae report. Carcinoma of the maxillary sinus manifested by temporomandibular joint pain dysfunction syndrome. J Oral Med 1966;21:127–131.
252. Shapshay SM, Elber E, Strong MS. Occult tumors of the infratemporal fossa: Report of seven cases appearing as preauricular facial pain. Arch Otolaryngol 1976;102:535–538.
253. Sharav Y, Feinsod M. Nasopharyngeal tumor initially manifested as myofascial pain dysfunction syndrome. Oral Surg Oral Med Oral Pathol 1977;44:54–77.
254. DelBalso AM, Pyatt RS, Busch RF, Hirokawa R, Fink CS. Synovial cell sarcoma of the temporomandibular joint. Computed tomographic findings. Arch Otolaryngol 1982;108:520–522.
255. Roistacher SL, Tanenbaum D. Myofascial pain associated with oropharyngeal cancer. Oral Surg Oral Med Oral Pathol 1986;61:459–462.
256. Christiansen EL, Thompson JR, Appleton SS. Temporomandibular joint pain/dysfunction overlying more insidious diseases: Report of two cases. J Oral Maxillofac Surg. 1987;45:335–337.
257. Cohen SG, Quinn PD. Facial trismus and myofascial pain associated with infections and malignant disease. Report of five cases. Oral Surg Oral Med Oral Pathol 1988;65:538–544.
258. Epstein JB, Jones CK. Presenting signs and symptoms of nasopharyngeal carcinoma. Oral Surg Oral Med Oral Pathol Oral Radiol Endod 1993;75:31–36.
259. Grace EG, North AF. Temporomandibular joint dysfunction and orofacial pain caused by parotid gland malignancy: Report of case. J Am Dent Assoc 1988;116:348–350.
260. Malins TJ, Farrow A. Facial pain due to occult parotid adenoid cystic carcinoma. J Oral Maxillofac Surg 1991;49:1127–1129.
261. Raustia AM, Oikarinen KS, Luotonen J, Salo T, Pyhtinen J. Parotid gland carcinoma simulating signs and symptoms of craniomandibular disorders--A case report. Cranio 1993;11:153–156.

262. Halfpenny W, Verey A, Bardsley V. Myxoma of the mandibular condyle. A case report and review of the literature. Oral Surg Oral Med Oral Pathol Oral Radiol Endod 2000;90:348–353.
263. Kondoh T, Seto K, Kobayashi K. Osteoma of the mandibular condyle: Report of a case with a review of the literature. J Oral Maxillofac Surg 1998;56:972–979.
264. Silvennoinen U, Raustia AM, Lindqvist C, Oikarinen K. Occlusal and temporomandibular joint disorders in patients with unilateral condylar fracture. A prospective one-year study. Int J Oral Maxillofac Surg 1998;27:280–285.
265. Ellis E 3rd, Throckmorton G. Facial symmetry after closed and open treatment of fractures of the mandibular condylar process. J Oral Maxillofac Surg 2000; 58:719–728.
266. Khawaja SN, Crow H, Gonzalez Y. Goldenhar syndrome and pain-related temporomandibular disorders. A case report. N Y State Dent J 2016;82:21–24.
267. Cabanillas-Aquino AG, Rojas-Yauri MC, Atoche-Socola KJ, Arriola-Guillén LE. Assessment of craniofacial and dental characteristics in individuals with treacher collins syndrome. A review. J Stomatol Oral Maxillofac Surg 2021;122:511–515.
268. Mense S. Physiology of nociception in muscles. In: Fricton JR, Awad EA (eds). Advances in Pain Research and Therapy. New York: Raven, 1990:67–85.
269. Mense S. Considerations concerning the neurobiological basis of muscle pain. Can J Physiol Pharmacol 1991;69:610–616.
270. Mense S. Nociception from skeletal muscle in relation to clinical muscle pain. Pain 1993;54:241–289.
271. Layzer RB. Muscle pain, cramps and fatigue. In: Engle AG, Franzini-Armstrong C (eds). Myology: Basic and Clinical, vol 2, ed 2. New York: McGraw-Hill, 1994: 1754–1786.
272. Grassi C, Passatore M. Action of the sympathetic system on skeletal muscle. Ital J Neurol Sci 1988; 9:23–28.
273. Passatore M, Grassi C, Filippi GM. Sympathetically-induced development of tension in jaw muscles: The possible contraction of intrafusal muscle fibres. Pflugers Arch 1985;405:297–304.
274. McNulty WH, Gevirtz RN, Hubbard DR, Berkoff GM. Needle electromyographic evaluation of trigger point response to a psychological stressor. Psychophysiology 1994;31:313–316.
275. Mense S. The pathogenesis of muscle pain. Curr Pain Headache Rep 2003;7:419–425.
276. Gonzales R, Coderre TJ, Sherbourne CD, Levine JD. Postnatal development of neurogenic inflammation in the rat. Neurosci Lett 1991;127:25–27.
277. Cairns BE. Pathophysiology of TMD pain--Basic mechanisms and their implications for pharmacotherapy. J Oral Rehabil 2010;37:391–410.
278. Wolfe F, Clauw DJ, Fitzcharles MA, et al. 2016 revisions to the 2010/2011 fibromyalgia diagnostic criteria. Semin Arthritis Rheum 2016;46:319–329.
279. Wolfe F, Clauw DJ, Fitzcharles MA, et al. The American College of Rheumatology preliminary diagnostic criteria for fibromyalgia and measurement of symptom severity. Arthritis Care Res (Hoboken) 2010;62:600–610.
280. List T, Jensen RH. Temporomandibular disorders: Old ideas and new concepts. Cephalalgia 2017;37:692–704.
281. Apfelberg DB, Lavey E, Janetos G, Maser MR, Lash H. Temporomandibular joint diseases. Results of a ten-year study. Postgrad Med 1979;65:167–169, 171–172.
282. Okeson JP, Hayes DK. Long-term results of treatment for temporomandibular disorders: An evaluation by patients. J Am Dent Assoc 1986;112:473–478.
283. Garefis P, Grigoriadou E, Zarifi A, Koidis PT. Effectiveness of conservative treatment for craniomandibular disorders: A 2-year longitudinal study. J Orofac Pain 1994;8:309–314.
284. Polonowita AD, Thomson WM, Thorburn DN. Clinical efficacy of a simplified approach to managing chronic temporomandibular disorders: Evidence from a 1-year case series. Oral Surg Oral Med Oral Pathol Oral Radiol 2019;128:227–234.
285. Skeppar J, Nilner M. Treatment of craniomandibular disorders in children and young adults. J Orofac Pain 1993;7:362–369.
286. Vichaichalermvong S, Nilner M, Panmekiate S, Petersson A. Clinical follow-up with different disc positions. J Orofac Pain 1993;7:61–67.
287. Poluha RL, Canales GT, Costa YM, Grossmann E, Bonjardim LR, Conti PCR. Temporomandibular joint disc displacement with reduction: A review of mechanisms and clinical presentation. J Appl Oral Sci 2019;27:e20180433.
288. Murakami K, Kaneshita S, Kanoh C, Yamamura I. Ten-year outcome of nonsurgical treatment for the internal derangement of the temporomandibular joint with closed lock. Oral Surg Oral Med Oral Pathol Oral Radiol Endod 2002;94:572–575.
289. Schmitter M, Zahran M, Duc JMP, Henschel V, Rammelsberg P. Conservative therapy in patients with anterior disc displacement without reduction using 2 common splints: A randomized clinical trial. J Oral Maxillofac Surg 2005;63:1295–1303.
290. Rasmussen OC. Clinical findings during the course of temporomandibular arthropathy. Scand J Dent Res 1981;89:283–288.

291. Rasmussen OC. Temporomandibular arthropathy. Int J Oral Surg 1983;12:365–397.
292. de Leeuw R, Boering G, Stegenga B, de Bont LG. Clinical signs of TMJ osteoarthrosis and internal derangement 30 years after nonsurgical treatment. J Orofac Pain 1994;8:18–24.
293. de Leeuw R, Boering G, van der Kuijl B, Stegenga B. Hard and soft tissue imaging of the temporomandibular joint 30 years after diagnosis of osteoarthrosis and internal derangement. J Oral Maxillofac Surg 1996;54:1270–1280.
294. Scholte AM, Steenks MH, Bosman F. Characteristics and treatment outcome of diagnostic subgroups of CMD patients: Retrospective study. Community Dent Oral Epidemiol 1993;21:215–220.
295. Rammelsberg P, LeResche L, Dworkin SF, Mancl Lloyd. Longitudinal outcome of temporomandibular disorders: A 5-year epidemiological study of muscle disorders defined by research diagnostic criteria for temporomandibular disorders. J Orofac Pain 2003; 17:9–20.
296. Linton SJ, Hellsing AL, Andersson D. A controlled study of the effects of an early intervention on acute musculoskeletal pain problems. Pain 1993;54:353–359.
297. List T, Helkimo M. Acupuncture and occlusal splint therapy in the treatment of craniomandibular disorders. II. A 1-year follow-up study. Acta Odontol Scand 1992;50:375–385.
298. Roberts AH, Kewman DG, Mercier L, Hovell M. The power of nonspecific effects in healing: Implications for psychosocial and biological treatments. Clin Psych Rev 1993;13:375–391.
299. Greene CS, Laskin DM. Splint therapy for the myofascial pain--Dysfunction (MPD) syndrome: A comparative study. J Am Dent Assoc 1972;84:624–628.
300. Flor H, Fydrich T, Turk DC. Efficacy of multidisciplinary pain treatment centers: A meta-analytic review. Pain 1992;49:221–230.
301. Aggarwal VR, Fu Y, Main CJ, Wu J. The effectiveness of self-management interventions in adults with chronic orofacial pain: A systematic review, meta-analysis and meta-regression. Eur J Pain 2019;23: 849–865.
302. Durham J, Al-Baghdadi M, Baad-Hansen L, et al. Self-management programmes in temporomandibular disorders: Results from an international Delphi process. J Oral Rehabil 2016;43:929–936.
303. Danzig WN, VanDyke AR. Physical therapy as an adjunct to temporomandibular joint therapy. J Prosthet Dent 1983;49:96–99.
304. Ohrbach R. Biobehavioral therapy. In: Laskin DM, Greene CS, Hylander WL (eds). Temperomandibular Disorders: An Evidence-Based Approach to Diagnosis and Treatment. Chicago: Quintessence, 2006:391–403.
305. Cannistraci AJ, Fritz G. Dental applications of biofeedback. In: Basmajiam JV (ed). Biofeedback: Principles and Practice for Clinicians, ed 3. Philedelphia: Williams & Wilkins 1989:297–310.
306. Erlandson PM Jr, Poppen R. Electromyographic biofeedback and rest position training of masticatory muscles in myofascial pain-dysfunction patients. J Prosthet Dent 1989;62:335–338.
307. Florjanski W, Malysa A, Orzeszek S, et al. Evaluation of Biofeedback Usefulness in Masticatory Muscle Activity Management–A Systematic Review. J Clin Med. 2019;8:766.
308. Integration of Behavioral and Relaxation Approaches into the Treatment of Chronic Pain and Insomnia [Proceedings of National Institutes of Health Technology Assessment Conference Statement, 16–18 Oct 1995]. Bethesda, MD: National Institutes of Health, 1995.
309. Jokubauskas L, Baltrušaitytė A. Efficacy of biofeedback therapy on sleep bruxism: A systematic review and meta-analysis. J Oral Rehabil 2018;45:485–495.
310. Bussadori SK, Motta LJ, Horliana ACRT, Santos EM, Martimbianco ALC. The current trend in management of bruxism and chronic pain: An overview of systematic reviews. J Pain Res 2020;13:2413–2421.
311. Saito-Murakami K, Sato M, Otsuka H, Miura H, Terada N, Fujisawa M. Daytime masticatory muscle electromyography biofeedback regulates the phasic component of sleep bruxism. J Oral Rehabil 2020;47:827–833.
312. Turk DC, Zaki HS, Rudy TE. Effects of intraoral appliance and biofeedback/stress management alone and in combination in treating pain and depression in patients with temporomandibular disorders. J Prosthet Dent 1993;70:158–164.
313. Randhawa K, Bohay R, Côté P, et al. The effectiveness of noninvasive interventions for temporomandibular disorders: A systematic review by the Ontario Protocol for Traffic Injury Management (OPTIMa) Collaboration. Clin J Pain 2016;32:260–278.
314. de Freitas RFCP, Ferreira MÂF, Barbosa GAS, Calderon PS. Counselling and self-management therapies for temporomandibular disorders: A systematic review. J Oral Rehabil 2013;40:864–874.
315. Dionne RA. Pharmacologic approaches. In: Laskin DM, Greene CS, Hylander WL (eds). Temperomandibular Disorders: An Evidence-Based Approach To Diagnosis And Treatment. Chicago: Quintessence, 2006:347–357.

316. Kalso E, Edwards JE, Moore AR, McQuay HJ. Opioids in chronic non-cancer pain: Systematic review of efficacy and safety. Pain 2004;112:372–380.
317. Els C, Jackson TD, Kunyk D, et al. Adverse events associated with medium- and long-term use of opioids for chronic non-cancer pain: An overview of Cochrane Reviews. Cochrane Database Syst Rev 2017;10:CD012509.
318. Von Korff M, Merrill J, Rutter C, Sullivan M, Campbell C, Weisner C. Time-scheduled vs. pain-contingent opioid dosing in chronic opioid therapy. Pain 2011; 152:1256–1262.
319. Häggman-Henrikson B, Alstergren P, Davidson T, et al. Pharmacological treatment of oro-facial pain - Health technology assessment including a systematic review with network meta-analysis. J Oral Rehabil 2017;44:800–826.
320. Mycek MJ, Harvey RA, Champe PC. Pharmacology, ed 2. Philadelphia: Lippincott-Raven, 1997.
321. Roth SH. Coming to terms with nonsteroidal anti-inflammatory drug gastropathy. Drugs 2012;72:873–879.
322. Freedberg DE, Kim LS, Yang YX. The risks and benefits of long-term use of proton pump inhibitors: Expert review and best practice advice from the American Gastroenterological Association. Gastroenterology 2017;152:706–715.
323. Hamad AM, Sutcliffe AM, Knox AJ. Aspirin-induced asthma: Clinical aspects, pathogenesis and management. Drugs 2004;64:2417–2432.
324. Chang RW, Tompkins DM, Cohn SM. Are NSAIDs safe? Assessing the risk-benefit profile of nonsteroidal anti-inflammatory drug use in postoperative pain management [epub ahead of print 26 Nov 2020]. Am Surg doi:10.1177/0003134820952834.
325. Ungprasert P, Cheungpasitporn W, Crowson CS, Matteson EL. Individual non-steroidal anti-inflammatory drugs and risk of acute kidney injury: A systematic review and meta-analysis of observational studies. Eur J Intern Med 2015;26:285–291.
326. Wenneberg B, Kopp S, Gröndahl HG. Long-term effect of intra-articular injections of a glucocorticosteroid into the TMJ: A clinical and radiographic 8-year follow-up. J Craniomandib Disord 1991;5:11–18.
327. Vallon D, Akerman S, Nilner M, Petersson A. Long-term follow-up of intra-articular injections into the temporomandibular joint in patients with rheumatoid arthritis. Swed Dent J 2002;26:149–158.
328. Moldez MA, Camones VR, Ramos GE, Padilla M, Enciso R. Effectiveness of intra-articular injections of sodium hyaluronate or corticosteroids for intracapsular temporomandibular disorders: A systematic review and meta-analysis. J Oral Facial Pain Headache 2018 32:53–66.
329. Goiato MC, da Silva EVF, de Medeiros RA, Túrcio KHL, Dos Santos DM. Are intra-articular injections of hyaluronic acid effective for the treatment of temporomandibular disorders? A systematic review. Int J Oral Maxillofac Surg 2016;45:1531–1537.
330. Chung PY, Lin MT, Chang HP. Effectiveness of platelet-rich plasma injection in patients with temporomandibular joint osteoarthritis: A systematic review and meta-analysis of randomized controlled trials. Oral Surg Oral Med Oral Pathol Oral Radiol 2019; 127:106–116.
331. Bousnaki M, Bakopoulou A, Koidis P. Platelet-rich plasma for the therapeutic management of temporomandibular joint disorders: A systematic review. Int J Oral Maxillofac Surg 2018;47:188–198.
332. Soares A, Andriolo RB, Atallah AN, da Silva EMK. Botulinum toxin for myofascial pain syndromes in adults. Cochrane Database Syst Rev 2014;7:CD007533.
333. Khalifeh M, Mehta K, Varguise N, Suarez-Durall P, Enciso R. Botulinum toxin type A for the treatment of head and neck chronic myofascial pain syndrome: A systematic review and meta-analysis. J Am Dent Assoc 2016;147:959–973.
334. Patel J, Cardoso JA, Mehta S. A systematic review of botulinum toxin in the management of patients with temporomandibular disorders and bruxism. Br Dent J 2019;226:667–672.
335. Mujakperuo HR, Watson M, Morrison R, Macfarlane TV. Pharmacological interventions for pain in patients with temporomandibular disorders. Cochrane Database Sys Rev 2010;10:CD004715.
336. Herman CR, Schiffman EL, Look JO, Rindal DB. The effectiveness of adding pharmacologic treatment with clonazepam or cyclobenzaprine to patient education and self care for the treatment of jaw pain upon awakening: A randomized clinical trial. J Orofac Pain 2002;16:64–70.
337. Dionne R. Pharmacologic treatments for temporomandibular disorders. Oral Surg Oral Med Oral Pathol Oral Radiol Endod 1997;83:134–142.
338. Arnold L, Palmer R, Gendreau RM, Chen W. Relationships among pain, depressed mood, and global status in fibromyalgia patients: Post hoc analyses of a randomized, placebo-controlled trial of milnacipran. Psychosomatics 2012;53:371–379.
339. Ganzberg S. Pain management part II: Pharmacologic management of chronic orofacial pain. Anesth Prog 2010;57:114–118.
340. Pettengill CA, Reisner-Keller L. The use of tricyclic antidepressants for the control of chronic orofacial pain. Cranio 1997;15:53–56.
341. Mohamed SE, Christensen LV, Penchas J. A randomized double-blind clinical trial of the effect of amitriptyline on nocturnal masseteric motor activity (sleep bruxism). Cranio 1997;15:326–332.

342. Raigrodski AJ, Mohamed SE, Gardiner DM. The effect of amitriptyline on pain intensity and perception of stress in bruxers. J Prosthodont 2001;10:73–77.
343. Cascos-Romero J, Vazquez-Delgado E, Vazquez-Rodríguez E, Gay-Escoda C. The use of tricyclic antidepressants in the treatment of temporomandibular joint disorders: Systematic review of the literature of the last 20 years. Med Oral Patol Oral Cir Bucal 2009;14:E3–E7.
344. Plesh O, Curtis D, Levine J, McCall WD Jr. Amitriptyline treatment of chronic pain in patients with temporomandibular disorders. J Oral Rehabil 2000;27:834–841.
345. Dos Santos Calderon P, Tabaquim MLM, Oliveira LC, Camargo APA, Netto TCR, Conti PCR. Effectiveness of cognitive-behavioral therapy and amitriptyline in patients with chronic temporomandibular disorders: A pilot study. Braz Dent J 2011;22:415–421.
346. Alajbeg IZ, Boric Brakus R, Brakus I. Comparison of amitriptyline with stabilization splint and placebo in chronic TMD patients: A pilot study. Acta Stomatol Croat 2018;52:114–122.
347. Porporatti AL, Costa YM, Réus JC, et al. Placebo and nocebo response magnitude on temporomandibular disorder-related pain: A systematic review and meta-analysis. J Oral Rehabil 2019;46:862–882.
348. Gebhardt S, Heinzel-Gutenbrunner M, König U. Pain relief in depressive disorders: A meta-analysis of the effects of antidepressants. J Clin Psychopharmacol 2016;36:658–668.
349. Patetsos E, Horjales-Araujo E. Treating chronic pain with SSRIs: What do we know? Pain Res Manag 2016;2016:2020915.
350. Banzi R, Cusi C, Randazzo C, Sterzi R, Tedesco D, Moja L. Selective serotonin reuptake inhibitors (SSRIs) and serotonin-norepinephrine reuptake inhibitors (SNRIs) for the prevention of migraine in adults. Cochrane Database Syst Rev 2015;4:CD002919.
351. Garrett AR, Hawley JS. SSRI-associated bruxism: A systematic review of published case reports. Neurol Clin Pract 2018;8:135–141.
352. Johansson Cahlin B, Samuelsson N, Dahlström L. Utilization of pharmaceuticals among patients with temporomandibular disorders: A controlled study. Acta Odontol Scand 2006;64:187–192.
353. Haviv Y, Rettman A, Aframian D, Sharav Y, Benoliel R. Myofascial pain: An open study on the pharmacotherapeutic response to stepped treatment with tricyclic antidepressants and gabapentin. J Oral Facial Pain Headache 2015;29:144–151.
354. Singh JA, Noorbaloochi S, MacDonald R, Maxwell LJ. Chondroitin for osteoarthritis. Cochrane Database Syst Rev 2015;1:CD005614.
355. Hochberg MC, Martel-Pelletier J, Monfort J, et al. Combined chondroitin sulfate and glucosamine for painful knee osteoarthritis: A multicentre, randomised, double-blind, non-inferiority trial versus celecoxib. Ann Rheum Dis 2016;75:37–44.
356. Nguyen P, Mohamed SE, Gardiner D, Salina T. A randomized double-blind clinical trial of the effect of chondroitin sulfate and glucosamine hydrochloride on temporomandibular joint disorders: A pilot study. Cranio 2001;19:130–139.
357. Thie NM, Prasad NG, Major PW. Evaluation of glucosamine sulfate compared to ibuprofen for the treatment of temporomandibular joint osteoarthritis: A randomized double blind controlled 3 month clinical trial. J Rheumatol 2001;28:1347–1355.
358. Cahlin BJ, Dahlström L. No effect of glucosamine sulfate on osteoarthritis in the temporomandibular joints--A randomized, controlled, short-term study. Oral Surg Oral Med Oral Pathol Oral Radiol Endod 2011;112:760–766.
359. Zhu X, Sang L, Wu D, Rong J, Jiang L. Effectiveness and safety of glucosamine and chondroitin for the treatment of osteoarthritis: A meta-analysis of randomized controlled trials. J Orthop Surg Res 2018;13:170.
360. Cömert Kiliç S. Does glucosamine, chondroitin sulfate, and methylsulfonylmethane supplementation improve the outcome of temporomandibular joint osteoarthritis management with arthrocentesis plus intraarticular hyaluronic acid injection. A randomized clinical trial. J Craniomaxillofac Surg 2021;49:711–718.
361. McPherson ML, Cimino NM. Topical NSAID formulations. Pain Med 2013;14(suppl 1):S35–S39.
362. Argoff CE. Topical Analgesics in the Management of Acute and Chronic Pain. Mayo Clin Proc 2013;88:195–205.
363. Senye M, Mir CF, Morton S, Thie NM. Topical nonsteroidal anti-inflammatory medications for treatment of temporomandibular joint degenerative pain: A systematic review. J Orofac Pain 2012;26:26–32.
364. Mena M, Dalbah L, Levi L, Padilla M, Enciso R. Efficacy of topical interventions for temporomandibular disorders compared to placebo or control therapy: A systematic review with meta-analysis. J Dent Anesth Pain Med 2020;20:337–356.
365. Tchivileva IE, Ohrbach R, Fillingim RB, et al. Effect of comorbid migraine on propranolol efficacy for painful TMD in a randomized controlled trial. Cephalalgia 2021;41:839–850.
366. Slade GD, Fillingim RB, Ohrbach R, et al. COMT genotype and efficacy of propranolol for TMD pain: A randomized trial. J Dent Res 2021;100:163–170.
367. Srebro D, Vuckovic S, Milovanovic A, Kosutic J, Vujovic KS, Prostran M. Magnesium in pain research: State of the art. Curr Med Chem 2017;24:424–434.

368. Bujalska-Zadrożny M, Tatarkiewicz J, Kulik K, Filip M, Naruszewicz M. Magnesium enhances opioid-induced analgesia - What we have learnt in the past decades? Eur J Pharm Sci 2017;99:113–127.
369. Carr AC, McCall C. The role of vitamin C in the treatment of pain: New insights. J Transl Med 2017;15:77.
370. Martin KR, Reid DM. Is there role for vitamin D in the treatment of chronic pain? Ther Adv Musculoskelet Dis 2017;9:131–135.
371. Yildiz S, Tumer MK, Yigit S, Nursal AF, Rustemoglu A, Balel Y. Relation of vitamin D and BsmI variant with temporomandibular diseases in the Turkish population. Br J Oral Maxillofac Surg 2021;59:555–560.
372. Kui A, Buduru S, Labunet A, Balhuc S, Negucioiu M. Vitamin D and temporomandibular disorders: What do we know so far? Nutrients 2021;13:1286.
373. Li XI, Dong Z, Zhang F, Dong J, Zhang Y. Vitamin E slows down the progression of osteoarthritis. Exp Ther Med 2016;12:18–22.
374. de Melo LA, Bezerra de Medeiros AK, Campos MFTP, Machado de Resende CMB, Barbosa GAS, Oliveira de Almeida E. Manual therapy in the treatment of myofascial pain related to temporomandibular disorders: A systematic review. J Oral Facial Pain Headache 2020;34:141–148.
375. Calixtre LB, Moreira RFC, Franchini GH, Alburquerque-Sendín F, Oliveira AB. Manual therapy for the management of pain and limited range of motion in subjects with signs and symptoms of temporomandibular disorder: A systematic review of randomised controlled trials. J Oral Rehabil 2015;42:847–861.
376. Paço M, Peleteiro B, Duarte J, Pinho T. The effectiveness of physiotherapy in the management of temporomandibular disorders: A systematic review and meta-analysis. J Oral Facial Pain Headache 2016;30: 210–220.
377. Schmidt JE, Carlson CR, Usery AR, Quevedo AS. Effects of tongue position on mandibular muscle activity and heart rate function. Oral Surg Oral Med Oral Pathol Oral Radiol Endod 2009;108:881–888.
378. Møystad A, Krogstad BS, Larheim TA. Transcutaneous nerve stimulation in a group of patients with rheumatic disease involving the temporomandibular joint. J Prosthet Dent 1990;64:596–600.
379. McNeely ML, Olivo SA, Magee DJ. A systematic review of the effectiveness of physical therapy interventions for temporomandibular disorders. Phys Ther 2006;86:710–725.
380. Olivo SA, Bravo J, Magee DJ, Thie NMR, Major PW, Flores-Mir C. The association between head and cervical posture and temporomandibular disorders: A systematic review. J Orofac Pain 2006;20:9–23.
381. Valdés C, Astaburuaga F, Falace D, Ramirez V, Manns A. Effect of tongue position on masseter and temporalis electromyographic activity during swallowing and maximal voluntary clenching: A cross-sectional study. J Oral Rehabil 2014;41:881–889.
382. Valdés C, Gutiérrez M, Falace D, Astaburuaga F, Manns A. The effect of tongue position and resulting vertical dimension on masticatory muscle activity. A cross-sectional study. J Oral Rehabil 2013;40:650–656.
383. Armijo-Olivo S, Pitance L, Singh V, Neto F, Thie N, Michelotti A. Effectiveness of manual therapy and therapeutic exercise for temporomandibular disorders: Systematic review and meta-analysis. Phys Ther 2016;96:9–25.
384. Lindfors E, Magnusson T, Ernberg M. Effect of therapeutic jaw exercises in the treatment of masticatory myofascial pain: A randomized controlled study. J Oral Facial Pain Headache 2020;34:364–373.
385. Kraus SL. Physical therapy management of TMD. In: Kraus SL (ed). Temporomandibular Disorders, ed 2. New York: Churchill Livingstone, 1994:161–215.
386. Haketa T, Kino K, Sugisaki M, Takaoka M, Ohta T. Randomized clinical trial of treatment for TMJ disc displacement. J Dent Res 2010;89:1259–1263.
387. Okeson JP. Management of Temporomandibular Disorders and Occlusion, ed 7. St Louis: Mosby, 2013.
388. Wright E. Manual of Temporomandibular Disorders, ed 3. Hoboken: Wiley-Blackwell, 2014.
389. Minagi S, Nozaki S, Sato T, Tsuru H. A manipulation technique for treatment of anterior disc displacement without reduction. J Prosthet Dent 1991;65:686–691.
390. Saranya B, Ahmed J, Shenoy N, Ongole R, Sujir N, Natarajan S. Comparison of transcutaneous electric nerve stimulation (TENS) and microcurrent nerve stimulation (MENS) in the management of masticatory muscle pain: A comparative study. Pain Res Manag 2019;2019:8291624.
391. Mohl ND, Ohrbach RK, Crow HC, Gross AJ. Devices for diagnosis and treatment of temporomandibular disorders: Part III, Thermography, ultrasound, electrical stimulation, and EMG biofeedback. J Prosthet Dent 1990;63:472–477.
392. Ziskin MC, McDiarmid T, Michlovitz SL. Therapeutic ultrasound. In: Michlovitz SL (ed). Thermal Agents in Rehabilitation, ed 2. Philidelphia: FA Davis, 1990: 134–169.
393. Hartley A. Ultrasound, A Monograph. Chattanooga Group, 1991:1–35.
394. Mannheimer JS. Therapeutic modalities. In: Kraus SL (ed). TMJ Disorders: Management of the Craniomandibular Complex. London: Churchill Livingstone, 1988:311–337.

395. Cameron MH, Monroe LG. Relative transmission of ultrasound by media customarily used for phonophoresis. Phys Ther 1992;72:142–148.
396. van der Windt DAWM, van der Heijden GJMG, van den Berg SGM, Riet GT, de Winter AF, Bouter LM. Ultrasound therapy for musculoskeletal disorders: A systematic review. Pain 1999;81:257–271.
397. Hussain H, Crow H, Gonzalez Y, McCall WD Jr. Immediate effect of continuous ultrasound vs sham ultrasound for bilateral masseter myalgia: A double-blinded trial. J Oral Facial Pain Headache 2018;32: 304–308.
398. Ebadi S, Henschke N, Forogh B, et al. Therapeutic ultrasound for chronic low back pain. Cochrane Database Syst Rev 2020;7:CD009169.
399. Lark MR, Gangaros LP Sr. Iontophoresis: An effective modality for the treatment of inflammatory disorders of the temporomandibular joint and myofascial pain. Cranio 1990;8:108–119.
400. Reid KI, Dionne RA, Sicard-Rosenbaum L, Lord D, Dubner RA. Evaluation of iontophoretically applied dexamethasone for painful pathologic temporomandibular joints. Oral Surg Oral Med Oral Pathol 1994; 77:605–609.
401. Schiffman EL, Braun BL, Lindgren BR. Temporomandibular joint iontophoresis: A double-blind randomized clinical trial. J Orofac Pain 1996;10(2):157–165.
402. Jaeger B, Reeves JL. Quantification of changes in myofascial trigger point sensitivity with pressure algometer following passive stretch. Pain 1986;27: 203–210.
403. Koole P, Zonnenberg AJJ, Koole R. Spray and stretch technique and its effects on mouth opening. J Prosthet Dent 2020;123:455–460.
404. Carlson CR, Okeson JP, Falace DA, Nitz AJ, Lindroth JE. Reduction of pain and EMG activity in the masseter region by trapezius trigger point injection. Pain 1993;55:397–400.
405. Hong CZ. Lidocaine injection versus dry needling to myofascial trigger point. The importance of the local twitch response. Am J Phys Med Rehabil 1994;73: 256–263.
406. Scicchitano J, Rounsefell B, Plilowsky I. Baseline correlates of the response to the treatment of chronic localized myofascial pain syndrome by injection of local anesthetic. J Psychosom Res 1996;40:75–85.
407. Hong CZ. Treatment of myofascial pain syndrome. Curr Pain Headache Rep 2006;10:345–349.
408. Zink W, Graf BM. Local anesthetic myotoxicity. Reg Anesth Pain Med 2004;29:333–340.
409. Ge HY, Fernández-de-Las-Peñas C, Yue SW. Myofascial trigger points: Spontaneous electrical activity and its consequences for pain induction and propagation. Chin Med 2011;6:13.
410. Sabatke S, Scola RH, Paiva ES, Kowacs PA. Injection of trigger points in the temporal muscles of patients with miofascial syndrome. Arq Neuropsiquiatr 2015;73:861–866.
411. Montes-Carmona JF, Gonzalez-Perez LM, Infante-Cossio P. Treatment of localized and referred masticatory myofascial pain with botulinum toxin injection. Toxins (Basel) 2020;13:6.
412. Fernandes AC, Duarte Moura DM, Da Silva LGD, De Almeida EO, Barbosa GAS. Acupuncture in temporomandibular disorder myofascial pain treatment: A systematic review. J Oral Facial Pain Headache 2017;31:225–232.
413. Jung A, Shin BC, Lee MS, Sim H, Ernst E. Acupuncture for treating temporomandibular joint disorders: A systematic review and meta-analysis of randomized, sham-controlled trials. J Dent 2011;39:341–350.
414. Wu JY, Zhang C, Xu YP, et al. Acupuncture therapy in the management of the clinical outcomes for temporomandibular disorders A PRISMA-compliant meta-analysis. Medicine (Baltimore) 2017;96:e6064.
415. Mackler LS, Collender SL. Therapeutic uses of light in rehabilitation. In: Michlovitz SL (ed). Thermal Agents in Rehabilitation. Philidelphia: FA Davis, 1996:255–277.
416. Petrucci A, Sgolastra F, Gatto R, Mattei A, Monaco A. Effectiveness of low-level laser therapy in temporomandibular disorders: A systematic review and meta-analysis. J Orofac Pain 2011;25:298–307.
417. Marini I, Gatto MR, Bonetti GA. Effects of superpulsed low-level laser therapy on temporomandibular joint pain. Clin J Pain 2010;26:611–616.
418. Öz S, Gökçen-Röhlig B, Saruhanoglu A, Tuncer EB. Management of myofascial pain: Low-level laser therapy versus occlusal splints. J Craniofac Surg 2010;21:1722–1728.
419. Tunér J, Hosseinpour S, Fekrazad R. Photobiomodulation in temporomandibular disorders. Photobiomodul Photomed Laser Surg 2019;37:826–836.
420. Klasser GD, Greene CS, Lavigne GJ. Oral appliances and the management of sleep bruxism in adults: A century of clinical applications and search for mechanisms. Int J Prosthodont 2010;23:453–462.
421. Riley P, Glenny AM, Worthington HV, et al. Oral splints for patients with temporomandibular disorders or bruxism: A systematic review and economic evaluation. Health Technol Assess 2020;24:1–224.
422. Zhang C, Wu JY, Deng DL, et al. Efficacy of splint therapy for the management of temporomandibular disorders: A meta-analysis. Oncotarget 2016;7:84043–84053.
423. Zhang SH, He KX, Lin CJ, et al. Efficacy of occlusal splints in the treatment of temporomandibular disorders: A systematic review of randomized controlled trials. Acta Odontol Scand 2020;78:580–589.

424. Clark GT. A critical evaluation of orthopedic interocclusal appliance therapy: Design, theory and overall effectiveness. J Am Dent Assoc 1984;108:359–364.
425. Dao TT, Lavigne GJ. Oral splints: The crutches for temporomandibular disorders and bruxism? Crit Rev Oral Biol Med 1998;9:345–361.
426. Türp JC, Komine F, Hugger A. Efficacy of stabilization splints for the management of patients with masticatory muscle pain: A qualitative systematic review. Clin Oral Investig 2004;8:179–195.
427. Forssell H, Kalso E, Koskela P, Vehmanen R, Puuka P, Alanen P. Occlusal treatments in temporomandibular disorders: A qualitative systematic review of randomized controlled trials. Pain 1999;83:549–560.
428. Forssell H, Kalso E. Application of principles of evidence based medicine to occlusal treatment for temporomandibular disorders: Are there lessons to be learned? J Orofac Pain 2004;18:9–22.
429. Ebrahim S, Montoya L, Busse J, Carrasco-Labra A, Guyatt GH, Medically Unexplained Syndromes Research Group. The effectiveness of splint therapy in patients with temporomandibular disorders: A systematic review and meta-analysis. J Am Dent Assoc 2012;143:847–857.
430. Eliassen M, Hjortsjö C, Olsen-Bergem H, Bjørnland T. Self-exercise programmes and occlusal splints in the treatment of TMD-related myalgia-Evidence-based medicine? J Oral Rehabil 2019;46:1088–1094.
431. Alkhutari AS, Alyahya A, Rodrigues Conti PC, Christidis N, Al-Moraissi EA. Is the therapeutic effect of occlusal stabilization appliances more than just placebo effect in the management of painful temporomandibular disorders? A network meta-analysis of randomized clinical trials [epub ahead of print 16 Oct 2020]. J Prosthet Dent doi:10.1016/j.prosdent.2020.08.015.
432. Abbott DM, Bush FM. Occlusions altered by removable appliances. J Am Dent Assoc 1991;122:79–81.
433. Brown DT, Gaudet EL Jr, Phillips C. Changes in vertical tooth position and face height related to long term anterior repositioning splint therapy. Cranio 1994;12:19–22.
434. Greene CS, Laskin DM. Long-term evaluation of treatment for myofascial pain-dysfunction syndrome: A comparative analysis. J Am Dent Assoc 1983;107: 235–238.
435. Ekberg E, Vallon D, Nilner M. Treatment outcome of headache after occlusal appliance therapy in a randomized controlled trial among patients with temporomandibular disorders of mainly arthrogenous origin. Swed Dent J 2002;26:115–124.
436. Linde C, Isacsson G, Jonsson BG. Outcome of 6-week treatment with transcutaneous electric nerve stimulation compared with splint on symptomatic temporomandibular joint disk displacement without reduction. Acta Odontol Scand 1995;53:92–98.
437. Ekberg EC, Nilner M. Treatment outcome of short- and long-term appliance therapy in patients with TMD of myogenous origin and tension-type headache. J Oral Rehabil 2006;33:713–721.
438. Ström D, Behrenth E, Ekman K, Johansson A, Unell L, Carlsson GE. Management of tinnitus and jaw-muscle tenderness using an intraoral appliance and acupuncture. Swed Dent J 2013;37:105–110.
439. Kuttila M, Le Bell Y, Savolainen-Niemi E, Kuttila S, Alanen P. Efficiency of occlusal appliance therapy in secondary otalgia and temporomandibular disorders. Acta Odontol Scand 2002;60:248–254.
440. Saha FJ, Pulla A, Ostermann T, Miller T, Dobos G, Cramer H. Effects of occlusal splint therapy in patients with migraine or tension-type headache and comorbid temporomandibular disorder: A randomized controlled trial. Medicine (Baltimore) 2019;98:e16805.
441. Okeson JP. The effects of hard and soft splints on nocturnal bruxism. J Am Dent Assoc 1987;114:788–791.
442. Shi C, Wang HY. Influence of an occlusal splint on integrated electromyography of the masseter muscles. J Oral Rehabil 1991;18:253–256.
443. Jokubauskas L, Baltrušaitytė A, Pileičikienė G. Oral appliances for managing sleep bruxism in adults: A systematic review from 2007 to 2017. J Oral Rehabil 2018;45:81–95.
444. Carlson N, Moline D, Huber L, Jacobsen J. Comparison of muscle activity between conventional and neuromuscular splints. J Prosthet Dent 1993;70:39–43.
445. Kirk WS Jr. Magnetic resonance imaging and tomographic evaluation of occlusal appliance treatment for advanced internal derangement of the temporomandibular joint. J Oral Maxillofac Surg 1991;49:9–12.
446. Chung SC, Kim HS. The effect of stabilization splint on the TMJ closed lock. Cranio 1993;11:95–101.
447. Tecco S, Festa F, Salini V, Epifania E, D'Attilio M. Treatment of joint pain and joint noises associated with a recent TMJ internal derangement: A comparison of an anterior repositioning splint, a full-arch maxillary stabilization splint, and an untreated control group. Cranio 2004;22:209–219.
448. Kircos LT, Ortendahl DA, Mark AS, Arakawa M. Magnetic resonance imaging of the TMJ disc in asymptomatic volunteers. J Oral Maxillofac Surg 1987;45:852–854.
449. Al-Moraissi EA, Farea R, Qasem KA, Al-Wadeai MS, Al-Sabahi ME, Al-Iryani GM. Effectiveness of occlusal splint therapy in the management of temporomandibular disorders: Network meta-analysis of randomized controlled trials. Int J Oral Maxillofac Surg 2020; 49:1042–1056.

450. Truelove E, Huggins KH, Manci L, Dworkin SF. The efficacy of traditional, low-cost and nonsplint therapies for temporomandibular disorder. A randomized controlled trial. J Am Dent Assoc 2006;137:1099–1107.
451. Wright EF. Using soft splints in your dental practice. Gen Dent 1999;47:506–510.
452. Klasser GD, Greene CS. Oral appliances in the management of temporomandibular disorders. Oral Surg Oral Med Oral Pathol Oral Radiol Endod 2009;107(2):212–223.
453. Ingerslev H. Functional disturbances of the masticatory system in school children. J Dent Child 1983;50: 446–450.
454. Shankland WE. Nociceptive trigeminal inhibition—Tension supression system: A method of preventing migraine and tension headaches. Compend Contin Educ Dent 2002;23:105–108.
455. Lukic N, Saxer T, Hou MY, Wojcyńska AZ, Gallo LM, Colombo V. Short-term effects of NTI-tss and Michigan splint on nocturnal jaw muscle activity: A pilot study [epub ahead of print 25 Dec 2020]. Clin Exp Dent Res doi:10.1002/cre2.371.
456. Shankland WE. Nociceptive trigeminal inhibition—Tension supression system: A method of preventing migraine and tension headaches. Compend Contin Educ Dent 2001;22:1075–1080.
457. Magnusson T, Adiels AM, Nilsson HL, Helkimo M. Treatment effect on signs and symptoms of temporomandibular disorders--Comparison between stabilization splint and a new type of splint (NTI). A pilot study. Swed Dent J 2004;28:11–20.
458. Hasanoglu Erbasar GN, Alpaslan C, Eroglu Inan G. Can an NTI-tss device be effective as a first-line therapy in patients with TMD myofascial pain? J Oral Rehabil 2017;44:589–593.
459. Stapelmann H, Türp J. The NTI-tss device for the therapy of bruxism, temporomandibular disorders, and headache - where do we stand? A qualitative systematic review of the literature. BMC Oral Health 2008;29:22.
460. Greene CS, Menchel HF. The use of oral appliances in the management of temporomandibular disorders. Oral Maxillofac Surg Clin North Am 2018;30:265–277.
461. Gelb ML, Gelb H. Gelb appliance: Mandibular orthopedic repositioning therapy. Cranio Clin Int 1991;1: 81–98.
462. Anderson GC, Schulte JK, Goodkind RJ. Comparative study of two treatment methods for internal derangements of the TMJ. J Prosthet Dent 1985;53:392–397.
463. Bereznicki T, Barry E, Wilson NHF. Unintended changes to the occlusion following the provision of night guards. Br Dent J 2018;225:715–722.
464. Clark GT. The TMJ repositioning appliance: A technique for construction, insertion, and adjustment. Cranio 1986;4:37–46.
465. Clark GT. Treatment of jaw clicking with temporomandibular repositioning: Analysis of 25 cases. J Craniomandibular Pract 1984;2:263–270.
466. Tallents RH, Katzberg RW, Macher DJ, Roberts CA. Use of protrusive splint therapy in anterior disc displacement of the temporomandibular joint: A 1- to 3-year follow-up. J Prosthet Dent 1990;63:336–341.
467. Eberhard D, Bantleon HP, Steger W. The efficacy of anterior repositioning splint therapy studied by magnetic resonance imaging. Eur J Orthod 2002;24: 343–352.
468. Simmons HC 3rd, Gibbs SJ. Anterior repositioning appliance therapy for TMJ disorders: Specific symptoms relieved and relationship to disk status on MRI. Cranio 2005;23:89–99.
469. Orenstein ES. Anterior repositioning appliances when used for anterior disc displacement with reduction--A critical review. Cranio 1993;11:141–145.
470. Santacatterina A, Paoli M, Peretta R, Bambace A, Beltrame A. A comparison between horizontal splint and repositioning splint in the treatment of 'disc dislocation with reduction'. Literature meta-analysis. J Oral Rehabil 1998;25:81–88.
471. Okeson JP. Long-term treatment of disk-interference disorders of the temporomandibular joint with anterior repositioning occlusal splints. J Prosthet Dent 1988; 60:611–616.
472. Summer JD, Westesson PL. Mandibular repositioning can be effective in treatment of reducing TMJ disc displacement. A long-term clinical and MR imaging follow-up. Cranio 1997;15:107–120.
473. Widmalm SE. Use and abuse of bite splints. Compend Contin Educ Dent 1999;20:249–254, 256, 258–259.
474. Greene CS, Obrez A. Treating temporomandibular disorders with permanent mandibular repositioning: Is it medically necessary? Review. Oral Surg Oral Med Oral Pathol Oral Radiol 2015;119:489–498.
475. Helkimo E, Westling L. History, clinical findings, and outcome of treatment of patients with anterior disc displacement. Cranio 1987;5:269–276.
476. List T, Axelsson S. Management of TMD: Evidence from systematic reviews and meta-analyses. J Oral Rehabil 2010;37:430–451.
477. Luther F, Layton S, McDonald F. Orthodontics for treating temporomandibular joint (TMJ) disorders. Cochrane Database Syst Rev 2010;7:CD006541.
478. De Boever JA, Carlsson GE, Klineberg IJ. Need for occlusal therapy and prosthodontic treatment in the management of temporomandibular disorders. Part II: Tooth loss and prosthodontic treatment. J Oral Rehabil 2000;27:647–659.

479. Pullinger A, Seligman DA, Gornbein JA. A multiple logistic regression analysis of the risk and relative odds of temporomandibular disorders as a function of common occlusal features. J Dent Res 1993;72: 968–979.
480. Stohler CS, Zarb GA. On the management of temporomandibular disorders: A plea for a low-tech, high-prudence therapeutic approach. J Orofac Pain 1999; 13:255–261.
481. Athanasiou AE, Melsen B, Eriksen J. Concerns, motivation and experiences of orthognathic surgery patients: A retrospective study of 152 patients. Int J Adult Orthod Orthognath Surg 1989;2:47–55.
482. Ochs MW, La Banc JP, Dolwick MF. The diagnosis and management of concomitant dentofacial deformity and temporomandibular disorder. Oral Maxillofac Surg Clin North Am 1990;2:669–690.
483. Magnusson T, Ahbort G, Svartz K. Function of the masticatory system in 20 patients with mandibular hypo- or hyperplasia after correction by sagittal split osteotomy. Int J Oral Maxillofac Surg 1990;19:289–293.
484. Al-Moraissi EA, Wolford LM, Perez D, Laskin DM, Ellis E 3rd. Does orthognathic surgery cause or cure temporomandibular disorders? A systematic review and meta-analysis. J Oral Maxillofac Surg 2017;75: 1835–1847.
485. Bouloux G, Koslin MG, Ness G, Shafer D. Temporomandibular joint surgery. J Oral Maxillofac Surg 2017;75:e195–e223.
486. Laskin DM. Arthroscopy versus arthrocentesis for treating internal derangements of the temporomandibular joint. Oral Maxillofac Surg Clin North Am 2018;30:325–328.
487. Nitzan DW, Price A. The use of arthrocentesis for the treatment of osteoarthritis of the temporomandibular joints. J Oral Maxillofac Surg 2001;59:1154–1159.
488. Trieger N, Hoffman CH, Rodriguez E. The effect of arthrocentesis of the temporomandibular joint in patients with rheumatoid arthritis. J Oral Maxillofac Surg 1999;57:537–540.
489. Al-Belasy FA, Dolwick MF. Arthrocentesis for the treatment of temporomandibular joint closed lock: A review article. Int J Oral Maxillofac Surg 2007;36:773–782.
490. Monje-Gil F, Nitzan D, González-Garcia R. Temporomandibular joint arthrocentesis. Review of the literature. Med Oral Patol Oral Cir Bucal 2012;17:e575–581.
491. Bergstrand S, Ingstad HK, Møystad A, Bjørnland T. Long-term effectiveness of arthrocentesis with and without hyaluronic acid injection for treatment of temporomandibular joint osteoarthritis. J Oral Sci 2019;61:82–88.
492. Al-Moraissi EA, Wolford LM, Ellis E 3rd, Neff A. The hierarchy of different treatments for arthrogenous temporomandibular disorders: A network meta-analysis of randomized clinical trials. J Craniomaxillofac Surg 2020;48:9–23.
493. Blaustein D, Heffez L. Diagnostic arthroscopy to the temporomandibular joint. Part II. Arthroscopic find ings of arthographically diagnosed disc displacement. Oral Surg Oral Med Oral Pathol 1988;65:135–141.
494. Ohnuki T, Fukuda M, Nakata A, et al. Evaluation of the position, mobility, and morphology of the disc by MRI before and after four different treatments for temporomandibular joint disorders. Dentomaxillofac Radiol 2006;35:103–109.
495. Loureiro Sato FR, Tralli G. Arthroscopic discopexy technique with anchors for treatment of temporomandibular joint internal derangement: Clinical and magnetic resonance imaging evaluation. J Craniomaxillofac Surg 2020 May;48:501–507.
496. Undt G, Murakami K, Rasse M, Ewers R. Open versus arthroscopic surgery for internal derangement of the temporomandibular joint: A retrospective study comparing two centres' results using the Jaw Pain and Function Questionnaire. J Craniomaxillofac Surg 2006;34:234–241.
497. Politi M, Sembronio S, Robiony M, Costa F, Toro C, Undt G. High condylectomy and disc repositioning compared to arthroscopic lysis, lavage, and capsular stretch for the treatment of chronic closed lock of the temporomandibular joint. Oral Surg Oral Med Oral Pathol Oral Radiol Endod 2007;103:27–33.
498. Al-Moraissi EA. Arthroscopy versus arthrocentesis in the management of internal derangement of the temporomandibular joint: A systematic review and meta-analysis. Int J Oral Maxillofac Surg 2015;44: 104–112.
499. Haigler MC, Abdulrehman E, Siddappa S, Kishore R, Padilla M, Enciso R. Use of platelet-rich plasma, platelet-rich growth factor with arthrocentesis or arthroscopy to treat temporomandibular joint osteoarthritis: Systematic review with meta-analyses. J Am Dent Assoc 2018;149:940–952.e2.
500. Buckley MJ, Merrill RG, Braun TW. Surgical management of internal derangement of the temporomandibular joint. J Oral Maxillofac Surg 1993;51(suppl 1):20–27.
501. Anderson DM, Sinclair PM, McBride KM. A clinical evaluation of temporomandibular joint disk plication surgery. Am J Orthod Dentofac Orthop 1991;100: 156–162.
502. Hall HD, Nickerson JW, McKenna SJ. Modified condylotomy for treatment of the painful temporomandibular joint with a reducing point. J Oral Maxillofac Surg 1993;51:133–142.

503. Trumpy IG, Lyberg T. Surgical treatment of internal derangement of the temporomandibular joint: Long-term evaluation of three techniques. J Oral Maxillofac Surg 1995;53:740–746.
504. Krug J, Jirousek Z, Suchmová H, Cermáková E. Influence of discoplasty and discectomy of the temporomandibular joint on elimination of pain and restricted mouth opening. Acta Medica (Hradec Kralove) 2004; 47:47–53.
505. Silver CM. Long-term results of meniscectomy of the temporomandibular joint. Cranio 1984;3:46–57.
506. Eriksson L, Westesson PL. Long-term evaluation of meniscectomy of the temporomandibular joint. J Oral Maxillofac Surg 1985;43:263–269.
507. Hall HD. The role of discetomy for treating internal derangements of the temporomandibular joint. Oral Maxillofac Surg Clin North Am 1994;6:287–294.
508. Takaku S, Sano T, Yoshida M. Long-term magnetic resonance imaging after temporomandibular joint discectomy without replacement. J Oral Maxillofac Surg 2000;58:739–745.
509. Dimitroulis G. The use of dermis grafts after discectomy for internal derangement of the temporomandibular joint. J Oral Maxillofac Surg 2005;63:173–178.
510. Nickerson JW, Veaco NS. Condylotomy in surgery of the temporomandibular joint. Oral Maxillofac Surg Clin North Am 1989;1:303–327.
511. Nickerson JW. The role of condylotomy in the management of temporomandibular joint disorders. In: Worthington P, Evans J (eds). Controversies in Oral and Maxillofacial Surgery. Philadelphia: Saunders, 1994.
512. Hall HD. A technique to improve predictability of condylar position with modified condylotomy. Oral Surg Oral Med Oral Pathol Oral Radiol Endod 1999; 88:127–128.
513. Hall HD, Navarro EZ, Gibbs SJ. Prospective study of modified condylotomy for treatment of nonreducing disk displacement. Oral Surg Oral Med Oral Pathol Oral Radiol Endod 2000;89:147–158.
514. Hall HD, Navarro EZ, Gibbs SJ. One- and three-year prospective outcome study of modified condylotomy for treatment of reducing disc displacement. J Oral Maxillofac Surg 2000;58:7–17.
515. Johnson NR, Roberts MJ, Doi SA, Batstone MD. Total temporomandibular joint replacement prostheses: A systematic review and bias-adjusted meta-analysis. Int J Oral Maxillofac Surg 2017;46:86–92.
516. Zou L, He D, Ellis E. A comparison of clinical follow-up of different total temporomandibular joint replacement prostheses: A systematic review and meta-analysis. J Oral Maxillofac Surg 2018;76:294–303.
517. Elledge R, Mercuri LG, Attard A, Green J, Speculand B. Review of emerging temporomandibular joint total joint replacement systems. Br J Oral Maxillofac Surg 2019;57:722–728.
518. Springer BD, Sotile WM. The psychology of total joint arthroplasty. J Arthroplasty 2020;35:S46–S49.

9

Cervical Spinal Disorders and Associated Headaches

Key points

- Structures of the cervical spine can give rise to orofacial pain and headache disorders.
- A screening examination of the cervical spine is recommended if there is coexisting neck pain and temporomandibular disorder (TMD) pain.
- Specific and individualized interventions consisting of exercises, manual therapy, postural correction, and a home exercise program can assist the clinician in effectively managing cervical spinal disorders to reduce pain, restore function, and prevent recurrence of complaints.
- Referral is recommended when cervical spine involvement is suspected in the development of orofacial pain complaints.

Disorders of the musculoskeletal structures of the cervical spine can contribute to the development and perpetuation of orofacial pain complaints and various headaches. Therefore, the clinician should be able to distinguish different types of neck pain, understand the mechanisms of concurrent cervical spinal pain and orofacial pain, perform a screening evaluation of the cervical spine, and initiate appropriate referral for further evaluation and comprehensive management when indicated.

Defining Cervical Spine Disorders

Cervical spine disorders (CSDs) encompass a wide variety of disorders involving the musculoskeletal structures, discs, and nerves of the cervical spine. The most common symptoms of a CSD are neck pain and movement limitations. Head movements or sustained head postures usually aggravate the pain. Although neck pain may be a feature of virtually every disorder or disease of the upper quadrant, it is only rarely a symptom of a serious pathology such as a tumor or infection. Pain originating in the neck can radiate toward the head, trunk, or upper limbs.

Subclassification of CSDs includes an extensive list of diagnostic terms, such as *cervicalgia*, *cervical sprain/strain*, *discogenic disease*, and *facet syndrome*.[1] In the absence of pathology or systemic disease, neck pain is usually referred to as *nonspecific*. For the most common types of neck pain, the Neck Pain Task Force introduced a classification system to facilitate communication among health care professionals (Box 9-1).[2,3] This classification system differs from earlier classification systems for neck pain and lower back pain in that the decision for further assessment and treatment depends not only on the clinical signs, but also on the presence of disability.[4,5]

This chapter presents common CSDs that may be associated with orofacial pain or headaches and provides questionnaires to rate the level of disability related to neck pain. Together, these tools will assist the clinician to assess whether the cervical spine is involved in the patients' orofacial pain complaints and whether referral for additional assessments or treatment is indicated.

Box 9-1 Neck Pain Task Force classification system for neck pain[2]

Grade I
- Neck pain without signs of pathology, low disability
- Likely to respond to minimal intervention, such as reassurance and pain control
- Does not require intensive investigations or ongoing treatment

Grade II
- Neck pain without signs of pathology, high disability
- Requires pain relief and early activation aimed at preventing long-term disability

Grade III
- Neck pain with neurologic signs
- Might require investigation and, occasionally, more invasive treatments

Grade IV
- Neck pain with signs of pathology, such as fracture, infection, myelopathy, neoplasm, or systemic disease
- Requires prompt investigation and treatment

Note: This chart provides an overview of the classification system. For the full description, see the original report.[3]

Epidemiology of CSDs

Most people will experience some neck pain in their lifetimes, but for the majority, neck pain will not seriously interfere with daily activities.[2] One-year prevalence estimates of neck pain range from 30% to 50% in the general population, while 1-year incidence estimates of neck pain with associated disability range from 2% to 15%.[2] The annual rate of resolution of neck pain is estimated around 37%, and another 33% report improvement.[6] The prevalence of neck pain increases with age up to the fifth decade and then decreases.[2,7] Women are more likely than men to develop neck pain, more likely to suffer from persistent neck problems and less likely to experience resolution.[2,6,7] Between 50% and 85% of those who experience neck pain at one point will report neck pain again 1 to 5 years later.[8–10] In office workers, dentists, and professional drivers, higher prevalence of neck pain is reported as compared to other occupations.[11-14] Low satisfaction with the workplace environment, low work task variation, keyboard position close to the body, and self-perceived medium/high muscular tension are reported as risk factors for office workers for the development of neck pain.[14]

Relationship Between CSDs and Orofacial Pain

Many studies have reported the coexistence of TMDs and CSD symptoms.[15-17] In a large study of the general Dutch population, complaints of neck pain were twice as prevalent in patients with TMD pain (71% to 85%) compared to persons without TMD pain (39%).[18] A case-control study on adolescent TMD patients also revealed a prevalence for neck pain over twice that in controls of the same age and sex.[19] Both studies also found strong associations with headache, back pain, and widespread pain. In addition, a strong relationship was found between neck disability and jaw disability.[20] A recent review has emphasized neuronal convergence of the trigeminal and cervical spine sensory pathways as well as central sensitization processes as being mainly responsible for the association between TMD and CSD.[16] This affects pain management in these patients, and consequently, multidisciplinary approaches are warranted for patients with comorbid conditions.[16,20]

Peripheral and central sensitization

Sensitization of the nervous system occurs when persistent nociceptive facilitation exceeds its inhibitory capacity. In this situation, a spectrum of neuroplastic changes occurs, such as lowered nerve thresholds, enlarged receptive fields, and changed gene expression. *Peripheral sensitization* refers to the situation of increased responsiveness and reduced threshold of peripheral neurons.[21] *Central sensitization* refers to the increased responsiveness of nociceptive neurons in the central nervous system to their afferent input.[22] Patients may have *allodynia* (pain caused by stimuli that normally would not be perceived as painful) and *hyperalgesia* (exaggerated pain responses to painful stimuli). For more details on sensitization, see chapter 1.

Craniofacial pain is mediated by the upper cervical nerves; the sinuvertebral nerves of C1 to C3; and cranial nerves V, VII, IX, X, XI, and XII. Additional innervation is provided by sympathetic afferents that course with the first two thoracic nerves synapsing in the trigeminal nucleus, as well as parasympathetic afferents traveling with cranial nerves VII and IX.[23] Afferents of the cervical spinal nerves and the trigeminal nerve converge in the trigeminal spinal nuclei.[23] Consequently, nociceptive input from cervical structures can be referred to the orofacial region, and vice versa. Several experimental studies have demonstrated this mechanism. For example, Piovesan et al[24] showed that after painful stimulation of the greater occipital nerve, the participants experienced pain not only in the innervation area of that nerve but also into the projection area of the trigeminal nerve (ophthalmic division, V1 distribution). In another study,[25] glutamate-evoked pain in the splenius capitis muscle (innervated by C3 and C4) caused referral of pain to the temporal region. Even though glutamate injections into the masseter muscle (innervated by the mandibular division of the trigeminal nerve, V3) did not result in referral of pain to the neck region in that particular study, other studies have provided evidence for a bidirectional relationship in convergence of afferents from the trigeminal and upper cervical neural systems.[26-29]

Genetics

For both experimental pain and clinical pain, evidence for the contribution of genetic factors to individual differences in pain is evolving.[30] For TMD pain, there is culminating evidence for a genetic predisposition.[31] In 2011, Maixner et al[32] presented a model for the development of TMD pain that proposed TMD pain to be influenced by psychologic distress and pain amplification (eg, allodynia, hyperalgesia, and central sensitization), which in turn are subject to genetic regulation and environmental input. The mechanisms contributing to pain amplification are thought to relate to a decreased function in pain inhibition as well as increased function of pain-facilitating pathways. An example of such a pain inhibitory system is the serotonergic system. A recent study has been able to replicate earlier findings that a polymorphic variant (ie, the CC genotype) of the 5-hydroxytryptamine receptor 2A (*5HTR2A*) gene is more prevalent in TMD pain patients than in controls.[33] The serotonin receptor is suggested to have antinociceptive effects. Lower serotoninergic activity (eg, by less active postsynaptic receptors) may therefore lead to a decreased ability to stimulate the central descending analgesic system and result in higher levels of pain.[34] Another candidate gene for involvement in musculoskeletal pain is the catechol-O-methyltransferase (*COMT*) gene. Variants of this gene are reported to be associated with fibromyalgia, neck pain, and TMD pain.[30,35-37]

Biomechanical relationship

The cranium and the mandible both have muscular and ligament attachments to the cervical area, forming a functional system called the *craniocervical mandibular system* or *stomatognathic system*. Because of this close functional coupling, changes in the activity of the neck muscles and head position influence the activity of the masticatory muscles and jaw function, and vice versa.[38] When the mandible is at rest, its position is determined by the viscoelasticity of the muscles and the postural muscle tone acting on the mandible.[38] With an upright head position, the relaxed mandible maintains a fairly constant distance from the maxilla of approximately 2 to 5 mm.[39] When the head is held in a forward position, the condyles are pulled slightly downward during open-close movements.[40] Jaw opening and closing movements, as during eating, are accompanied by respective extension and flexion of the head, and several neck muscles are coactivated during jaw clenching.[41-43]

As a result of these cranio-cervico-mandibular relationships and the coexistence of TMDs and CSDs, poor head posture (mostly a forward head posture) and overload of the cervical spinal musculature have been suggested as etiologic factors for TMDs.[44,45] Clinical studies investigating such relationships, however, show contradictory results.[46] Even though some authors have reported small differences in head posture between TMD patients and healthy controls, the clinical relevance of these differences has been disputed, and other studies did not even find differences in head posture between TMD patients and controls.[20,47–49] So although there

Box 9-2 Red flags for serious pathology in neck pain patients with no exposure to blunt trauma[2]

- Pathologic fractures (eg, resulting from decreased bone density caused by osteoporosis or corticosteroid treatment)
- Neoplasms (eg, previous history of cancer, unexplained weight loss)
- Failure to improve after a month of evidence-based therapy
- Cervical myelopathy
- Systemic diseases (eg, inflammatory arthritis)
- Infections
- Intractable pain or tenderness over the vertebral body
- Prior neck surgery

is vast evidence showing the functional coupling between the musculoskeletal structures of the cervical spine and the masticatory system, there is only weak evidence for a direct biomechanical mechanism (eg, the effect of poor head posture on the masticatory system) as a cause for TMDs.[17,46]

Conclusion

There is solid evidence supporting the comorbid relationship between TMD and CSD. Pain mechanisms (ie, central sensitization and neuronal convergence) are the most likely explanation for the comorbid presentation of these disorders,[6] which in turn are subject to genetic regulation and environmental input.[32] These imposed challenges in clinical practice favor an integrated approach to the management of TMD patients with comorbid CSD. Therefore, a multidisciplinary approach including an assessment of the cervical spine by a physical therapist is highly recommended for these patients.

Screening of the Cervical Spine

As described in Box 9-1, the Task Force on Neck Pain introduced a four-grade classification system of neck pain severity. Because few major differences were found between trauma-related neck pain and neck pain with a nontraumatic etiology, the classification is recommended for all individuals who seek clinical care for neck pain.[2] To use the classification system, information is needed on serious pathology, disability, and signs of nerve compression.

Serious pathology

For patients without exposure to blunt trauma, the Task Force on Neck Pain suggests ruling out serious pathology based on existing recommendations for the lumbar spine (Box 9-2).[2,50] The presence of such red flags should prompt the clinician to seek additional evaluation and care for these patients. Although a full discussion is beyond the scope of this chapter, the Canadian C-Spine and NEXUS protocols provide an overview of screening protocols for neck pain patients seeking emergency medical care, mostly following a trauma.[51]

Table 9-1 Testing procedures of manual provocation tests for cervical radiculopathy[57]

Name	Description	Positive test outcome
Spurling test*	The patient is seated. The neck is passively bent sideways toward the symptomatic side, and overpressure (approximately 7 kg) is applied to the patient's head.	Symptom reproduction
Neck distraction test*	The patient is supine. The neck is passively flexed to a position of comfort, and a gradual force of distraction (up to 14 kg) is applied to the patient's head.	Symptom reduction or elimination
Valsalva maneuver	The patient is seated and instructed to take a deep breath and hold it while attempting to exhale for 2 to 3 seconds.	Symptom reproduction
Upper limb tension test*	The patient is supine. A sequence of movements is passively performed to elongate the median nerve: depression of the scapula, abduction and external rotation of the shoulder, extension of the elbow, supination of the forearm, and dorsiflexion/extension of the wrist.	Symptom reproduction

*Note: Passive evaluation of the neck should not be attempted unless the clinician has had specific training in this technique.

Disability

Several reliable and valid self-assessment questionnaires are available to determine the level of disability in neck pain patients, including the Neck Disability Index[52,53] and the Neck Bournemouth Questionnaire.[54] Within this framework, the Graded Chronic Pain Scale (GCPS)[55] is of special interest because it is a universal system that can be used for any pain condition (eg, neck pain, headache, or temporomandibular pain), it is easy to use, and it is the most commonly used system to rate disability in scientific publications on TMD patients. In this system, disability is rated on a scale from 0 to 4, with GCPS grades 3 and 4 representing patients with high disability. According to the Task Force on Neck Pain, patients experiencing such pain-related disability require further assessment and treatment to prevent long-term disability (see Box 9-1).

Signs of nerve compression

Nerve compression or entrapment is suspected in patients with neck pain that radiates to the arm (for a detailed description of this condition, see "Radiculopathy" section below). Neck pain from this origin is caused by an irritation of the cervical nerve root, mostly due to prolonged compression. In typical cases, the irradiating pain closely follows the area innervated by the affected nerve root. When nerve compression is suspected, a cluster of clinical provocation tests is recommended, such as the Spurling test, traction/neck distraction, Valsalva maneuver, and upper limb tension test.[56] A summary of the testing procedures is presented in Table 9-1. These diagnostic procedures have high predictive value when compared with gold standards of nerve conduction/magnetic resonance imaging and myelography.[2] The Spurling test, traction/neck distraction, and Valsalva maneuver have

Table 9-2 Diagnostic procedures for the management of neck pain

Name	Description	Positive test outcome
Range of motion	Active and passive* range of motion is observed during flexion, extension, rotation, and side bending head movements.	Limited or irregular movements and/ or reproduction of neck pain
Palpation	Important cervical muscles or muscle groups to evaluate are the sternocleidomastoid, suboccipital, paravertebral (scalenes), posterior deep cervical, and upper trapezius muscles.	Symptom reproduction
Resistance tests	Dynamic (head movements against a slight manual resistance) and static (strong manual resistance while no movement occurs) resistance tests are performed in the same directions as described by range of motion.	Symptom reproduction (more dynamic than static pain is indicative of arthrogenous pain; more static than dynamic pain is indicative of myogenous pain)

*Note: Passive evaluation of the neck should not be attempted unless the clinician has had specific training in this technique.

high specificity, so positive test results might be suggestive of nerve compression when they are consistent with the history and other physical findings. The upper limb tension test, on the other hand, has high sensitivity, so a negative result is highly suggestive of the absence of nerve compression.

In the absence of acute trauma and symptoms of serious pathology, the use of diagnostic procedures such as routine imaging, anesthetic facet or medial branch blocks, or surface electromyography for the diagnosis of nerve compression is not supported by the literature.[2]

Additional diagnostic procedures for neck pain

The clinical physical examination of the neck, like that for back pain, is generally better at ruling out a radiculopathy than at diagnosing other specific etiologic conditions for neck pain.[2] Still, a screening clinical examination usually includes a chronologic history (including past and current treatments, functional limitations, and successful pain modifiers), assessment of the active and passive range of motion, palpation of the cervical spine and associated muscles, and dynamic and static resistance tests of the neck.[58-59] Additional studies are needed for the validity of these diagnostic procedures, but evidence is growing, and they are widely used and considered to provide useful information for prognosis and management (eg, options for treatment or evaluation of outcome).[59-62] It is recommended to cluster findings of multiple tests because this increases the diagnostic value.[63]

It is beyond the scope of this chapter to describe a thorough examination of the cervical spine, but a short overview of the most common clinical tests for neck pain is provided in Table 9-2. If further evaluation of the cervical region is indicated, patients should be referred to an appropriately trained clinician (eg, a physical therapist with specialized training in the craniocervical region). Similar to other musculoskeletal disorders, such as TMDs and back pain, the finding of degenerative changes in the neck on imaging has not been shown to always be associated with neck pain.[2]

Common CSDs

While it is important for the clinician to be aware of cervical etiologic factors that can contribute to the presence or perpetuation of orofacial pain, cervical disorders should not be managed in the dental setting. Orofacial pain patients with a CSD should be referred to a physical therapist with specialized training in the craniocervical region (eg, a physical therapist registered by the Physical Therapy Board of Craniofacial and Cervical Therapeutics [PTBCCT] or a cervical spine specialist) for thorough evaluation and treatment.[64] The remainder of this chapter highlights some of the more common CSDs that can contribute to the experience of orofacial pain and headaches and includes their codes according to the International Classification of Headache Disorders, 3rd edition (ICHD-3)[65] and the *International Classification of Diseases, Tenth Revision (ICD-10)* and *Eleventh Revision (ICD-11)*. This overview should be considered a description of possible causes of neck pain, allowing pattern recognition but not claiming criteria for objective diagnoses. In most cases, the below-mentioned CSDs fulfill the criteria for grade I or II of the Neck Pain Task Force classification system.[2]

Cervicalgia (*ICD-10* M54.2; *ICD-11* ME84.0)

Cervicalgia is a broad term covering pain in the neck and represents the most common neck pain complaints. Although the pain may originate from any cervical structure, discomfort is primarily felt in the suboccipital area and sternocleidomastoid (SCM) and upper trapezius muscles, with possible referral to the frontal, temporoparietal, occipital, vertex, and orbital regions. The Task Force on Neck Pain defined *neck pain* as symptoms "located in the anatomical region of the neck with or without radiation to the head, trunk, and upper limbs."[66] Treatment of cervicalgia includes conservative techniques such as cervical physical therapy. In a systematic review, evidence supports the recommendations from the Neck Pain Task Force that mobilization, manipulation, and clinical massage are effective interventions for the management of neck pain.[67] No evidence was found to support the use of electro-acupuncture, strain-counterstrain, relaxation massage, and other passive physical modalities (heat, cold, diathermy, hydrotherapy, and ultrasound). The evidence for the effectiveness of such multimodal approaches in the short, intermediate, and long term is growing and has been translated into clinical practice guidelines.[68–70]

Sprain and strain of cervical spine (*ICD-10* S13.4; *ICD-11* NA23.4Y)

The most frequent traumatic spinal injury encountered in medical practice is a sprain or strain of the cervical spine following a motor vehicle accident, also known as a *flexion/extension injury*, *acceleration-deceleration injury*, and *whiplash-associated disorder* (WAD).[71] Similar to cervicalgia, or common neck pain, WADs are usually classified as grade I or II. Neck symptoms without or with only minor interference with activities in daily life (ADL) would be considered grade I, and neck symptoms with substantial interference with ADL are grade II. Grade III is reserved for those patients with neurologic signs (radiculopathy), and grade IV for those with major structural pathology in the anterior, posterior, or lateral structures of the cervical spine, as well as parts of the shoulder girdle.[71–75] The incidence of resultant neck pain and postural changes is significant.[70,71,73,74] Patients with a WAD have significantly more signs and symptoms of TMDs when compared with healthy controls, as well as compared with neck-pain patients without a traumatic onset of their complaints.[76–80] However, when other physical pain complaints are accounted for, the higher prevalence of TMD pain is found to be merely part of a more general widespread pain disorder in WAD patients.[80]

The onset of neck pain following acute trauma may occur immediately or with a delay of up to 2 days. It may occur as an ache or stiffness in the neck. Pain referral to sites distant from the original injury is common, as is the presence of headache, dizziness, tinnitus, dysphagia, and visual disturbances.[81,82] Most patients show recovery after a whiplash trauma in the first 3 months. Thereafter, little improvement is seen. Because a large proportion of patients (up to 50%) will not recover completely, WAD is a therapeutic challenge.[71,83,84] Prognostic indicators to assess the risk of poor recovery are high scores on the Neck Disability Index, age of 40 years or older, and signs of hyperarousal.[83,85]

For grades I and II, treatment primarily consists of rest, relative immobilization (ie, act as usual but temporarily prevent extreme movements and exercises), and, when necessary, anti-inflammatory drugs or muscle relaxants until the patient is pain free and has regained full mobility of the cervical spine. When recovery is delayed (ie, complaints are still present after 3 to 6 weeks), referral for further therapy should be considered. In that case, conservative treatments including active exercise, manual techniques, and physical therapy can be useful to reduce pain and increase cervical range of motion.[86] Neck-specific exercise, particularly with a behavioral approach, is found to have a more positive impact on health-related quality of life than physical activity prescription in chronic WAD grades II and III.[87,88] Historically, cervical collars were frequently prescribed to immobilize the neck in WAD patients. Several studies have evaluated the additional effect of soft collars on WAD patients and found that soft collars in combination with other interventions resulted in delayed recovery in terms of pain and range of motion.[89] Therefore, the use of soft collars is no longer recommended to prevent inactivity of the cervical spine.[89]

Cervical osteoarthritis (*ICD-10* M47.8; *ICD-11* FA0Z)

With increasing age, degenerative changes can occur in the vertebral body, adjacent uncinate processes (joints of Luschka), posterior facet areas, and intervertebral discs.[90–92] Degenerative changes include inflammation of the joint linings with osteophyte formation, along with bony and cartilaginous exostoses. The most common regions of degenerative changes of the intervertebral disc are in the area of C5 to C6 and C6 to C7.[92,93] Osteoarthritis (OA) of the synovial joints is more commonly found in the more mobile upper cervical segments.[90]

OA is common in individuals over the age of 50 years. By the seventh decade of life, 75% of individuals display signs and symptoms of OA, and it is generally considered that 100% of individuals will develop signs and symptoms of OA during the course of a normal lifetime.[91] As the elasticity of tissues decreases with age, there is a concomitant loss of range of motion, the neck becomes less resilient, and muscle strength declines. Early subjective complaints of OA include occasional episodes of neck pain triggered by activity. These episodes often resolve in a couple of days with little more than rest (ie, act as usual but temporarily prevent extreme movements and exercises). More advanced symptoms include stiffness, limitation of movements, crepitus, and chronic neck pain. Progressive degeneration can lead to narrowing of the intervertebral spaces and may result in radiculopathy. However, no association between degenerative changes on imaging and neck pain has been found, indicating that degenerative changes without pain and vice versa are common findings.[2]

Mild and moderate stages of cervical OA will normally respond to comprehensive physical therapy management, including mobilization, exercise, and transcutaneous electrical nerve stimulation, with or without medication.[94,95] However, once osteoarthritic changes have reached the point of neural compression and radiculopathy (grade III or IV of the Task Force on Neck Pain), multidisciplinary treatment is warranted, including a referral to a medical specialist (eg, a neurologist or an orthopedist).[92]

Radiculopathy (*ICD-10* M54.1; *ICD-11* 8B93.Z)

Radiculopathy is a pain and/or sensorimotor deficit syndrome caused by compression of a nerve root. The most common causes for cervical radiculopathy are osteoarthritic changes of the uncovertebral joints, zygapophyseal joints or intervertebral disc herniation.[92,96] Patient complaints related to radiculopathy in the cervical region range from neck pain, numbness, and/or tingling in the upper extremity to electric-type pains or even weakness.[96,97]

The cervical spinal nerves are named corresponding to the vertebral body below the nerve.[22] Radicular pain from the C2 nerve roots can manifest itself as eye and/or ear pain and headache.[96] In addition, involvement of the C1 to C3 nerve roots may be accompanied by suboccipital or occipital headaches, neck pain, or pain referred to the shoulder girdle region.[96]

Many cases of cervical radiculopathy, even with neurological symptoms, will resolve spontaneously and can initially be managed conservatively.[97] If symptoms of cervical radiculopathy persist for longer than 4 to 6 weeks, or there is earlier evidence of abnormal neurology, such as lower-limb symptoms, referral for imaging or medical specialist assessment should be considered. Further reading may include guidelines such as *The Clinical Guideline for the Diagnosis and Treatment of Cervical Radiculopathy from Degenerative Disorders*.[98]

If space-occupying lesions or malignant processes have been ruled out as the source of the pain, comprehensive noninvasive treatment may include physical therapy.[98] There is widespread indication that prolonged use of a cervical collar leads to deconditioning of the neck musculature and tissue damage; hence, such use should be avoided.[96] Active interventions with education, instructions in proper postural techniques, and therapeutic exercises are more favored.[99,100]

Cervical dystonia (*ICD-10* G24.3; *ICD-11* 8402.0Y)

Cervical dystonia, or *spasmodic torticollis*, is a condition characterized by sustained contractions of the neck muscles and sometimes the shoulder muscles.[101] The head is typically tilted laterally, bending toward the affected muscle and rotated toward the opposite side. It may be spasmodic (clonic) or permanent (tonic). Bilateral SCM involvement will yield the head in an extended position (retrocollis) and is often associated with dysphagia (problems with swallowing) and vocal disturbances.[102] It can be a primary (idiopathic) or secondary condition. Secondary cervical dystonia can be a consequence of a disease process (eg, Wilson disease), or may be linked to the use of medication (eg, neuroleptics) or excessive toxin introduction into the body (eg, carbon monoxide poisoning).[102] Structural lesions, primarily of the basal ganglia, such as trauma or vascular insults, can also be a cause.[102] Cervical dystonia is one of the most common forms of focal dystonia, occurring in approximately 5 per 100,000 individuals in the general population.[103] A recent meta-analysis revealed no significant differences between men and women, with a prevalence of 6.5 per 100,000 in women and 5.0 per 100,000 in men.[103] Cervical dystonias usually develop from age 45 years (ie, late-onset).[102] Although pain is not the dominant complaint of patients with other types of dystonia, cervical dystonia is an exception, with 75% of the patients reporting neck pain.[102] The usual treatment for torticollis is botulinum toxin injection.[104] Usually, these injections need to be readministered every couple of months. A relatively common side effect of botulinum injections is dysphagia, especially in case of bilateral SCM injections. The dysphagia is usually mild (severe in less than 5% of cases) and disappears gradually after 2 to 3 weeks.[104] Studies as to the additional effects of behavioral interventions in cervical dystonia are scarce and usually of low methodologic quality. The limited data indicate, however, that behavioral therapies including cognitive behavioral and relaxation exercises could have a beneficial effect for enabling individuals to manage their dystonia.[104] In addition, preliminary results suggest that kinesiotaping may be useful in treating pain in patients with cervical dystonia.[105]

Occipital neuralgia (ICHD 13.4; *ICD-10* G52.8; *ICD-11* 8A85)

Occipital neuralgia is a primary headache disorder characterized by paroxysms of sharp, shooting occipital pain that last for seconds to minutes. The pain is associated with dysesthesia and/or allodynia in the area and tenderness over the affected nerve branches.[65] The pathogenesis is unknown, and most cases are considered idiopathic. In some cases, head trauma or nerve entrapment has been suggested as a cause of occipital neuralgia.[106] The differential diagnosis includes migraine, cluster headache, hemicrania continua, tension-type headache, and temporal arteritis involving the occipital artery.[106] Occipital referral of pain from the atlantoaxial or upper zygapophyseal joints, resulting in cervicogenic headache, should also be considered in the differential diagnosis, as should neoplasms or other destructive lesions affecting the spine or occiput.[106,107]

Initial conservative treatment including physical therapy directed at alleviating secondary muscle tension and improving posture is often an effective approach.[107] Low-dose antiepileptic drugs and tricyclic antidepressants may reduce acute pain, while refractory cases may respond to pulse radiofrequency or occipital nerve stimulation.[106]

Head or facial pain attributed to inflammation of the stylohyoid ligament (ICHD 11.8)

This type of head or facial pain, previously called *Eagle syndrome*, is a rare condition that is caused by inflammation of the stylohyoid ligament.[108] The pain is generally perceived in the oropharynx, neck, and/or face, but some patients experience a more diffuse headache. This type of headache is usually unilateral, with neck, pharyngeal, and/or facial pain that is provoked by turning the head. Examination should include palpation of the stylohyoid ligament and/or provocation tests, such as turning the head in ipsilateral as well as contralateral directions. Radiographic examination will reveal an elongated or calcified stylohyoid process and/or stylohyoid ligament.[109] Pain is significantly improved by local injection of local anesthetics or by styloidectomy.[108] Treatment may consist of pharmacologic management with analgesics or anti-inflammatory agents and/or surgical excision via either an intraoral or extraoral approach.[110–112]

Cervicogenic headache (ICHD 11.2.1; *ICD-10* G44.841; *ICD-11* 8A84.Y)

Cervicogenic headache is described as a "headache which is caused by a disorder of the cervical spine and its bony, disc and/or soft tissue elements, usually but not invariably accompanied by neck pain."[65] To classify this type of headache, there should be evidence of a cervical disorder or lesion with a known ability to cause headache. In addition, at least three of the following criteria should be present: *(1)* headache has developed in temporal relation to the onset of the cervical disorder or lesion, *(2)* headache has significantly improved or resolved in parallel with improvement in or resolution of the cervical disorder or lesion, *(3)* cervical range of motion is reduced and headache is made significantly worse by provocative maneuvers, and *(4)* headache is abolished following diagnostic blockade of a cervical structure or its nerve supply.[65] Features that tend to distinguish this type of headache from migraine and tension-type headache (while not unique for cervicogenic headache) include side-locked pain, provocation of the typical headache by digital pressure on neck muscles and by head movement, and posterior-to-anterior radiation of pain.[65,113] It should be noted that the coexistence of headache and neck pain does not automatically imply a causal relationship. Manipulative therapy and exercise can reduce the symptoms of cervicogenic headache.[114]

In the ICHD, the condition formerly known as *neck-tongue syndrome* is now encompassed by the less specific diagnosis of *cervicogenic headache*.[65,115] The understanding of the neck-tongue syndrome pathology involving C2 nerve root entrapment by subluxation of the atlantoaxial joint is better accounted for by cervicogenic headache than by its previous classification as a cranial neuralgia. It is a rare disorder characterized by abrupt unilateral pain in the neck or occiput with associated abnormal sensation involving the ipsilateral tongue and precipitated by sudden neck movements.[115] It has a duration of seconds to minutes.[115] The proposed mechanism for neck-tongue syndrome involves subluxation of the atlantoaxial joint, producing neck pain and irritation of the C2 nerve.[116] In the absence of pathologic findings, the disorder appears benign, and it is treated conservatively. Reported treatments, mostly from case reports, involve nonsteroidal anti-inflammatory drugs, antiepileptics, antidepressants, corticosteroids, muscle relaxants, injections of local anesthetics, cervical collars for immobilization, and postural correction with patient education.[115,117]

References

1. Scientific approach to the assessment and management of activity-related spinal disorders. A monograph for clinicians. Report of the Quebec Task Force on Spinal Disorders. Spine 1987;12(7 suppl):S1–S59.
2. Haldeman S, Carroll L, Cassidy JD. Findings from the Bone and Joint Decade 2000 to 2010 Task Force on Neck Pain and Its Associated Disorders. J Occup Environ Med 2010;52:424–427.
3. Haldeman S, Carroll L, Cassidy JD, Schubert J, Nygren A, Bone and Joint Decade 2000-2010 Task Force on Neck Pain and Its Associated Disorders. The Bone and Joint Decade 2000-2010 Task Force on Neck Pain and Its Associated Disorders: Executive summary. Spine 2008;33(4 suppl):S5–S7.
4. Abenhaim L, Rossignol M, Valat JP, et al. The role of activity in the therapeutic management of back pain. Report of the International Paris Task Force on Back Pain. Spine 2000;25(4 suppl):1S–33S.
5. Merskey H, Bogduk N. Classification of chronic pain. Descriptions of chronic pain syndromes and definitions of pain terms. Task Force on Taxonomy of the International Association for the Study of Pain, ed 2. Seattle: IASP Press, 1994.
6. Côté P, Cassidy DJ, Carroll LJ, Kristman V. The annual incidence and course of neck pain in the general population: A population-based cohort study. Pain 2004;112:267–273.
7. Bovim G, Schrader H, Sand T. Neck pain in the general population. Spine 1994;19:1307–1309.
8. Carroll LJ, Hogg-Johnson S, Côté P, et al. Course and prognostic factors for neck pain in workers: Results of the Bone and Joint Decade 2000-2010 Task Force on Neck Pain and Its Associated Disorders. Spine 2008; 33(4 suppl):S93–100.
9. Carroll LJ, Holm LW, Hogg-Johnson S, et al. Course and prognostic factors for neck pain in whiplash-associated disorders (WAD): Results of the Bone and Joint Decade 2000-2010 Task Force on Neck Pain and Its Associated Disorders. Spine 2008;33(4 suppl):S83–S92.
10. Carroll LJ, Hogg-Johnson S, van der Velde G, et al. Course and prognostic factors for neck pain in the general population: Results of the Bone and Joint Decade 2000-2010 Task Force on Neck Pain and Its Associated Disorders. Spine 2008;33(4 suppl):S75–S82.
11. Abiodun-Solanke IMF, Agbaje JO, Ajayi DM, Arotiba JT. Prevalence of neck and back pain among dentists and dental auxiliaries in South-western Nigeria. Afr J Med Med Sci 2010;39:137–142.

12. Lalumandier JA, McPhee SD, Parrott CB, Vendemia M. Musculoskeletal pain: Prevalence, prevention, and differences among dental office personnel. Gen Dent 2001;49:160–166.
13. Rehn B, Nilsson T, Lundström R, Hagberg M, Burström L. Neck pain combined with arm pain among professional drivers of forest machines and the association with whole-body vibration exposure. Ergonomics 2009;52:1240–1247.
14. Jun D, Zoe M, Johnston V, O'Leary S. Physical risk factors for developing non-specific neck pain in office workers: A systematic review and meta-analysis. Int Arch Occup Environ Health 2017;90:373–410.
15. Visscher CM, Lobbezoo F, de Boer W, van der Zaag J, Naeije M. Prevalence of cervical spinal pain in craniomandibular pain patients. Eur J Oral Sci 2001;109:76–80.
16. Costa YM, Conti PC, de Faria FA, Bonjardim LR. Temporomandibuler disorders and painful comorbidities: clinical associations and underlying mechanisms. Oral Surg Oral Med Oral Pathol Oral Radiol 2017;123:288–297.
17. Armijo Olivo S, Magee DJ, Parfitt M, Major P, Thie NM. The association between the cervical spine, the stomatognathic system, and craniofacial pain: A critical review. J Orofac Pain 2006;20:271–287.
18. Visscher CM, Ligthart L, Schuller AA, et al. Comorbid disorders and sociodemographic variables in temporomandibular pain in the general Dutch population. J Oral Facial Pain Headache 2015;29:51–59.
19. Nilsson I-M, List T, Drangsholt M. Headache and co-morbid pains associated with TMD pain in adolescents. J Dent Res 2013;92:802–807.
20. Armijo-Olivo S, Magee D. Cervical musculoskeletal impairments and temporomandibular disorders. J Oral Maxillofac Res 2013;3:e4.
21. Mannion RJ, Woolf CJ. Pain mechanisms and management: A central perspective. Clin J Pain 2000;16(3 suppl):S144–S156.
22. Loeser JD, Butler SH, Chapman CR, Turk DC. Bonica's Management of Pain, ed 3. Baltimore: Lippincott Williams & Wilkins, 2001.
23. Drake RL, Vogl AW, Mitchell AWM, Tibbitts RM, Richardson PE. Gray's Atlas of Anatomy E-Book, ed 2. Philadelphia: Churchill Livingstone, 2015.
24. Piovesan EJ, Kowacs PA, Tatsui CE, Lange MC, Ribas LC, Werneck LC. Referred pain after painful stimulation of the greater occipital nerve in humans: Evidence of convergence of cervical afferences on trigeminal nuclei. Cephalalgia 2001;21:107–109.
25. Svensson P, Wang K, Arendt-Nielsen L, Cairns BE, Sessle BJ. Pain effects of glutamate injections into human jaw or neck muscles. J Orofac Pain 2005;19:109–118.
26. Ge HY, Wang K, Madeleine P, Svensson P, Sessle BJ, Arendt-Nielsen L. Simultaneous modulation of the exteroceptive suppression periods in the trapezius and temporalis muscles by experimental muscle pain. Clin Neurophysiol 2004;115:1399–1408.
27. Bartsch T, Goadsby PJ. Increased responses in trigeminocervical nociceptive neurons to cervical input after stimulation of the dura mater. Brain 2003;126:1801–1813.
28. Busch V, Jakob W, Juergens T, Schulte-Mattler W, Kaube H, May A. Functional connectivity between trigeminal and occipital nerves revealed by occipital nerve blockade and nociceptive blink reflexes. Cephalalgia 2006;26:50-55.
29. Mørch CD, Hu JW, Arendt-Nielsen L, Sessle BJ. Convergence of cutaneous, musculoskeletal, dural and visceral afferents onto nociceptive neurons in the first cervical dorsal horn. E J Neurosci 2007;26:142–154.
30. Fillingim RB, Wallace MR, Herbstman DM, Ribeiro-Dasilva M, Staud R. Genetic contributions to pain: A review of findings in humans. Oral Dis 2008;14:673–682.
31. Visscher CM, Lobbezoo F. TMD pain is partly heritable. A systematic review of family studies and genetic association studies. J Oral Rehabil 2015;42:386–399.
32. Maixner W, Diatchenko L, Dubner R, et al. Orofacial pain prospective evaluation and risk assessment study: The OPPERA study. J Pain 2011;12(11 suppl):T4–T11.e1–e2.
33. de Freitas LVS, Lopes ACP, Piatto VB, Maniglia JV. Association of temporomandibular dysfunction with the 102T-C polymorphism in the serotonin receptor gene in Brazilian patients. Arch Med Sci 2013;9:1013–1018.
34. Bardin L, Tarayre JP, Malfetes N, Koek W, Colpaert FC. Profound, non-opioid analgesia produced by the high-efficacy 5-HT(1A) agonist F 13640 in the formalin model of tonic nociceptive pain. Pharmacology 2003;67:182–194.
35. McLean SA, Diatchenko L, Lee YM, et al. Catechol O-methyltransferase haplotype predicts immediate musculoskeletal neck pain and psychological symptoms after motor vehicle collision. J Pain 2011;12:101–107.
36. Diatchenko L, Slade GD, Nackley AG, et al. Genetic basis for individual variations in pain perception and the development of a chronic pain condition. Hum Mol Genet 2005;14:135–143.
37. Michelotti A, Liguori R, Toriello M, et al. Catechol-O-methyltransferase (COMT) gene polymorphisms as risk factor in temporomandibular disorders patients from Southern Italy. Clin J Pain 2014;30:129–133.

38. Woda A, Pionchon P, Palla S, Piochon P. Regulation of mandibular postures: Mechanisms and clinical implications. Crit Rev Oral Biol Med 2001;12:166–178.
39. Lawrence ES, Razook SJ. Nonsurgical management of mandibular disorders. In: Kraus SL (ed). Temporomandibular Disorders, ed 2. New York: Churchill Livingstone, 1994.
40. Visscher CM, Huddleston Slater JJ, Lobbezoo F, Naeije M. Kinematics of the human mandible for different head postures. J Oral Rehabil 2000;27:299–305.
41. Eriksson PO, Häggman-Henrikson B, Nordh E, Zafar H. Co-ordinated mandibular and head-neck movements during rhythmic jaw activities in man. J Dent Res 2000;79:1378–1384.
42. Häggman-Henrikson B, Eriksson P-O. Head movements during chewing: Relation to size and texture of bolus. Dent Res 2004;83:864–868.
43. Guo S-X, Li B-Y, Zhang Y, et al. An electromyographic study on the sequential recruitment of bilateral sternocleidomastoid and masseter muscle activity during gum chewing. J Oral Rehabil 2017;44:594–601.
44. Mannheimer JS, Rosenthal RM. Acute and chronic postural abnormalities as related to craniofacial pain and temporomandibular disorders. Dent Clin North Am 1991;35:185–208.
45. Manfredini D. Current Concepts on Temporomandibular Disorders. Chicago: Quintessence, 2010.
46. Olivo SA, Bravo J, Magee DJ, Thie NMR, Major PW, Flores-Mir C. The association between head and cervical posture and temporomandibular disorders: A systematic review. J Orofac Pain 2006;20:9–23.
47. Armijo-Olivo S, Rappoport K, Fuentes J, et al. Head and cervical posture in patients with temporomandibular disorders. J Orofac Pain 2011;25:199–209.
48. Visscher CM, De Boer W, Lobbezoo F, Habets LL, Naeije M. Is there a relationship between head posture and craniomandibular pain? J Oral Rehabil 2002; 29:1030–1036.
49. Hackney J, Bade D, Clawson A. Relationship between forward head posture and diagnosed internal derangement of the temporomandibular joint. J Orofac Pain 1993;7:386–390.
50. Nordin M, Carragee EJ, Hogg-Johnson S, et al. Assessment of neck pain and its associated disorders: Results of the Bone and Joint Decade 2000-2010 Task Force on Neck Pain and Its Associated Disorders. Spine 2008;33(4 suppl):S101–S122.
51. Stiell IG, Clement CM, McKnight RD, et al. The Canadian C-spine rule versus the NEXUS low-risk criteria in patients with trauma. N Engl J Med 2003;349:2510–2518.
52. Vernon H, Mior S. The Neck Disability Index: A study of reliability and validity. J Manipulative Physiol Ther 1991;14:409–415.
53. Lemeunier N, da Silva-Oolup S, Olesen K. et al. Reliability and validity of self-reported questionnaires to measure pain and disability in adults with neck pain and its associated disorders: Part 3—A systematic review from the CADRE Collaboration. Eur Spine J 2019;28: 1156–1179.
54. Bolton JE, Humphreys BK. The Bournemouth Questionnaire: A short-form comprehensive outcome measure. II. Psychometric properties in neck pain patients. J Manipulative Physiol Ther 2002;25:141–148.
55. Von Korff M, Ormel J, Keefe FJ, Dworkin SF. Grading the severity of chronic pain. Pain 1992;50:133–149.
56. Rubinstein SM, Pool JJM, van Tulder MW, Riphagen II, de Vet HC. A systematic review of the diagnostic accuracy of provocative tests of the neck for diagnosing cervical radiculopathy. Eur Spine J 2007;16:307–319.
57. Wainner RS, Fritz JM, Irrgang JJ, Boninger ML, Delitto A, Allison S. Reliability and diagnostic accuracy of the clinical examination and patient self-report measures for cervical radiculopathy. Spine 2003;28:52–62.
58. Visscher CM, Lobbezoo F, Naeije M. A reliability study of dynamic and static pain tests in temporomandibular disorder patients. J Orofac Pain 2007;21:39–45.
59. Visscher CM, Lobbezoo F, de Boer W, van der Zaag J, Verheij JGC, Naeije M. Clinical tests in distinguishing between persons with or without craniomandibular or cervical spinal pain complaints. Eur J Oral Sci 2000;108:475–483.
60. Humphreys BK, Delahaye M, Peterson CK. An investigation into the validity of cervical spine motion palpation using subjects with congenital block vertebrae as a 'gold standard.' BMC Musculoskelet Disord 2004;5:19.
61. Schneider GM, Jull G, Thomas K, et al. Derivation of a clinical decision guide in the diagnosis of cervical facet joint pain. Arch Phys Med Rehabil 2014;95: 1695–1701.
62. Mansfield M. Physical examination for the diagnosis of cervical facet joint pain: A systematic review. Int J Ther Rehabil 2014;21(suppl 7):S8.
63. De Hertogh WJ, Vaes PH, Vijverman V, De Cordt A, Duquet W. The clinical examination of neck pain patients: The validity of a group of tests. Man Ther 2007;12:50–55.
64. Kraus S. Temporomandibular disorders, head and orofacial pain: Cervical spine considerations. Dent Clin North Am 2007;51:161–193.
65. Headache Classification Committee of the International Headache Society (IHS). The international classification of headache disorders, 3rd edition. Cephalalgia 2018;38:1–211.

66. Guzman J, Haldeman S, Carroll LJ, et al. Clinical practice implications of the Bone and Joint Decade 2000-2010 Task Force on Neck Pain and Its Associated Disorders: From concepts and findings to recommendations. J Manipulative Physiol Ther 2009;32(2 suppl):S227–S243.
67. Wong JJ, Shearer HM, Mior S et al. Are manual therapies, passive physical modalities, or acupuncture effective for the management of patients with whiplash-associated disorders or neck pain and associated disorders? An update of the Bone and Joint Decade Task Force on Neck Pain and Its Associated Disorders by the OPTIMa collaboration. Spine J 2015;16:1598–1630.
68. Côté P, Wong JJ, Sutton D, et al. Management of neck pain and associated disorders: A clinical practice guideline from the Ontario Protocol for Traffic Injury Management (OPTIMa) Collaboration. Eur Spine J 2016;25:2000–2022.
69. Gross AR, Paquin JP, Dupont G, et al. Exercises for mechanical neck disorders: A Cochrane review update. Man Ther 2016;24:25–45.
70. Gross A, Langevin P, Burnie SJ, et al. Manipulation and mobilisation for neck pain contrasted against an inactive control or another active treatment. Cochrane Database Syst Rev 2015;23:CD004249.
71. McClune T, Burton AK, Waddell G. Whiplash associated disorders: A review of the literature to guide patient information and advice. Emerg Med J 2002; 19:499–506.
72. Barnsley L, Lord S, Bogduk N. Whiplash injury. Pain 1994;58:283–307.
73. Cusick JF, Pintar FA, Yoganandan N. Whiplash syndrome: Kinematic factors influencing pain patterns. Spine 2001;26:1252–1258.
74. Kumar S, Ferrari R, Narayan Y. Looking away from whiplash: Effect of head rotation in rear impacts. Spine 2005;30:760–768.
75. Rao SK, Wasyliw C, Nunez DB. Spectrum of imaging findings in hyperextension injuries of the neck. Radiographics 2005;25:1239–1254.
76. Klobas L, Tegelberg A, Axelsson S. Symptoms and signs of temporomandibular disorders in individuals with chronic whiplash-associated disorders. Swed Dent J 2004;28:29–36.
77. Eriksson P-O, Häggman-Henrikson B, Zafar H. Jaw-neck dysfunction in whiplash-associated disorders. Arch Oral Biol 2007;52:404–408.
78. Carroll LJ, Ferrari R, Cassidy JD. Reduced or painful jaw movement after collision-related injuries: A population-based study. J Am Dent Assoc 2007;138:86–93.
79. Grönqvist J, Häggman-Henrikson B, Eriksson PO. Impaired jaw function and eating difficulties in whiplash-associated disorders. Swed Dent J 2008; 32:171–177.
80. Visscher C, Hofman N, Mes C, Lousberg R, Naeije M. Is temporomandibular pain in chronic whiplash-associated disorders part of a more widespread pain syndrome? Clin J Pain 2005;21:353–357.
81. Treleaven J, Jull G, Sterling M. Dizziness and unsteadiness following whiplash injury: Characteristic features and relationship with cervical joint position error. J Rehabil Med 2003;35:36–43.
82. Malik H, Lovell M. Soft tissue neck symptoms following high-energy road traffic accidents. Spine 2004;29:E315–E317.
83. Ritchie C, Sterling M. Recovery pathways and prognosis after whiplash injury. J Orthop Sports Phys Ther 2016;46:851–861.
84. Dehner C, Hartwig E, Strobel P, et al. Comparison of the relative benefits of 2 versus 10 days of soft collar cervical immobilization after acute whiplash injury. Arch Phys Med Rehabil 2006;87:1423–1427.
85. Ritchie C, Hendrikz J, Kenardy J, Sterling M. Derivation of a clinical prediction rule to identify both chronic moderate/severe disability and full recovery following whiplash injury. Pain 2013;154:2198–2206.
86. Wiangkham T, Duda J, Haque S, Madi M, Rushton A. The effectiveness of conservative management for acute whiplash associated disorder (WAD) II: A systematic review and meta-analysis of randomised controlled trials. PLoS One 2015;10:e0133415.
87. Ludvigsson LM, Peterson G, Peolsson A. The effect of three exercise approaches on health-related quality of life, and factors associated with its improvement in chronic whiplash-associated disorders: analysis of a randomized controlled trial. Qual Life Res 2019;28: 357–368.
88. Rosenfeld M, Seferiadis A, Carlsson J, Gunnarsson R. Active intervention in patients with whiplash-associated disorders improves long-term prognosis: A randomized controlled clinical trial. Spine 2003;28: 2491–2498.
89. Schnabel M, Ferrari R, Vassiliou T, et al. Randomised, controlled outcome study of active mobilisation compared with collar therapy for whiplash injury. Emerg Med J 2004;21:306–310.
90. Bland JH, Boushey DR. The cervical spine, from anatomy and physiology to clinical care. In: Berthoz A, Vidal PP, Graf W (eds). The Head-Neck Sensory Motor System. New York: Oxford University, 1992.
91. Christian C. Medical management of cervical spine diseases. In: Camins MB, O'Leary PF (eds). Disorders of the Cervical Spine. Baltimore: Williams & Wilkins, 1992:147–155.

92. Nguyen C, Sanchez K, Roren A, et al. Anatomical specificities of the degenerated cervical spine: a narrative review of clinical implications, with special focus on targeted spinal injections. Ann Phys Rehabil Med 2016; 59:276–281.
93. Abdulkarim JA, Dhingsa R, Finlay DB. Magnetic resonance imaging of the cervical spine: Frequency of degenerative changes in the intervertebral disc with relation to age. Clin Radiol 2003;58:980–984.
94. Mannheimer JS. Prevention and restoration of abnormal upper quarter posture. In: Gelb H (ed). New Concepts in Craniomandibular and Chronic Pain Management. London: Mosby-Wolfe, 1994:277–323.
95. Mannheimer JS, Lampe GN. Clinical Transcutaneous Electrical Nerve Stimulation. Philadelphia: FA Davis, 1984.
96. Caridi JM, Pumberger M, Hughes AP. Cervical radiculopathy: A review. HSS J 2011;7:265–272.
97. McCartney S, Baskerville R, Blagg S, McCartney D. Cervical radiculopathy and cervical myelopathy: Diagnosis and management in primary care. Br J Gen Pract 2018;68:44–46.
98. Bono CM, Ghiselli G, Gilbert TJ, et al. An evidence-based clinical guideline for the diagnosis and treatment of cervical radiculopathy from degenerative disorders. Spine J 2011;11:64–72.
99. Dreyer SJ, Boden SD. Nonoperative treatment of neck and arm pain. Spine 1998;23:2746–2754.
100. Jette DU, Jette AM. Physical therapy and health outcomes in patients with spinal impairments. Phys Ther 1996;76:930–941.
101. Patel S, Martino D. Cervical dystonia: From pathophysiology to pharmacotherapy. Behav Neurol 2013;26:275–282.
102. Geyer HL, Bressman SB. The diagnosis of dystonia. Lancet Neurol 2006;5:780–790.
103. Steeves TD, Day L, Dykeman J, Jette N, Pringsheim T. The prevalence of primary dystonia: A systematic review and meta-analysis. Mov Disord 2012;27:1789–1796.
104. Contarino MF, Van Den Dool J, Balash Y, et al. Clinical practice: Evidence-based recommendations for the treatment of cervical dystonia with botulinum toxin. Front Neurol 2017;8:35.
105. Pelosin E, Avanzino L, Marchese R, et al. Kinesiotaping reduces pain and modulates sensory function in patients with focal dystonia: A randomized crossover pilot study. Neurorehabil Neural Repair 2013; 27:722–731.
106. Dougherty C. Occipital neuralgia. Curr Pain Headache Rep 2014;18:411.
107. Vanelderen P, Lataster A, Levy R, Mekhail N, van Kleef M, Van Zundert J. 8. Occipital neuralgia. Pain Pract 2010;10:137–144.
108. Smania N, Corato E, Tinazzi M, Montagnana B, Fiaschi A, Aglioti SM. The effect of two different rehabilitation treatments in cervical dystonia: Preliminary results in four patients. Funct Neurol 2003;18:219–225.
109. Beder E, Ozgursoy OB, Karatayli Ozgursoy S, Anadolu Y. Three-dimensional computed tomography and surgical treatment for Eagle's syndrome. Ear Nose Throat J 2006;85:443–445.
110. Beder E, Ozgursoy OB, Karatayli Ozgursoy S. Current diagnosis and transoral surgical treatment of Eagle's syndrome. J Oral Maxillofac Surg 2005;63:1742–1745.
111. Mendelsohn AH, Berke GS, Chhetri DK. Heterogeneity in the clinical presentation of Eagle's syndrome. Otolaryngol Head Neck Surg 2006;134:389–393.
112. Cheifetz I. Intraoral treatment of Eagle's syndrome. J Oral Maxillofac Surg 2006;64:749.
113. Sjaastad O, Fredriksen TA. Cervicogenic headache: Criteria, classification and epidemiology. Clin Exp Rheumatol 2000;18(2 suppl 19):S3–S6.
114. Jull G, Trott P, Potter H, et al. A randomized controlled trial of exercise and manipulative therapy for cervicogenic headache. Spine 2002;27:1835–1843.
115. Hu N, Dougherty C. Neck-tongue syndrome. Curr Pain Headache Rep 2016;20:27.
116. Bogduk N. An anatomical basis for the neck-tongue syndrome. J Neurol Neurosurg Psychiatry 1981;44: 202–208.
117. Borody C. Neck-tongue syndrome. J Manipulative Physiol Ther 2004;27:e8.

10

Extracranial and Systemic Causes of Head and Facial Pain

Key points

- Clinicians managing patients with orofacial pain should inquire about local and systemic symptoms to exclude systemic diseases.
- Several systemic conditions cause head and facial pain; therefore, the pain may be a symptom of a serious underlying condition.
- Because pain can be primary or referred, it is necessary to identify and treat the underlying cause and refer to a specialist if necessary.

Although head or facial pain frequently arises from the dental or other masticatory structures, it may also originate from any of the tissues and organs of the head and neck, or it may be a manifestation of a systemic disease. In the case of head or facial pain associated with a serious or life-threatening illness, timely recognition and treatment are crucial. When the cause of head or facial pain is not readily apparent, nonmasticatory, extracranial, and systemic pain sources should be considered. This chapter briefly summarizes these pain sources based on the current classification format of the International Headache Society (IHS)—International Classification of Headache Disorders, 3rd edition (ICHD-3),[1] and the *International Classification of Diseases, Tenth Revision (ICD-10)* and *Eleventh Revision (ICD-11)*—and provides lists of associated disorders and symptoms for easy reference. For further information and treatment guidelines, the reader is referred to other chapters in the text or to standard medical references.

Pain Stemming from Tissues or Organs in the Head and Neck

Cranial bones (ICHD 11.1)

Most lesions that affect the bones of the skull are nonpainful.[2] Although it is unusual for pain to arise from the cranial bones, when it does, it is derived from nociceptors of the underlying periosteum. Lesions of the skull most likely to produce a headache are those that are rapidly expansile or aggressively osteoclastic or those that have an inflammatory component.[3] Included in this group of lesions are osteomyelitis, multiple myeloma, sickle cell disease, Paget disease, osteopetrosis, mastoiditis, petrous apicitis, eosinophilic granuloma, Langerhans cell histiocytosis, osteoblastoma, immunoglobulin G4–related disease, non-Hodgkin lymphoma, and metastatic tumors.[4–10]

Eyes (ICHD 11.3.x)

Patients with eye pain will most often have obvious ocular signs accompanying the pain, making the diagnosis relatively straightforward. However, there are instances of headache or facial pain originating in the eyes without obvious ocular signs. Ocular pain may be either primary or referred (Box 10-1). Primary pain arises from the ophthalmic division of the trigeminal nerve (V1), although the maxillary division (V2) supplies most of the lower eyelid through its infraorbital branch.[11] The retina and optic nerve are not capable of nociception, but the cornea, conjunctiva, iris, extraocular muscles, dural sheath of the optic nerve, and periorbital area are supplied with pain-sensing nociceptors. Pain may be perceived as originating in the orbit by stimulation of the optic nerve at any point along its path from the cornea to the cortex. Possible stimuli include tumors of the orbit or paranasal sinuses, cavernous sinus diseases (inflammation, thrombosis, tumors), carotid aneurysms, and intracranial tumors.[12] Facial, cervical, and pericranial muscles are common sources of pain that may be referred to the orbit or periorbital areas.[13]

Ocular pain associated with inflammation is often accompanied by photophobia and conjunctival injection. Pain with eye movement can be due to optic neuritis. Refractive errors may also cause eye pain or headache. Although headache is often accompanied by ocular or periorbital pain, in the absence of ocular or periocular findings, it should be assumed the pain is not due to a primary ocular disorder, and further investigations should be performed.[14] Metastatic tumors to the orbit may present with diplopia (49%), pain (42%), and vision loss (30%) as the most common symptoms. Breast carcinoma (29%), melanoma (20%), and prostatic cancer (13%) are the most common cancers that metastasize to the orbit.[15] Orbital infarctions secondary to sickle cell disease cause acute periorbital pain, proptosis, ophthalmoplegia, and

Box 10-1 Head and facial pain arising from the eyes

Primary pain
- Acute glaucoma (ICHD 11.3.1)
- Convergence disorders (heterophoria or heterotropia; ICHD 11.3.3)
- Ocular inflammation (ICHD 11.3.4)
- Corneal diseases
- Painful ophthalmoplegia
- Superior orbital fissure syndrome
- Orbital tumors
- Metastatic tumors
- Orbital schwannomas
- Orbital lymphomas

Referred pain
- Saccular aneurysms (ICHD 6.3.1)
- Cavernous sinus inflammation
- Carotid-cavernous fistula (ICHD 6.3.3)
- Carotid artery dissection (ICHD 6.5.1)
- Myofascial pain
- Orbital apex syndrome
- Parasellar syndrome

visual impairment.[16,17] Orbital schwannomas are benign, well-encapsulated, slowly progressive tumors that may cause symptoms of proptosis, blurred vision, pain, eyelid swelling, diplopia, or headache.[18] Orbital lymphomas can present with proptosis, eyelid lesions, tearing, chemosis, decreased visual acuity, ptosis, pain, squint, and optic nerve compression.[19]

Ears (ICHD 11.4)

About 50% of earaches (otalgia) are due to structural lesions of the external or middle ear.[20] The remainder of earaches involve referred pain arising from disorders such as toothache and pharyngeal, laryngeal, cervical, and temporomandibular disorders (TMDs).[21,22] Sensory innervations of the ear are supplied by numerous cranial nerves, including branches of the 5th, 7th, 9th, and 10th cranial nerves, in addition to branches from the lesser occipital and greater auricular nerves originating from the spinal nerves C2 and C3. Hence, pain originating in the regions that supply these numerous nerve branches may be perceived as pain in or around the ears.

Primary painful disorders of the ear can originate in the auricle, external auditory canal, tympanic membrane, middle ear, or temporal bone (Box 10-2). The common causes of primary otalgia include otitis externa, otitis media, foreign body, and barotrauma.[23] Primary otalgia may also be accompanied by other symptoms, including vertigo, hearing loss, or tinnitus.[24] Benign lesions originating in the temporomandibular joint (TMJ) have been reported to present as masses in the external auditory canal. These lesions include pigmented villonodular synovitis, nodular fasciitis, foramen tympanicum herniation with salivary fistula, fibroepithelial polyp, superficial angiomyxoma, and giant cell tumor. Symptoms include TMJ pain, hearing loss, and otalgia.[25]

The prevalence of otologic signs and symptoms in adult patients with TMD is high. The most common symptoms in patients with TMD are ear fullness, earache, and tinnitus.[26] Tinnitus is the perception of sound in the absence of an external source and affects 30% of people older than 55 years.[27] It can be classified as subjective (only heard by the patient), objective (also heard by the examiner), pulsatile, non-pulsatile, and primary (no identifiable cause) versus secondary (with an underlying cause). Subjective non-pulsatile tinnitus, typically described as a ringing, buzzing, hissing, or roaring, is by far the most common type of tinnitus, accounting for 90% of all cases. It is most commonly related to high-frequency hearing loss from acoustic trauma and presbycusis (hearing loss due to aging). It is very rarely caused by ear conditions (eg, Ménière disease, otosclerosis, cholesteatoma), medications, neurologic conditions (eg, multiple sclerosis), autoimmune conditions (systemic lupus erythematous, rheumatoid arthritis), and endocrine conditions (eg, diabetes).[28] Pulsatile tinnitus is often described as a heartbeat or a "whooshing" noise, and vascular etiologies are the most common cause, ranging from cardiovascular (hypertension, valvular heart disease, carotid artery stenosis) to neoplasms (paraganglioma, vestibular schwannoma) and muscular myoclonus (eg, palate); therefore, imaging studies are essential in the diagnostic workup.[29]

In a cohort of patients with chronic tinnitus in the absence of hearing loss, a significant portion of patients had somatic disorders, most commonly TMD. Tinnitus was found to be significantly more prevalent especially in young women, who most commonly reported a pulsatile tinnitus aggravated by loud sounds and stress.[30] This tinnitus—particularly pulsatile tinnitus—caused a moderate impact on quality of life, although daily activities could still be performed.[31] It has been proposed that tinnitus with TMD complaints could constitute a distinct subtype that is amenable to treatment.[32]

It is also very important to note the facial symptoms or headaches associated with vestibular schwannomas, also known as *acoustic neuromas* (ANs). ANs are the most common tumors of the cerebellopontine angle, and they account for more than 90% of the primary tumors, the remaining tumors being meningiomas (3%), primary cholesteatomas (2.5%), and facial nerve schwannomas (1%).[33] ANs are benign, slowly growing neoplasms (averaging 2 mm/year) originating in the nerve sheath of the oculovestibular nerve (8th cranial nerve). ANs consist of Schwann cells in a collagenous matrix, and they arise mainly from the vestibular division of the 8th cranial nerve. Their growth occurs in three phases, with compression of *(1)* the internal auditory canal, *(2)* the cistern, and *(3)* the brain stem. The most common symptoms are sensorineural hearing loss (60% to 97%), tinnitus (50% to 66%), disequilibrium (46% to 59%) and numbness or tingling of the face (33%), headache (19% to 29%), and trigeminal nerve disturbances (hypesthesia, paresthesia and neuralgia) (12% to 45%).[34] Decreased facial sensation or corneal reflex result from the compression of the trigeminal nerve, usually with tumors larger than 3 cm. Compression of the fourth ventricle can also lead to ataxia and increased intracranial pressure (eg, headaches).[35] If the facial nerve is involved, some patients will complain of hypoesthesia of the posterior meatal wall, called the *Hitselberger sign*.[36]

Box 10-2 Head and facial pain arising from the ears

Primary pain

- Otitis externa
- Herpes zoster oticus
- Cellulitis/chondritis of the auricle
- Foreign body
- Otitis media
- Cholesteatoma (ICHD 11.4)
- Mastoiditis
- Gradenigo syndrome
- Barotrauma
- Ramsey Hunt syndrome
- Temporal bone tumors

Referred pain

- Temporomandibular disorders
- Myofascial pain
- Toothache
- Auriculotemporal syndrome
- Carotid artery dissection (ICHD 6.5.1)
- Red ear syndrome
- Sinus infections
- Pharyngitis or tonsillitis
- Cervical spine arthritis
- Pigmented villonodular synovitis
- Nodular fasciitis
- Foramen of Huschke herniation
- Fibroepithelial polyp
- Superficial angiomyxoma
- Giant cell tumor
- Oropharyngeal and laryngeal tumors

Nose/paranasal sinus complex (ICHD A11.5)

The nasal cavity is surrounded by the paranasal sinuses, which include the maxillary, ethmoid, frontal, and sphenoid sinuses. Sensory innervation of the nasal/paranasal sinus complex is supplied by the first and second divisions of the trigeminal nerve.[15] One of the functions of the sinuses is dependent upon ciliary action that actively transports mucous and debris to the ostia to allow drainage into the middle meatus of the nasal cavity. If the ostia become blocked due to inflammation or obstruction, fluid and bacteria accumulate, and this leads to a sinus infection. Acute rhinosinusitis—unlike the chronic rhinosinusitis, which lasts longer than 12 weeks—is typically sudden in onset, lasts up to 4 weeks, and resolves spontaneously or with antibiotic treatment if necessary. The symptoms of acute or chronic rhinosinusitis commonly include nasal discharge (anterior, posterior, or both), nasal obstruction, nasal congestion, facial pressure and pain, alteration in the sense of smell, cough, fever, halitosis, fatigue, dental pain, pharyngitis, otalgia, and headache.[37]

In a study of the symptoms of acute sinusitis, maxillary toothache was highly specific (93%), but only 11% of patients with sinusitis actually had pain from the tooth.[38] Headache had a sensitivity of 68% but a specificity of only 30%. "Sinus headache" is a term that is nonspecific and often confused with migraine and tension-type headache because of similarity in the location of the headache. Some studies have shown that up to 90% of sinus headaches are actually migraines (migraine with sinus symptoms).[39,40] No precise clinical definition exists for what constitutes a sinus headache, which has always been a diagnostic dilemma. Thus, patients may self-treat or receive treatment for rhinosinusitis, while migraine remains undiagnosed.[41]

Other sinus-related conditions that are often considered to cause headache are not sufficiently validated as causes of headache. These include deviation of nasal septum, hypertrophy of turbinates, atrophy of sinus membranes, and nasal mucosal contact points (located between the septum and structures of the lateral nasal wall).[1,42] The location of pain often provides clues as to which of the sinuses is primarily involved. For example, maxillary sinusitis may cause infraorbital or cheek discomfort, ethmoid rhinosinusitis may cause tenderness over the lacrimal region, frontal sinusitis characteristically causes pain in the forehead over the orbits, and pain due to sphenoid sinusitis radiates to the occiput and vertex areas.[43] Box 10-3 is a list of painful disorders of the nose and paranasal sinus complex.

Salivary glands

There are three pairs of major salivary glands: the parotid, submandibular, and sublingual glands. The sensory innervation to the parotid gland is supplied by the auriculotemporal nerve, a branch of the trigeminal nerve (V3), while the secretory fibers are derived from the glossopharyngeal nerve via the auriculotemporal nerve as well. Both the submandibular and sublingual glands derive their sensory nerve supply from the lingual nerve (branch of V3), while the parasympathetic input is via the chorda tympani, a branch of the facial nerve originating in the middle ear.[44] Pain originating in the salivary glands is typically inflammatory, infectious, traumatic, or neoplastic in origin. Common salivary gland disorders that are accompanied by pain include sialadenitis, sialolithiasis, epidemic parotitis, and tumors. Diagnosis of salivary gland pain is usually not difficult due to accompanying signs or symptoms of the affected gland. For example, in a salivary gland duct blockage or infection, the patient often presents with moderate to severe pain occurring while eating in conjunction with swelling and tenderness of the affected gland. Purulent exudate associated with fever, malaise, and foul taste may also occur. Other clinical

Box 10-3 Head and facial pain arising from the nose and paranasal sinus complex

Primary pain
- Acute or chronic rhinosinusitis (ICHD 11.5)
- Nasal polyposis
- Hypertrophic turbinates
- Nasal vestibulitis
- Septal deviation
- Septal abscess/hematoma
- Wegener granulomatosis
- Sarcoidosis
- Sinonasal tumors

Referred pain
- Toothache
- TMDs
- Myofascial pain
- Migraine
- Tension-type headache
- Pharyngeal pain

signs include a raised earlobe in the case of a parotid swelling, tenderness when palpating the gland, inflammation of the overlying skin, enlarged cervical lymphadenopathy, and, very rarely, weakness of a branch of the facial nerve. Sublingual gland swellings present with a raised floor of the mouth along with obstruction or swelling of the sublingual caruncle.[45] It is noteworthy to mention first-bite syndrome, mostly caused by surgeries of the parapharyngeal space. Patients will experience excruciating pain in the ipsilateral parotid gland region at the first bite of each meal, but this pain improves with subsequent mastication. This syndrome is thought to be due to an imbalance between the sympathetic and parasympathetic impulses. There is no consensus on the best treatment for first-bite syndrome, although symptoms tend to improve with time.[46] Intraparotid injections of botulinum toxin type A have been shown to decrease the severity of the symptoms.[47]

10-4 Head and facial pain arising from the throat

Primary pain
- Streptococcal pharyngitis
- Nonstreptococcal bacterial pharyngotonsillitis
- Peritonsillar abscess
- Viral pharyngitis
- Mononucleosis
- Laryngopharyngeal reflux
- Mucositis (primary and secondary)
- Allergic rhinitis with postnasal drip
- Chronic mouth breathing
- Foreign body
- Epiglottitis
- Muscle tension dysphonia
- Vocal cord granuloma
- Granulomatous diseases (rheumatoid arthritis, gout)
- Glossopharyngeal neuralgia
- Pemphigus
- Kawasaki disease
- Tumors
- Pharyngeal and laryngeal candidiasis
- Deep space neck infection (retropharyngeal/parapharyngeal/prevertebral space infections)

Referred pain
- TMDs
- Myofascial pain
- Gastroesophageal reflux disease
- Cardiac pain

Throat

The throat, or pharynx, is divided into the nasopharynx, oropharynx, and hypopharynx. The sensory supply to the pharyngeal tissues occurs via branches of the glossopharyngeal and vagus nerves.[48] Because of the significant overlap of innervations to these structures, throat pain is often poorly localized, and referred otalgia is common.[20] Painful disorders of the throat can be developmental, infectious, inflammatory, neuropathic, or neoplastic in origin.[49] Box 10-4 contains a list of the most common painful throat disorders.

Pain Stemming from Systemic Diseases

Oromandibular dystonia (*ICD-10* G24.4; *ICD-11* 8A02.0)

Oromandibular dystonia is an uncommon motor disorder that may contribute to orofacial pain. It is one form of focal dystonia that affects the orofacial region and involves the jaw-opening muscles (lateral pterygoid muscles and anterior bellies of the digastric muscles), tongue muscles, facial muscles (especially orbicularis ori and buccinator muscles), and platysma. Dystonia is characterized by an involuntary, repetitive, sustained muscle contraction. The sustained contraction results in an abnormal posturing of a structure and subsequent pain.[50-52] Oromandibular dystonias are often disabling and affect patients' overall quality of life and are associated with difficulty chewing food,[53] speech difficulty,[54] drooling, and social embarrassment.[51]

Multiple sclerosis (*ICD-10* G35; *ICD-11* 8A40)

Multiple sclerosis (MS) is a systemic inflammatory autoimmune disease that is characterized by demyelinating lesions and plaques within the central nervous system (CNS). Although the etiology and pathogenesis of MS remain unclear, the current literature illustrates that the cause of MS is multifactorial and includes genetic predisposition together with environmental factors such as exposure to infectious agents, vitamin deficiencies, childhood obesity, and smoking. These agents are able to trigger a cascade of events in the immune system that lead to neuronal cell death accompanied by nerve demyelination and neuronal dysfunction.[55,56] The onset of MS symptoms is most often during the second to fourth decade of life, with an average age of onset of 30 years. This is younger than that of trigeminal neuralgia (TN), which has an average age of onset of between 50 and 60 years.[57] In patients with MS, secondary TN occurs at approximately 15 times the prevalence of that in the general population,[58] and is most likely due to lesions in the intrapontine trigeminal tract or root-entry zone.[59–61] In MS, up to 31% of TN is bilateral, a rate much higher than TN in the non-MS population.[62] Treatment of TN pain in MS patients is similar to that in non-MS patients with TN (see chapter 6).

Lyme disease (*ICD-10* A69.20; *ICD-11* 1C1G)

Lyme disease is a multisystem infection, geographically localized, caused by the tick-borne spirochete *Borrelia burgdorferi* and characterized by a red rash called *erythema migrans* at the site of the tick bite, which is often accompanied by flu-like symptoms. The early systemic dissemination of the infection primarily involves spreading of the erythema migrans to other cutaneous locations; the heart, most commonly causing otherwise unexplained conduction block; and the nervous system. In the late stages, the infection is localized to joints, causing swelling, arthralgia, and arthritis.[63] Only 10% to 15% of untreated patients develop symptomatic nervous system involvement, which may present as a triad of cranial neuropathy, painful radiculopathy, or lymphocytic meningitis with episodic headaches and neck stiffness. Although any cranial nerve can be involved, the most common neurologic manifestation is facial nerve palsy, reported in 8.4% of patients.[64–66] The disorder itself is indistinguishable from Bell palsy in other circumstances, except that in Lyme disease it is bilateral in up to 20% to 25% of affected individuals.[67] Involvement of nerves supplying the extraocular muscles can cause diplopia. Involvement of the 5th cranial nerve can cause hypoesthesia or pain and headaches; vestibulocochlear and 7th cranial nerve involvement can result in hearing changes or vertigo. The optic nerve is rarely involved.[67–69]

Bruxism (*ICD-10* G47.63; *ICD-11* DA0E)

An international consensus position paper defined *bruxism* as a repetitive jaw-muscle activity characterized by clenching or grinding of the teeth and/or by bracing or thrusting of the mandible. Bruxism has two distinct circadian manifestations: it can occur during sleep (sleep bruxism) or during wakefulness (awake bruxism).[70] Recently, a revision of the consensus definition was made, and two separate definitions were proposed[71]:

- Sleep bruxism (SB) is a masticatory muscle activity during sleep that is characterized as rhythmic (phasic) or non-rhythmic (tonic) and is not a movement disorder or a sleep disorder in otherwise healthy individuals.
- Awake bruxism (AB) is a masticatory muscle activity during wakefulness that is characterized by repetitive or sustained tooth contact and/or by bracing or thrusting of the mandible and is not a movement disorder in otherwise healthy individuals.

Based on this definition, bruxism is considered a behavior and not a disorder. However, in certain clinical conditions, it may become a risk factor or a sign of a pathologic condition.[72] Moreover, in some individuals, it may play a protective role. For instance, in gastroesophageal reflux disease (GERD) patients, it has been suggested that SB can stimulate saliva production to neutralize the harmful effect of acid reflux on oral structures. Similarly, a protective role of jaw muscle activity has been proposed to facilitate the opening of the upper airway in sleep breathing disordered patients.[73,74] Other sleep comorbidities associated with SB include insomnia, periodic limb movement, or rapid eye movement disorders.[75] To date, further studies are needed to fully elucidate the shared physiologic or pathophysiologic mechanisms between these comorbidities.

Box 10-5 Clinical features of sleep bruxism*

Self-report from patient or sleep partner

Sleep
- Sleep partner complains of grinding noise (occasionally tapping noise with oromandibular myoclonus)

Waking in the morning
- Patient reports jaw muscle discomfort or fatigue
- Temporal headache of short duration
- Difficulty in jaw opening, jaw stiffness, TMJ noise
- Tooth hypersensitivity to cold stimuli (eg, food, beverage, or air)

Clinical observations

Visual inspection
- Tooth wear, fracture, and cervical defects
- Tongue indentation

Digital palpation
- Masseter muscle hypertrophy during voluntary clenching (bilateral)
- Jaw muscle tenderness (masseter, temporalis) and TMJ pain

Miscellaneous
- Dental restoration failure or fracture (eg, crown, denture, inlay, implant)
- Occlusal trauma
- Tongue biting (observed in oromandibular myoclonus)

*Adapted with permission from Kato and Lavigne.[76]

The prevalence of bruxism among the general population presents a high variability due to the lack of standardized diagnostic methods. Even though laboratory polysomnography (PSG) or electromyography (EMG) studies are considered the gold standard for the diagnosis of bruxism, in clinical settings, the diagnosis is often based on self-reported questionnaires and clinical examination (Box 10-5).[76] Hence, a Standardized Tool for the Assessment of Bruxism (STAB) has been proposed as a multidimensional evaluation system that would include instrumental assessment, self-report, clinical examination, risk factors, and comorbidities.[77]

The prevalence of SB, based on the subjective report of grinding noises during sleep, has been reported to be 5% to 8% in adults, 10% to 20% in children, and 3% in the elderly.[78–82] Although AB is a distinctive entity from SB, there appears to be overlap in some individuals, with AB affecting 20% of the population.[83,84]

Even though, certain musculoskeletal signs and symptoms are associated to some extent with SB (see Box 10-5),[76] a strong positive association between musculoskeletal pain and SB has not yet been demonstrated.[85,86] In contrast, AB seems to be positively associated with masticatory muscle pain.[87]

Studies investigating the physiology of sleep bruxism reveal a cascade of events involving sympathetic cardiac activation, leading to microarousal prior to the SB episodes. This cascade of events includes temporary increases in sympathetic tone, heart rate, α and δ electroencephalogram (EEG) activity, infrahyoid muscle activity, and respiratory activity[88] (see chapter 11). Based on the limited scientific evidence, the pathophysiology of AB may be associated with anxiety-related personalities, suggesting an involvement of the limbic portion of the basal ganglia.[89]

The risk factors that have been reported to be associated with bruxism include the use of alcohol, nicotine, caffeine, recreational drugs (eg, heroin, methamphetamine, and MDMA), medications (ie, selective seratonin reuptake inhibitors, phenethylamines, and anticonvulsants), and anxiety.[79,88,90–94] Other comorbidities that have been reported include neurologic disorders (ie, encephalitis, Parkinson disease, epilepsy, traumatic brain injury, and stroke) and endocrine disorders such as hyperthyroidism.[77,95]

Connective tissue diseases

Connective tissue diseases are the result of systemic autoimmune dysfunction and dysregulation involving one or multiple organs. This section discusses more common connective tissue diseases, such as systemic lupus erythematosus, rheumatoid arthritis, Sjögren syndrome, and systemic sclerosis. Other less common connective tissue diseases, such as dermatomyositis, polymyositis, and mixed connective tissue diseases, may also contribute to orofacial pain and dysfunction.[96]

Systemic lupus erythematosus (*ICD-10* M32.9; *ICD-11* A440)

Systemic lupus erythematosus (SLE) is a multiorgan connective tissue disease related to abnormal production of autoantibodies, multisystem inflammation, and vasculopathy. In 2019, the European League Against Rheumatism (EULAR) and the American College of Rheumatology (ACR) developed the new classification for SLE. The EULAR/ACR 2019 criteria include clinical and immunologic findings. An elevated amount of antinuclear antibodies is required to be classified as SLE in addition to a score of 10 points out of a list of 21 symptoms and clinical tests. The clinical criteria include but are not limited to the presence of fever, rash, oral ulcers, or synovitis (in at least two joints), and clinical tests including but not limited to biopsy-proven lupus nephritis, positive lupus anticoagulant, or low complement.[97] TMJ pain, locking, and crepitation have been reported in systemic lupus erythematosus patients. Similarly, trigeminal neuropathy has been reported to develop as an initial presentation or gradually with this disease.[96–98]

Rheumatoid arthritis (*ICD-10* M06.9; *ICD-11* FA20)

Rheumatoid arthritis is a chronic, systemic inflammatory disease in which pro-inflammatory cytokines destroy articular cartilage and subchondral bone.[96] In a subset of patients (40%), systemic involvement can affect extra-articular organs resulting in the following conditions: pericarditis, pleuritis, Felty syndrome, vasculitis (eg, major cutaneous vasculitis, scleritis, episcleritis, retinal vasculitis, or vasculitis affecting other organs), glomerulonephritis, amyloidosis, keratoconjunctivitis sicca, xerosotomia, secondary Sjögren syndrome, pulmonary fibrosis, bronchiolitis obliterans organizing pneumonia, cervical myelopathy, subcutaneous rheumatoid nodules, and rheumatoid nodules in other locations.[99] The diagnosis of rheumatoid arthritis is based on the 2010 EULAR/ACR classification criteria, and there are updated guidelines for its treatment.[100] Half of rheumatoid arthritis patients have TMJ pain and swelling, jaw stiffness, and limited mouth opening.[101] However, involvement of the TMJ typically occurs later in this disease process as compared to other joints.[102] TMJ pain and crepitus occur within 2 years of general symptom onset.[103,104] Fibrous and bony ankylosis may occur with disease progression.[105] Imaging of the TMJ with computed tomography (CT) or magnetic resonance imaging (MRI) scans may reveal joint effusion, synovial proliferation, marrow edema, altered disc morphology and displacement, and condylar abnormalities, namely erosions, flattening, sclerosis, subchondral cysts, and osteophytes.[106,107] Class II malocclusion involving heavy posterior contacts and anterior open bite occur in advanced cases of condylar destruction.[108]

Juvenile idiopathic arthritis (*ICD-10* M08.9; *ICD-11* FA24)

Juvenile idiopathic arthritis (JIA) is an autoimmune condition of unknown etiology that encompasses all forms of chronic arthritis (> 6 weeks) starting before the age of 16 years.[109] Systemic JIA is characterized by an autoinflammatory phenotype including fever, rash, lymphadenopathies, and marked systemic inflammation, among other symptoms.[110] The diagnosis of JIA, based on the International League of Associations for Rheumatology (IALR) classification (not formally validated but essentially developed by consensus), subdivides patients into seven subcategories.[109,111] However, there is currently a new proposed diagnostic criteria being considered by the Pediatric Rheumatology International Trials Organization (PRINTO).[110]

The involvement of the TMJ is a common problem in children with JIA. Morphologic changes of the TMJ have been found in 70% of patients and can lead to craniomandibular growth disturbances (eg, micrognathia or facial asymmetry), and dental malocclusions if left untreated.[112,113]

The prevalence of TMD such as TMJ pain and functional limitation has been estimated to be around 40% in children and adolescents with JIA versus 11.3% in healthy controls.[112,114,115] TMD is more prevalent particularly in JIA patients with polyarticular course, cervical spine involvement, longer duration of the disease, and female sex.[116]

It is worth emphasizing the importance of an early diagnosis of JIA, because the introduction of disease-modifying antirheumatic drugs has dramatically improved the prognosis of the disease, preventing the development of craniofacial deformities when the TMJs are involved.[113]

Sjögren syndrome (*ICD-10* M35.00; *ICD-11* 4A43.2)

Sjögren syndrome is characterized by chronic inflammation of exocrine glands, affecting primarily the lacrimal and salivary glands. The decrease in exocrine secretions is caused by autoreactive lymphocytic infiltrates replacing epithelium, causing keratoconjunctivitis sicca and hyposalivation.[96] The diagnosis of primary Sjögren syndrome is based on the 2016 EULAR/ACR classification criteria based on the weighted sum of five items: *(1)* anti-Sjögren-syndrome-related antigen A antibody positivity and *(2)* focal lymphocytic sialadenitis with a focus score of ≥ 1 foci/4 mm², each scoring 3; *(3)* an abnormal ocular staining score of ≥ 5 (or van Bijsterveld score of ≥ 4); *(4)* a Schirmer test result of ≤ 5 mm/5 min; *(5)* and an unstimulated salivary flow rate of ≤ 0.1 mL/min, each scoring 1. Patients who have a total score of ≥ 4 along with signs and symptoms of Sjögren syndrome fulfill the criteria.[117]

Peripheral neuropathy including trigeminal neuropathy characterized by facial numbness and paresthesia has been reported.[118,119] Signs of TMDs such as jaw joint sounds, tenderness of the masticatory muscles, and limited range of jaw movement were more common in Sjögren syndrome.[120] Similarly, the prevalence of headache was 78.1% among Sjögren syndrome patients, with migraine (54%) and tension-type headache (24.1%) being the most common types.[121]

Systemic sclerosis (*ICD-10* M34; *ICD-11* A442)

Systemic sclerosis is characterized by abnormal fibrosis and subsequent damage and dysfunction of the skin, vasculature, and internal organs.[96] Microstomia secondary to limited mouth opening from fibrosis is a known orofacial manifestation.[122–124] The diagnosis of systemic sclerosis is based on the joint 2013 classification criteria of the EULAR/ACR. Essentially, the diagnosis of systemic sclerosis may be established based on skin thickening of the fingers extending proximal to the metacarpophalangeal joints. Alternatively, seven additive items of varying weights may apply, including skin thickening of the fingers, fingertip lesions, telangiectasia, abnormal nailfold capillaries, interstitial lung disease or pulmonary arterial hypertension, Raynaud phenomenon, and disease-related autoantibodies.[125] TMJ pain and swelling secondary to synovitis have been noted among systemic sclerosis patients.[126] Patients with systemic sclerosis often complain of muscle pain with chewing, headache, and difficulty with mouth opening.[127] Erosion of the coronoid process, condyle, angle of the mandible, and ramus may also be noted on radiographs.[128,129] Trigeminal neuropathy involving pain and sensory loss has been reported, as have symptoms consistent with trigeminal neuralgia.[130,131] There are also reports of giant cell arteritis (GCA) in patients with systemic sclerosis.[132]

Fibromyalgia (*ICD-10* M79.7; *ICD-11* MG30.01)

Fibromyalgia is a pain disorder likely neurogenic in origin presenting as chronic widespread allodynia and/or hyperalgesia. It is postulated that *fibromyalgia* may in fact be a misnomer as it merely represents the severe end of the chronic widespread pain spectrum for which no cause can be identified. There is also debate on whether individuals diagnosed with fibromyalgia or chronic widespread pain need to be classified as such, as both conditions are treated similarly.[133]

Although its pathophysiology remains an enigma, there is substantial evidence of central nervous system (CNS) involvement leading to augmented nociceptive and sensory processing, as demonstrated by quantitative sensory testing, neurofunctional imaging alterations,[134] CNS neurotransmitter imbalance, and a decreased conditioned pain modulation system. Additionally, the hypothalamic pituitary axis and sympathetic nervous system have also been implicated, because stress enhances the pain experience in fibromyalgia patients.[135] Lastly, recent evidence has begun to explore the potential role of the peripheral nervous system and chronic systemic inflammation in fibromyalgia.[135,136]

Current clinical diagnostic criteria for fibromyalgia from the ACR exclude counting tender points as previously required.[137] Fibromyalgia symptoms include pain for at least 3 months involving the right and left side of the body, above and below the waist, and in the axial skeleton (scored with the widespread pain index) as well as CNS-mediated somatic symptoms such as fatigue, sleep disturbances, and cognitive disturbances (scored with the symptom severity index).[138] The most common comorbidities for fibromyalgia are mood and anxiety disorders.

Other overlapping pain conditions include irritable bowel syndrome, tension-type headache, migraine, interstitial cystitis, prostadynia, vulvodynia, chronic pelvic pain, and TMDs.[139]

There have been numerous studies suggesting a relationship between TMDs and fibromyalgia. Up to 75% to 80% of fibromyalgia patients present with signs and symptoms consistent with TMDs.[140] One study showed that 53% of fibromyalgia patients reported face pain, of which 71% fulfilled the Research Diagnostic Criteria for TMDs.[141] Practitioners treating orofacial pain patients should inquire about pains in other areas of the body to exclude fibromyalgia as an etiology.

Lymphatic system

The lymphatic system is composed of an extensive network of small lymphatic capillaries, larger lymphatic vessels, and lymph nodes. The lymphatic system functions as a supplementary drainage system that collects interstitial fluid, protein, and cells and returns them to circulation. In the head and neck, lymph nodes are grouped into chains, located both within subcutaneous tissues and in deeper tissues associated with muscle and fascial planes. The lymph chains include the occipital, preauricular, postauricular, parotid, buccal, mandibular, submandibular, submental, superficial cervical, internal jugular, spinal accessory, and supraclavicular lymph nodes.

In health, lymph nodes generally are not palpable. *Lymphadenopathy*, which is an alteration in lymph node size, number, and consistency, may indicate pathology, possibly due to a drug reaction, infection, immunologic disorder, or malignancy.[142,143] Infective causes may be local or systemic and include bacterial, fungal, and viral disease. Inflammatory lymphadenopathy may also be of a noninfective nature from disorders such as sarcoidosis or connective tissue disease. Neoplastic enlargement can be due to primary lymph node disease or metastatic disease.

In the head and neck, the most common node to be enlarged is the jugulodigastric node. This node is located just inferior and anterior to the angle of the mandible. Enlarged nodes that are soft, freely movable, and tender are likely inflammatory. Nodes that are firm or rubbery, fixed to underlying tissue, or matted together and nontender are likely neoplastic. The differential diagnoses of nonpainful lymphadenopathies include tuberculosis, Hodgkin lymphoma, non-Hodgkin lymphoma, leukemia, and plasmacytoma. Most pain disorders associated with the lymphatic system occur secondary to a regional acute inflammatory process (Box 10-6).

Blood vessels

Vascular disease may be a source of head and facial pain (Box 10-7). Orofacial pain is a common presenting symptom of GCA (also known as *temporal arteritis* and described in chapter 4; *ICD-10* M31.6; *ICD-11* 4A44.2), a condition caused by granulomatous inflammation of the temporal artery or other branches of the aortic arch. It is found predominantly in people over the age of 50 years, often in the seventh and eighth decade of life. There appears to be an association between GCA and polymyalgia rheumatica, an inflammatory rheumatic condition that affects individuals over the age of 50 years. Temporal artery biopsies of polymyalgia rheumatica patients without clinical characteristics of GCA showed expression of cytokines (a marker for inflammation) without overt vasculitis.[144] GCA is characterized by a swollen, tender superficial temporal artery, headache, hip and shoulder girdle pain, and constitutional symptoms.[145] A prominent feature of the disease is jaw claudication, affecting 30% to 40% of patients. Jaw clandication is characterized by an aching cramp in the masseter or temporalis muscles produced by jaw function, and it can

Box 10-6 Etiology of head and neck lymphadenopathy*

I. Infectious diseases

- Viral: Infectious mononucleosis (Epstein-Barr virus, cytomegalovirus), infectious hepatitis, herpes simplex, human herpes virus 6, varicella zoster virus, rubella, measles, adenovirus, human immunodeficiency virus
- Bacterial: *Streptococcus*, *staphylococcus*, cat-scratch disease, brucellosis, tularemia, chancroid, tuberculosis, atypical mycobacterial infection, primary and secondary syphilis, diphtheria, leprosy
- Fungal: Histoplasmosis, coccidioidomycosis, paracoccidioidomycosis
- Chlamydial: Lymphogranuloma venereum, trachoma
- Parasitic: Toxoplasmosis, leishmaniasis, trypanosomiasis, filariasis
- Rickettsial: Scrub typhus, rickettsialpox

II. Immunologic diseases

- Rheumatoid arthritis
- Mixed connective tissue disease
- Systemic lupus erythematosus
- Dermatomyositis
- Sjögren syndrome
- Serum sickness
- Drug hypersensitivity
- Primary biliary cirrhosis
- Graft-vs-host disease
- Silicone-associated
- Periodic fever, aphthous stomatitis, pharyngitis, cervical adenitis (PFAPA)

III. Malignant diseases

- Hematologic (Hodgkin or non-Hodgkin lymphoma, acute lymphoblastic leukemia, chronic lymphoblastic leukemia, hairy cell leukemia, malignant histiocytosis, T-cell lymphoma, multiple myeloma with amyloidosis)
- Metastatic from primary sites

IV. Lipid storage diseases

- Gaucher
- Niemann-Pick
- Tangier

V. Endocrine diseases

- Hyperthyroid
- Thyroiditis
- Adrenal insufficiency

VI. Other disorders

- Castleman disease (giant lymph node hyperplasia)
- Sarcoidosis
- Dermatopathic lymphadenitis
- Lymphomatoid granulomatosis
- Kikuchi disease (histiocytic necrotizing lymphadenitis)
- Kawasaki disease (mucocutaneous lymph node syndrome)
- Langerhans cell histiocytosis
- Severe hypertriglyceridemia

*Adapted with permission from Parisi and Glick.[143]

easily be confused with TMD. Another feature of the disease is an erythrocyte sedimentation rate of at least 50 mm/h, an elevated C-reactive protein level > 2.45 mg/dL, and platelet counts > 400,000. C-reactive protein level is a more sensitive marker than the erythrocyte sedimentation rate, while the combination of both improves specificity.[146,147] GCA is considered a medical emergency because of the high risk of irreversible blindness that can occur due to inflammation of the posterior ciliary arteries with anterior ischemic optic neuropathy and cerebrovascular accidents.[148] A positive temporal artery biopsy provides the most definitive evidence of GCA, with an estimated sensitivity of 77%.[149] However, early treatment should be initiated if GCA is suspected even before the results of the biopsy are available. Treatment involves prednisolone, 40 to 60 mg daily for 4 to 6 weeks and then gradually tapered as symptoms improve over 12 to 24 months.[150]

Box 10-7 Head and facial pain arising from blood vessels

Primary pain

- Subarachnoid hemorrhage (ICHD 6.2.2)
- Unruptured vascular malformation (ICHD 6.3)
- Saccular aneurysm (ICHD 6.3.1)
- Arteriovenous malformation (ICHD 6.3.2)
- Giant cell arteritis (ICHD 6.4.1)
- Primary intracranial angiitis (ICHD 6.4.2)
- Systemic lupus erythematosus (ICHD 6.4.3)
- Carotid or vertebral artery dissection (ICHD 6.5.1)
- Postcarotid endarterectomy (ICHD 6.5.2)
- Cerebral venous thrombosis (ICHD 6.6)
- Arterial hypertension (ICHD 10.3)

Vertebro-basilar artery syndrome (*ICD-10* G45.0; *ICD-11* 8B10.Y)

Vertebral artery (VA) involvement can contribute to various cervicogenic headaches. Syndromes with similar symptoms include VA compression syndrome (*ICD-10* M47.12; *ICD-11* 8B42) and benign paroxysmal positional vertigo (*ICD-10* H81.13; *ICD-11* AB31.2). The major extracranial region of the VA is protected by the vertebral canal and the surrounding soft tissue structures; however, there is vulnerability from the second cervical vertebrae to the foramen magnum.[151,152] VA injury in the suboccipital region can occur from severe cervical spine trauma, such as a fracture of the atlas, or iatrogenically during surgery.[153] Red flags immediately necessitate further testing to rule out VA involvement; these include disorientation, nausea, vomiting, visual disturbances, dizziness, or vertigo that occur simply by changing from a non-weight-bearing (supine) position to a weight-bearing position (ie, sitting or standing).[154] An experienced physician or physical therapist should perform the assessment, which can be curtailed in favor of neurologic and radiologic testing if any of the above red flags reoccur or intensify during the evaluative process. Active cervical spine range of movement and provocation testing into positions of rotation, side-bending, and extension can be used to stretch, narrow, or kink the ipsilateral and/or contralateral VA; however, this must be performed with great caution, and the reliability is questionable unless performed by an experienced clinician.[155] The delineation between labyrinthine and VA involvement should also be considered. The trained dentist can auscultate the carotid and subclavian arteries for bruits (also known as a *vascular murmur*, which is an audible vascular sound associated with turbulent blood flow) with the patient in a seated position and the head in neutral, but further testing in positions of cervical rotation and extension to each side should be designated to others.[156]

Box 10-8 Head and facial pain arising from systemic disease

- Anemia
- Adrenal insufficiency
- Arthritides
  - Rheumatoid arthritis
  - Osteoarthritis
  - Psoriatic arthritis
  - Systemic lupus erythematosus
- Chronic pulmonary failure with hypercapnia
- Diabetes mellitus
- Fibromyalgia
- Hashimoto thyroiditis
- Herpes zoster
- HIV/AIDS
- Hypertension/pheochromocytoma
- Infectious mononucleosis
- Ischemic heart disease
- Lyme disease
- Menopause
- Menstruation
- Metastatic malignancies
- Multiple sclerosis
- Primary malignancies
- Renal failure (uremia)/dialysis

Box 10-9 Signs or symptoms suggestive of systemic disease

- Chest pain
- Chronic fatigue
- Extreme hunger or thirst
- Fever
- Generalized aches and pains
- Malaise
- Palpitations
- Shortness of breath
- Skin lesions
- Tachycardia
- Unintentional weight loss or gain

Barré-Liéou syndrome (*ICD-10* M53.0)

Barré-Liéou syndrome was named after Jean-Alexander Barré, professor of neurology, who in 1926 first described the posterior cervical sympathetic syndrome. This rare syndrome was caused by cervical degenerative joint disease, resulting in occipital headaches accompanied by orofacial pain, tinnitus, dizziness, visual disturbances, and tiredness. Hence, Barré-Liéou syndrome is arguably the first description of cervicogenic headache, linking headache to degenerative joint disease of the cervical spine (see chapter 9).[157]

His proposed posterior cervical sympathetic syndrome was later rejected.[158] However, more recent studies have provided evidence to support his initial hypothesis on the involvement of the sympathetic nervous system in the pathophysiology of cervicogenic dizziness. Furthermore, it has been hypothesized that the use of sympatholytic agents might be useful as an adjuvant treatment for the sympathetic symptoms associated with cervical degenerative joint disease.[159]

In summary, even though the use of the eponym Barré-Liéou syndrome remains controversial, further studies are needed to elucidate the possible involvement of the sympathetic nervous system and to study the effectiveness of spinal interventions in patients with degenerative cervical joint disease and associated systemic symptoms.

Other systemic causes of head and facial pain

There are many systemic diseases and disorders that are accompanied by headache or facial pain. Included among these are metabolic and endocrine disorders, infectious disease, autoimmune disease, cardiovascular disease, renal disease, and pulmonary disease. Box 10-8 lists some of the more common of these systemic diseases. It is beyond the scope of this chapter to discuss these many entities; however, the practitioner should remain alert to include systemic disease in a differential diagnosis when facial pain is accompanied by systemic signs or symptoms.[160] Symptoms that may suggest systemic disease are listed in Box 10-9.[161,162] In these instances, head or facial pain is merely an accompanying symptom of a potentially serious underlying disease, and the clinician must guard against the trap of attempting to treat the facial pain when a much more serious underlying problem is present.[34,163] In these situations, referral to the appropriate health clinician must be considered. In addition to these disorders, the reader is referred to chapter 4 for a discussion of other worrisome constitutional symptoms.

References

1. Headache Classification Committee of the International Headache Society (IHS) The International Classification of Headache Disorders, 3rd edition. Cephalgia 2018;38:1–211.
2. Göbel H. Headache from cranial bone. In: Gebhart GF, Schmidt RF (eds). Encyclopedia of Pain. Berlin/Heidelberg: Springer, 2013.
3. Göbel H, Edmeads JG. Disorders of the skull and cervical spine. In: Olesen J, Goadsby PJ, Ramadan NM, Tfelt-Hansen P, Welch KMA (eds). The Headaches, ed 3. Philadelphia: Lippincott Williams & Wilkins, 2006:1003–1011.
4. Arends S, Coebergh JA, Kerkhoffs JL, van Gils A, Koppen H. Severe unilateral headache caused by skull bone infarction with epidural haematoma in a patient with sickle cell disease. Cephalalgia 2011;31:1325–1328.
5. Dlouhy BJ, Menezes AH. Osteopetrosis with Chiari I malformation: Presentation and surgical management. J Neurosurg Pediatr 2011;7:369–374.
6. Loh JK, Su YF, Hwang SL, Chai CY, Howng SL, Lieu AS. Eosinophilic granuloma of the occipital bone in an adult: A case report. Kaohsiung J Med Sci 2011;27:76–79.
7. Muzumdar D, Balasubramaniam S, Jhawar S, Goel A. Massive benign osteoblastoma of the suboccipital bone and foramen magnum region. Pediatr Neurosurg 2010;46:232–237.
8. Soni CR, Kumar G, Sahota P, Miller DC, Litofsky NS. Metastases to Meckel's cave: Report of two cases and comparative analysis of malignant tumors with meningioma and schwannoma of Meckel's cave. Clin Neurol Neurosurg 2010;112:927–932.
9. Singh AD, Soneja M, Memon SS, Vyas S. Interesting case of base of skull mass infiltrating cavernous sinuses. BMJ Case Rep 2016:bcr2016217669.
10. Bhatoe HS, Ambastha R. Primary non Hodgkin's lymphoma of the cranial vault in a child. J Neurooncol 2016;126:209–211.
11. Beck RW, Smith CH. Trigeminal nerve. In: Duane TD, Jaeger EA (eds). Biomedical Foundations in Ophthalmology. Philadelphia: Harper & Row, 1983:1–16.
12. Orcutt JC. Ocular and periocular pain. In: Loeser JD (ed). Bonica's Management of Pain. Philadelphia: Lippincott Williams & Wilkins, 2001:925–935.
13. Jaeger B. Overview of head and neck region. In: Simons DG, Travell JG, Simons LS (eds). Travell & Simons' Myofascial Pain and Dysfunction: The Trigger Point Manual. Baltimore: Williams & Wilkins, 1999:237–277.
14. Lajmi H, Choura R, Ben Achour B, Doukh M, Amin Z, Hmaied W. Headache associated with refractive errors: Characteristics and risk factors [epub ahead of print 20 Jan 2021]. Rev Neurol (Paris) doi:10.1016/j.neurol.2020.10.008.
15. Valenzuela AA, Archibald CW, Fleming B, et al. Orbital metastasis: Clinical features, management and outcome. Orbit 2009;28:153–159.
16. Ganesh A, Al-Zuhaibi S, Pathare A, et al. Orbital infarction in sickle cell disease. Am J Ophthalmol 2008;146:595–601.
17. Peleg A, Heran MK, White VA, Chang WY, Rootman J. Malignant lymphoproliferative disorders extending into the orbit from the paranasal sinuses. Orbit 2009;28:80–87.
18. Pointdujour-Lim R, Lally SE, Shields JA, Eagle RC Jr, Shields CL. Orbital schwannoma: Radiographic and histopathologic correlation in 15 cases. Ophthalmic Plast Reconstr Surg 2018;34:162–167.
19. Briscoe D, Safieh C, Ton Y, Shapiro H, Assia EI, Kidron D. Characteristics of orbital lymphoma: A clinicopathological study of 26 cases. Int Ophthalmol 2018;38:271–277.
20. Göbel H, Baloh RW. Disorders of ear, nose, and sinus. In: Olesen J, Goadsby PJ, Ramadan NM, Tfelt-Hansen P, Welch KMA (eds). The Headaches, ed 3. Philadelphia: Lippincott Williams & Wilkins, 2006:1019–1027.
21. Simons DG, Travell JG, Simons LS (eds). Travell & Simons' Myofascial Pain and Dysfunction: The Trigger Point Manual. Baltimore: Williams & Wilkins, 1999.
22. Wright EF. Referred craniofacial pain patterns in patients with temporomandibular disorder. J Am Dent Assoc 2000;131:1307–1315.

23. Earwood JC, Rogers TS, Rathjen NA. Ear pain: Diagnosing common and uncommon causes. Am Fam Physician 2018;97:20–27.
24. Dray TG, Weymuller EA. Pain in the ear, midface, and aerodigestive tract. In: Loeser JD (ed). Bonica's Management of Pain. Philadelphia: Lippincott Williams & Wilkins, 2001:936–947.
25. Williams RA, Jackler RK, Corrales CE. Benign temporomandibular joint lesions presenting as masses in the external auditory canal. Otol Neurotol 2017;38:563–571.
26. Porto De Toledo I, Stefani FM, et al. Prevalence of otologic signs and symptoms in adult patients with temporomandibular disorders: A systematic review and meta-analysis. Clin Oral Investig 2017;21:597–605.
27. Shargorodsky J, Curhan GC, Farwell WR. Prevalence and characteristics of tinnitus among US adults. Am J Med 2010;123:711–718.
28. Kircher MT, Standring RT, Leonetti JP. Neuroradiologic assessment of pulsatile tinnitus. Otolaryngol Head Neck Surg 2008;139:144.
29. Tunkel DE, Bauer CA, Sun GH, et al: Clinical practice guideline: Tinnitus. Otolaryngol Head Neck Surg 2014;151(2 suppl):S1–S40.
30. Edvall NK, Gunan E, Genitsaridi E, et al. Impact of temporomandibular joint complaints on tinnitus-related distress. Front Neurosci 2019;13:879.
31. Moreira de Lacerda AB, Facco C, Zeigelboim BS, Cristoff K, Neto JS, Fonseca VR. The impact of tinnitus on the quality of life in patients with temporomandibular dysfunction. Int Tinnitus J 2016;20:24–30.
32. Ralli M, Greco A, Boccassini A, et al. Subtyping patients with somatic tinnitus: Modulation of tinnitus and history for somatic dysfunction help identify tinnitus patients with temporomandibular joint disorders. PLoS One 2018;13(8):e0202050.
33. Brackmann DE, Bartels LJ. Rare tumors of the cerebellopontine angle. Otolaryngol Head Neck Surg (1979) 1980;88:555–559.
34. Matsuka Y, Fort ET, Merrill RL. Trigeminal neuralgia due to an acoustic neuroma in the cerebellopontine angle. J Orofac Pain 2000;14:147–151.
35. House WF. Translabyrinthine approach. In: House WF, Leutje CM, Doyle KJ (eds). Acoustic Tumors. San Diego: Singular Publishing, 1997:171–176.
36. Hitselberger WE, House WE. Acoustic neuroma diagnosis. External auditory canal hypesthesia as an early sign. Arch Otolaryngol 1966;83:218–221.
37. Lanza DC, Kennedy DW. Adult rhinosinusitis defined. Otolaryngol Head Neck Surg 1997;117:S1–S7.
38. Williams JW Jr, Simel DL, Roberts L, Samsa GP. Clinical evaluation for sinusitis. Making the diagnosis by history and physical examination. Ann Intern Med 1992;117:705–710.
39. Schreiber CP, Hutchinson S, Webster CJ, Ames M, Richardson MS, Powers C. Prevalence of migraine among patients with history of self-reported or physician-diagnosed "sinus" headache. Arch Intern Med 2004;164:1769–1772.
40. Eross E, Dodick D, Eross M. The sinus, allergy and migraine study (SAMS). Headache 2007;47:213–224.
41. Gryglas A. Allergic rhinitis and chronic daily headaches: Is there a link? Curr Neurol Neurosci Rep 2016;16(4):33.
42. Cady RK, Schreiber CP. Sinus problems as a cause of headache refractoriness and migraine chronification. Curr Pain Headache Rep 2009;13:319–325.
43. Hadley JA, Schaefer SD. Clinical evaluation of rhinosinusitis: History and physical examination. Otolaryngol Head Neck Surg 1997;117:S8–S11.
44. Bradley PJ. Tumors of the salivary gland. In: Jones AS, Phillips DE, Hilgers FJ (eds). Diseases of the Head and Neck, Nose and Throat. London: Arnold, 1998:329–346.
45. Ram S, Kumar SK, Clark GT. Using oral medications, infusions and injections for differential diagnosis of orofacial pain. J Calif Dent Assoc 2006;34:645–654.
46. Wong EH, Farrier JN, Cooper DG. First-bite syndrome complicating carotid endarterectomy: A case report and literature review. Vasc Endovascular Surg 2011;45:459–461.
47. Ghosh A, Mirza N. First bite syndrome: Our experience with intraparotid injections with botulinum toxin type A. Laryngoscope 2016;126:104–107.
48. Sharp J, Watkinson JC. Surgical anatomy of the head and neck. In: Jones AS, Phillips DE, Hilgers FJ (eds). Diseases of the Head and Neck, Nose and Throat. London: Arnold, 1998:11–23.
49. Chan TV. The patient with sore throat. Med Clin North Am 2010;94:923–943.
50. Balasubramaniam R, Ram S. Orofacial movement disorders. Oral Maxillofac Surg Clin North Am 2008;20:273–285.
51. Clark GT, Ram S. Orofacial movement disorders. Oral Maxillofac Surg Clin North Am 2016;28:397–407.
52. Sude A, Matsumoto J, Kaimal S, Petersen A, Nixdorf DR. Temporomandibular disorder-related characteristics and treatment outcomes in oromandibular dystonia patients in two different clinical settings: A cross-sectional study. J Oral Rehabil 2021;48:542–550.
53. Bakke M, Baram S, Dalager T, Biernat HB, Møller E. Oromandibular dystonia, mental distress and orofacial dysfunction-A follow-up 8–10 years after start of treatment with botulinum toxin. J Oral Rehabil 2019;46:441–449.

54. Page AD, Siegel LH, Baylor CR, Adams SG, Yorkston KM. The consequences of oromandibular dystonia on communicative participation: A qualitative study of the insider's experiences. Am J Speech Lang Pathol 2019;28(2S):771–783.
55. Ghasemi N, Razavi S, Nikzad E. Multiple sclerosis: Pathogenesis, symptoms, diagnoses and cell-based therapy. Cell J 2017;19:1–10.
56. McGinley MP, Goldschmidt CH, Rae-Grant AD. Diagnosis and treatment of multiple sclerosis: A review. JAMA 2021;325:765–779.
57. Bendtsen L, Zakrzewska JM, Heinskou TB, et al. Advances in diagnosis, classification, pathophysiology, and management of trigeminal neuralgia. Lancet Neurol 2020;19:784–796.
58. Laakso SM, Hekali O, Kurdo G, Martola J, Sairanen T, Atula S. Trigeminal neuralgia in multiple sclerosis: Prevalence and association with demyelination. Acta Neurol Scand 2020;142:139–144.
59. Cruccu G, Biasiotta A, Di Rezze S, et al. Trigeminal neuralgia and pain related to multiple sclerosis. Pain 2009;143:186–191.
60. Aboud T, Schuster NM. Pain management in multiple sclerosis: A review of available treatment options. Curr Treat Options Neurol 2019;21(12):62.
61. Swinnen C, Lunskens S, Deryck O, Casselman J, Vanopdenbosch L. MRI characteristics of trigeminal nerve involvement in patients with multiple sclerosis. Mult Scler Relat Disord 2013;2:200–203.
62. O'Connor AB, Schwid SR, Herrmann DN, Markman JD, Dworkin RH. Pain associated with multiple sclerosis: Systematic review and proposed classification. Pain 2008;137:96–111.
63. Halperin JJ. Nervous system Lyme disease. J R Coll Physicians Edinb 2010;40:248–255.
64. Steere AC, Strle F, Wormser GP, et al. Lyme borreliosis. Nat Rev Dis Primers 2016;2:16090.
65. Murphy MA, Szabados EM, Mitty JA. Lyme disease associated with postganglionic Horner syndrome and Raeder paratrigeminal neuralgia. J Neuroophthalmol 2007;27:123–124.
66. Schwartz AM, Hinckley AF, Mead PS, Hook SA, Kugeler KJ. Surveillance for Lyme disease—United States, 2008–2015. MMWR Surveill Summ 2017; 66:1–12.
67. Halperin JJ. A neurologist's view of Lyme disease and other tick-borne infections. Semin Neurol 2019;39: 440–447.
68. Halperin JJ. Nervous system Lyme disease. Clin Lab Med 2015;35:779–795.
69. Lantos PM, Rumbaugh J, Bockenstedt LK, et al. Clinical practice guidelines by the Infectious Diseases Society of America, American Academy of Neurology, and American College of Rheumatology: 2020 guidelines for the prevention, diagnosis, and treatment of Lyme disease. Neurology 2021;96:262–273.
70. Lobbezoo F, Ahlberg J, Glaros AG, et al. Bruxism defined and graded: An international consensus. J Oral Rehabil 2013;40:2–4.
71. Lobbezoo F, Ahlberg J, Raphael KG, et al. International consensus on the assessment of bruxism: Report of a work in progress. J Oral Rehabil 2018;45:837–844.
72. Svensson P, Lavigne G. Clinical bruxism semantics beyond academic debates: Normo- and patho-bruxism as a new proposal. J Oral Rehabil 2020;47: 547–548.
73. Balasubramian R, Klasser GD, Cistulli PA, Lavigne GJ. The link between sleep bruxism, sleep disordered breathing and temporomandibular disorders. JDSM 2014;1(1):27–37.
74. Manfredini D, Guarda-Nardini L, Marchese-Ragona R, Lobbezoo F. Theories on possible temporal relationships between sleep bruxism and obstructive sleep apnea events. An expert opinion. Sleep Breath 2015;19:1459–1465.
75. Lobbezoo F, Lavigne GJ, Kato T, de Almeida FR, Aarab G. The face of dental sleep medicine in the 21st century. J Oral Rehabil 2020;47:1579–1589.
76. Kato T, Lavigne GJ. Sleep bruxism: A sleep-related movement disorder. Sleep Med Clin 2010;5:9–35.
77. Manfredini D, Ahlberg J, Aarab G. Towards a standardized tool for the assessment of bruxism (STAB)-Overview and general remarks of a multidimensional bruxism evaluation system. J Oral Rehabil 2020; 47:549–556.
78. Lavigne GJ, Montplaisir JY. Restless legs syndrome and sleep bruxism: Prevalence and association among Canadians. Sleep 1994;17:739–743.
79. Ohayon MM, Li KK, Guilleminault C. Risk factors for sleep bruxism in the general population. Chest 2001; 119:53–61.
80. Laberge L, Tremblay RE, Vitaro F, Montplaisir J. Development of parasomnias from childhood to early adolescence. Pediatrics 2000;106:67–74.
81. Ng DK, Kwok KL, Cheung JM, et al. Prevalence of sleep problems in Hong Kong primary school children: A community-based telephone survey. Chest 2005;128: 1315–1323.
82. Khoury S, Carra MC, Huynh N, Montplaisir J, Lavigne JG. Sleep bruxism-tooth grinding prevalence, characteristics and familial aggregation: A large cross-sectional survey and polysomnographic validation. Sleep 2016;39:2049–2056.
83. Wetselaar P, Vermaire EJH, Lobbezoo F, Schuller AA. The prevalence of awake bruxism and sleep bruxism in the Dutch adult population. J Oral Rehabil 2019; 46:617–623.
84. Ahlberg J, Piirtola M, Lobbezoo F, et al. Correlates and genetics of self-reported sleep and awake bruxism in a nationwide twin cohort. J Oral Rehabil 2020;47: 1110–1119.

85. Manfredini D, Lobbezoo F. Sleep bruxism and temporomandibular disorders: A scoping review of the literature. J Dent 2021;111:103711.
86. Santiago V, Raphael K. Absence of joint pain identifies high levels of sleep masticatory muscle activity in myofascial temporomandibular disorder. J Oral Rehabil 2019;46:1161–1169.
87. Baad-Hansen L, Thymi M, Lobbezoo F, Svensson P. To what extent is bruxism associated with musculoskeletal signs and symptoms? A systematic review. J Oral Rehabil 2019;46:845–861.
88. Lavigne GJ, Khoury S, Abe S, Yamaguchi T, Raphael K. Bruxism physiology and pathology: An overview for clinicians. J Oral Rehabil 2008;35:476–494.
89. Ella B, Ghorayeb I, Burbaud P, Guehl D. Bruxism in movement disorders: A comprehensive review. J Prosthodont 2017;26:599–605.
90. de Baat C, Verhoeff M, Ahlberg J, et al. Medications and addictive substances potentially inducing or attenuating sleep bruxism and/or awake bruxism. J Oral Rehabil 2021;48:343–54.
91. Bertazzo-Silveira E, Kruger CM, De Toledo IP, et al. Association between sleep bruxism and alcohol, caffeine, tobacco, and drug abuse: A systematic review. J Am Dent Assoc 2016;147:859–866.e4.
92. Castroflorio T, Bargellini A, Rossini G, Cugliari G, Deregibus A. Sleep bruxism and related risk factors in adults: A systematic literature review. Arch Oral Biol 2017;83:25–32.
93. Feu D, Catharino F, Quintão CCA, Almeida MA de O. A systematic review of etiological and risk factors associated with bruxism. J Orthod 2013;40:163–171.
94. Polmann H, Domingos FL, Melo G, et al. Association between sleep bruxism and anxiety symptoms in adults: A systematic review. J Oral Rehabil 2019;46:482–491.
95. Burke DJ, Seitz A, Aladesuru O, Robbins MS, Ch'ang JH. Bruxism in acute neurologic illness. Curr Pain Headache Rep 2021;25:41.
96. Klasser GD, Balasubramaniam R, Epstein J. Topical review-connective tissue diseases: Orofacial manifestations including pain. J Orofac Pain 2007;21:171–184.
97. Aringer, M, Costenbader, K, Daikh, D et al. 2019 European League Against Rheumatism/American College of Rheumatology classification criteria for systemic lupus erythematosus. Ann Rheum Dis 2019;78:1151–1159.
98. Nascimento IS, Bonfá E, de Carvalho JF, et al. Clues for previously undiagnosed connective tissue disease in patients with trigeminal neuralgia. J Clin Rhemotol 2010;16:205–208.
99. Myasoedova E, Crowson CS, Turesson C, Gabriel SE, Matteson EL. Incidence of extraarticular rheumatoid arthritis in Olmest County, Minnesota, in 1995–2007 versus 1985–1994: A population-based study. J Rheumatol 2011;38:983–989.
100. Aletaha D, Neogi T, Silman AJ, et al. 2010 rheumatoid arthritis classification criteria: An American College of Rheumatology/European League Against Rheumatism collaborative initiative. Ann Rheum Dis 2010;69:1580–1588.
101. Lin YC, Hsu ML, Yang JS, Liang TH, Chou SL, Lin HY. Temporomandibular joint disorders in patients with rheumatoid arthritis. J Chin Med Assoc 2007;70:527–534.
102. Delantoni A, Spyropoulou E, Chatzigiannis J, Papademitriou P. Sole radiographic expression of rheumatoid arthritis in the temporomandibular joints: A case report. Oral Surg Oral Med Oral Pathol Oral Radiol Endod 2006;102:e37–e40.
103. Kroese JM, Kopp S, Lobbezoo F, Alstergren P. TMJ Pain and crepitus occur early whereas dysfunction develops over time in rheumatoid arthritis. J Oral Facial Pain Headache 2020;34:398–405.
104. Chin Jen Sem JP, van der Leeden M, Visscher CM, et al. Prevalence, course, and associated factors of pain in the temporomandibular joint in early rheumatoid arthritis: Results of a longitudinal cohort study. J Oral Facial Pain Headache 2017;31:233–239.
105. Cordeiro PC, Guimaraes JP, de Souza VA, et al. Temporomandibular joint involvement in rheumatoid arthritis patients: Association between clinical and tomographic data. Acta Odontol Latinoam 2016;29:123–129.
106. Hirahara N, Kaneda T, Muraoka H, Fukuda T, Ito K, Kawashima Y. Characteristic magnetic resonance imaging findings in rheumatoid arthritis of the temporomandibular joint: Focus on abnormal bone marrow signal of the mandibular condyle, pannus, and lymph node swelling in the parotid glands. J Oral Maxillofac Surg 2017;75:735–741.
107. Mupparapu M, Oak S, Chang YC, Alavi A. Conventional and functional imaging in the evaluation of temporomandibular joint rheumatoid arthritis: A systematic review. Quintessence Int 2019;50:742–753.
108. Malliari M, Bakopoulou A, Koidis P. First diagnosis of rheumatoid arthritis in a patient with temporomandibular disorder: A case report. Int J Prosthodont 2015;28:124–126.
109. Petty RE, Southwood TR, Manners P, et al. International League of Associations for Rheumatology classification of juvenile idiopathic arthritis: Second revision, Edmonton, 2001. J Rheumatol 2004;31:390–392.

110. Martini A, Ravelli A, Avcin T, et al. Toward new classification criteria for juvenile idiopathic arthritis: First steps, Pediatric Rheumatology International Trials Organization International Consensus. J Rheumatol 2019;46:190–197.
111. Petty RE, Southwood TR, Baum J, et al. Revision of the proposed classification criteria for juvenile idiopathic arthritis: Durban, 1997. J Rheumatol 1998;25:1991–1994.
112. Collin M, Hagelberg S, Ernberg M, Hedenberg-Magnusson B, Christidis N. Temporomandibular joint involvement in children with juvenile idiopathic arthritis-Symptoms, clinical signs and radiographic findings. J Oral Rehabil 2022;49:37–46.
113. Glerup M, Stoustrup P, Matzen LH, et al. Longterm outcomes of temporomandibular joints in juvenile idiopathic arthritis: 17 Years of followup of a Nordic juvenile idiopathic arthritis cohort. J Rheumatol 2020;47:730–738.
114. Fischer J, Skeie MS, Rosendahl K, et al. Prevalence of temporomandibular disorder in children and adolescents with juvenile idiopathic arthritis - a Norwegian cross- sectional multicentre study. BMC Oral Health 2020;20:282.
115. Skeie MS, Gil EG, Cetrelli L, et al. Oral health in children and adolescents with juvenile idiopathic arthritis - A systematic review and meta-analysis. BMC Oral Health 2019;19:285.
116. Frid P, Nordal E, Bovis F, et al. Temporomandibular joint involvement in association with quality of life, disability, and high disease activity in juvenile idiopathic arthritis. Arthritis Care Res (Hoboken) 2017;69:677–686.
117. Shiboski CH, Shiboski SC, Seror R, et al. 2016 American College of Rheumatology/European League Against Rheumatism classification criteria for primary Sjögren's syndrome: A consensus and data-driven methodology involving three international patient cohorts. Ann Rheum Dis 2017;76:9–16.
118. Font J, Ramos-Casals M, de la Red G, et al. Pure sensory neuropathy in primary Sjögren's syndrome. Long-term prospective follow-up and review of the literature. J Rheumatol 2003;30:1552–1557.
119. Mori K, Iijima M, Koike H, et al. The wide spectrum of clinical manifestations in Sjögren's syndrome-associated neuropathy. Brain 2005;128(Pt 11):2518–2534.
120. Crincoli V, Di Comite M, Guerrieri, M, et al. Orofacial manifestations and temporomandibular disorders of Sjögren syndrome: An observational study. Int J Med Sci 2018;15:475–483.
121. Gökçay F, Oder G, Celebisoy N, Gökçay A, Sirin H, Kabasakal Y. Headache in primary Sjögren's syndrome: A prevalence study. Acta Neurol Scand 2008;118:189–192.
122. Spackman GK. Scleroderma: What the general dentist should know. Gen Dent 1999;47:576–579.
123. Scardina GA, Messina P. Systemic sclerosis: Description and diagnostic role of the oral phenomena. Gen Dent 2004;52:42–47.
124. Wada T, Ram S. Limited mouth opening secondary to diffuse systemic sclerosis. Case Rep Dent 2013;2013:937487.
125. Van den Hoogen F, Khanna D, Fransen J, et al. 2013 classification criteria for systemic sclerosis: An American College of Rheumatology/European League against Rheumatism collaborative initiative. Arthritis Rheum 2013;65:2737–2747.
126. Ramon Y, Samra H, Oberman M. Mandibular condylosis and apertognathia as presenting symptoms in progressive systemic sclerosis (scleroderma). Pattern of mandibular bony lesions and atrophy of masticatory muscles in PSS, presumably caused by affected muscular arteries. Oral Surg Oral Med Oral Pathol 1987;63:269–274.
127. Crincoli V, Fatone L, Fanelli M, et al. Orofacial manifestations and temporomandibular disorders of systemic scleroderma: An observational study. Int J Mol Sci 2016;17:1189.
128. Chaffee NR. CREST syndrome: Clinical manifestations and dental management. J Prosthodont 1998;7:155–160.
129. Wood RE, Lee P. Analysis of the oral manifestations of systemic sclerosis (scleroderma). Oral Surg Oral Med Oral Pathol 1988;65:172–178.
130. Nadeau SE. Neurologic manifestations of connective tissue disease. Neurol Clin 2002;20:151–178.
131. Fischoff DK, Sirois D. Painful trigeminal neuropathy caused by severe mandibular resorption and nerve compression in a patient with systemic sclerosis: Case report and literature review. Oral Surg Oral Med Oral Pathol Oral Radiol Endod 2000;90:456–459.
132. Hupp SL. Giant cell arteritis associated with progressive systemic sclerosis. J Clin Neuroophthalmol 1989;9:126–130.
133. On AY, Aykanat D, Atamaz FC, Eyigor C, Kocanogullari H, Oksel F. Is it necessary to strictly diagnose fibromyalgia syndrome in patients with chronic widespread pain? Clin Rheumatol 2015;34:1473–1479.
134. Jensen KB, Srinivan P, Spaeth R et al. Overlapping structural and functional brain changes in patients with long-term exposure to fibromyalgia pain. Arthritis Rheum 2013;65:3293–3303.
135. Sluka KA, Clauw DJ. Neurobiology of fibromyalgia and chronic widespread pain. Neuroscience 2016;338:114–129.
136. Sánchez-Domínguez B, Bullón P, Román-Malo L, et al. Oxidative stress, mitochondrial dysfunction and, inflammation common events in skin of patients with fibromyalgia. Mitochondrion 2015;21:69–75.

137. Wolfe F, Clauw DJ, Fitzcharles MA, et al. The American College of Rheumatology preliminary diagnostic criteria for fibromyalgia and measurement of symptom severity. Arthritis Care Res (Hoboken) 2010;62:600–610.
138. Mease PJ, Arnold LM, Crofford LJ, et al. Identifying the clinical domains of fibromyalgia: Contributions from clinician and patient Delphi exercises. Arthritis Rheum 2008;59:952–960.
139. Arnold LM, Clauw DJ, McCarberg BH, FibroCollaborative. Improving the recognition and diagnosis of fibromyalgia. Mayo Clin Proc 2011;86:457–464.
140. Ayouni I, Chebbi R, Hela Z, Dhidah M. Comorbidity between fibromyalgia and temporomandibular disorders: A systematic review. Oral Surg Oral Med Oral Path Oral Radiol 2019;128:33–42.
141. Balasubramaniam R, de Leeuw R, Zhu H, Nickerson RB, Okeson JP, Carlson CR. Prevalence of temporomandibular disorders in fibromyalgia and failed back syndrome patients: A blinded prospective comparison study. Oral Surg Oral Med Oral Pathol Oral Radiol Endod 2007;104:204–216.
142. Scully C, Porter S. Orofacial disease: Update for the dental clinical team: II. Cervical lymphadenopathy. Dent Update 2000;27:44–47.
143. Parisi E, Glick M. Cervical lymphadenopathy in the dental patient: A review of clinical approach. Quintessence Int 2005;36:423–436.
144. Weyand CM, Hicok KC, Hunder GG, Goronzy JJ. Tissue cytokine patterns in patients with polymyalgia rheumatica and giant cell arteritis. Ann Intern Med 1994; 121:484–491.
145. Wall M, Corbett JJ. Arteritis. In: Olesen J, Goadsby PJ, Ramadan NM, Tfelt-Hansen P, Welch KMA (eds). The Headaches, ed 3. Philadelphia: Lippincott Williams & Wilkins, 2006:901–910.
146. Kermani TA, Schmidt J, Crowson CS, et al. Utility of erythrocyte sedimentation rate and C-reactive protein for the diagnosis of giant cell arteritis. Semin Arthritis Rheum 2012;41:866–871.
147. Borchers AT, Gershwin ME. Giant cell arteritis: A review of classification, pathophysiology, geoepidemiology and treatment. Autoimmun Rev 21012;11: A544–554.
148. Simon S, Nihan J, Hissaria P. Diagnosis and management of giant cell arteritis: Major review. Clin Experiment Ophthalmol 2021;49:169–185.
149. Rubenstein E, Maldini C, Gonzalez-Chiappe S, Chevret S, Mahr A. Sensitivity of temporal artery biopsy in the diagnosis of giant cell arteritis: A systematic literature review and meta-analysis. Rheumatology (Oxford) 2020;59:1011–1020.
150. Salvarani C, Hunder GG. Giant cell arteritis with low erythrocyte sedimentation rate: frequency of occurrence in a population-based study. Arthritis Rheum 2001;45:140–145.
151. Zaina C, Grant R, Johnson C, Dansie B, Taylor J, Spyropolous P. The effect of cervical rotation on blood flow in the contralateral vertebral artery. Man Ther 2003;8:103–109.
152. Mitchell JA. Changes in vertebral artery blood flow following normal rotation of the cervical spine. J Manipulative Physiol Ther 2003;26:347–351.
153. Ramamurti P, Weinreb J, Fassihi SC, Rao R, Patel S. Vertebral artery injury in the cervical spine: Anatomy, diagnosis, and management. JBJS Rev 2021;9: e20.00118.
154. Sakaguchi M, Kitagawa K, Hougaku H, et al. Mechanical compression of the extracranial vertebral artery during neck rotation. Neurology 2003;61:845–847.
155. Mitchell J. Is mechanical deformation of the suboccipital vertebral artery during cervical spine rotation responsible for vertebrobasilar insufficiency? Physiother Res Int 2008;13:53–66.
156. Strupp M, Planck JH, Arbusow V, Steiger HJ, Brückmann H, Brandt T. Rotational vertebral artery occlusion syndrome with vertigo due to "labyrinthine excitation." Neurology 2000;54:1376–1379.
157. Gorelov V. J-A Barré's historic article «On posterior cervical sympathetic syndrome»: A translation from French. Cephalalgia 2020;40:1261–1265.
158. Foster CA, Jabbour P. Barré-Lieou syndrome and the problem of the obsolete eponym. J Laryngol Otol 2007;121:680–683.
159. Devaraja K. Approach to cervicogenic dizziness: A comprehensive review of its aetiopathology and management. Eur Arch Otorhinolaryngol 2018;275: 2421–2433.
160. Sarlani E, Balciunas BA, Grace EG. Orofacial Pain-- Part II: Assessment and management of vascular, neurovascular, idiopathic, secondary, and psychogenic causes. AACN Clin Issues 2005;16:347–358.
161. Gladstone J, Bigal ME. Headaches attributable to infectious diseases. Curr Pain Headache Rep 2010; 14:299–308.
162. Celle ME, Carelli V, Fornarino S. Secondary headache in children. Neurol Sci 2010;31(suppl 1):S81–S82.
163. Trumpy IG, Lyberg T. Temporomandibular joint dysfunction and facial pain caused by neoplasms. Report of three cases. Oral Surg Oral Med Oral Pathol 1993;76:149–152.

11

Sleep and Orofacial Pain

Key Points

- Sleep is a vital physiologic activity that normally occupies approximately one-third of an individual's life.
- There is a bidirectional relationship between pain and sleep. Sleep disturbances and sleep disorders can lead to pain disorders and can negatively impact pain management, and acute and chronic pain conditions can disturb sleep.
- Clinicians should be acutely aware that many patients presenting with orofacial pain frequently suffer from sleep disorders.
- When sleep disorders are suspected in orofacial pain patients, clinicians should understand their role in screening and how to make the most appropriate referrals for accurate diagnosis and comprehensive care.

The relationship between pain and sleep has been extensively studied. Approximately one-third of patients with temporomandibular disorders (TMDs) report poor sleep quality or unrefreshed feelings on awakening. Patients with orofacial pain frequently have associated sleep disturbances, including sleep fragmentation, insomnia, restless legs, periodic limb movements, and obstructive sleep apnea (OSA). Several quantitative sleep variables (eg, total sleep time, slow-wave sleep, sleep stage duration, sleep arousal, presence of disordered breathing events, and periodic limb movements during sleep) characterize the pain-related disruption of sleep. It is widely accepted that poor sleep leads to pain disorders, including TMD,[1] and that pain disorders can impact sleep quality. It is therefore essential for dental practitioners involved in the clinical management of orofacial pains to understand and recognize the presence of sleep disorders and to evaluate the role of concomitant musculoskeletal pain, headaches, neuropathic pain, and comorbid conditions (eg, fatigue, depression, and anxiety). Clinicians should work closely with physicians and refer patients to the appropriate provider in sleep medicine for further evaluation of a suspected sleep disorder, such as insomnia (*The International Classification of Diseases, Tenth Revision* [*ICD-10*] G47.0; *The International Classification of Diseases, Eleventh Revision* [*ICD-11*] 7A0Z), sleep apnea (*ICD-10* G47.3; *ICD-11* 7A41), or periodic limb movements (*ICD-10* G47.61; *ICD-11* 7A81). Dental practitioners will also intervene in the management of specific sleep disorders such as snoring, OSA, and sleep bruxism. The aim of this chapter is to provide an overview of the current understanding of pain and sleep interactions; to discuss evidence-based and empirical knowledge to help clinicians recognize, diagnose, and manage poor sleep in patients with chronic orofacial pain conditions; and to discuss the role of the dental practitioner in the management of sleep disorders.

Sleep Overview

Functions of sleep

Sleep is a natural physiologic activity that is necessary for life and species survival. It is a cyclic process, and a period of rest for the body and mind. During sleep, there is disengagement from the environment and partial interruption of bodily functions. It is, however, a state that is easy to reverse through exposure to external stimuli. Sleep has multiple functions, including recovery from fatigue, memory consolidation, homeostasis, heart and muscle tissue repair, and brain function at cellular and network levels. Its duration is variable from individual to individual.[2] Most human adults sleep between 6 and 9 hours per night; below or above this range, individuals tend to report more pain.[3,4] Adolescents tend to have an irregular circadian sleep schedule (*ICD-10* G47.23; *ICD 11* 7A60) that may predispose them to some pains. Secretion of growth hormone is greatest during sleep. Without enough sleep, humans tend to be less functional and to report cognitive problems, mood alterations, immune dysfunction, and somatic pain-related complaints within 3 to 4 days.[5,6] In addition to the abovementioned functions, sleep also appears to allow for the removal of waste metabolites in the brain.[7] Biologic activity causes the production of metabolic breakdown products in the central nervous system (CNS). The resultant buildup of proteins such as β-amyloid (Aβ), α-synuclein, and tau have been linked to neurodegenerative problems.[8–10]

In the peripheral tissues, the lymphatic system will return excess interstitial proteins to the circulation for elimination in the liver.[11] However, the brain lacks such a system and instead recirculates cerebral spinal fluid (CSF) through the brain, mixing it with interstitial fluid (ISF) to remove these proteins. This system has been described as the *glymphatic pathway* due to its dependence on glial water channels and its

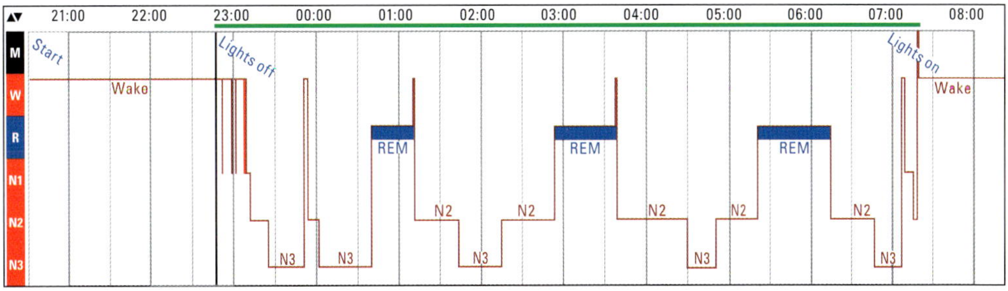

Fig 11-1 Normal hypnogram of a 50-year-old man, showing three complete sleep cycles. Registration began at 20:30 and finished at 8:30. Analysis time *(green line)* is shown from the time lights were turned off until they were turned back on. M, movement time; W, wake time; R, REM time. (Courtesy of Dr D. M. Laman, Department of Clinical Neurophysiology, Onze Lieve Vrouwe Gasthuis [OLVG], Amsterdam, The Netherlands.)

method of clearance being like the peripheral lymphatic system.

This pathway is partially dependent on the brain's arousal level.[12] During deep stages of sleep, the interstitial space volume will tend to expand, lowering the resistance to perivascular inflow, which results in a significant increase in the CSF-ISF fluid exchange and movement of the waste products into the perivascular spaces surrounding the large cerebral veins, ultimately leading to clearance in the cervical lymphatic vessels.[13] Evidence has also suggested that this process may be affected by sleep posture[12] and circadian periodicity.[14]

Sleep and wakefulness—Circadian rhythm

Sleep and wakefulness are under the regulation of a circadian process that lasts approximately 24 hours. Typically, sleep and wake cycles are regulated by an oscillatory behavior at the level of the hypothalamus suprachiasmatic nucleus in the higher regions of the CNS. Human sleep and wake rhythms are tuned by the sun and moon (ie, 24-hour light and dark cycle) as well as by external cues like sounds.[15,16]

Sleep architecture

Sleep is divided into two primary phases: rapid eye movement (REM or R) and non-REM (NREM or N) sleep. These two phases alternate cyclically during a typical night, with a total of three to five NREM to REM cycles, termed the *ultradian rhythm cycle*, in contrast to the 24-hour circadian cycle that is under the sun and moon time schedule. NREM sleep is further divided into light sleep (stages N1 and N2) and deep sleep (N3, formerly stages 3 and 4), also known as *delta sleep*, and dominated by slow-wave (frequency of 1 to 4 Hz and high amplitude waves) brain activity (Fig 11-1). REM sleep is often called *paradoxical sleep* because the CNS and the autonomic nervous system are highly active while all skeletal muscles are in a hypotonic state, as if the body were paralyzed.[15]

The typical length of each sleep state changes throughout the night. Stage N3 is more prevalent at the beginning of the night, while REM cycles are longer as sleep progresses toward the morning hours. As the person goes into sleep, electromyography (EMG) demonstrates a decrease in muscle tone, electrooculography (EOG) shows slow eye movements, and electro-

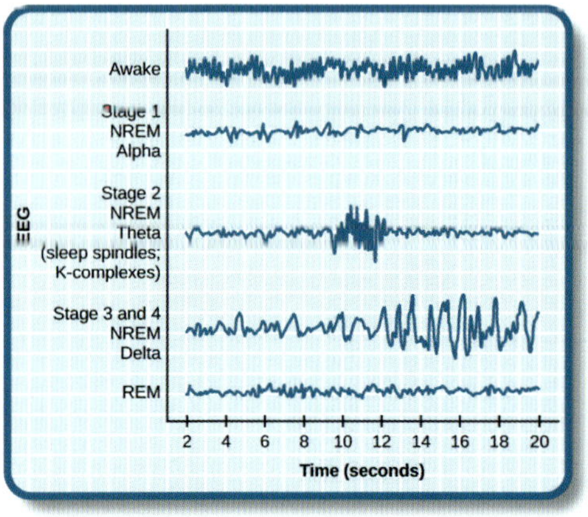

Fig 11-2 Brain wave activity seen in EEG, characteristic of wakefulness and of each sleep stage. Stage Wake: with alpha rhythmic pattern (frequency of 8 to 12 Hz and high-amplitude waves). Stage N1: characterized by waves of low voltage, mixed frequency pattern, predominantly of 4 to 7 Hz activity, and irregularly spaced bursts of slow waves. Stage N2: characterized by K complexes (very high amplitude biphasic waves lasting ≥ 0.5 seconds) and sleep spindles (burst-like trains of waves of 11 to 16 Hz with a total duration ≥ 0.5 seconds). Stage N3: characterized by high-amplitude slow waves; delta waves in the range of 0.5 to 2 Hz with amplitudes of equal to 75 microV. Stage REM: saw-tooth waves are seen, sharply contoured or triangular, of 2 to 6 Hz.

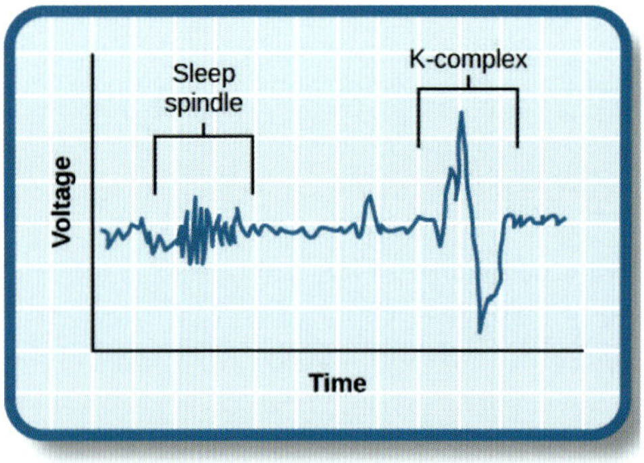

Fig 11-3 Sleep spindles and K-complexes characteristic of stage N2. K-complexes are defined by a negative sharp wave immediately followed by a positive wave (V-shaped) standing out from the background EEG, lasting 0.5 seconds. *Sleep spindles* are defined as distinct waves having frequencies of 11 to 16 Hz with a duration of ≥ 0.5 seconds.

encephalography (EEG) shows a change from an alpha rhythmic pattern (pre-sleep frequency of 8 to 12 Hz and high-amplitude waves) to a low voltage, mixed frequency pattern, indicating stage N1 (Fig 11-2). Other patterns on EEG that help confirm sleep consolidation and transition to stage N2 are K-complexes (well-defined, very high-amplitude biphasic waves lasting ≥ 0.5 seconds, potentially related to responses to environmental stimuli) and sleep spindles (burst-like trains of waves in the 11 to 16 Hz range with a total duration ≥ 0.5 seconds, potentially related to memory and learning; Fig 11-3). As stage N2 advances, high-amplitude slow waves start appearing, leading to transition into stage N3. REM sleep is characterized by very low EMG activity and very active EEG, resembling wakefulness. During normal healthy adult sleep, nociception is partially attenuated to preserve sleep continuity. The required intensity of the stimulus to wake up a person increases from stage N1 to N2 to N3, with overall lower response rates to noxious stimuli than during wakefulness. These thresholds vary during REM sleep.[3,17,18]

Sleep is associated with a partial physiologic deafferentation of sensory (ie, afferent) inputs into the CNS, and there is reduced neuronal activity at the thalamocortical network level with brief and transient reactivation of neural pathways from the brain stem to the cortex during arousal.[16–18] Duration spent in each sleep phase is approximately 2% to 5% in stage N1, 45% to 55% in N2, 10% to 20% in N3, and 20% to 25% in REM.

In healthy adults, most body movements (eg, of limbs and jaws) tend to occur within light sleep, more specifically in relation to sleep stage shifts, such as from deeper to lighter sleep or from any stage toward REM sleep. The occurrence of movements is periodic during sleep and follows a cyclic pattern. Such active periods, termed *arousals*, are normally occurring windows where the sleeping individual can readjust his or her body position, reset body temperature, and, if any harmful event is perceived, become fully awake (ie, a fight-or-flight reaction could be triggered). Sleep arousals will normally occur between 6 to 14 times per hour of sleep and last for approximately 3 to 10 seconds.[19,20]

Sleep disorders

A detailed review of the classification of sleep disorders is outlined by the International Classification of Sleep Disorders, 3rd edition (ICDS-3).[21] Understanding the differential diagnosis of sleep disorders is essential in the management of chronic orofacial pains. Patient evaluations should reflect the investigation of risk factors for sleep disorders, and appropriate coordination of care and referrals should be facilitated for patients when indicated. Additionally, the dental practitioner can play a key role in the management of specific sleep disorders such as snoring, OSA, and sleep bruxism.

Interactions Between Sleep and Pain

Epidemiology of sleep disorders in chronic pain

As with sleep, pain is a vital function necessary for human survival. Dysregulation of either function has not only the capacity to affect the other but ultimately interfere with optimum health. Approximately 10% to 25% of adults will experience some form of *chronic pain*, defined as persistent or recurrent pain lasting ≥ 3 months.[22–24] Recent data would suggest that 50% to 90% of people with chronic pain also report poor sleep, specifically regarding insomnia, sleep latency, sleep efficiency, and awakenings after sleep onset.[25–27]

Impact of nonrestorative sleep on pain and vice versa

Nonrestorative sleep is defined as an unrefreshed feeling on awakening, and it is present in about 10% of the general population, with a higher risk in older individuals. Nonrestorative sleep is a frequent complaint found in shift workers who work during the night, in patients who sleep more than 9 hours per night, and in those with insomnia-related symptoms or with fatigue and mood alterations.[3,5]

Patients with various chronic pain conditions, including TMDs, often report sleep to be of poor quality or nonrestorative. Patients suffering from trigeminal neuralgia or orofacial neuropathic pain will often report waking episodes during their sleep due to pain.[28] Indicators of poor sleep such as daytime sleepiness, frequent awakenings during the night, restless leg syndrome–related complaints, and signs of sleep related breathing disorders have been shown to be more prevalent in chronic pain patients.[29] Interestingly, the return of restorative sleep (ie, sleep that leaves the individual feeling refreshed, rested, and reenergized) appears to predict the resolution of chronic widespread pain in some individuals.[30]

Various models have been proposed regarding the relationship between sleep and pain.[30] It has been previously proposed that acute and chronic pain can interfere with sleep quality and disrupt its continuity. However, there is lack of prospective studies to confirm that pain leads to a sleep disorder, as this association is based on cross-sectional studies.[31] Longitudinal studies have shown that poor sleep leads to several pain disorders, including headaches,[32,33] fibromyalgia,[34] and musculoskeletal pain.[35] The Orofacial Pain Prospective Evaluation and Risk Assessment (OPPERA) study revealed that sleep quality is changed months before the novel onset of temporomandibular pain, independently from other variables, suggesting that impaired sleep may also yield orofacial pain.[1] Moreover, this interaction can be altered by personal variables such as endogenous pain modulation, inflammation, and comorbidities such as mood disorders, negative affect, and other states such as catastrophizing.[36]

Neurobiology and neurochemicals involved in sleep and pain

Several CNS structures have been shown to be adversely affected by both chronic pain conditions and prolonged sleep disturbances, including the hippocampus and prefrontal cortex.[37,38]

In addition, there are a number of neurotransmitters common to both sleep and pain. Dopaminergic pathways play a central role in both sleep modulation and endogenous analgesic mechanisms.[39] A decrease in dopamine availability may explain both sleep disturbances and impaired endogenous analgesic pathways seen in patients with chronic pain conditions. Serotonin (5-hydroxytryptamine [5-HT]) is involved in both descending pain inhibitory pathways and regulation of non-rapid eye movement (NREM or N) sleep.[40,41] Rapid eye movement (REM or R) sleep deprivation has been shown in animal models to decrease levels of 5-HT in the frontal cortex and hippocampus.[40,41] Serotonergic dysfunction has been postulated to result in disturbances of normal sleep-wake patterns as well as a dysfunction in endogenous analgesic mechanisms.[42] Gamma-aminobutyric acid (GABA) is an inhibitory neurotransmitter actively involved with the sleep-wake cycle. GABA also modulates ascending trigeminal and spinal sensory input in the thalamus. A deficiency may allow for hyperarousal from non-attenuated sensory input in chronic pain states.[43] Orexins (hypocretins) are neuropeptides synthesized in the lateral hypothalamus. There are two types: A and B. Orexins are primarily wake-promoting neurotransmitters but also play a role in other homeostatic functions such as appetite, hormone secretion, and autonomic regulation. In addition, new data suggests a role of orexins in migraine.[44] Adenosine is produced by the breakdown of adenosine triphosphate (ATP) and is generally considered an inhibitory neuromodulator shown to be important for both pain and sleep. Adenosine levels will increase during wakefulness and decrease during periods of sleep. High extracellular levels of adenosine will decrease neuronal activity in the CNS and promote the need for sleep via activation of the adenosine A1 receptors.[45] Stimulation of the A1 receptor in the CNS will result in antinociception while stimulation of the A2A receptor will result in nociception.[46] Caffeine will act as a competitive antagonist of adenosine at both the A1 and A2A receptors and results in a wake-promoting effect.[47] Caffeine appears to have a somewhat ambiguous role in pain presentations. The antinociceptive effects are thought to be due to an inhibition of cyclooxygenase activity as well as by adenosine receptor antagonism. Caffeine acts not only in the CNS but also in the periphery by blocking adenosine receptors on sensory afferents.[48] In migraine, it is postulated that caffeine, by blocking the A2A receptor, may affect the activation of calcitonin gene-related peptide (CGRP) receptors.[47] Melatonin, a hormone produced by the pineal gland, regulates the sleep/wake cycle and other circadian and seasonal rhythms. Secretion will increase with the onset of darkness then peak in the middle of the night before gradually decreasing toward the morning hours. Besides its hypnotic effects, melatonin is reported to possess analgesic effects via potentiation of GABA inhibition, modulation of 5-HT signaling, inhibition of pro-inflammatory cytokine production, inhibition of nitric oxide synthase, and antioxidant effects, among other effects.[49,50]

Polysomnography findings in chronic pain patients

Historically, much of the research related to disturbed sleep in patients with chronic pain has relied on subjective measures such as sleep diaries and questionnaires.[51] As seen in many studies that rely on retrospective recall, these measures are prone to inaccuracies and recall bias. In a recent meta-analysis of studies that included only polysomnography (PSG)-evaluated patients, it was found that chronic pain patients showed more time in sleep stage N1, less total sleep time, took longer to get to sleep, and spent more time awake as compared to healthy controls.[52] It was also noted that chronic pain patients tended to have more frequent arousals and awakenings along with more periodic limb movements per hour of sleep than the healthy controls. There were no significant differences seen in sleep stages N2, N3, and REM between the chronic pain patients and healthy controls.

Sleep and Pain: Clinical Relevance

Recent work has shown that as a group, the sleep quality of patients with TMDs is decreased as compared to healthy controls.[53,54] While the specific mechanisms involved are yet to be fully elucidated, animal studies have shown that pro-inflammatory mediators as well as the bone metabolism-related factor RANKL (receptor activator of nuclear factor kappa-B ligand) are increased after a period of sleep deprivation.[55] This may play a significant role in degenerative joint disease of the TMJs. Additional animal studies have shown that chronic sleep deprivation will alter the expression of myosin heavy chain isoforms of masseter muscle fibers and lead to a long-term alteration in the types of fibers present[56] as well as the production of acute inflammatory cells, congested vessels, fibrosis, and high cellularity in the fibers of the masseter and temporalis muscles leading to muscle atrophy not seen in the non–sleep deprived controls.[57]

Other factors may also contribute to the interaction between pain and poor sleep. For example, lifestyle, beliefs, difficulties in coping with anxiety, poor physical fitness, and chronic fatigue may be risk factors for insomnia, a condition found in 36% of patients with TMD.[58,59] In addition, sleep comorbidities like periodic limb movements and sleep-disordered breathing can exacerbate the interaction between pain and poor sleep (Fig 11-4). Periodic limb movements and sleep apnea/hypopnea have been reported in both TMD and chronic widespread pain/fibromyalgia patients with greater frequency than in controls.[59,60]

Patients with chronic widespread pain have a higher risk (odds ratio [OR] > 3) of reporting comorbid conditions such as fatigue, headache, gastrointestinal problems, and sleep disturbances as compared to healthy controls.[61] Orofacial pain patients also report more problems in coping with fatigue, psychologic distress, headaches, and abdominal pains.[59,62–64] Patients in a family medical practice who had hypertension, pain syndromes (eg, back pain, arthritis), and depression also had more sleep disturbance–related complaints.[29] Several sleep-related problems, such as sleepiness, dozing off during daily activity, frequent awakenings during the night, complaints related to restless legs syndrome, and signs of sleep-related breathing disturbances (eg, loud snoring and cessation of breathing suggestive of apnea) were higher in pain patients.[3,30,65] Likewise, a recent large-scale United States–based case-control study reported a high likelihood of self-reported OSA being associated with higher odds of chronic TMD (OR > 3).[66] While this is an important finding, the absence of polysomnographic confirmation of sleep-disordered breathing calls for a careful interpretation.[67]

Alteration of circadian rhythms can play a role in the clinical presentation of pain patients. A person who goes to sleep later every night

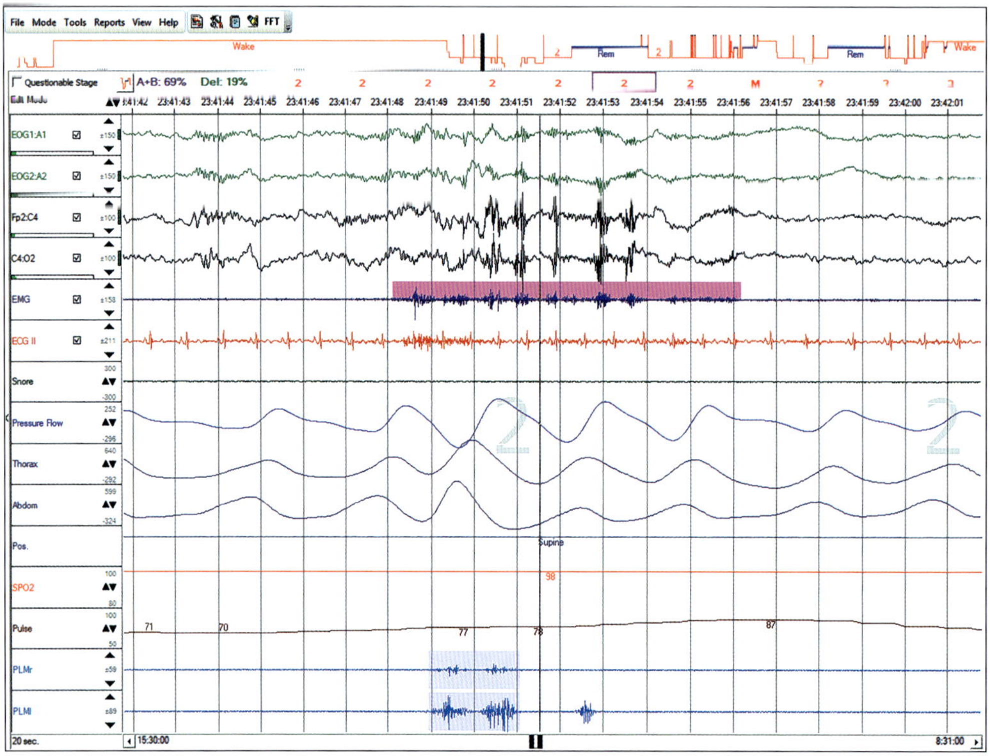

Fig 11-4 Example of a 20-second page of a polysomnographic recording. On top is the hypnogram of the total registration time. The *thick black line* represents the 20-second epoch shown in the rest of the image. On the left side are the various recording channels: EOG, eye movements (1, *left*; 2, *right*); FP2:C4 and C4:O2, long-distance EEG channels from front to back on the right side; EMG, electromyogram of the chin/jaw; ECG, electrocardiogram (electrodes placed near Erb's point, above the clavicle); snore, channel of the snore sensor; pressure flow, air flow sensor; thorax and abdom, thoracic and abdominal respiratory effort sensors channels; Pos, sleep position (in this case, supine); SPO_2, oxygen saturation measured at the fingertip; pulse, pulse rate; PLMr and PLMl, leg movements (right and left). An 8-second event of repetitive jaw-muscle activities is shown in the EMG (chin/jaw) channel *(pink area)* and in the EEG channels. At the same time or slightly before, the EEG shows signs of arousal (more fast activity), the respiration deepens and becomes more pronounced, the pulse increases, and independently, some repetitive leg movements lasting less than 1 second following the start of the arousal are shown in the PLM channels. (Courtesy of Dr D. M. Laman, Department of Clinical Neurophysiology, Onze Lieve Vrouwe Gasthuis [OLVG], Amsterdam, The Netherlands.)

may have a hard time waking up early. This sleep cycle is called *delayed sleep phase* (*ICD-10* G47.2; *ICD-11* 7A60). Conversely, a person who goes to sleep earlier every day may wake up earlier (*advanced sleep phase*; *ICD-10* G47.22; *ICD-11* 7A61).[4,65] Some gene expressions (eg, a tandem-repeat polymorphism in the coding region of the 5-repeat allele of the clock gene PER3 5/5 [period circadian protein homolog 3]) may explain vulnerability to sleep loss as cognitive frontal cortex dysfunction.[68,69] The role of circadian rhythm–related genes in cognitive function and fatigue is an area of ongoing investigation. The outcomes of this research may also provide better understanding of the interaction between chronic pain and sleep.

Box 11-1 Elements for assessment of orofacial pain and sleep complaints

- Identify the nature of the pain and sleep complaints. Ask the patient to keep a 24-hour diary, if possible, to monitor periods of pain exacerbation, time and duration of daily naps, sleep time, and wake time.
- Review medication type and dose, time of intake, and use of other treatments for pain or sleep complaints, such as physical therapy or cognitive behavioral therapy (CBT).
- Identify mood alterations (eg, depression, anxiety).
- Identify stressful life events or traumatic events.
- Identify poor sleep behavior or hygiene (eg, irregular sleep schedule; disrupted sleep environment; frequent use of caffeine, alcohol, or medications that alter sleep).
- Identify the extent of fatigue and/ or sleepiness (eg, falling asleep easily during daily activities or while watching TV, driving-related sleepiness) using the Epworth Sleepiness Scale.*
- Identify the risk of sleep-disordered breathing using the STOP-Bang or Berlin questionnaire or NoSAS scale.†
- Assess the risk of insomnia (ie, more than 20 to 30 minutes' delay in falling asleep, depending on nap habits, or difficulty resuming sleep after awakening during the night).
- Assess the presence of any periodic limb movements (eg, leg kicks that will increase sleep fragmentation above a cumulative threshold of events per hour of sleep).
- Assess if any snoring, alone or with sleep-disordered breathing (RERA upper airway resistance) or apnea/hypopnea (ie, cessation of breathing with reduced oxygenation with concomitant sleepiness), may contribute to increased sleep fragmentation and poor sleep quality complaints.
- Identify clinical risk factors associated with sleep-related breathing disorders, such as retrognathia, a deep and narrow palate and narrow arch, a large tongue, and large tonsils and adenoids.

*The Epworth Sleepiness Scale is an easy-to-use screening questionnaire to guide the clinician on the extent of daytime sleepiness; scores over 10 to 12 are suggestive of a sleep-related disorder and warrant medical evaluation.[70]

†The STOP-Bang or Berlin sleep questionnaire may help the clinician discern between simple snoring and sleep apnea.[71,72]

The NoSAS scale enables identification of individuals at risk for sleep-disordered breathing.[73]

See also the recent review on the use of sleep questionnaires for TMD patients.[67]

Normal adults usually fall asleep within 20 to 30 minutes of their going to bed. Insomnia may be suspected when sleep onset is longer than 20 to 30 minutes, occurring three to five times a week, or if spontaneous awakening is present during the night without the ability to resume sleeping.[21,65] About 10% of the general population suffers from chronic insomnia, but the prevalence is reported to be around 30% in chronic pain patients.[3] Importantly, clinicians should recognize and understand the influences of the above-described sleep comorbidities on the differential diagnoses and treatment planning for orofacial pain patients (Box 11-1).[67,70–73]

Sleep Bruxism

Of particular interest to the dental practitioner is the role of bruxism as it relates to orofacial pains. Bruxism tends to occur commonly, with an estimated prevalence between 8% to 31% in the general population.[74] It is important to note that bruxism is classified and defined according to its circadian presentation. An international consensus of experts has recently described sleep bruxism (SB; *ICD-10* G47.63; *ICD-11* 7A83) as a masticatory muscle activity during sleep that is characterized as rhythmic (phasic) or nonrhythmic (tonic), not to be considered a movement disorder or a sleep disorder in otherwise healthy individuals.[75]

About 50% to 80% of SB events are observed during recurrent arousal periods.[76,77] The majority of sleep arousals tend to occur in a repetitive and well-organized manner known as the *cyclic alternating pattern* (CAP).[78] CAP comprises an active phase A that is subdivided into three periods: A1 (dominated by slow-wave brain activity, which preserves sleep), A2 (the transition period between A1 and A3), and A3 (the period dominated by arousal).[17] Phase B of a CAP is the quiet period of sleep. Sleep bruxism tends to occur in CAP A2 and especially in A3, thereby providing a physiologic window to facilitate the onset of rhythmic movements during sleep.[79] Patients with other chronic pains and more specifically fibromyalgia (ie, chronic widespread pain) tend to present with 50% more phase A2 and A3 type CAP periods than healthy individuals.[17] Also of importance is the understanding that SB tends to occur in association with sleep-stage transitions and when arousal pressure is greater.

The frequently assumed association between TMD pain and SB remains controversial. In a recent scoping review, the authors concluded that previous conclusions from the articles included in their study have largely been dependent on the assessment mechanism of SB. Interestingly, they found that questionnaire-based studies did in fact report a positive association between TMDs and sleep bruxism, while instrumental-based studies (EMG, PSG) found no significant correlation between the two.[80] Interestingly, in a recent study of 77 patients with various TMD diagnoses who underwent PSG and were assessed for SB, none of the TMD diagnoses were found to occur more frequently in the SB group as compared to the non-SB group.[81]

Of note, TMD patients have been shown to have more respiratory effort-related arousals (RERAs) and higher jaw-muscle tone over the course of the night.[82,83] This may suggest that TMD patients have a propensity to maintain a type of hyperarousal level during the entire night; in other words, similar to insomnia patients and unlike good sleepers, they are not able to relax in a healthy manner.[83,84] In addition, factors like trait anxiety and an imbalance in the autonomic cardiac activity during sleep may be concomitantly associated factors in patients with TMDs.[85,86]

The role of sleep-disordered breathing (SDB) in the genesis of SB is another topic of recent controversy. While SDB may play a role in some SB manifestations, a recent systematic review concluded that to date, there is insufficient evidence to support a conclusive cause and effect relationship between the two.[87]

As some pharmacotherapeutic agents can impact SB, it is important for the dental practitioner to become familiar with over-the-counter, prescription, and even recreational agents that may have an effect, both as it pertains to the induction or aggravation as well as the attenuation of sleep.[88]

Screening, Referral, and Management Considerations

It is the responsibility of the orofacial pain provider to screen for any sleep disorders that, if present, could be negatively impacting treatment outcomes. In fact, it is estimated that 5.9 million U.S. adults have OSA, with up to 80% remaining undiagnosed.[89] Additionally, when indicated, the appropriate referral should be facilitated for further evaluation, diagnosis, and any necessary treatments. Management strategies for sleep disorders will vary depending on the diagnosis and should be patient centered. Box 11-2 outlines how to approach management of sleep-related disturbances in orofacial pain patients.[3,29]

Box 11-2 Management of sleep-related disturbances in orofacial pain patients*

- Review the patient's sleep hygiene to provide basic empirical advice on features such as the following:
  - Wake-sleep cycle (eg, regular bedtime and awakening schedule)
  - Sleep environment (eg, dark, cool, quiet bedroom; if the partner snores, use of ear plugs or sleeping in a different room may help)
  - Lifestyle habits (eg, avoidance of intense exercise, coffee, smoking, alcohol, and intense or troubling discussions 3 to 6 hours before sleep)
- Advise the patient on the benefits of regular mild exercise (eg, walking).
- Consider the benefits of physical therapy and CBT.
- Consider short-term pharmacologic methods:
  - Analgesics alone or combined with muscle relaxants (eg, methocarbamol) or with sleep aids (eg, diphenhydramine)
  - Muscle relaxants or sedatives (eg, cyclobenzaprine, temazepam)
  - Hypnotics or antidepressants (eg, zolpidem, trazodone, amitriptyline, duloxetine)
  - Other medications (eg, gabapentin, pregabalin)
- Consider the possibility of complementary medicine approaches (eg, melatonin, yoga, acupuncture, meditation, valerian, lavender).
- Consider oral appliances for patients with snoring and/or obstructive sleep apnea and sleep bruxism.
- If there is any evidence of sleepiness with sleep apnea/hypopnea or other medical conditions, arrange a consultation with a specialist in sleep medicine.

*Low on evidence for sleep and TMDs.

Sleep hygiene

Sleep hygiene involves recommendations regarding personal habits and practices as well as environmental factors that could interfere with the quality and duration of sleep. Avoiding exercising late, caffeine and other stimulants, alcohol, or any significant external stimuli in the bedroom and maintaining a consistent sleep-wake schedule will facilitate the necessary relaxation to initiate sleep. Developing rituals to practice before sleep to separate sleep from any stressors may also be beneficial. Sleep hygiene by itself might not be sufficient as a sole therapy for insomnia. It is, however, an important initial step in management, as it is a readily available, noninvasive measure that can be easily implemented clinically while facilitating referral to a sleep specialist.[90]

Cognitive behavioral therapy (CBT)

The American Academy of Sleep Medicine recommends that cognitive behavioral therapy (CBT) be used as a first line of treatment for the management of insomnia based on a large body of evidence of improvement of clinical outcomes. CBT-I involves a combination of strategies with education about sleep regulation plus stimulus control instructions and sleep restriction therapy. It can also include sleep hygiene education, relaxation training, and other counter-arousal methods. CBT has been used to aid in the management of pain conditions as well as sleep disturbances[91–93] with reported benefits on both pain intensity and quality of sleep. The type of CBT known to improve pain is different than CBT used to manage insomnia or poor sleep behavior. It seems logical that merging both pain and insomnia CBT methods might yield the best results, but to date there have not been enough studies supporting CBT use in patients suffering from both orofacial pain and poor sleep or insomnia.[94] Of note is a recent randomized controlled trial that failed to demonstrate any benefit from progressive muscle relaxation and sleep hygiene measures on sleep bruxism.[95]

Pharmacotherapy

The goals of pharmacotherapy in chronic orofacial pain and sleep disturbances will vary depending on the diagnosis and individual patient characteristics, with the common objective of reducing pain and improving sleep. Sedatives, hypnotics, antidepressants, and anticonvulsants may be beneficial and are frequently prescribed. Mild analgesics are commonly used alone or in combination with a muscle relaxant or other sleep inducer, but this practice is also not yet based on sound evidence for orofacial pain conditions. Benzodiazepines, acting on GABA A receptors in the CNS, tend to shorten sleep latency and increase sleep duration in most individuals. They are anxiolytic and sedating and have shown to be beneficial for rheumatoid arthritis,[96] chronic TMD pain,[97,98] and SB.[99] Cyclobenzaprine, used commonly in the management of fibromyalgia[100,101] and other musculoskeletal pains, is also frequently used in the management of TMDs. It has shown to be beneficial in decreasing morning TMD pain while improving subjective sleep quality.[102] Duloxetine, a selective serotonin and norepinephrine reuptake inhibitor (SSRI), is approved by the U.S. Food and Drug Administration (FDA) for the treatment of widespread pain/fibromyalgia and shows a slight improvement in sleep quality. More established medications, such as tricyclic antidepressants (eg, amitriptyline or trazodone), have mild to moderate positive effects on both pain and sleep. The positive effects of amitriptyline have been documented for the management of orofacial neuropathic pains[103] as well as chronic tension-type headache.[104] Gabapentin, pregabalin, and sodium oxybate also appear to improve pain and sleep quality and continuity.[105] The use of opioids in the management of chronic pain is still common despite the potential for tolerance and addiction, as well as the development of opioid-induced hyperalgesia. Opioid use in headache patients has been shown to be a risk factor for medication overuse headache.[106] In addition, the risk of respiratory depression associated with opioid use is of significant concern in patients with sleep-disordered breathing. Cannabis and its pharmacologically active constituents, the phytocannabinoids, have previously been reported to have sedative properties and provide subjective improvements in sleep.[107] A recent review did find that the use of tetrahydrocannabinol (THC) and its derivatives, alone or in combination with cannabidiol CBD, may subjectively improve sleep.[108] However, it should be noted that randomized controlled trails are needed to better elucidate the potential benefits weighed against potential adverse outcomes. Of note, an even more recent review found that users of cannabis for sleep were more likely than non-users to report both short and long sleep durations.[109] These extremes were experienced even more in heavy cannabis users. Apart from duloxetine, none of the listed agents has approval from the FDA for the combination of sleep and pain management. Their use is thus off-label, and clinicians prescribing such medications must take responsibility for such use.

Oral appliances

Patients with sleep breathing disorders such as snoring and OSA may benefit from oral appliances (OA) or mandibular advancement devices (MAD). Continuous positive airway pressure (CPAP) is currently the gold standard treatment for sleep apnea and is also offered as a first line of treatment, with the ability to effectively reduce apnea-hypopnea index for a large number of patients, especially with mild to moderate severity.[110] Additionally, OAs provide equivalent benefit in terms of quality of life, cognitive, and functional outcomes compared to CPAP, and they appear to have greater treatment compliance.[111] OAs function by keeping the upper airway patentduring sleep and preventing oropharyngeal tissue collapse. They help decrease the number of apneic events and blood oxygen desaturations, helping in turn with sleep continuity, excessive daytime sleepiness, quality of life, and health outcomes such as stroke, heart disease, and diabetes. Orofacial pain patients should be routinely screened for sleep breathing disorders and referred to the appropriate sleep medicine provider for diagnosis when indicated.

Pediatric OSA

OSA can occur in children in the same manner as in adults. Risk factors that are known to contribute to pediatric OSA include large size of lymphoid tissue, obesity, and other anatomical variables such as retrognathia and maxillary hypoplasia. It is recommended that all children have a clinical risk assessment and that physicians be involved in the diagnosis and treatment planning of OSA. Several treatments are available to address pediatric OSA, including weight reduction, watchful waiting, adenotonsillectomy, medications to improve nasal breathing, rapid maxillary expansion (RME), maxillary or mandibular advancement appliances, and CPAP in severe cases.[112,113]

Myofunctional therapy

Myofunctional therapy teaches people exercises to help improve tongue positioning, nasal breathing, and the tonicity of oropharyngeal muscles, and it is used in the management of OSA with beneficial effects. More studies are needed to better understand its effectiveness.[114]

References

1. Sanders AE, Akinkugbe AA, Bair E, et al. Subjective sleep quality deteriorates before development of painful temporomandibular disorder. J Pain 2016;17:669–677.
2. Hirshkowitz M. Normal human sleep: An overview. Med Clin North Am 2004;88:551–565, vii.
3. Lavigne GJ, Smith MT, Denis R, Zucconi M. Pain and sleep. In: Kryger MH, Roth T, Dement WC, (eds). Principles and Practice of Sleep Medicine. Philadelphia: Saunders, 2011:1442–1451.
4. Lavigne G, Morin C, Carra MC. The nature of sleep. In: Lavigne GJ, Cistulli PA, Smith MT (eds). Sleep Medicine for Dentists: A Practical Overview. Chicago: Quintessence, 2009:3–10.
5. Haack M, Mullington JM. Sustained sleep restriction reduces emotional and physical well-being. Pain 2005;119:56–64.
6. Haack M, Sanchez E, Mullington JM. Elevated inflammatory markers in response to prolonged sleep restriction are associated with increased pain experience in healthy volunteers. Sleep 2007;30:1145–1452.
7. Hauglund NL, Pavan C, Nedergaard M. Cleaning the sleeping brain–The potential restorative function of the glymphatic system. Curr Opin Physiol 2020;15:15–16.
8. Cirrito JR, Yamada KA, Finn MB, et al. Synaptic activity regulates interstitial fluid amyloid-beta levels in vivo. Neuron 2005;48:913–922.
9. Larson ME, Sherman MA, Greimel S, et al. Soluble alpha-synuclein is a novel modulator of Alzheimer's disease pathophysiology. J Neurosci 2012;32:10253–10266.
10. Yamada K, Cirrito JR, Stewart FR, et al. In vivo microdialysis reveals age-dependent decrease of brain interstitial fluid tau levels in P301S human tau transgenic mice. J Neurosci 2011;31:13110–13117.
11. Aukland K, Reed RK. Interstitial-lymphatic mechanisms in the control of extracellular fluid volume. Physiol Rev 1993;73:1–78.
12. Lee H, Xie L, Yu M, et al. The effect of body posture on brain glymphatic transport. J Neurosci 2015;35:11034–11044.
13. Xie L, Kang H, Xu Q, et al. Sleep drives metabolite clearance from the adult brain. Science 2013;342:373–377.
14. Hablitz LM, Plá V, Giannetto M, et al. Circadian control of brain glymphatic and lymphatic fluid flow. Nat Commun 2020;11:4411.
15. Amzica F, Lavigne G. Sleep neurobiology. In: Lavigne GJ, Cistulli PA, Smith MT (eds). Sleep Medicine for Dentists: A Practical Overview. Chicago: Quintessence, 2009:11–19.

16. Krueger JM, Rector DM, Roy S, Van Dongen HPA, Belenky G, Panksepp J. Sleep as a fundamental property of neuronal assemblies. Nat Rev Neurosci 2008;9:910–919.
17. Parrino L, Zucconi M, Terzano MG. Sleep fragmentation and arousal in the pain patient. In: Lavigne GJ, Sessle BJ, Choinière M, Soja PJ (eds). Sleep and Pain. Seattle: International Association for the Study of Pain, 2007:213–234.
18. Peever JH, Sessle BJ. Sensory and motor processing during sleep and wakefulness. In: Kryger MH, Roth T, Dement WC (eds). Principles and Practice of Sleep Medicine. Philadelphia: Saunders, 2017:239–249.
19. Carra MC, Rompré PH, Kato T, et al. Sleep bruxism and sleep arousal: An experimental challenge to assess the role of cyclic alternating pattern. J Oral Rehabil 2011;38:635–642.
20. Zou G, Xu J, Zhou S, et al. Functional MRI of arousals in nonrapid eye movement sleep. Sleep 2020;43:zsz218.
21. International Classification of Sleep Disorders, ed 3. American Academy of Sleep Medicine, 2014.
22. Scholz J, Finnerup NB, Attal N, et al. The IASP classification of chronic pain for *ICD-11*: Chronic neuropathic pain. Pain 2019;160:53–59.
23. Goldberg DS, McGee SJ. Pain as a global public health priority. BMC Public Health 2011;11:770.
24. Henderson JV, Harrison CM, Britt HC, Bayram CF, Miller GC. Prevalence, causes, severity, impact, and management of chronic pain in Australian general practice patients. Pain Med 2013;14:1346–1361.
25. Cheatle MD, Foster S, Pinkett A, Lesneski M, Qu D, Dhingra L. Assessing and managing sleep disturbance in patients with chronic pain. Anesthesiol Clin 2016;34:379–393.
26. de Tommaso M, Delussi M, Vecchio E, Sciruicchio V, Invitto S, Livrea P. Sleep features and central sensitization symptoms in primary headache patients. J Headache Pain 2014;15:64.
27. Ødegård SS, Sand T, Engstrøm M, Zwart JA, Hagen K. The impact of headache and chronic musculoskeletal complaints on the risk of insomnia: Longitudinal data from the Nord-Trøndelag health study. J Headache Pain 2013;14:24.
28. Benoliel R, Eliav E, Sharav Y. Self-reports of pain-related awakenings in persistent orofacial pain patients. J Orofac Pain 2009;23:330–338.
29. Alattar M, Harrington JJ, Mitchell CM, Sloane P. Sleep problems in primary care: A North Carolina Family Practice Research Network (NC-FP-RN) study. J Am Board Fam Med 2007;20:365–374.
30. Lavigne GJ, Nashed A, Manzini C, Carra MC. Does sleep differ among patients with common musculoskeletal pain disorders? Curr Rheumatol Rep 2011;13:535–542.
31. Finan PH, Goodin BR, Smith MT. The association of sleep and pain: An update and a path forward. J Pain 2013;14:1539–1552.
32. Boardman HF, Thomas E, Millson DS, Croft PR. The natural history of headache: Predictors of onset and recovery. Cephalalgia 2006;26:1080–1088.
33. Odegård SS, Sand T, Engstrøm M, Stovner LJ, Zwart JA, Hagen K. The long-term effect of insomnia on primary headaches: A prospective population-based cohort study (HUNT-2 and HUNT-3). Headache 2011;51:570–580.
34. Mork PJ, Nilsen TIL. Sleep problems and risk of fibromyalgia: Longitudinal data on an adult female population in Norway. Arthritis Rheum 2012;64:281–284.
35. Nitter AK, Pripp AH, Forseth KØ. Are sleep problems and non-specific health complaints risk factors for chronic pain? A prospective population-based study with 17 year follow-up. Scand J Pain 2012;3:210–217.
36. Herrero Babiloni A, De Koninck BP, Beetz G, De Beaumont L, Martel MO, Lavigne GJ. Sleep and pain: Recent insights, mechanisms, and future directions in the investigation of this relationship. J Neural Transm (Vienna) 2020;127:647–660.
37. Barad MJ, Ueno T, Younger J, Chatterjee N, Mackey S. Complex regional pain syndrome is associated with structural abnormalities in pain-related regions of the human brain. J Pain 2014;15:197–203.
38. Spiegelhalder K, Regen W, Baglioni C, Riemann D, Winkelman JW. Neuroimaging studies in insomnia. Curr Psychiatry Rep 2013;15:405.
39. Finan PH, Smith MT. The comorbidity of insomnia, chronic pain, and depression: Dopamine as a putative mechanism. Sleep Med Rev 2013;17:173–183.
40. Millan MJ. Descending control of pain. Prog Neurobiol 2002;66:355–474.
41. Whitney MS, Shemery AM, Yaw AM, Donovan LJ, Glass JD, Deneris ES. Adult brain serotonin deficiency causes hyperactivity, circadian disruption, and elimination of siestas. J Neurosci 2016;36:9828–9842.
42. Wei H, Pertovaara A. 5-HT(1A) receptors in endogenous regulation of neuropathic hypersensitivity in the rat. Eur J Pharmacol 2006;535:157–165.
43. Merrill R. Orofacial pain and sleep. Sleep Med Clin 2010;5:131–144.
44. Hoffmann J, Supronsinchai W, Akerman S, et al. Evidence for orexinergic mechanisms in migraine. Neurobiol Dis 2015;74:137–143.
45. Porkka-Heiskanen T, Alanko L, Kalinchuk A, Stenberg D. Adenosine and sleep. Sleep Med Rev 2002;6:321–332.

46. Giffin NJ, Kowacs F, Libri V, Williams P, Goadsby PJ, Kaube H. Effect of the adenosine A1 receptor agonist GR79236 on trigeminal nociception with blink reflex recordings in healthy human subjects. Cephalalgia 2003;23:287–292.
47. Ribeiro JA, Sebastião AM. Caffeine and adenosine. J Alzheimers Dis 2010;20(suppl 1):S3–S15.
48. Baratloo A, Rouhipour A, Forouzanfar MM, Safari S, Amiri M, Negida A. The role of caffeine in pain management: A brief literature review. Anesth Pain Med 2016;6:e33193.
49. Dodick DW, Eross EJ, Parish JM, Silber M. Clinical, anatomical, and physiologic relationship between sleep and headache. Headache 2003;43:282–292.
50. Peres MFP. Melatonin, the pineal gland and their implications for headache disorders. Cephalalgia 2005;25:403–411.
51. Menefee LA, Cohen MJ, Anderson WR, Doghramji K, Frank ED, Lee H. Sleep disturbance and nonmalignant chronic pain: A comprehensive review of the literature. Pain Med 2000;1:156–172.
52. Mathias JL, Cant ML, Burke ALJ. Sleep disturbances and sleep disorders in adults living with chronic pain: A meta-analysis. Sleep Med 2018;52:198–210.
53. Benoliel R, Zini A, Zakuto A, et al. Subjective sleep quality in temporomandibular disorder patients and association with disease characteristics and oral health-related quality of life. J Oral Facial Pain Headache 2017;31:313–322.
54. Rener-Sitar K, John MT, Pusalavidyasagar SS, Bandyopadhyay D, Schiffman EL. Sleep quality in temporomandibular disorder cases. Sleep Med 2016; 25:105–112.
55. Geng W, Wu G, Huang F, et al. Sleep deprivation induces abnormal bone metabolism in temporomandibular joint. Int J Clin Exp Med 2015;8:395–403.
56. Cao R, Huang F, Wang P, et al. Chronic sleep deprivation alters the myosin heavy chain isoforms in the masseter muscle in rats. Br J Oral Maxillofac Surg 2015; 53:430–435.
57. Yujra VQ, Antunes HKM, Mônico-Neto M, et al. Sleep deprivation induces pathological changes in rat masticatory muscles: Role of toll like signaling pathway and atrophy. J Cell Biochem 2018;119:2269–2277.
58. Davies KA, Macfarlane GJ, Nicholl BI, et al. Restorative sleep predicts the resolution of chronic widespread pain: Results from the EPIFUND study. Rheumatology (Oxford) 2008;47:1809–1813.
59. Smith MT, Wickwire EM, Grace EG, et al. Sleep disorders and their association with laboratory pain sensitivity in temporomandibular joint disorder. Sleep 2009;32:779–790.
60. Okura K, Lavigne GJ, Huynh N, Manzini C, Fillipini D, Montplaisir JY. Comparison of sleep variables between chronic widespread musculoskeletal pain, insomnia, periodic leg movements syndrome and control subjects in a clinical sleep medicine practice. Sleep Med 2008;9:352–361.
61. Rohrbeck J, Jordan K, Croft P. The frequency and characteristics of chronic widespread pain in general practice: a case-control study. Br J Gen Pract 2007; 57:109–115.
62. de Leeuw R, Studts JL, Carlson CR. Fatigue and fatigue-related symptoms in an orofacial pain population. Oral Surg Oral Med Oral Pathol Oral Radiol Endod 2005;99:168–174.
63. Gonçalves DA, Camparis CM, Speciali JG, Franco AL, Castanharo SM, Bigal ME. Temporomandibular disorders are differentially associated with headache diagnoses: A controlled study. Clin J Pain 2011;27: 611–615.
64. Macfarlane TV, Blinkhorn AS, Davies RM, Ryan P, Worthington HV, Macfarlane GJ. Orofacial pain: Just another chronic pain? Results from a population-based survey. Pain 2002;99:453–458.
65. Lavigne G, Heinzer R, Cistulli P, Smith M. Classification of sleep disorders. In: Lavigne GJ, Cistulli P, Smith MT (eds). Sleep Medicine for Dentists: A Practical Overview. Chicago: Quintessence, 2009:21–31.
66. Sanders AE, Essick GK, Fillingim R, et al. Sleep apnea symptoms and risk of temporomandibular disorder: OPPERA cohort. J Dent Res 2013;92(7 suppl):70S–77S.
67. Sommer I, Lavigne G, Ettlin DA. Review of self-reported instruments that measure sleep dysfunction in patients suffering from temporomandibular disorders and/or orofacial pain. Sleep Med 2015;16:27–38.
68. Vandewalle G, Archer SN, Wuillaume C, et al. Functional magnetic resonance imaging-assessed brain responses during an executive task depend on interaction of sleep homeostasis, circadian phase, and PER3 genotype. J Neurosci 2009;29:7948–7956.
69. Dijk DJ, Archer SN. PERIOD3, circadian phenotypes, and sleep homeostasis. Sleep Med Rev 2010;14:151–160.
70. Johns MW. A new method for measuring daytime sleepiness: The Epworth sleepiness scale. Sleep 1991;14:540–545.
71. Chung F, Yegneswaran B, Liao P, et al. STOP questionnaire: A tool to screen patients for obstructive sleep apnea. Anesthesiology 2008;108:812–821.
72. Netzer NC, Stoohs RA, Netzer CM, Clark K, Strohl KP. Using the Berlin Questionnaire to identify patients at risk for the sleep apnea syndrome. Ann Intern Med 1999;131:485–491.

73. Marti-Soler H, Hirotsu C, Marques-Vidal P, et al. The NoSAS score for screening of sleep-disordered breathing: A derivation and validation study. Lancet Respir Med 2016;4:742–748.
74. Manfredini D, Winocur E, Guarda-Nardini L, Paesani D, Lobbezoo F. Epidemiology of bruxism in adults: A systematic review of the literature. J Orofac Pain 2013;27:99–110.
75. Manfredini D, Ahlberg J, Lobbezoo F. Bruxism definition: Past, present, and future - What should a prosthodontist know? [epub ahead of print 4 Mar 2021]. J Prosthet Dent doi: 10.1016/j.prosdent.2021.01.026.
76. Bader G, Kampe T, Tagdae T. Body movement during sleep in subjects with long-standing bruxing behavior. Int J Prosthodont 2000;13:327–333.
77. Sjöholm TT, Polo OJ, Alihanka JM. Sleep movements in teethgrinders. J Craniomandib Disord 1992;6:184–191.
78. Terzano MG, Mancia D, Salati MR, Costani G, Decembrino A, Parrino L. The cyclic alternating pattern as a physiologic component of normal NREM sleep. Sleep 1985;8:137–145.
79. Carra MC, Macaluso GM, Rompré PH, et al. Clonidine has a paradoxical effect on cyclic arousal and sleep bruxism during NREM sleep. Sleep 2010;33:1711–1716.
80. Manfredini D, Lobbezoo F. Sleep bruxism and temporomandibular disorders: A scoping review of the literature. J Dent 2021;111:103711.
81. Wieckiewicz M, Smardz J, Martynowicz H, Wojakowska A, Mazur G, Winocour E. Distribution of temporomandibular disorders among sleep bruxers and non-bruxers—A polysomnographic study. J Oral Rehabil 2020;47:820–826.
82. Dubrovsky B, Raphael KG, Lavigne GJ, et al. Polysomnographic investigation of sleep and respiratory parameters in women with temporomandibular pain disorders. J Clin Sleep Med 2014;10:195–201.
83. Raphael KG, Janal MN, Sirois DA, et al. Masticatory muscle sleep background electromyographic activity is elevated in myofascial temporomandibular disorder patients. J Oral Rehabil 2013;40:883–891.
84. Quartana PJ, Wickwire EM, Klick B, Grace E, Smith MT. Naturalistic changes in insomnia symptoms and pain in temporomandibular joint disorder: A cross-lagged panel analysis. Pain 2010;149:325–331.
85. Manfredini D, Fabbri A, Peretta R, Guarda-Nardini L, Lobbezoo F. Influence of psychological symptoms on home-recorded sleep-time masticatory muscle activity in healthy subjects. J Oral Rehabil 2011;38:902–911.
86. Eze-Nliam CM, Quartana PJ, Quain AM, Smith MT. Nocturnal heart rate variability is lower in temporomandibular disorder patients than in healthy, pain-free individuals. J Orofac Pain 2011;25:232–239.
87. da Costa Lopes AJ, Cunha TCA, Monteiro MCM, Serra-Negra JM, Cabral LC, Simamoto PC Jr. Is there an association between sleep bruxism and obstructive sleep apnea syndrome? A systematic review. Sleep Breath 2020;24:913–921.
88. de Baat C, Verhoeff M, Ahlberg J, et al. Medications and addictive substances potentially inducing or attenuating sleep bruxism and/or awake bruxism. J Oral Rehabil 2021;48:343–354.
89. Peppard PE, Young T, Barnet JH, Palta M, Hagen EW, Hla KM. Increased prevalence of sleep-disordered breathing in adults. Am J Epidemiol 2013;177:1006–1014.
90. Edinger JD, Arnedt JT, Bertisch SM, et al. Behavioral and psychological treatments for chronic insomnia disorder in adults: An American Academy of Sleep Medicine clinical practice guideline. J Clin Sleep Med 2021;17:255–262.
91. Smith MT, Haythornthwaite JA. How do sleep disturbance and chronic pain inter-relate? Insights from the longitudinal and cognitive-behavioral clinical trials literature. Sleep Med Rev 2004;8:119–132.
92. Vitiello MV, McCurry SM, Shortreed SM, et al. Cognitive-behavioral treatment for comorbid insomnia and osteoarthritis pain in primary care: The lifestyles randomized controlled trial. J Am Geriatr Soc 2013; 61:947–956.
93. Pigeon WR, Moynihan J, Matteson-Rusby S, et al. Comparative effectiveness of CBT interventions for co-morbid chronic pain and insomnia: A pilot study. Behav Res Ther 2012;50:685–689.
94. Tang NKY, Lereya ST, Boulton H, Miller MA, Wolke D, Cappuccio FP. Nonpharmacological treatments of insomnia for long-term painful conditions: A systematic review and meta-analysis of patient-reported outcomes in randomized controlled trials. Sleep 2015;38:1751–1764.
95. Valiente López M, van Selms MKA, van der Zaag J, Hamburger HL, Lobbezoo F. Do sleep hygiene measures and progressive muscle relaxation influence sleep bruxism? Report of a randomised controlled trial. J Oral Rehabil 2015;42:259–265.
96. Walsh JK, Muehlbach MJ, Lauter SA, Hilliker NA, Schweitzer PK. Effects of triazolam on sleep, daytime sleepiness, and morning stiffness in patients with rheumatoid arthritis. J Rheumatol 1996;23:245–252.
97. Harkins S, Linford J, Cohen J, Kramer T, Cueva L. Administration of clonazepam in the treatment of TMD and associated myofascial pain: A double-blind pilot study. J Craniomandib Disord 1991;5:179–186.
98. Singer E, Dionne R. A controlled evaluation of ibuprofen and diazepam for chronic orofacial muscle pain. J Orofac Pain 1997;11:139–146.

99. Saletu A, Parapatics S, Saletu B, et al. On the pharmacotherapy of sleep bruxism: Placebo-controlled polysomnographic and psychometric studies with clonazepam. Neuropsychobiology 2005;51:214–225.
100. Santandrea S, Montrone F, Sarzi-Puttini P, Boccassini L, Caruso I. A double-blind crossover study of two cyclobenzaprine regimens in primary fibromyalgia syndrome. J Int Med Res 1993;21:74-80.
101. Carette S, Bell MJ, Reynolds WJ, et al. Comparison of amitriptyline, cyclobenzaprine, and placebo in the treatment of fibromyalgia. A randomized, double-blind clinical trial. Arthritis Rheum 1994;37:32–40.
102. Herman CR, Schiffman EL, Look JO, Rindal DB. The effectiveness of adding pharmacologic treatment with clonazepam or cyclobenzaprine to patient education and self-care for the treatment of jaw pain upon awakening: A randomized clinical trial. J Orofac Pain 2002;16:64–70.
103. Sharav Y, Singer E, Schmidt E, Dionne RA, Dubner R. The analgesic effect of amitriptyline on chronic facial pain. Pain 1987;31:199–209.
104. Ashina S, Bendtsen L, Jensen R. Analgesic effect of amitriptyline in chronic tension-type headache is not directly related to serotonin reuptake inhibition. Pain 2004;108:108–114.
105. Hindmarch I, Dawson J, Stanley N. A double-blind study in healthy volunteers to assess the effects on sleep of pregabalin compared with alprazolam and placebo. Sleep 2005;28:187–193.
106. Diener HC, Katsarava Z, Limmroth V. Headache attributed to a substance or its withdrawal. Handb Clin Neurol 2010;97:589–599.
107. Walsh Z, Callaway R, Belle-Isle L, et al. Cannabis for therapeutic purposes: Patient characteristics, access, and reasons for use. Int J Drug Policy 2013;24:511–516.
108. Kuhathasan N, Dufort A, MacKillop J, Gottschalk R, Minuzzi L, Frey BN. The use of cannabinoids for sleep: A critical review on clinical trials. Exp Clin Psychopharmacol 2019;27:383–401.
109. Diep C, Tian C, Vachhani K, et al. Recent cannabis use and nightly sleep duration in adults: a population analysis of the NHANES from 2005 to 2018. Reg Anesth Pain Med 2022;47:100–104.
110. Ramar K, Dort LC, Katz SG, et al. Clinical practice guideline for the treatment of obstructive sleep apnea and snoring with oral appliance therapy: An update for 2015. J Clin Sleep Med 2015;11:773–827.
111. Schwartz M, Acosta L, Hung YL, Padilla M, Enciso R. Effects of CPAP and mandibular advancement device treatment in obstructive sleep apnea patients: A systematic review and meta-analysis. Sleep Breath 2018;22:555–568.
112. Venekamp RP, Hearne BJ, Chandrasekharan D, Blackshaw H, Lim J, Schilder AGM. Tonsillectomy or adenotonsillectomy versus non-surgical management for obstructive sleep-disordered breathing in children. Cochrane Database Syst Rev 2015(10):CD011165.
113. Behrents RG, Shelgikar AV, Conley RS, et al. Obstructive sleep apnea and orthodontics: An American Association of Orthodontists White Paper. Am J Orthod Dentofacial Orthop 2019;156:13–28.e1.
114. Rueda JR, Mugueta-Aguinaga I, Vilaró J, Rueda-Etxebarria M. Myofunctional therapy (oropharyngeal exercises) for obstructive sleep apnoea. Cochrane Database Syst Rev 2020;11:CD013449.

12

Axis II: Biobehavioral Considerations

Key Points

- The biobehavioral model of pain is the foundation for clinical assessment and pain management.
- Core biobehavioral principles include multifactorial assessment; the role of learning in the patient's history; and the interplay between biologic, psychologic, and social factors.
- It is necessary to screen for biobehavioral risk factors including pain, distress, and pain-related disability as part of a comprehensive pain history. Be sure to note red and yellow flags for patient care.
- A comprehensive pain history includes pain location and intensity, limitations in use and movement, and parafunctional activities involving the masticatory system; modifying factors that lead to variations in symptom severity include pain-related disability, psychologic distress, sleep dysfunction, posttraumatic stress disorder (PTSD), and alcohol and drug abuse.
- The most common psychiatric disorders encountered in the orofacial pain practice include depression, anxiety, PTSD, somatic symptom disorders, and personality disorders. The use of initial screening instruments can help identify the presence of depression, anxiety, PTSD, and somatic symptom disorders and alert the dentist of the need for referral to a mental health care provider.
- Following referral to mental health care providers, the clinician should expect a summary report detailing a comprehensive evaluation and treatment plan targeting skills acquisition that is provided in a timely manner.
- The standard of care for orofacial pain is integrated care among health care professionals.

Foundation of the Biobehavioral Model

Scientific advances have been made in understanding modulatory control of ascending and descending neural circuits involved in pain processing, including the role of glial cells and gut microbiome influences on neural functioning. Variables such as emotion, cognition (including attention and expectations), and behavior are now understood to play very important roles in pain transmission, awareness, and suffering. Because emotions, cognitions, and behaviors can facilitate or inhibit orofacial pain, it is necessary to adopt a biobehavioral model of disease. Behavioral factors encompass a broad spectrum of behavioral science theory and techniques for change. Examples of behavioral science theory include principles of learning, cognitions and memory, interpersonal processes, family systems, and social learning; techniques for change may be relaxation training, interpersonal psychotherapy, biofeedback, cognitive therapy, and breathing training. When behavioral factors are discussed in the context of how they contribute to the functioning of biologic systems, it is appropriate to use the term *biobehavioral.*

As discussed in chapter 1, Engel[1] noted that the biomedical model, with its focus on patho-biology, does not fully explain the development of disease states. Therefore, he introduced the term *biopsychosocial* to describe the complex interactions between the biology, psychologic states, and social conditions that bring about and/or maintain function or dysfunction. The term *biobehavioral* is parallel to the word *biomedical*, and both concepts are subsumed in Engel's biopsychosocial model. While the term *biopsychosocial* is often used because it is more globally accepted, *biobehavioral* calls attention to behavioral factors as they contribute to the functioning of biologic systems, and *biobehavioral* forms an important contrast to *biomedical* in terms of how levels or types of evaluations and treatments are implemented.

Adopting the biobehavioral model of orofacial pain requires that linear, unidirectional models of causation and of treatment be replaced with a bidirectional approach to understanding disease etiology and delivering treatment.[2,3] Whether the practitioner provides dental or psychologic treatment, a mechanistic linear model (eg, identify the cause, treat the cause, observe recovery) for understanding orofacial pain conditions is an incomplete model that will yield incomplete, inappropriate, and misdirected clinical care. Unless behavioral, psychologic, and social dimensions of the patient's presenting complaints and current adaptive strategies are jointly addressed in the treatment plan, effective management of the pain condition will likely not be achieved, especially in chronic pain conditions. This multidisciplinary philosophy of treatment does not necessarily require a multispecialty clinic with dentists, psychologists, physical therapists, and physicians; instead, it requires individual practitioners themselves to possess a worldview that embraces the biobehavioral perspective. From there, appropriate integration of diverse treatment strategies can be implemented instantaneously through direct care or through referral as patient circumstances, the symptom picture, and the case conceptualization evolve over the course of treatment as well as over the course of the disorder.

Pain is a complex phenomenon influenced by multiple biologic, psychologic, and social factors. The sensation of pain is evoked when nociception reaches thalamo-cortical basal ganglia circuitry in the brain; however, because pain is a personalized perceptual experience, it can be modified by factors other than the intensity of the nociceptive stimuli themselves. For example, excitatory factors that could amplify the pain experience include fear, anxiety, attention, and expectations of pain. Conversely, reports of pain may reduce as a result of self-confidence, positive emotional states, relaxation, and belief that the pain is manageable.[4] Importantly, these modifying factors not only affect the perceptual aspects of what defines pain at any moment for an individual; they also contribute to descending modulation. These examples highlight the concept that nociception is the result of a dynamic balance between peripheral input and ongoing central nervous system (CNS) regulation of that input at the level of the dorsal horn entry into the CNS. For the trigeminal system, there is additional complexity due to convergence in the subnucleus caudalis (analog of the dorsal horn in the spinal cord) from cutaneous, tooth pulp, visceral, and neck and masticatory muscle afferents.

The biobehavioral approach to orofacial pain disorders involves assessing not only the underlying behavioral and psychologic disturbances but also the physiologic disturbances that may be associated with the pain condition. The patient may need to learn new skills for managing these disturbances and should be able to rely on the health care provider for help. The need for skill acquisition can range from simple to complex, and the latter may involve referral to a mental health care professional. Effective symptom management, both physical and psychologic, may be elusive for many patients, especially those whose pain has become chronic (ie, lasting longer than 3 to 6 months). These patients may have adopted coping patterns to maintain some level of functioning, but their efforts should be assessed by the clinician to ensure they remain in the patient's best interest. Certain coping strategies, while perhaps successful in the early stage of an illness, may eventually contribute to the development of maladaptive patterns that extend beyond the pain condition and into multiple aspects of daily life. For example, a patient who stops engaging in pleasurable daily activities because of pain on movement may be prone to depression. When maladaptive patterns emerge, it is important that the clinician be prepared to recognize and manage them appropriately, because failure to do so will likely prolong suffering (ie, an individual's negative emotional reaction to pain) and prevent effective symptom management. It is also possible that maladaptive coping patterns were being used before the onset of the pain condition and may have intensified the problem. Such coping patterns may also be associated with the variety of psychopathologic conditions (which are discussed in later sections of this chapter). The psychopathology may be actively preexisting, it may be subclinical until the onset of the intractable problem, or it may be emergent in response to a new illness.

The biobehavioral perspective introduces a model whereby the assessment process includes an interview component that focuses not only on the biologic aspects of the presenting condition but also on the psychosocial processes, thus providing a broader perspective from which to understand and conceptualize treatment for a patient's presenting pain symptoms. It is rare that pain reports are based solely on psychologic or so-called psychogenic factors.[5] It is equally rare, however, to find that pain—especially chronic pain of at least 3 to 6 months duration—is not influenced by psychologic and social factors to some degree. Such factors may also account for the individual differences in response to similar levels of pain. Because there can be substantial individual variability in response to painful conditions and a variety of social factors (eg, modeling, litigation, compensation), the reported intensity of pain may not necessarily be linked to an individual's expressed reaction to the pain. It is common for both clinicians and patients to be confused regarding the relative nature of reported pain intensities; one reaction is to dismiss such reports as "subjective" (often with the intended meaning of *irrelevant or imaginary*). The relative nature of pain intensity does not diminish its validity; rather, it requires the clinician's active interpretation to make it meaningful. In short, it is the task of the clinician to understand the patient story and to make sense of the pain reports from the person seeking care.

For many chronic pain conditions, it may be difficult to predict treatment outcomes without knowing the full psychosocial history of the patient. Learning to manage one's orofacial pain conditions for extended periods of time can help patients considerably, but ongoing biobehavioral issues may either promote or prevent the use of such skills for symptom management, leading to the common pattern of remission-relapse. The reality is that "curing" pain is often not a viable clinical treatment goal, whereas learning to manage pain with the physical and psychologic tools developed and refined through the practice of science can be a viable goal. A major long-term goal is finding the dynamic balance of input and CNS control at the dorsal horn level. Stress reactivity is one of the most easily recognized factors that often contributes to relapse; managing that reactivity can be one of the most difficult skills to master. To prevent relapse as a result of stress, patients should work toward experiential understanding of *allostasis,* another example of a dynamic balance among systems.

In recognition of these complexities, Dworkin et al[6–9] proposed several models for capturing the dimensions of pain over time. Inherent in these models is the simultaneous consideration of both the physical status and the biobehavioral status for every patient. For assessment of both types of status to be equally useful in the clinic, reliable assessment methods are needed for the physical examination (using an operationalized framework) and the biobehavioral screening (using standardized, validated instruments). Extensive research has demonstrated the value of these core components in terms of clinical trials and modeling disease progression and response to treatment.[10–13] The current versions of diagnostic and biobehavioral assessments are emerging from structured assessments whose reliability and validity has been demonstrated through well-established research.[10,14–17] A recent development has been the Orofacial Pain Prospective Evaluation and Risk Assessment (OPPERA) studies that place due recognition on the genetic underpinnings of neural plasticity, behavioral factors, and all their interactions in shaping risk for developing a pain disorder.[18–36] A primary overarching conclusion from the OPPERA studies is that temporomandibular disorders (TMDs) are seldom a simple localized condition and are far more often a result of complex multiple risk determinants.[37] Consistent with that conclusion, the biobehavioral model for the clinical care of patients with pain disorders is intended to encompass all aspects of neurobiology associated with health and disease. For example, when a patient tells her doctor that she is depressed, she is informing him or her of the state of her brain and how the resulting depressive behavior is recursively further shaping that brain state. Assuming that reliable and valid methods are used for the assessment, this type of information gathered via self-report instruments and interviews is no less valuable than that obtained from a clinical examination.

Implementing a Biobehavioral Framework: Dual-Axis Coding

A multiaxial nosology has been created, implemented, and refined on a broad scale to recognize behavioral and psychologic dimensions in the etiology of orofacial pain disorders. Similar to the development of axial coding systems for psychiatric disorders created by the American Psychiatric Association[38] and pain disorders developed by the International Association for the Study of Pain, the Research Diagnostic Criteria for Temporomandibular Disorders (RDC/TMD) were developed by a group of scientists and clinicians in 1992.[39] Axis I focuses on the physical nature of the disease and includes the variety of orofacial pain conditions discussed in earlier chapters of this text. Axis II focuses on the patient's adaptation to the pain experience and pain-related disability that may result from the pain itself. It also uses standardized and validated methods to assess the extent to which

Table 12-1 Axis II assessment Instruments

Domain	Instrument	No. of items	Level of screening		
			Ultra-brief	Brief	Comprehensive
Based on DC/TMD recommendations					
Pain location	Pain manikin drawing	1	Yes	Yes	Yes
Pain intensity	Graded chronic pain scale	3	Yes	Yes	Yes
Pain disability	Graded chronic pain scale	4	Yes	Yes	Yes
Distress	PHQ-4	4	Yes	Yes	Yes
	PHQ-9 Depression	9			Yes
	GAD-7 Anxiety	7			
Physical symptoms	PHQ-15	15			Yes
Limitation	Jaw functional limitation scale	8 or 20		Yes (8)	Yes (20)
Parafunction	Oral behaviors checklist	21		Yes	Yes
Other instruments for pain-relevant constructs					
Sleep	Pittsburgh Sleep Quality Index	18			Yes
	PROMIS—Sleep	43			Yes
PTSD	PTSD Checklist	17			Yes
Alcohol use	AUDIT-C	3			Yes
Stress	Perceived Stress Scale	10			Yes
Catastrophizing	Pain Catastrophizing Questionnaire	14			Yes

PHQ-4, Patient Health Questionnaire 4; PHQ-9, Patient Health Questionnaire 9; GAD-7, Generalized Anxiety Disorder 15; PHQ-15, Patient Health Questionnaire 15; PROMIS, Patient-Reported Outcome Measures Information System; AUDIT-C, Alcohol Use Disorders Identification Test.

the orofacial pain condition is associated with psychologic distress, disability, or impairment in functioning (ie, significant disruption in normal activities; Table 12-1).

The RDC/TMD Axis II was an attempt to codify the emotional sequelae and functional limitations that accompanied chronic orofacial pain conditions and to determine whether there is a need to refer patients to additional providers. Psychiatrists or clinical psychologists may perform a formal assessment of cognitive, emotional, and behavioral sources of disruption and normal functioning due to or associated with the pain problem. This coding system was refined with the Diagnostic Criteria for Temporomandibular Disorders (DC/TMD) project to update the RDC/TMD, but the two-axis coding strategy has remained a central feature of the nosologic framework.[39,40] The two-axis approach has been expanded to also include five domains, common across all chronic pain conditions[41] and also applied to TMDs.[42] These axes are diagnostic criteria, common features, comorbidities, consequences, and putative mechanisms, and while their primary purpose is to facilitate more comprehensive research, they also serve as a reminder of the complex domains associated with pain disorders. The five-domain perspective also highlights the relative efficiency of a two-axis approach for routine clinical use.

In 2010, an international consensus workshop[10] agreed on the minimal basic components that should be assessed for a sufficient biobehavioral evaluation: pain, physical function, overuse behaviors, comorbid physical symptoms, and emotional and psychosocial function. Another workshop[43] clarified the distinction between what is needed for initial screening, what is needed for more comprehensive assessment in a clinical setting, and what might be of value in a specialist biobehavioral setting. Ongoing workshops sponsored by the International Network for Orofacial Pain and Related Disorders Methodology (INfORM; previously, International RDC/TMD Consortium) continue to develop Axis II assessment strategies. Recent workshops highlighted the benefits of assessing pain-related disability and psychologic status in both general and specialist dental practice[44] and examined the barriers to implementing the biopsychosocial model in dental care settings.[45]

It is the responsibility of the clinician to judge the level of complexity of the patient's clinical presentation and to decide whether the treatment plan should include additional resources outside the scope of the dental practice. The task is not to develop a psychiatric diagnosis (eg, major depression secondary to the loss of a spouse) but to develop a treatment plan that includes appropriate care for the unique features of the presenting patient. There are various self-report instruments that have demonstrated reliability and validity in identifying potential psychologic dysfunction that can interfere with pain management from the physical medicine perspective, and these can be used to augment the screening. Standardized instruments provide the clinician with an actuarial approach to decision-making. This will ensure more information is gathered than the limited amount provided by the initial interview and prevent inherent clinician-based personal biases from clouding clinical judgments.[46] Health care providers can have difficulty making accurate judgments of the psychologic status of pain patients and may tend to over-report psychopathology.[47,48] These results suggest that the use of screening instruments may help improve the accuracy and efficiency of clinical decision-making in the orofacial pain setting.

Brief Screening for Biobehavioral Factors

It is necessary for clinicians to conduct an assessment of biobehavioral factors in the initial consultation session.[40,49–51] In terms of which factors should be evaluated, the extent of the assessment should depend on the setting (eg, general dental or medical office, orofacial pain specialist office, research clinic, psychologist office) and the purpose (eg, initial screening, more in-depth evaluation by the orofacial pain specialist, comprehensive evaluation by a consulting psychologist) of the evaluation. The selection of the extent of the biobehavioral focus implies that the clinician understands the importance of biobehavioral factors in the patient's presentation and the contexts in which the patient evaluations occur. When it comes to the first line of screening, however, the critical dimensions include *(1)* some means of assessing multiple pain conditions or complaints in addition to the orofacial pain that generated the initial clinical visit, *(2)* pain intensity and pain-related disability, and *(3)* psychologic distress.[10,16,50,52,53]

One of the strongest and most consistent predictors of the onset of a new orofacial pain condition is the presence of other ongoing pain complaints.[37] The presence of other significant pain locations affects TMD-examination findings as well as the reporting of symptom severity of all TMD-related symptoms.[54] Even though direct studies are still needed, piecing together the evidence across the life-course of painful TMDs suggests that multiple pain conditions also appear to be a strong predictor of the transition from acute pain to chronic pain.[24,34,55] Presence of multiple pain complaints can be assessed with a drawing of the full human body (*pain manikin*), front and back, where the patient can note areas of ongoing pain. Among individuals with chronic painful TMDs, only about 22% will have no other body locations affected by significant pain,[56] while the other 78% will report significant pains affecting nearly every part of the body more adversely than is found in individuals with primary headache or irritable bowel syndrome.[57] Other initial strategies for assessing multiple pain conditions include using a checklist or specific questions concerning pain in other regions of the body.

Both the intensity of pain and the impact of the pain on functioning can be obtained with the Graded Chronic Pain Scale (GCPS).[58] This brief, eight-item screening instrument includes an assessment of number of pain days in the last 6 months; current pain intensity, worst pain intensity, and average pain intensity using the scale of 0 to 10 (where 0 represents "no pain" and 10 represents "pain as bad as can be"); and four questions concerning disability related to the pain. When averaged together, the pain intensity items provide an overall index of pain intensity. Based on the intensity and disability ratings, patients can be classified into one of five categories, grades 0 to IV. Grade 0 represents being pain-free, grade I represents low intensity of pain and low disability, grade II represents high intensity of pain and low disability, grade III represents moderately limiting disability, and grade IV represents severely limiting disability. Pain intensity is not considered in grades III and IV because poor functional status, as represented by the disability grade, becomes substantially more important than pain intensity. The GCPS is recommended for regular use in the orofacial pain setting because it is a reliable, valid, and brief screening tool for pain and pain-related disability. The 30-day version, as included in the DC/TMD protocol, provides assessment concurrent with the time period typically used for diagnosis, while the original 6-month version most likely provides a better estimate regarding disability and has better concordance with high-impact chronic pain.[59,60] High self-rated levels of pain, interference, and impact, along with low ability to control pain, suggest the need for further biobehavioral evaluation and appropriate referral for consultation.[58,61]

The more common forms of distress presenting in the orofacial pain clinic include depression and anxiety, ranging from mild symptoms to severe disorders.[61] Depression and anxiety are described in detail in later sections of this chapter to provide a broader understanding of these conditions within the context of the orofacial pain setting. The immediate concerns of the clinician are to screen patients and identify those who need further consultation and care by a qualified mental health provider. While there are a variety of screening instruments, a very brief measure for screening distress is the Patient Health Questionnaire 4 (PHQ-4),[62] which assesses both depression and anxiety. The PHQ-4 is a four-item measure that evaluates functioning over the past 2 weeks, with the scale ranging from 0, meaning "not at all" to 3, meaning "nearly every day." The instrument includes an additional item that assesses the impact on functioning due to any of the symptoms in the four items. The PHQ-4 requires about 1 minute for administration. This brief instrument yields a rating of normal, mild, moderate, or severe distress. Any nonnormal rating, particularly if accompanied by a report of very or extremely difficult with regard to functioning, is an indication for further evaluation by a qualified mental health provider. This instrument is ideally suited for the screening of distress in the orofacial pain environment.

Several other standardized screening questionnaires are available for depression and anxiety that can enable the clinician to make informed decisions about the need for more extensive diagnostic decision-making and treatment planning.[63–65] In clinical settings, the choice of one instrument over another is far less important than knowing the instrument and knowing the distribution of scores in one's clinical population.

The Jaw Functional Limitations Scale (JFLS) is recommended as a primary assessment tool for evaluating the impact of pain on the core functions of the masticatory system.[66] Functional limitation refers to the patient's appraisal regarding how extensive functioning is limited. The JFLS may be administered as a 20-item instrument yielding three subscales (masticatory limitation, job mobility limitation, and verbal and emotional expressiveness limitation) or as an eight-item global limitation scale. The information obtained from the patient at the initial evaluation should be consistent with any physical diagnosis, and when it is not, other questions should be raised in the clinical interview. For example, reported severe limitation in both mastication and jaw mobility simultaneous with minimum clinical signs may point toward catastrophizing and/or symptom amplification, or it may point toward an incomplete understanding of what has happened to the patient. In contrast, minimal limitation despite severe reported pain and significant clinical signs may indicate a patient who was trying to overcompensate. Assessment instruments also provide important functional evidence in situations when the provider must demonstrate treatment efficacy.

The clinician should consider whether the screening assessment should also address oral behaviors. The Oral Behaviors Checklist (OBC)[67,68] is a 21-item scale that was developed during the DC/TMD validation study to identify common oral behaviors associated with TMDs. This scale provides the clinician with the patient's perspective on a broad sample of oral behaviors (eg, chewing gum, clenching teeth, pressing tongue forcibly against teeth) that may influence orofacial pain. It has demonstrated acceptable validity and reliability for the measurement of oral behaviors over time. Such behaviors are strong contributors toward initial onset of a painful TMD,[29] and the behaviors continue to increase after TMD onset.[55] When pain becomes chronic, it is strongly associated with a very high extent of oral parafunctional behaviors, with the suggestion that the behaviors at that stage are likely both contributing factors for pain persistence as well as reactive to pain.[24]

Utilizing this brief comprehensive screening battery (eg, the pain manikin, GCPS, PHQ-4, JFLS, and OBC) provides the clinician with initial data to guide case conceptualization and treatment planning. However, there may be circumstances where there is insufficient time or resources to use all these measures. In these cases, it is recommended to at least perform an ultra-brief screening comprising the pain manikin, GCPS, and PHQ-4.

Comprehensive Evaluation of Biobehavioral Factors

In addition to depression and anxiety, studies have identified the important roles of sleep disturbances, somatic awareness, catastrophizing, perceived distress, and PTSD as strong predictors of distress and pain in orofacial pain patients.[24,28,29,32,35,37,69–72] There are brief, reliable paper and pencil screening instruments available to assess sleep (eg, Pittsburgh Sleep Quality Index, Patient-Reported Outcome Measures Information sleep instruments), somatic awareness (eg, SCL90-R, Pennebaker Inventory of Limbic Languidness), perceived stress (Perceived Stress Scale), catastrophizing (Pain Catastrophizing Scale), and PTSD (PTSD Checklist). These represent a large set of constructs that can be productively assessed in individuals with pain when time for assessment and interpretation is available. However, time is more often limited. Consequently, even within the comprehensive

Box 12-1 Red and yellow flags for referral of orofacial pain patients

Red flag—Refer immediately

- Suicidal thoughts or plans

Yellow flag—Proceed with caution and consider referral

- Alcohol or drug use
- Persistent beliefs about pain
- Illness behaviors
- Problems in compensation or claims
- Time off work
- Problems at work
- Overprotection from family members
- Lack of social support
- Chronicity of pain
- Functional limitations
- Discrepancies in findings
- Overuse of medications
- Inappropriate behavior, expectations, or responsiveness to prior treatment

Axis II assessment battery of the DC/TMD protocol, only a small number of the above constructs are recommended for routine assessment: Clinicians may use the PHQ-9 for a more detailed screening for depression, the Generalized Anxiety Disorder 7 (GAD-7) for anxiety, and the PHQ-15 for evaluation of physical symptoms.

Many clinicians may find the information for these instruments helpful in the processes of evaluation and treatment planning. Overall, it is important that dentist and other health care clinicians be able to recognize maladaptive coping mechanisms and direct patients to appropriate evaluation and treatment programs to address these dysfunctions. Stressful life events—such as conflicts in home or work relationships, financial problems, and cultural readjustment—may contribute to illness and chronic pain.[7,73,74] Environmental stressors may heighten tensions, insecurities, and dysphoric affects that may in turn lead to increased adverse loading (eg, through clenching or grinding of the teeth) of the masticatory system as stress is converted to muscle tension and increased parafunctional behavior.[75,76] Stressors will not always lead to increases in muscle tension, and increases in muscle tension will not always create pain, but it is a distinct possibility to consider when evaluating an individual's clinical presentation. The use of a pain manikin, the GCPS, and the PHQ-4 serves as an acceptable initial minimum screening for all orofacial pain patients to determine if they should be referred for further evaluation by qualified mental health care providers.

In addition to pain-relevant biobehavioral constructs, Turner and Dworkin[50] noted the value of screening for prolonged and/or excessive use of opiate medications, benzodiazepines, alcohol, and other addictive medications. Clinicians can screen for these problems in the course of their initial evaluation interview. When screening for alcohol use, one instrument is the Alcohol Use Disorders Identification Test (AUDIT-C).[77] This three-item questionnaire is a reliable means of identifying whether an individual should be referred for careful evaluation of alcohol abuse.

Health care providers working with patients with chronic back pain use a strategy in the initial evaluation process to identify red and yellow flags: *Red flags* are those presenting a potentially serious condition for which immediate attention is needed, and *yellow flags* represent potential psychologic or social barriers to full recovery (Box 12-1). Clinicians in the orofacial pain setting should also use a red and yellow flag identification strategy when implementing a biobehavioral approach. Red flags in the psychosocial history of the orofacial pain patient demand immediate attention; these primarily focus on signs of suicide. The most common signs of potential suicide include talking about suicide, either generally or specifically, and/or actual plans for taking one's own life (suicidal ideation) and hopelessness. There are other warning signs for suicide, including persistent and despairing mood, significant weight loss or gain, change in appetite, withdrawal, and social isolation, and change in sleep pattern—all symptoms that are associated with depression as well. Any patient who presents with thoughts about suicide, plans for suicide, or hopelessness should be evaluated for risk assessment as soon as possible by qualified mental health care professionals.

Yellow flags for treatment may include persistent beliefs about pain, illness behaviors, problems and compensation/claims, time off from work, problems at work, overprotection from family members, or lack of social support. Additional factors include chronicity of pain, extensive functional limitations, discrepancy in findings, overuse of medication, inappropriate behavior (often including items from the first list, but not exclusively), inappropriate expectations, and inappropriate responsiveness to any prior treatment[43,78] (see Box 12-1). Any of these issues can interfere with treatment, and the orofacial pain specialist needs to be wary of initiating treatment in individuals with these concerns. When possible, a careful and thorough evaluation should be performed by a psychologist, psychiatrist, psychiatric nurse practitioner, or other appropriately trained mental health care provider before treatment begins.

Psychiatric Disorders

Orofacial pain patients, particularly those with a history of significant pain over 3 months in duration, may experience significant psychologic distress that complicates the management of their presenting complaints. A distinction can be drawn between the role of pain psychology and the use of diagnostic psychiatric disorders in a clinical setting for orofacial pain. One difference is that pain psychology places emphasis on dimensional assessment rather than classification (diagnosis). Furthermore, pain psychology is interested in the detailed integration of specific domains of functioning known to be important in the pain patient's experience and the incorporation of the biobehavioral domain into the clinical arena and decision-making. This approach to patient management focuses on the identification of problem areas that lend themselves to structured, empirically supported therapies (eg, cognitive behavioral therapy) that will facilitate referrals when needed. Pain clinicians will encounter patients whose functioning is severely compromised; knowing when to refer to a mental health care provider benefits the patient and the clinician alike. The description of mental states provided by the classic psychiatric disorders captures the many ways in which human systems undergo dysregulation. Recognizing these signs of dysregulation is essential in patients so that the foundations of a dual-axis classification system can be better understood and applied clinically.

Although many mental conditions can be influenced by or result from orofacial pain disorders, only a select group is addressed in this chapter. This section highlights the more common mental disorders that clinicians are likely to encounter; the comprehensive evaluation of psychologic status should be conducted by appropriately trained mental health care providers.[79] Gatchel et al among others[80–82] have reported that the most frequently occurring problems include major depression, anxiety disorders, and personality disorders. The other disorders presented in this chapter have a much lower frequency of recurrence, but orofacial pain clinicians should be aware of them in order to make a successful referral for definitive diagnosis and treatment. For a description of other mental conditions, the reader is encouraged to review the current *Diagnostic and Statistical Manual of Mental Disorders, Fifth Edition* (*DSM-5*).[38] Each disorder is accompanied by its codes from the *DSM-5* and/or *The International Classification of Diseases, Tenth Revision* (*ICD-10*) and *11th Revision* (*ICD-11*). Please note that as of January 1, 2022, the *ICD-11* codes will be used in place of the *ICD-10* codes.

Major depressive disorder (*DSM-5* 296.2x; *ICD-10* F32; *ICD-11* 6A70.3)[38]

Major depression has been identified as one of the most common mental disorders occurring in the orofacial pain environment.[81] Clinical data suggest that almost one-third of patients presenting for treatment of orofacial pain may be experiencing symptoms consistent with a diagnosis of depression.[83] The diagnosis of major depression requires at least five of the following symptoms over a 2-week period, with at least one of the symptoms being depressed mood or loss of interest or pleasure:

- Depressed mood most of the day
- Decreased interest or pleasure in all or most daily activities
- Weight loss or change in appetite
- Insomnia or hypersomnia
- Daily psychomotor agitation or retardation
- Fatigue or loss of energy
- Feelings of worthlessness or guilt
- Reduced ability to think or concentrate
- Thoughts of death or suicide

When the symptoms cause distress and impair functioning and are not due to a medical condition or substance use, the diagnosis of major depression is likely. Major depression is a serious, potentially life-threatening condition, and referral to appropriate health care providers for effective treatment is essential in addition to care for the pain disorder itself.

Anxiety disorders

Generalized anxiety disorder (*DSM-5* 300.02; *ICD-10* F41.1; *ICD-11* 6B00)[38]

Generalized anxiety disorder (GAD) is diagnosed when an individual has persistent and excessive anxiety or worry for a period of 6 months or longer. The person who is experiencing GAD is not able to control the feelings of anxiety or worry, and at least three of the following symptoms are present: restlessness, fatigue, difficulty concentrating, irritability, muscle tension, and sleep disturbance. In addition, the symptoms cause significant impairment of interpersonal functioning or work performance, and the anxiety and worry are not associated with another mental disorder (eg, obsessive-compulsive disorder), substance use (drugs or alcohol), or other medical condition. It is estimated that between 10% and 30% of the orofacial pain population may be experiencing GAD.[81] Anxiety is particularly important to identify during the acute phase of the pain disorder because it leads to nonadaptive behaviors, which may promote chronicity.[4] Referral for treatment of GAD may be delayed based on whether treatment of the orofacial pain condition itself may begin to alter symptoms.

Panic disorder (*DSM-5* 300.01; *ICD-10* F41.0; *ICD-11* 6B01)[38]

Although much less common than GAD, *panic disorder* involves a sudden, intense onset of fear and terror that is often accompanied by thoughts of impending disaster. It can include chest pain, palpitations, and shortness of breath, which can be so severe that the individuals may feel as though they are dying. Individuals having a panic attack report sensations of choking or smothering and are afraid of losing control of their thoughts. Panic disorder is diagnosed when a panic attack has occurred and when at least one of the following criteria are present for at least 1 month: persistent concern about having another attack, worry about the implications or consequences of the attack, and a notable change in behavior related to the attacks or fear thereof. In addition, the panic attacks must not be due to a medical condition or substance use. Even though panic disorder is uncommon, it is a condition that requires immediate attention and coping skills. Therefore, if panic disorder is suspected, appropriate referral should be made immediately.

Posttraumatic stress disorder (*DSM-5* 309.81; *ICD-10* F43.1; *ICD-11* 6B40)[38]

Considerable professional interest and burgeoning public concern have focused on the sequalae of traumatic experiences. It is now well recognized that physical and sexual abuse are implicated in the etiology of a broad spectrum of physical and emotional symptoms. The essential feature of PTSD is the onset of characteristic symptoms following exposure to a traumatic event either involving direct personal experience or the witnessing of such an event. Traumatic events usually involve actual or threatened death or serious injury or a threat to one's physical and psychologic integrity. Typical symptoms include persistent reexperiencing of the traumatic event, persistent avoidance of stimuli associated with the trauma and numbing of general responsiveness, and persistent symptoms of increased arousal. The full symptom picture must be present for more than 1 month, and the disturbance must cause clinically significant distress or impairment in daily functioning. For children, sexually traumatic events may include developmentally inappropriate sexual experiences without threatening or actual violence or injury. The disorder may be especially severe or long lasting when the traumatic experience has been created by deliberate human intent (eg, torture or rape) as contrasted with naturally occurring disasters. The likelihood of developing this disorder may increase as the intensity of and physical proximity to the event increases.

Psychologic reexperiencing of the traumatic event may occur in several ways, commonly as recurrent and intrusive recollections, distressing dreams, and, in rare instances, brief dissociative states or flashbacks during which components of the events are relived and the person behaves as though experiencing the event at that moment. Intense psychologic distress or physiologic reactions often occur when the person is exposed to triggering events that resemble or symbolize an aspect of the traumatic event (eg, entering an elevator for a person who may have been assaulted or raped in an elevator; or any intraoral pain or manipulation for individuals who may have been sexually violated or traumatized in the mouth).

Typically, individuals suffering from this condition make deliberate efforts to avoid thoughts, feelings, or conversations about the traumatic event and, in some instances, may develop amnesia for important aspects of the traumatic experience. Diminished psychologic responsiveness, referred to as *psychic numbing* or *emotional anesthesia*, may be accompanied by markedly diminished interest in previously enjoyed activities and markedly reduced capacity for emotional responsiveness. The individual has persistent symptoms of anxiety or increased arousal that were not present before the trauma; the arousal symptoms are frequently associated with sleep disturbance, nightmares, hypervigilance, and an exaggerated startle response. This increased arousal is often accompanied by activation of the autonomic nervous system as measurable by electrocardiography, electromyography, and sweat gland activity. In younger children, distressing dreams of the event may change into generalized nightmares. Rather than having a sense of reliving the past as a memory, for example, a child involved in a motor vehicle accident may reenact scenes of toy cars crashing, or sexually traumatized children may depict genital contact occurring between toy animals.

It should be emphasized that not all psychopathology occurring in individuals exposed to extreme stress should necessarily be attributed to PTSD. Symptoms of avoidance, numbing, and increased arousal that are present before exposure to the stressor require consideration of other diagnostic alternatives (eg, a mood disorder or an anxiety disorder). *Acute stress disorder* is distinguished from PTSD because the symptoms appear and subsequently resolve within four weeks of the trauma. *Adjustment disorder* is the appropriate diagnosis for situations in which the response to stress does not meet the criteria for PTSD or when the stressor itself is not judged to be that threatening.

A significant proportion of orofacial pain patients are likely to meet lifetime criteria for having experienced PTSD.[70,71] This relatively high rate of occurrence is consistent with other data, suggesting that exposure to traumatic life events is common among orofacial pain patients and patients with other pain conditions as well.[70,84] It is therefore necessary that clinicians have an awareness of the signs and symptoms of PTSD and are able to make appropriate referrals for treatment. The characteristics of this disorder (ie, autonomic activation, perceptual distortion, and denial of one's own needs) may prevent significant therapeutic gains unless the underlying disorder is addressed.

Substance use disorders (*DSM-5* 295-301; *ICD-10* F10-19; *ICD-11* 6C42)[38]

It is not uncommon for patients with orofacial pain to have ongoing or previous substance-related disorders. These disorders include dependence, abuse, intoxication, and withdrawal. *Substance dependence* is defined as a pattern of substance use that leads to clinically significant impairment or distress. The term *substance abuse* refers to a pattern of substance use that has significant negative consequences, such as failure to meet obligations at work, school, or home; behaviors that are physically hazardous like driving a car when impaired; legal problems; or interpersonal problems related to the continued substance use. *Substance intoxication* refers to the reversible signs and symptoms associated with the intake of the substance that can produce physical, behavioral, or psychologic changes. *Withdrawal* refers to substance-specific physical, behavioral, or psychologic changes that occur with the reduction or stoppage of a substance that has been used over a period of time.

Clinicians should also be familiar with the terms *addiction* and *pseudoaddiction*. *Addiction* involves one or more of the following characteristics: impaired control over drug use, compulsive use of drug(s), continued use despite harm, and craving. A person with an addiction often does not take medications according to prescription or schedule, has multiple visits to multiple practitioners, and likely reports on a frequent basis that personal prescriptions have been lost or stolen. It is important to distinguish addiction from pseudoaddiction in chronic pain patients.[85,86] *Pseudoaddiction* looks like addiction in that the same behaviors are typically present, but the patient has identifiable nociception (eg, cancer pain, neuropathic pain, postsurgical pain) that is undermedicated, so the patient is constantly searching for effective treatment to control the pain. When such a person is given adequate medication, the addiction-like behavior ceases. Distinguishing addiction from pseudoaddiction requires good knowledge of the patient by the clinician and is greatly facilitated by careful history taking, comprehensive and standardized physical examinations, and use of biobehavioral assessment instruments. In the case of pseudoaddiction in particular, progress notes should clearly document the contingent nature of the medication seeking along with the appropriateness of the medication to the identified or suspected nociception.

These disorders can occur within broad classes of substances that include alcohol, amphetamines or similar compounds, caffeine, cannabis, cocaine, hallucinogens, inhalants, nicotine, opioids, phencyclidine or similar compounds, and sedatives/hypnotics/anxiolytics. The clinician must be alert to potential abuse disorders and be able to develop a treatment plan that is in the best interests of the patient and clinician. Unless the clinician has specialty training in the management of addiction disorders, the appropriate standard of care is referral to a health care provider who does have specialty training. It is important to develop rapport with patients who have problems with substance abuse in order to foster successful referral.

Sleep disorders[38]

Sleep disorders are common in patients with chronic pain, and there are two major sleep disorders the clinician is likely to encounter: *primary insomnia* (*DSM-5* 780.52; *ICD-10* F51.0; *ICD-11* 7A00) and *breathing-related sleep disorders* (eg, sleep apnea, *DSM-5* 3237; *ICD-10* G47.3; *ICD-11* 7A41). Other sleep disorders, such as narcolepsy or night terrors, are not as common in the chronic pain environment. *Primary insomnia* involves difficulty in initiating or maintaining sleep, and it must have persisted for at least 1 month. The sleep problem results in distress or difficulties in the individual's life that could include interpersonal or work-related issues. For primary insomnia to be diagnosed, it must be clear that depression, anxiety, or medication/substance use is not contributing to the disruptions in sleep. Primary insomnia can be managed with behavioral medicine strategies playing primary roles. Cognitive-behavioral treatment of insomnia can be an especially powerful tool to address sleep disruptions in an orofacial pain patient.[87]

Breathing-related sleep disorders involve being sleepy or experiencing insomnia as a result of a breathing problem that disrupts regular sleep. The breathing problem is usually the result of either obstructive or central sleep apnea, but it can be the result of central alveolar hypoventilation syndrome or sleep-related hypoxemia disorder. These latter conditions represent medical disorders that merit immediate referral to physicians trained in sleep medicine. Breathing-related sleep disorders require medical evaluation, and biobehavioral approaches should also be considered when appropriate for interventions.

Somatic symptom and related disorders[38]

Clinicians should recognize and appreciate somatic symptoms and related disorders because they represent an extremely important group of mental conditions in which the patient reports somatic complaints and yet has no physical evidence of organic disease. Somatic symptoms and related disorders are subdivided into the following categories: somatic symptoms disorder, illness anxiety disorder, conversion disorder, factitious disorder, unspecified somatic symptom and related disorders, other specified somatic symptoms and related disorders, and psychologic factors affecting other medical conditions.

Somatic symptom disorder (*DSM-5* 300.82; *ICD-10* F45.0; *ICD-11* 6C20)

The essential features of somatic symptom disorder are recurrent and multiple somatic complaints of at least several years duration for which treatment has been sought contrasting with significant disarray or distress in the person's life for which no treatment has been sought. Clinical characteristics include preoccupation with somatic complaints, amplification of symptoms, denial of difficulty in life, and the high level of treatment seeking for somatic complaints accompanied by poor adherence and compliance to that treatment. The disorder classically begins before age 30 years and has a chronic but fluctuating course. Historically, this condition was previously referred to as *hysteria* or *Briquet syndrome*, and the history of medicine clearly demonstrates that its presentation is anchored into the current values and beliefs of the host culture.[88] Complaints are often presented in a dramatic, vague, or exaggerated manner or are a part of a complicated dental and/or medical history in which many physical diagnoses have been considered. The individuals frequently receive dental care from a number of practitioners, sometimes simultaneously. Complaints often extend to multiple organ systems. The term *hypochondriasis* is no longer used in the diagnostic nosology because approximately 75% of hypochondriasis patients match the diagnostic criteria for somatic symptom disorder while the remaining 25% have elevated levels of anxiety such that they are more appropriately diagnosed with *illness anxiety disorder* (*DSM-5* 300.7; *ICD-10* F45.212; *ICD-11* 6B23.z).

To diagnose somatic symptom disorder, there must be a history of the report of somatic symptoms that are distressing, along with thoughts, feelings, and/or behaviors that are out of proportion with the symptoms, and an inordinate amount of time and energy must be devoted to addressing these health concerns. Individuals with this disorder, for example, complain of abdominal bloating and nausea, while vomiting, diarrhea, and food intolerance are less frequent symptoms. It should be emphasized that the unexplained symptoms in somatic symptom disorder are not intentionally feigned or produced.

Because of the highly restrictive character of the required symptom pattern, somatic symptom disorder is not common, but somatic symptom disorder as a style or as a major characteristic about a person is fairly common in the orofacial pain population.[89] For example, the so-called somatization scale scores on the Symptom Checklist-90R (SCL-90R) have a significant relationship with the number of muscles reported as tender during an RDC/TMD examination.[90] These clinical data highlight the necessary attention needed to consider somatic symptom disorder as a way of coping among patients in an orofacial pain practice.

Anxiety and depressed mood are common, and suicide threats or attempts, antisocial behavior, and occupational, interpersonal, and marital difficulties frequently accompany somatization. The clinical course is typically chronic but fluctuating in nature and rarely remits spontaneously. Through seeking numerous evaluations, diagnostic tests, and multiple trials on medication and frequently submitting unwillingly to unnecessary surgery, these patients often experience iatrogenic complications both in and out of the hospital.

The differential diagnosis necessitates ruling out physical disorders that present with vague, multiple, and confusing somatic symptoms. In addition, schizophrenia with multiple somatic delusions, dysthymic disorder, GAD, panic disorder, and conversion disorder need to be excluded from the specific diagnostic classification. Because pathophysiology has yet to be fully identified, myofascial pain could qualify as a disorder without clear organic pathology for clinicians; according to the description presented here, such a patient would qualify for a diagnosis of at least somatic symptom disorder as a style of coping. Before neuropathic mechanisms were suspected to underlie burning mouth disorder types of conditions, *somatization* was a diagnostic label unfortunately applied to such individuals for many years. Because many chronic pain disorders do not have obvious pathology responsible for the inferred nociception, distinguishing such functional disorders from somatic symptom disorder is neither conceptually nor procedurally simple, but it is critically important for both the patient and clinician. These disorders may include nonspecific lower back pain and irritable bowel syndrome, for example, and they represent at least a disorder of psychophysiologic dysregulation. The distinction is also not clinically simple, but a comprehensive history and attention to the biobehavioral screening and identified yellow flags (see Box 12-1) are an excellent and essential starting point. In recognition of the complexity associated with pain disorders, the term *complex overlapping pain conditions* has been recommended by the National Institutes of Health[91] in order to identify a frequent constellation of symptoms and burden on individuals with multiple pain conditions and to help distinguish such conditions from somatic symptoms disorders.

Conversion disorder (functional neurologic symptom disorder) (*DSM-5* 300.11; *ICD-10* F44.x; *ICD-11* 6B60.z)

Patients with conversion disorder present with a loss of or alteration in physical functioning that suggests a physical disorder but instead is an expression of psychologic conflict or need. The disturbance is not under voluntary control and cannot be explained by any physical disorder or known pathophysiologic mechanism. Conversion disorder is not diagnosed when conversion symptoms are limited to pain (see somatoform pain disorder) or to a circumscribed disturbance in sexual functioning.

Factitious disorder (*DSM-5* 300.19; *ICD-10* F678.1; *ICD-11* 6D5Z)

Factitious means not real, genuine, or natural. *Factitious disorders* are therefore characterized by physical and/or psychologic symptoms that are produced by the individual and are under voluntary control. The judgment that the patient is willfully creating the symptoms is based, in part, on the patient's ability to simulate illness in such a way as to avoid detection. However, such acts also have a compulsive quality because the individual is unable to refrain from a particular behavior even if its dangers are known. These conditions should therefore be considered *voluntary* only in the sense that they are deliberate and purposeful but not in the sense that the patient adopts or sustains the pathologic behavior intentionally. The presence of factitious psychologic or physical symptoms does not preclude the coexistence of true psychologic or physical illness.

Factitious disorder is distinguished from acts of malingering. Whereas in *malingering,* the patient is in pursuit of obvious and recognizable benefits through willful falsification, in a factitious disorder, there is no apparent goal other than to assume the patient role. An act of malingering may be considered adaptive under certain conditions, but a diagnosis of factitious disorder implies psychopathology (often a severe personality disturbance). According to the *DSM-5,* malingering is not considered a mental illness.

Unspecified somatic symptom and related disorder (*DSM-5* 300.82; *ICD-10* F45.9; *ICD-11* 6C20.z)

The essential feature of unspecified somatic symptom and related disorder is one or more physical complaints that persist for 6 months or longer. These symptoms cannot be fully explained either by any known physical condition or by the direct effects of an incident or substance (eg, the effects of injury, substance use, or medication side effects). Alternatively, the physical complaints or resultant impairment are grossly in excess of what would be expected from the history, physical examination, or laboratory findings. The symptoms must cause clinically significant distress or impairment in social, occupational, or other areas of adaptive functioning. This is a residual category for those persistent somatic form presentations that do not meet the full criteria for other somatic symptoms disorders.

Psychologic factors affecting other medical conditions (*DSM-5* 316; *ICD-10* F54; *ICD-11* 6E40.2)

When the primary presenting complaint is a medical (ie, physical) condition influenced by one or more psychologic or behavioral states, psychologic factors affecting other medical conditions can be diagnosed. Typically, the diagnosis will link the psychologically related issues with the physical condition, as in the example, "stress and anger toward significant other affecting masticatory muscle pain." The issues identified must be contributing to the disorder by *(1)* having a close connection in terms of time between the beginning of the physical condition and the onset of the psychologic behavioral factors, *(2)* interfering with the treatment of the condition, *(3)* increasing health risk, or

(4) increasing physiologic activation that brings on or intensifies the physical condition.

This diagnostic category provides the practitioner with the means to codify a comorbid psychologic condition that may be contributing to the patient's capacity to manage a medical problem. Because chronic pain complaints represent a complex interaction between psychologic and physiologic factors, the use of this diagnostic category is common. This label also may be more acceptable to some patients than other labels of psychiatric conditions.

Personality disorders[38]

Generally speaking, a *personality disorder* is a long-term pattern of thinking and acting that is significantly different from that of the general population and results in significant consequences to the individual or those around the individual. These abnormal patterns may manifest as exaggerations or dysfunction of certain dimensions of personality. For example, it is normal to have occasional moments of not trusting another person, but it is abnormal to live with a consistent pattern of suspiciousness and mistrust. An orofacial pain condition is most likely to appear after the individual has already been displaying a pattern of thoughts and behaviors characteristic of a personality disorder. These patterns, however, may or may not have interfered with daily functioning prior to the development of the orofacial pain condition. Recent data suggest that a significant number of orofacial pain patients have coexisting personality disorders.[81,82]

There are three basic groups of personality disorders that share common clinical presentations (Table 12–2). *Cluster A* includes odd or eccentric disorders and schizotypal disorders. *Cluster B* includes emotional, dramatic, or unpredictable disorders like antisocial, borderline, or histrionic disorders. *Cluster C* includes anxious and fearful disorders like avoidant, dependent, and obsessive-compulsive disorders.[38]

Cluster A

Within Cluster A, *paranoid personality disorder* describes an individual who does not trust others and is very suspicious. These patients may overinterpret what the clinician says or may be unforgiving of others for perceived injury or insult. Patients with *schizoid personality disorder* are detached from others and have very limited emotional expression. A person with this disorder has few, if any, close friends or family and usually does things alone. The *schizotypal personality disorder* shares the features of detachment and limited emotional expression but is also characterized by substantial distortions of thought and very unusual behavior. Thought distortions including magical thinking, belief in telepathy, and weird fantasies. Unusual behaviors might involve acting out the use of "special powers" or listening to "voices for direction."

Cluster B

Within Cluster B, the *antisocial personality disorder* is characterized by little or no regard for the rights of others. The diagnosis of this personality disorder involves the individual committing crimes, lying, not planning ahead, being irritable and aggressive to the point of getting into fights, disregarding the safety of self and others, being irresponsible, and/or not expressing remorse or sorrow for behavior that hurts others. In short, the antisocial personality involves behavior that is self-centered and does not conform to the general rules and expectations of society.

Borderline personality disorder represents a repeated pattern of instability of relationships and impulsivity in action. The instability takes the form of leaving and entering relationships in a recurrent pattern as well as frequent changes in the nature of the relationship. The patient

Table 12-2 Personality disorders

Disorder	*DSM-5* code	*ICD-10* code	*ICD-11* code
Cluster A: Odd or eccentric disorders			
Paranoid	301.0	F60.0	6D10.Z
Schizoid	302.20	F60.1	6D10.Z
Schizotypical	301.22	F60.3	6A22
Cluster B: Emotional, dramatic, or unpredictable disorders			
Antisocial	301.71	F60.2	6D10.Z
Borderline	301.83	F60.3	6D10.Z
Histrionic	301.50	F60.4	6D10.Z
Narcissistic	301.81	F60.81	6D10.Z
Cluster C: Anxious and fearful disorders			
Avoidant	301.82	F60.6	6D10.Z
Dependent	301.6	F60.7	6D10.Z
Obsessive-compulsive	3-1.4	F60.5	6D10.Z

with borderline personality disorder often has an inordinate fear of being abandoned and exhibits extremes of thinking. For example, the relationship with the health care provider may involve the patient holding the provider in the highest regard and later accusing him or her of incompetency. These patients exhibit impulsive, self-destructive behavior such as substance abuse, unsafe sex, binge eating, and reckless driving, and they engage in repeated threats and gestures of self-harm, including suicide. There is also marked emotional instability and intense, inappropriate anger. The borderline personality can also manifest as paranoid thoughts or dissociative symptoms. The person with borderline personality disorder can present an extremely difficult case management challenge to the unwary practitioner.

Histrionic personality disorder is characterized as pronounced emotional expression and attention seeking. Patients with this disorder can be provocative and sexually seductive and easily suggestible, and they may perceive relationships as more intimate than they really are. In other words, they think and act in ways that are inconsistent with boundaries normally maintained by orofacial pain patients. Patients with *narcissistic personality disorder* act in a grandiose manner and have an intense need to be admired by others while displaying little empathy. These individuals expect the clinician to respond to their needs at all hours, including during the weekend.

Cluster C

Cluster C personality disorders involve patients who are overly anxious or afraid as a predominant feature of their everyday experience. *Avoidant personality disorder* is associated with feeling socially inhibited and inadequate and being overly sensitive to any criticism. Patients with *dependent personality disorder* have a pervasive need to be taken care of, so there is excessive clinging and fear of being abandoned. These individuals will continue to seek care for their orofacial pain condition despite lack of improvement over time or even when harmed by treatment. Moreover, they may continue to seek care despite any reasonable interpretation of having improved substantially. With *obsessive-compulsive personality disorder*, the patient's day-to-day life is ruled by a drive for perfection, orderliness, and being in control. There is limited openness to new ideas, and rules, details, and lists are very important. Individuals with obsessive-compulsive personality disorder do not like to work with others, keep everything they have owned (even worthless items), and hoard their resources in the event that something happens in the future.

This last cluster of personality disorders can present a very real challenge to effective orofacial pain management. Patients can be so intently focused on personal criticism, symptom improvement, or support from providers that anxiety and nervousness interfere with obtaining positive treatment outcomes. Body dysmorphic disorder, which has been reclassified into the category of obsessive-compulsive personality disorder, is particularly relevant to the orofacial pain clinician because it causes the individual to experience extreme anxiety over a real or imagined physical flaw. For example, this diagnostic category could be applied to a patient who is convinced that there is a slight angle of the canine tooth that is responsible for his or her pain condition.

Consultation and Referral Strategies

Chronic orofacial pain management requires a multidisciplinary team that includes competent mental health care providers. Development of professional relationships with such providers should be a high priority for clinicians practicing in this field because it facilitates the implementation of informed referrals when necessary. Patients may present with red or yellow flags prompting more extensive evaluation or the need for skills training or psychotherapy related to cognitive, behavioral, or emotional issues.

One effective approach for making a referral focuses on the patient's need for assistance with stress management. This strategy helps alleviate a patient's concerns about "being crazy" or being labeled as having a psychiatric disorder. The clinician should reassure the patient with statements such as the following to assuage any concerns:

- The referral is intended to address better ways of managing the consequences of pain.
- All pain is real.
- The relationship with the referring provider will continue through and beyond any referral therapy.
- The patient's physical status will continue to be monitored to detect any change that would warrant a different direction and treatment.
- The referral is not in any way a suggestion that the patient is "crazy."

Another effective strategy is to focus on getting help for physical self-regulation skills training. Patients will often be much more willing to visit with a mental health care provider when the referral focuses on learning how to better manage stress or learning new skills for controlling physical functioning. Biofeedback or diaphragmatic breathing training and their grounded focus on physical self-regulation are topics dentists often discuss with their patients when arranging referrals.

Axis II Evaluation as a Part of Any Evaluation

The assessment of Axis II status must be a standard and routine part of the clinician's initial evaluation of the patient, even if only a brief assessment is used. Self-report screening instruments can be administered through a mailed packet or forms completed while the patient is in the reception area; however, the interview portion is best deferred until the clinician has obtained enough pain and health history to form a matrix within which biobehavioral aspects can be anchored and appropriately interpreted. This part of the evaluation includes the range of biobehavioral factors and their interconnection with a standard pain history and typical review of systems, past medical history, and any family or social history. In addition, the clinician needs time to build rapport and trust with the patient before asking questions about personal functioning, and such questions need to fit into the overall sequence of information gathering. For example, everyone experiences stress (ie, the sense of being threatened or overwhelmed by events or common daily hassles), so it is not enough to simply identify that a patient experiences stress, or even how often and to what extent. The stress experience has to be anchored into the pain and health histories for temporal and causal relationships to be identified, and thus the pain and health histories need to be first explored and understood. This part of an interview is often referred to as the *causal reasoning* portion.[92] The goal is to bring different parts together into a coherent network.

When a patient is referred to a mental health care provider for evaluation, the clinician can expect that the mental health care provider will perform a complete assessment and provide appropriate feedback in a timely manner. Typically, the evaluation can be performed within a 50- to 75-minute period and will include a review of the presenting complaints and history of onset from the perspective of the mental health care provider. The mental health care provider will also likely assess conditions that intensify or reduce the complaints as well as typical antecedents and consequences. It is not uncommon for the clinician to explore a typical day in the life of the patient. Pain cognitions, operant and respondent behavioral factors, activity management, and methods of coping are common features of a pain psychology evaluation. This may be followed by a careful review of the physical history including medication use; sleep issues; nicotine, caffeine, and alcohol use; and physical activity level. Mental status, mood, and ongoing emotional state are then assessed along with risks of harm to self and harm to others. This is typically followed by a review of any psychiatric history or hospitalizations. Then the current social support system, marital history, work history, and exposure to significant stressors or trauma are reviewed, as well as other relevant issues related to the patient's presentation (eg, spiritual or religious issues, compensation issues, legal issues). The data should be summarized in a readable report with appropriate recommendations for the clinician.

Biobehavioral Care: Integrated Care as the Standard of Care

While acute pain patients may respond to treatment in a linear and perhaps even dose-dependent manner, chronic pain patients typically do not. Even an acute pain patient with an obvious etiology and disorder may not respond to treatment in a linear manner if preinjury risk factors (eg, significant oral parafunctional behaviors, fear of reinjury) are present; in fact, the simple injury may result in further activation of those preinjury factors. Unless the initial evaluation sufficiently encompasses both the physical and the biobehavioral domains, the clinician will not know or suspect if there are other factors that might interfere with treatment response. Furthermore, that level of assessment must be maintained at each follow-up as indicated based on patient response to treatment; otherwise, the poor treatment response can be accompanied by more physical treatments, medications, surgical referrals, and so forth.

Chronic orofacial pain conditions share features with other pain disorders across the domains of pain, psychologic characteristics, quantitative sensory testing, and health status; the reporting of symptoms of orofacial pains is similarly affected by the presence of other conditions.[54,56,57,93–95] Orofacial pain conditions seldom exist in isolation of other potent contributors to these disorders, and as noted above regarding the importance of comorbid pain conditions, most individuals with a chronic orofacial pain condition will have other pain disorders that need simultaneous consideration in the overall patient management protocol. With additional pain disorders come further challenges to the pain processing system, such as maintaining sufficient coping responses to nociceptive drive.[5] Additional forms of dysregulation occur, such as the dopaminergic regulatory system involved in learning and motivated behavior or maintaining allostasis in the face of life's inevitable challenges to the self.[96–98] As a consequence, the individual patient's engagement in and response to any treatment is challenged, and the pain processing system itself undergoes maladaptive changes.[99] The implication for comprehensive assessment is becoming increasingly clearer and more imperative for all stages of the health care system, whether in the office of the non-specialist dentist or pain-specialist dentist, or in the office of the non-specialist mental health provider or the pain-specialist mental health provider.[45] Psychologic therapies have a clear role in improving pain and how it impacts the functioning of the CNS.[100] Placing a priority on imaging of the TMJs for a presumed painful TMD with negative history of painful clicking or mechanical locking of the joint, for example, to the exclusion of an initial sufficient dual-axis evaluation as outlined within the DC/TMD and in this chapter is, given the available evidence, a strategy that does not adequately address the centrality of pain. Integration of care is clearly necessary.

If the patient's response to treatment cannot be expected to unfold in a linear manner, then the clinician must link the outcomes assessment goals for the primary physical domain with biobehavioral processes. This means that biobehavioral assessment is ongoing—at every follow-up visit, if necessary—just as physical assessment is. When properly done, this ongoing dual-axis assessment allows both the patient and clinician to see whether the patient is responding appropriately to current treatment; if not, the direction for additional treatments or consultations should be evident to both the patient and the clinician.

In conclusion, the biobehavioral aspect of care must be viewed as central to patient care, not an optional add-on. For example, if physical exercises are part of the treatment but the patient's mobility is not improving, then the clinician should query this outcome. Considerations include inadequate assessment of the physical condition and incorrect execution of the exercises. Other possible causes should also be considered, such as depression, poor time management, avoidance behavior, personality disorder, and a passive coping style, among others. Without an adequate initial biobehavioral assessment, these possible causes of poor treatment outcome cannot be adequately interpreted and managed.

Biobehavioral models used in pain medicine across all disorders emphasize the partnership between provider and patient and the critical role that patient behavior plays in managing pain. Orofacial pain management can be likened to the management of hypertension in that it is enhanced through the simultaneous implementation of multiple treatments. For hypertension, these treatments include stress reduction, exercise, weight control, sodium restriction, relaxation training and biofeedback, and medications. Similarly, for a myofascial pain disorder, multiple self-administered treatments are effective: short-term analgesics and thermal agents; and longer-term stretching, parafunctional behavior control, relaxation/diaphragmatic breathing training and biofeedback, and stress reduction. Each of these management strategies, from medication to stress reduction, is ultimately about behavioral self-regulation. For a patient to develop mastery in behavioral self-regulation, a biobehavioral model is needed to integrate all aspects of evaluation and treatment into an understandable framework.

It is also recognized that the development and implementation of new behavioral and cognitive strategies to influence biologic outcomes is a challenge because these new strategies often introduce significant demands for change. Change is difficult even in the best of circumstances, not to mention when a person is experiencing profound discomfort and distress in regions mediated by the trigeminal nerve. The well-known Prochaska theoretical model for change includes the phases of precontemplation, contemplation, preparation, action, and maintenance.[101,102] While this model offers a conceptual framework for understanding patient status and monitoring the acquisition of new patterns of acting and thinking, the practical business of change is often not so straightforward. This model has been pursued in addressing behavioral change for pain conditions, for example, degenerative joint disease,[103] and the observational data accord with routine clinical observation: People vary across the phases identified in the stages of change. The implication is that the success of any treatment requiring adherence, compliance, and ultimately change on the patient's part must be gauged by where the patient is in that process of change as well as by the correct matching of that treatment to the clinical problem. Alcohol addiction is among the most difficult behaviors to overcome; yet Miller has shown that implementing enduring change is possible even within a brief time window when providers help patients clarify their goals, develop effective skills, and engage in discussion regarding the advantages of new behaviors and their confidence in performing those behaviors.[104] The challenge for orofacial pain clinicians is to gain the necessary training and practical skills to become effective change agents for their patients or to have other health professionals on the team who have those skills. The establishment of durable behavioral and cognitive changes that exert positive influence on physiologic functioning is a major contributor to the effective long-term management of orofacial pain conditions.

References

1. Engel GL. The need for a new medical model: A challenge for biomedicine. Science 1977;196:129–136.
2. Rothman KJ, Greenland S. Causation and causal inference in epidemiology. Am J Public Health 2005;95 (suppl 1):S144–S150.
3. National Academies of Sciences Engineering and Medicine. Temporomandibular Disorders: Priorities for Research and Care. Washington, DC: National Academies, 2020.
4. Carlson CR. Psychological factors associated with orofacial pain. Dent Clin North Am 2007;51:145–160.
5. Doleys DM. Pain: Dynamics and Complexities. New York: Oxford, 2014.
6. Dworkin SF, Von Korff MR, LeResche L. Epidemiologic studies of chronic pain: A dynamic-ecologic perspective. Ann Behav Med 1992;14:3–11.
7. Dworkin SF. Illness behavior and dysfunction: Review of concepts and application to chronic pain. Can J Physiol Pharmacol 1991;69:662–671.
8. Dworkin SF, LeResche L. Research diagnostic criteria for temporomandibular disorders: Review, criteria, examinations and specifications, critique. J Craniomandib Disord 1992;6:301–355.
9. Dworkin SF, Massoth DL. Temporomandibular disorders and chronic pain: Disease or illness? J Prosthet Dent 1994;72:29–38.
10. Ohrbach R, List T, Goulet J-P, Svensson P. Recommendations from the International Consensus Workshop: Convergence on an orofacial pain taxonomy. J Oral Rehabil 2010;37:807–812.
11. Dworkin SF, Turner JA, Mancl L, et al. A randomized clinical trial of a tailored comprehensive care treatment program for temporomandibular disorders. J Orofac Pain 2002;16:259–276.
12. Dworkin SF, Huggins KH, Wilson L, et al. A randomized clinical trial using research diagnostic criteria for temporomandibular disorders-axis II to target clinic cases for a tailored self-care TMD treatment program. J Orofac Pain 2002;16:48–63.
13. Gatchel RJ, Stowell AW, Wildenstein L, Riggs R, Ellis EI. Efficacy of an early intervention for patients with acute temporomandibular disorder-related pain: A one-year outcome study. J Am Dent Assoc 2006;137: 339–347.

14. Dworkin SF, Sherman JJ, Mancl L, Ohrbach R, LeResche L, Truelove E. Reliability, validity, and clinical utility of RDC/TMD Axis II scales: Depression, non-specific physical symptoms, and graded chronic pain. J Orofac Pain 2002;16:207–220.
15. Ohrbach R, Turner JA, Sherman JJ, et al. Research diagnostic criteria for temporomandibular disorders. IV: Evaluation of psychometric properties of the Axis II measures. J Orofac Pain 2010;24:48–62.
16. Truelove E, Pan W, Look JO, et al. The Research diagnostic criteria for temporomandibular disorders. III: Validity of Axis I diagnoses. J Orofac Pain 2010;24: 35–47.
17. Schiffman EL, Ohrbach R, Truelove EL, et al. The research diagnostic criteria for temporomandibular disorders. V: Methods used to establish and validate revised Axis I diagnostic algorithms. J Orofac Pain 2010;24:63–78.
18. Maixner W, Diatchenko L, Dubner R, et al. Orofacial pain prospective evaluation and risk assessment study—The OPPERA study. J Pain 2011;12(suppl 11):T4–T11.e1–e2.
19. Greenspan JD, Slade GD, Bair E, et al. Pain sensitivity risk factors for chronic TMD: Descriptive data and empirically identified domains from the OPPERA case-control study. J Pain 2011;12(suppl 11):T61–T74.
20. Maixner W, Greenspan JD, Dubner R, et al. Potential autonomic risk factors for chronic TMD: Descriptive data and empirically identified domains from the OPPERA case-control study. J Pain 2011;12(suppl 11):T75–T91.
21. Slade GD, Bair E, By K, et al. Study methods, recruitment, sociodemographic findings, and demographic representativeness in the OPPERA study. J Pain 2011;12(suppl 11):T12–T26.
22. Smith S, Maixner D, Greenspan JD, et al. Case-control association study of TMJD reveals genetic risk factors. J Pain 2011;12(suppl 11):T92–T101.
23. Fillingim RB, Slade GD, Diatchenko L, et al. Summary of findings from the oppera baseline case-control study: Implications and future directions. J Pain 2011;12(suppl 11):T102–T107.
24. Ohrbach R, Fillingim RB, Mulkey F, et al. Clinical findings and pain symptoms as potential risk factors for chronic TMD: Descriptive data and empirically identified domains from the OPPERA case-control study. J Pain 2011;12(suppl 11):T27–T45.
25. Bair E, Brownstein NC, Ohrbach R, et al. Study protocol, sample characteristics and loss-to-follow-up: the OPPERA prospective cohort study. J Pain 2013;14 (suppl 12):T2–T19.
26. Bair E, Ohrbach R, Fillingim RB, et al. Multivariable modeling of phenotypic risk factors for first-onset TMD: The OPPERA prospective cohort study. J Pain 2013;14(suppl 12):T102–T115.
27. Fillingim RB, Ohrbach R, Greenspan JD, et al. Psychosocial factors associated with development of TMD: The OPPERA prospective cohort study. J Pain 2013; 14(suppl 12):T75–T90.
28. Greenspan JD, Slade GD, Bair E, et al. Pain sensitivity and autonomic factors associated wtih development of TMD: The OPPERA prospective cohort study. J Pain 2013;14(suppl 12):T63–T74.
29. Ohrbach R, Bair E, Fillingim RB, et al. Clinical orofacial characteristics associated with risk of first-onset TMD: The OPPERA prospective cohort study. J Pain 2013; 14(suppl 12):T33–T50.
30. Slade G, Sanders A, Bair E, et al. Preclinical episodes of orofacial pain symptoms and their association with healthcare behaviors in the OPPERA prospective cohort study. Pain 2013;154:750–760.
31. Slade GD, Bair E, Greenspan JD, et al. Signs and symptoms of first-onset TMD and socio-demographic predictors of its development: The OPPERA prospective cohort study. J Pain 2013;14(suppl 12):T20–T32.
32. Smith SB, Mir E, Bair E, et al. Genetic variants associated with development of TMD and its intermediate phenotypes: the genetic architecture of TMD in the OPPERA prospective cohort study. J Pain 2013;14 (suppl 12):T91–T101.
33. Sanders AE, Essick GK, Fillingim R, et al. Sleep apnea symptoms and risk of temporomandibular disorder: OPPERA cohort. J Dent Res 2013;92(suppl 7):S70–S77.
34. Sanders AE, Slade GD, Bair E, et al. General health status and incidence of first-onset temporomandibular disorder: The OPPERA prospective cohort study. J Pain 2013;14(suppl 12):T51–T62.
35. Slade GD, Fillingim RB, Sanders AE, et al. Summary of findings from the OPPERA prospective cohort study of incidence of first-onset temporomandibualr disorder: Implications and future directions. J Pain 2013; 14(suppl 12):T116–T124.
36. Slade GD, Smith SB, Zaykin DV, et al. Facial pain with localized and widespread manifestations: Separate pathways of vulnerability. Pain 2013;154:2335–2343.
37. Slade GD, Ohrbach R, Greenspan JD, et al. Painful temporomandibular disorder: Decade of discovery from OPPERA studies. J Dent Res 2016;95:1084–1092.
38. American Psychiatric Association. Diagnostic and Statistical Manual of Mental Disorders, Fifth Edition. Arlington, VA: American Psychiatric Association, 2013.
39. Ohrbach R, Dworkin SF. The evolution of TMD diagnosis: Past, present, future. J Dent Res 2016;95:1093–1101.

40. Schiffman E, Ohrbach R, Truelove E, et al. Diagnostic criteria for temporomandibular disorders (DC/TMD) for clinical and research applications: Recommendations of the International RDC/TMD Consortium Network and Orofacial Pain Special Interest Group. J Oral Facial Pain Headache 2014;28:6–27.
41. Fillingim RB, Bruehl S, Dworkin RH, et al. The ACTTION-American Pain Society Pain Taxonomy (AAPT): An evidence-based and multidimensional approach to classifying chronic pain conditions. J Pain 2014;15:241–249.
42. Ohrbach R, Dworkin SF. AAPT diagnostic criteria for chronic painful temporomandibular disorders. J Pain 2019;20:1276–1292.
43. Cairns B, List T, Michelotti A, Ohrbach R, Svensson P. JOR-CORE recommendations on rehabilitation of temporomandibular disorders. J Oral Rehabil 2010;37:481–489.
44. Visscher CM, Baad-Hansen L, Durham J, et al. Benefits of implementing psychosocial assessment in dental practice. J Am Dent Assoc 2018;149:422–431.
45. Sharma S, Breckons M, Bronnimann-Lambelet B, et al. Challenges in the clinical implementation of a biopsychosocial model for assessment and management of orofacial pain. J Oral Rehabil 2019;47:87–100.
46. Dawes RM, Faust D, Meehl PE. Clinical versus actuarial judgement. Science 1989;243:1668–1674.
47. Epker J, Gatchel RJ, Ellis EI. A model for predicting chronic TMD: Practical application in clinical settings. J Am Dent Assoc 1999;130:1470–1475.
48. Oakley ME, McCreary CP, Flack VF, Clark GT, Solberg WK, Pullinger AG. Dentist's ability to detect psychological problems in patients with temporomandibular disorders and chronic pain. J Am Dent Assoc 1989;118:727–730.
49. Schiffman E, Ohrbach R. Executive summary of the diagnostic criteria for temporomandibular disorders for clinical and research applications. J Am Dent Assoc 2016;147:438–445.
50. Turner JA, Dworkin SF. Screening for psychosocial risk factors in patients with chronic orofacial pain: Recent advances. J Am Dent Assoc 2004;135:1119–1125.
51. Durham J, Raphael KG, Benoliel R, Ceusters W, Michelotti A, Ohrbach R. Perspectives on next steps in classification of oro-facial pain—Part 2: Role of psychosocial factors. J Oral Rehabil 2015;42:942–955.
52. Anderson GC, Gonzalez YM, Ohrbach R, et al. The research diagnostic criteria for temporomandibular disorders. VI: Future directions. J Orofacial Pain 2010;24:79–88.
53. Palla S. Biopsychosocial pain model crippled? J Orofacial Pain 2011;25:289–290.
54. Sharma S, Slade GD, Fillingim RB, Greenspan JD, Rathnayaka N, Ohrbach R. Attributes germane to temporomandibular disorders and their associations with five chronic overlapping pain conditions. J Oral Facial Pain Headache 2020;34:s57–s72e.
55. Ohrbach R, Slade GD, Bair E, et al. Premorbid and concurrent predictors of TMD onset and persistence. Eur J Pain 2020;24:145–158.
56. Slade GD, Greenspan JD, Fillingim RB, Maixner W, Sharma S, Ohrbach R. Overlap of five chronic pain conditions: Temporomandibular disorders, headache, back pain, irritable bowel syndrome, and fibromyalgia. J Oral Facial Pain Headache 2020;34:s15–s28.
57. Ohrbach R, Sharma S, Fillingim RB, Greenspan JD, Rosen JD, Slade G. Clinical characteristics of pain among five chronic overlapping pain conditions. J Oral Facial Pain Headache 2020;34:s29–s42.
58. Von Korff M, Ormel J, Keefe FJ, Dworkin SF. Grading the severity of chronic pain. Pain 1992;50:133–149.
59. Sharma S, Kallen MA, Ohrbach R. Graded chronic pain scale:Validation of 1-month reference frame. Clin J Pain 2021;38:119–131.
60. Von Korff M, DeBar LL, Krebs EE, Kerns RD, Deyo RA, Keefe FJ. Graded chronic pain scale revised: Mild, bothersome, and high-impact chronic pain. Pain 2020;161:651–661.
61. Dworkin SF. Psychosocial issues. In: Sessle B, Lavigne GJ, Lund JP, Dubner R (eds). Orofacial Pain: From Basic Science to Clinical Management. Chicago: Quintessence; 2001:115–127.
62. Kroenke K, Spitzer RL, Williams JB, Löwe B. An ultra-brief screening scale for anxiety and depression: The PHQ-4. Psychosomatics 2009;50:613–621.
63. Beck AT. Beck Anxiety Inventory. San Antonio, TX: The Psychological Corporation, 1993.
64. Spielberger CD. State-Trait Anxiety Inventory. Palo Alto, CA: Consulting Psychologists, 1983.
65. Beck AT, Steer RA, Brown GK. Beck depression inventory—II. San Antonio 1996;78:490–498.
66. Ohrbach R, Larsson P, List T. The jaw functional limitation scale: Development, reliability, and validity of 8-item and 20-item versions. J Orofacial Pain 2008;22:219–230.
67. Markiewicz MR, Ohrbach R, McCall WD, Jr. Oral behaviors checklist: Reliability of performance in targeted waking-state behaviors. J Orofacial Pain 2006;20:306–316.
68. Ohrbach R, Markiewicz MR, McCall WD, Jr. Waking-state oral parafunctional behaviors: Specificity and validity as assessed by electromyography. Eur J Oral Sci 2008;116:438–444.

69. Curran SL, Sherman JJ, Cunningham LL, Okeson JP, Reid KI, Carlson CR. Physical and sexual abuse among orofacial pain patients: Linkages with pain and psychologic distress. J Orofacial Pain 1995;10:221–228.
70. De Leeuw R, Bertoli E, Schmidt JE, Carlson CR. Prevalence of post-traumatic stress disorder symptoms in orofacial pain patients. Oral Surg Oral Med Oral Pathol Oral Radiol Endod 2005;99:558–568.
71. Sherman JJ, Carlson CR, Wilson JF, Okeson JP, McCubbin JA. Post-traumatic stress disorder among patients with orofacial pain. J Orofac Pain 2005;19:309–317.
72. Häggman-Henrikson B, Bechara C, Pishdari B, Visscher CM, Ekberg E. Impact of catastrophizing in patients with temporomandibular disorders—A systematic review. J Oral Facial Pain Headache 2020;34:379–397.
73. Dworkin SF, Burgess JA. Orofacial pain of psychogenic origin: Current concepts and classification. J Am Dent Assoc 1987;115:565–571.
74. Rugh JD, Davis SE. Temporomandibular disorders: Psychological and behavioral aspects. In: Sarnat BG, Laskin DM (eds). The Temporomandibular Joint: A Biological Basis for Clinical Practice. Philadelphia: WB Saunders, 1992:329–345.
75. Bertrand PM. Management of facial pain. Oral Maxillofacial Surgery Knowledge Update 2001;3:79–109.
76. Ohrbach R, Michelotti A. The role of stress in the etiology of oral parafunction and myofascial pain. In: Laskin D, Renapurkar SK (eds). Current Controversies in the Management of Temporomandibular Disorders: Oral and Maxillofacial Surgery Clinics of North America. Philadelphia: Elsevier, 2018:369–380.
77. Bush K, Kivlahan DR, McDonell MB, Fihn SD, Bradley KA. The AUDIT alcohol consumption questions (AUDIT-C): An effective brief screening test for problem drinking. Arch Intern Med 1998;158:1789–1795.
78. Durham J, Ohrbach R. Oral rehabilitation, disability and dentistry. J Oral Rehabil 2010;37:490–494.
79. Romano JM, Turner JA, Moore JE. Psychological Evaluation. In: Tollison CD (ed). Handbook of Chronic Pain Management. Philadelphia: Williams & Wilkins, 1989:38–51.
80. Gatchel RJ, Garofalo JP, Ellis E, Holt C. Major psychological disorders in acute and chronic TMD: An initial examination. J Am Dent Assoc 1996;127:1365–1374.
81. Kight M, Gatchel RJ, Wesley L. Temporomandibular disorders: Evidence for significant overlap with psychopathology. Health Psychol 1999;18:177–182.
82. Kinney RK, Gatchel RJ, Ellis E, Holt C. Major psychological disorders in chronic TMD patients: Implications for successful management. J Am Dent Assoc 1992;123:49–54.
83. Korszun A, Hinderstein B, Wong M, Peterson LJ. Comorbidity of depression with chronic facial pain and temporomandibular disorders. Oral Surg Oral Med Oral Pathol Oral Radiol Endod 1996;82:496–500.
84. Wurtele SK, Kaplan GM, Keairnes M. Childhood sexual abuse among chronic pain patients. Clin J Pain 1990;6:110–113.
85. Heit HA. The truth about pain management. The difference between a pain patient and an addicted patient. Eur J Pain 2001;5(suppl A):27–29.
86. Weissman DE. Understanding pseudoaddiction. J Pain Symptom Manage 1994;9:74.
87. Oltmanns JR, Carlson CR. Behavioral treatment of sleep problems for orofacial pain patients. Dental Sleep Practice 2018;(Fall):30–32.
88. Shorter E. From Paralysis to Fatigue: A History of Psychosomatic Illness in the Modern Era. New York: The Free Press, 1992.
89. Dworkin SF. Somatization, distress and chronic pain. Qual Life Res 1994;3,(suppl 1):S77–S83.
90. Wilson L, Dworkin SF, Whitney C, LeResche L. Somatization and pain dispersion in chronic temporomandibular disorder pain. Pain 1994;57:55–61.
91. Chronic Pain Research Alliance. Impact of Chronic Overlapping Pain Conditions on Public Health and the Urgent Need for Safe and Effective Treatment: 2015 Analysis and Policy Recommendations. chronicpainresearch.org/public/CPRA_WhitePaper_2015-FINAL-Digital.pdf. Accessed 10 November 2022.
92. Kassirer JP, Kopelman RI. Learning Clinical Reasoning. Baltimore: Williams and Wilkins, 1991.
93. Greenspan JD, Slade GD, Rathnayaka N, Fillingim RB, Ohrbach R, Maixner W. Experimental pain sensitivity in subjects wtih TMD and multiple other chronic pain conditions: The OPPERA Prospective Cohort Study. J Oral Facial Pain Headache 2020;34:s43–s56b.
94. Fillingim RB, Ohrbach R, Greenspan JD, et al. Associations of psychological factors with multiple chronic overlapping pain conditions. J Oral Facial Pain Headache 2020;34:s85–s100a.
95. Sanders A, Greenspan JD, Fillingim RB, Rathnayaka N, Ohrbach R, Slade G. Associations of sleep disturbance, atopy, and other health measures with chronic overlapping pain conditions. J Oral Facial Pain Headache 2020;34:s73–s84b.
96. Cahill CM, Walwyn W, Taylor AM, Pradhan AA, Evans CJ. Allostatic mechanisms of opioid tolerance beyond desensitization and downregulation. Trends Pharmacol Sci 2016;37:963–976.
97. Wise RA. Dopamine, learning and motivation. Nat Rev Neurosci 2004;5:483–494.

98. Chapman CR, Tuckett RP, Song CW. Pain and stress in a systems perspective: Reciprocal neural, endocrine, and immune interactions. J Pain 2008;9:122–145.
99. Galambos A, Szabó E, Nagy Z, et al. A systematic review of structural and functional MRI studies on pain catastrophizing. J Pain Res 2019;12:1155.
100. Cunningham NR, Kashikar-Zuck S, Coghill RC. Brain mechanisms impacted by psychological therapies for pain: Identifying targets for optimization of treatment effects. Pain Rep 2019;4:e767.
101. Prochaska JO, DiClemente CC. Transtheoretical therapy: Toward a more integrative model of change. Psychother Theory Res Pract 1982;19:276–288.
102. Prochaska JO, Johnson S, Lee P. The transtheoretical model of behavior change. In: Shumaker SA, Ockene JK, Riekert KA (eds). The Handbook of Health Behavior Change. New York: Springer, 2009:59–83.
103. Keefe FJ, Lefebvre JC, Kerns RD, et al. Understanding the adoption of arthritis self-management: Stages of change profiles among arthritis patients. Pain 2000;87:303–314.
104. Miller WR, Rollnick S. Motivational Interviewing: Helping People Change. New York: Guilford, 2013.

Index

Page numbers followed by "t" denote tables, "f" denote figures, and "b" denote boxes.

A

Index

D

Index

Index

N